Simple Health Secrets

Your Total Guide
to Living a
Disease-Free,
High-Energy,
All-Natural Life

D1441772

Reader's Digest

The Reader's Digest Association, Inc.
New York, NY/Montreal

A READER'S DIGEST BOOK
Supercharge Your Health
Copyright © 2009 The Reader's Digest Association, Inc.
Previously published in hardcover as *Disease Free*

Homemade
Copyright © 2007 The Reader's Digest Association, Inc.

PROJECT STAFF

Supercharge Your Health
Editor: Marianne Wait
Senior Art Director: Edwin Kuo
Designer: Erick Swindell
Writers: Debra Gordon, Timothy Gower, Sari Harrar,
Alice Kelly
Recipe Developer: Patsy Jamieson
Research Coordinator: Kristina Swindell
Copy Editor: Jane Sherman
Exercise Photography: © Jill Wachter
Food Photography: © Tara Donne
Medical Illustrations: © Bryan Christie Design
Angel and Devil Illustrations: Adam Raiti
Additional photography courtesy of Jupiter Images,
RD Publications, Veer, iStockphoto and Getty Images

Homemade
Editor: Don Earnest
Designer: Michele Laseau
Recipe Editor: Nancy Shuker
Writers: Kim Gayton Elliott, Jay Ansell, Beth Kalet,
Debra Gordon, Steven Schwartz, and Delilah Smittle
Illustrator: Masi + Monkey, Inc.
Layout: Edwin Kuo, Rachel Maloney
Copy Editor: Jeanette Gingold

READER'S DIGEST TRADE PUBLISHING
U.S. Project Editor: Kim Casey
Project Designer: Rich Kershner
Senior Art Director: George McKeon
Editor-in-Chief, Books & Home Entertainment: Neil Wertheimer
Associate Publisher, Trade Publishing: Rosanne McManus
President and Publisher, Trade Publishing: Harold Clarke

We are committed to both the quality of our products and the service we provide to our customers. We value your comments, so please feel free to contact us.

The Reader's Digest Association, Inc.
Adult Trade Publishing
44 South Broadway
White Plains, NY 10601

For more Reader's Digest products and information, visit our website: www.rd.com (in the United States)

Printed in China

1 3 5 7 9 10 8 6 4 2

NOTE TO READERS
The information in this book should not be substituted for, or used to alter, medical therapy without your doctor's advice. For a specific health problem, consult your physician for guidance. The mention of any products, retail businesses, or websites in this book does not imply or constitute an endorsement by the authors or by The Reader's Digest Association, Inc.

contents

BOOK 1

SUPERCHARGE Your Health

Proven Ways to Prevent Illness

The Reader's Digest Association, Inc.
New York, NY | Montreal

Chief Consultants

This book would not have been possible without the expertise and dedication of the following physicians, who helped ensure the quality of the information and advice in these pages and who share our goal of helping people everywhere acheive lifelong health. Don't forget to involve your own physician in your personal quest to remain disease free. If you're coping with a health issue already, make a separate appointment to talk about the steps you can take to prevent chronic illness. Then vow to do your part. As one doctor told us, "There is no one who can prevent disease in patients better than the patients themselves!"

Graham Colditz, MD, DrPH
Niess-Gain Professor in the School of Medicine, Department of Surgery
Associate Director Prevention and Control, Alvin J. Siteman Cancer Center
Washington University School of Medicine

Andrea Fagiolini, MD
Associate Professor of Psychiatry
University of Pittsburgh School of Medicine

Steven R. Feldman, MD, PhD
Professor of Dermatology, Pathology & Public Health Sciences
Wake Forest University Health Sciences

David R. Friedland MD, PhD
Associate Professor
Chief, Division of Otology and Neuro-otologic Skull Base Surgery
Department of Otolaryngology and Communication Sciences
Medical College of Wisconsin

Leonard G. Gomella, MD, FACS
The Bernard W. Godwin Professor of Prostate Cancer
Chairman, Department of Urology
Associate Director of Clinical Affairs, Jefferson Kimmel Cancer Center
Thomas Jefferson University

David L. Katz, MD
Associate Clinical Professor
Public Health and Medicine
Yale University School of Medicine

Robert B. Kelly, MD, MS
Associate Professor of Family Medicine
Case Western Reserve University School of Medicine

Wendy Klein, MD, FACP
Associate Professor Emeritus of Medicine, Obstetrics & Gynecology
Virginia Commonwealth University School of Medicine
Senior Deputy Director, VCU Institute for Women's Health

Michelle Lee, MD
Assistant Professor of Clinical Medicine
Columbia University

JoAnn E. Manson, MD, DrPH
Chief, Division of Preventive Medicine
Brigham and Women's Hospital
Professor of Medicine and the Elizabeth F. Brigham Professor of Women's Health
Harvard Medical School

Daniel Muller, MD, PhD
Associate Professor of Medicine (Rheumatology)
University Wisconsin-Madison

Gerard E. Mullin, MD
Division of Gastroenterology and Liver Disease
Johns Hopkins Hospital

Donald L. Price, MD
Professor of Pathology, Neurology, and Neuroscience
Director, Division of Neuropathology
Director, Alzheimer's Disease Research Center
The Johns Hopkins University School of Medicine

Dr. Christopher Randolph, MD
Associate Clinical Professor at Yale Division of Allergy

Elizabeth A. Stewart, MD
Professor of Obstetrics and Gynecology
Division of Reproductive Endocrinology
Mayo Clinic and Mayo Medical School

Special thanks to the American College of Preventive Medicine and its members for their participation.

Contents

disease preventing recipes

disease free living

Whoever said "life is short" didn't realize just how long you can live—and how well—when you stay illness free. Fortunately, the good life is also a healthy one.

A Whole New Way to Prevent Disease

What if we told you that it's well within your grasp to live an extra decade? We're not talking about 10 years of wheeling around an oxygen tank, withering away in a nursing home, or even popping multiple prescription medications to keep you going, but about really *living*. Traveling or learning another language. Pursuing a new hobby (one that keeps you young!) or extending a career. Playing with your great-grandchildren or fulfilling other dreams. If you stay disease free, it's not just possible—it's likely.

you hold the power

About half of all adults live with one or more chronic conditions. But the truth is that many of the diseases people face today are almost entirely preventable. In creating this book, Reader's Digest surveyed more than 100 physicians who specialize in preventive medicine and asked all sorts of questions relating to chronic diseases and how to avoid them. More than half of the doctors in our Disease Prevention Survey said they believe that at least 60 percent of chronic disease cases could be avoided entirely.

The power you hold to prevent disease and live a long, healthy life is nothing short of amazing. Consider this: A 2008 study of more than 2,000 men found that those who met just four criteria—they didn't smoke, they weren't overweight, they exercised regularly, and they consumed alcohol in moderation if at all—lived an average of 10 years longer than men who didn't fit at least one of these descriptions—and 10 good years at that! More than two-thirds of the men who lived to age 90 rated their late-life health as either excellent or very good. We're going to go out on a limb and surmise that the men who lived longer were also happier; you'll read more on the deep connection between health and emotional well-being a bit later.

The men in the study didn't do anything outrageous to protect themselves from disease, and you don't have to either, whether you're a man or a woman. In fact, doing just one thing—getting a half hour of exercise most days—could dramatically turn your health around and strengthen your resistance to disease. (By the way, the experts we polled told us that if you do only one thing for your health, besides quitting smoking, that should be it.) Is living longer and sidestepping crippling conditions like heart disease and cancer worth 30 minutes a day, the time it takes to watch the evening news or another sitcom rerun? That's up to you, of course—but it's hard to see how it isn't.

You may already practice some of the measures known to help prevent disease. Are you taking a daily aspirin on your doctor's advice? Did you get a flu shot this year? Have you scheduled your next colonoscopy? Studies confirm that each of these steps saves lives. In the 12 Steps to Total Prevention chapter, you'll learn about the measures rated in the Disease Prevention Survey as the top ones that keep disease at bay. Consider that chapter your overall "action guide" for living a healthier life. But first, a few fascinating highlights of the survey and our own research.

Your Life, Your Health

Our understanding of what causes chronic disease has radically changed over the past decade. Even as researchers discover more and more links between flawed genes and certain health conditions, it's clearer than ever that the underlying causes of most chronic diseases are lifestyle factors that we control.

say goodbye to these diseases

Doctors we polled say these eight diseases could be virtually *eliminated* with the right lifestyle measures.

- Chronic obstructive pulmonary disease
- Type 2 diabetes
- Emphysema
- Heart disease
- High blood pressure
- Lung cancer
- Obesity
- Stroke

Hang on just a minute, you may be thinking. What if I come from a long line of people who had cancer or heart attacks or diabetes? What good is eating salads and running around in a gym going to do if I was dealt a lousy hand of genes?

These are fair questions, but the science is incontrovertible: Genes may increase your risk for certain conditions, but lifestyle choices have a far greater impact on your health and longevity. Imagine the factors that determine your life span depicted in a pie chart. Studies of identical twins, who share identical genes, suggest that DNA dictates only 25 to 33 percent of how long you live, or one-quarter to one-third of the pie. The rest? That depends on how you live.

Unfortunately, or fortunately, depending on how you look at it, the way we live—what we eat, the amount of stress we're under, what we do or don't do with our leisure time—is the reason so many of us get sick as we get older.

The "New" Causes of Disease

In the Disease Prevention Survey, the number one cause of chronic disease wasn't bad genes. It wasn't even high cholesterol. It was something many people assume is relatively harmless: high blood pressure. There's a reason it's often called the silent killer. Fortunately, it's a condition that many doctors listed as one that could be entirely eliminated. If you have it and you haven't dealt with it, now's the time.

Also ranked above genes and high cholesterol was something you might find more or less right under your nose: intra-abdominal fat, the kind of fat that lies deep within the belly, padding internal organs and contributing to everything from diabetes to heart attacks. If you have a large waistline, you probably have this killer fat (see page 26 for details).

If you're overweight, there's a decent chance you have another high-ranking disease risk: insulin resistance, in which the body no longer effectively uses the hormone insulin to get blood sugar into muscle cells. Chalk up the current epidemic of insulin resistance to our sedentary ways and the foods we tend to favor, including potatoes, rice, white bread, and sugary carbs—all of which raise blood sugar quickly and essentially begin to wear out the insulin response. It's a huge step down the path to diabetes, but it's also turning out to contribute to heart attacks, cancer, and even Alzheimer's disease.

You may have noticed that all three of these root causes—high blood pressure, intra-abdominal fat, and insulin resistance—are linked with heart disease, the leading cause of death in the developed world. It's no wonder they ranked so high. And they have something else in common: their solutions. If all of us lost a little weight, got a little more exercise, and ate more fruits and vegetables, cases of all three conditions—and the diseases they cause or contribute to—would plummet.

You'll discover all six of the top root causes of disease starting on page 23.

The "New" Keys to Health

Many of the basic messages haven't changed; it's still important to exercise, eat more fruits and vegetables, and stop smoking.

In the results of the survey, however, we found a new health message that has nothing to do with food or exercise and everything to do with the people we share (or don't share) our lives with.

The experts who answered our survey—all of them steeped in the best available knowledge of how to prevent disease—told us loud and clear that having healthy relationships was extremely important to health. And these are *doctors* we're talking about. In the survey, 79 percent said that being socially isolated was the "utmost detriment" or "extremely detrimental" to health. And they rated "having happy interactions with friends and family" above "cutting most saturated fat from your diet" as prevention strategies!

Maybe one reason family and friends are so important is that they help combat stress and depression. We were shocked at how many doctors mentioned stress as a contributing factor in major disease; in fact, 83 percent said that living with uncontrolled stress was the "utmost detriment" or "extremely detrimental" to health. They ranked it as even more dangerous than being 30 pounds overweight. (It's no wonder then, that more than half of doctors said that meditating or practicing another stress-relief technique was extremely beneficial to health.) They ranked depression significantly higher than high cholesterol as a condition with the greatest potential for causing chronic disease.

What's going on here? Simply put, what happens in your mind and heart (the figurative one this time) affects your body in profound ways. Chronic stress lowers the immune system's ability to function effectively—it even makes vaccines less effective. It raises levels of so-called stress hormones, such as coritsol. High cortisol

surprising advice from the prevention experts

Staying healthy is not all about eating your vegetables (though that certainly helps). In the Disease Prevention Survey, these tidbits of verbatim advice leapt off the page and convinced us that health really does spring from a life well lived.

"Believe in something good."

"Focus on a higher sense of purpose."

"Develop your unique potential."

"Eat less, exercise more, and have fun.

"Love the ones you're with (spouse, children, extended family, faith family, neighbors, co-workers, community members)."

"Achieve balance in your life."

"Exercise every day, eat a well-balanced diet, maintain meaningful social interactions and relationships, and choose work that is important to you."

"Find meaning in your life."

"Get eight hours or more of sleep a day."

"Manage stress and enjoy your friends."

"Stay positive and have a family physician who helps you to prevent disease and improve health."

such as meditation and happy daily interactions with others. Some made a special point to tell us, in their own words, how important it is to find something meaningful or fulfilling to do in life or to believe in a higher power or higher sense of purpose—both of which take our minds off our worries and supply inspiration for daily life. It's not something your own doctor is likely to "prescribe" because today's physicians simply don't have time to delve into issues of emotional well-being with their patients, but it may be just as important as taking your medicines.

Take a look at your life for a minute. Do you have people you can turn to? Do you get up every day with a sense of optimism or purpose? Or do you dread your to-do list or feel nothing much at all because in truth, you lost the sense of what's possible many years ago? Our message to you: It's never too late to get interested in and excited about something new or to reach out and make personal connections with others. You'll enjoy more benefits than you ever expected.

levels can keep you up at night, but they can also raise blood pressure, contribute to high blood sugar, and increase intra-abdominal fat, that "killer" fat you read about earlier.

There's also the more obvious effect that stress, depression, and loneliness has on us every day. As one doctor told us, "Mental stress, conflict, etc., drive the majority of bad physical habits and practices"—in other words, getting too little sleep, being too sedentary, and eating too many calories, especially in the form of junk food.

Chronic stress also raises the risk of depression, and if you're depressed, chances are you're not going to exercise or eat well. Depression often goes hand in hand with a whole litany of diseases, from heart disease to cancer, and doctors aren't always sure which causes which. But they do know that having depression and a serious illness tends to make the symptoms of that illness worse.

Considering the dangers of stress and depression, it's little surprise that many doctors in the survey advocated relaxation techniques

Getting Yourself to Act

People who exercise and eat well tend to live a long time, often surviving their neighbors by up to a decade or longer. Which begs a question: Why don't more people follow these basic steps for a longer, better life? Sometimes it's hard to get started. But we think that choosing just one healthy habit to adopt, or one bad habit to quit, will make you feel good both physically and emotionally—good enough to want to choose another. On page 19, you'll take a quiz that will help you identify your good and bad habits, giving you plenty to choose from.

It also helps to stop and think about all the trouble you'll save yourself by preventing a disease rather than waiting until you need treatment.

Remember, Prevention Trumps Cure

When Ben Franklin quipped, "An ounce of prevention is worth a pound of cure," he was actually cautioning homeowners to protect their property against fire. But if your health goes up in flames, old Ben's words may ring true. When you get sick, you place yourself in the hands of the healthcare system, which does save lives—but it also makes some people sicker, not to mention poorer. Just think of the side effects caused by taking multiple prescription drugs and the dangers associated with a hospital stay, not to mention the expense and inconvenience of it all.

For many people, taking prescription drugs is as much a part of their daily routine as brushing their teeth. In the United States, 44 percent of the population uses at least one prescription medication. One person in six takes three or more. Drugs can be lifesavers, of course. Some, like aspirin and cholesterol-lowering statins, may even be part of your disease prevention plan. But virtually all drugs, even seemingly benign ones, can produce unwanted side effects.

One example is medications for high blood pressure, which afflicts about a billion people worldwide. Only about one-third of patients who receive prescription drugs for the condition are able to bring their blood pressure into the safe zone. One well-documented reason: Many patients quit taking their medications. Some can't afford them, but others can't tolerate the side effects, which can include dry cough, swollen extremities, erectile dysfunction, headache, dizziness, fatigue, nausea, vomiting, and others. One study found that nearly 70 percent of patients given blood pressure pills called calcium channel blockers developed unpleasant side effects.

Why not take steps now to avoid high blood pressure and avoid this predicament altogether?

Sometimes the drugs we take don't even work. A 2008 analysis found little scientific proof that widely used antidepressants such as fluoxetine

Then and Now

A century ago, people were most likely to die from an infectious disease. But improved hygiene and sanitation later prevented millions of premature deaths from contagions such as tuberculosis. Today the diseases that kill us are largely caused by the way we live.

TOP CAUSES OF DEATH IN 1900	TOP CAUSES OF DEATH TODAY
1. Pneumonia/influenza	1. Heart disease
2. Tuberculosis	2. Cancer
3. Diarrhea, enteritis, and ulceration of the intestines	3. Stroke
4. Diseases of the heart	4. Chronic lower respiratory diseases (such as chronic obstructive pulmonary disease and emphysema)
5. Intracranial lesions of vascular origin (caused by stroke)	5. Accidents
6. Nephritis (inflammation of the kidney)	6. Diabetes
7. Accidents	7. Alzheimer's disease
8. Cancer and other malignant tumors	8. Influenza/pneumonia
9. Senility	9. Nephritis, nephrotic syndrome, and nephrosis (kidney disease)
10. Diphtheria	10. Septicemia (blood infection)

Between 5 and 10 percent of hospital patients acquire one or more infections during their stays, and the risk of hospital-acquired infection is rising rapidly. Simple urinary tract infections are the most common variety, but medical centers are increasingly plagued by "super-bugs" such as MRSA (methicillin-resistant *Staphylococcus aureus*), the staph infection immune to standard antibiotics. It can cause pneumonia and other life-threatening infections.

These tidbits should make anyone skip the doughnuts and eat a bowl of bran cereal, jog an extra 10 minutes, and take other steps to avoid today's healthcare system—not to mention avoiding a truly traumatic event like a heart attack or stroke.

Decide If You Really Want to Be Healthy

That's right, good health is a goal you can either reach for or ignore. You need to decide for yourself whether or not your health is a priority. If you don't make any effort to eat well, exercise, or control stress, you've decided that it's not, even if you never thought about it that way. But it's never too late to change your mind!

When asked about other significant causes of chronic disease, one doctor wrote, "Foolish behavior, even when the patient knows better." Truer words were never spoken! Most of us have a pretty good idea what it takes to be healthy; we just don't always bother to do it.

What's the solution? We loved this suggestion from one doctor: "Rely on your inner strength to change your ways." The source of that strength will be different for everyone. Maybe your kids or grandkids make you want to live a longer, healthier life—think of them every time you're tempted to reach for a cigarette or order a plate of barbecued ribs. Maybe you can use the "you

(Prozac) and paroxetine (Paxil) offer any benefit to patients with moderate depression. Another recent study showed that the widely prescribed cholesterol-lowering medication ezetimibe (Zetia) does not keep arteries clear of heart-stopping plaque.

Meanwhile, exercise, a happy personal life, and a healthy diet can help prevent both depression and high cholesterol.

Medications may also cause the ultimate side effect, of course. Data from the FDA shows that the number of people who died from adverse effects of drug treatments rose 2.7-fold from 1998 to 2005.

And what if you get sick enough to land in the hospital? You may have heard the joke: A hospital is no place for a sick person. Only it's no joke. We've all heard stories of doctors amputating the wrong limb, but much more common are deaths caused by mistakes made by doctors, nurses, and other staffers. By some estimates, medical errors are the third leading cause of death in the United States. Nearly 800,000 hospital patients are injured or die each year from bad reactions to medications alone.

can do it" attitude that made you a success in your career to help transform your lifestyle. Or think of a friend or relative who has struggled with the difficulties of an ongoing illness or condition. You may know firsthand the toll that being sick takes on your mental health, your will to live, your wallet; that may be motivation enough to make a few changes in your life. Consider the health problems your parents experienced and maybe even died from and promise yourself that you won't suffer the same fate. Your health really is up to you.

The bulk of this book is geared toward helping you defend yourself against conditions you're particularly worried about or may be susceptible to. Following our advice in the 12 Steps to Total Prevention chapter will go a long, long way toward making you less disease prone. For even more protection from specific ailments that concern you, turn to the chapters on those ailments, and you'll find more detailed prevention strategies.

Working with Your Doctor

Prevention often gets short shrift in doctors' offices, so it's up to you to take charge.

"The healthcare system is focused on care of diseases after they have manifested themselves—care that is sometimes delivered too late," says Howard Koh, MD, professor and associate dean for public health practice at the Harvard School of Public Health. "There is far too little emphasis on preventing diseases in the first place." Our survey doctors loudly echoed that sentiment.

Studies show that many doctors fail to give even the most obvious prevention advice, like telling their overweight patients to lose weight or encouraging patients who smoke to quit. The fact is, doctors are paid to treat sick patients—and that's what they're mainly trained for. Even

keeping brain drain at bay

If you need another reason to eat right and exercise, remember this one: These habits will not only keep your body in shape but may also preserve your memory and mental clarity.

Take the oldest diet advice you've ever heard: Eat your vegetables. Researchers at Chicago's Rush Institute for Healthy Aging found that people over 65 who consume about four servings per day slow cognitive decline by 38 percent. The same researchers found that eating fish as infrequently as once a week may lower the risk of Alzheimer's disease by up to 60 percent.

Jogging, swimming, and other forms of aerobic exercise—essential to any disease prevention plan— appear to protect the brain, too. One study of nearly 19,000 women found that the most active participants were the least likely to show signs of memory loss or fuzzy thinking. Studying, reading, and other mental challenges are also linked to a lower risk of dementia. The same is true of coping effectively with emotional stress.

Need further motivation? In a recent study, UCLA researchers asked a group of volunteers to eat healthy diets, exercise, perform brain teasers and memory exercises, and practice stress-reduction techniques. After two weeks, the participants improved their scores on word tests, and MRI scans showed that their brains worked more efficiently. The study's lead author, Gary W. Small, MD, director of the UCLA Center on Aging, concludes, "Living a healthy lifestyle can have an impact."

if they wanted to give prevention advice—and many do—with office visits shorter than the time it takes to hard boil an egg, there just isn't time. According to a 2003 study published in the *American Journal of Public Health,* primary care doctors would need about 7 1/2 hours every day to provide their patients with all of the appropriate counseling, screening, and immunizations recommended by the US Preventive Services Task Force. Short of cloning themselves, that would leave doctors little time to tend to patients who are already sick. Thus, it's partially up to you to make sure your doctor is paying attention to prevention.

"It's a two-way street, says Laurel B. Yates, MD, of Boston's Brigham and Women's Hospital, lead author of the study involving men that we mentioned at the beginning of the chapter. Yes, your doctor should know about and practice the power of prevention, "but the patient must play a part in knowing the importance of preventive medicine and making sure it's on the agenda," says Dr. Yates.

Anytime you walk into your doctor's office, she says, you should have a list of questions or problems to discuss, with the pressing preventive issues at the top. Raise your concerns right away; never wait until the end of an appointment to start asking questions. Busy physicians become frustrated with patients who say "By the way, Doctor," with one foot out the door.

If you're already coping with a chronic condition, your doctor may need to spend most or all of an office visit discussing medications and other treatments. If you run out of time and don't get to talk about exercise, diet, or other protective steps you could be taking, advises Dr. Yates, schedule another office visit solely to discuss preventive medicine.

Make that an essential role. "Prevention is not a luxury," comments pioneering scientist Paul Talalay, MD, noting that rates of most chronic diseases are rising fast and could produce a healthcare crisis in the not-too-distant future.

Remember, though, prevention is mainly about the things you do outside the doctor's office—what you make for dinner, how much time you spend sitting in front of the TV, whether you're an angry or a happy person. And it's up to you to take charge. As one doctor from the Disease Prevention Survey put it, "Don't simply wait for health professionals to correct your health problems after they become obvious." As another told us, "There is no one who can prevent disease better in patients than the patients themselves!"

The old cliché is true—an ounce of prevention is indeed worth a pound of cure. If your goal is to stay healthy through the years—and to have lots more of them—then you have opened the right book.

vaccines for grownups

No matter how much you exercise and watch what you eat, any plan for disease-proofing your body needs a shot or two in the arm—literally, in some cases. The most obvious form of defense against disease you can seek in a doctor's office is a flu shot. In addition to the chills, aches, and other miserable symptoms brought on by influenza, the condition can lead to life-threatening complications such as pneumonia. A flu shot cuts your risk by up to 90 percent. If you haven't discussed vaccinations with your doctor in some time, don't assume that you're up to date. You may be eligible for one of several newer vaccines that have become available in recent years, which guard against conditions such as cervical cancer and shingles.

Quiz: Are You a Health Devil or Angel?

It's oh, so tempting to blame "bad genes" for whatever goes wrong with our health. But the truth is, in most cases it's the way we live our lives day to day that spells out what happens to our bodies—whether we stay "young for our age" or become burdened by this or that condition that slows us down and zaps our energy and zest for living.

In the Reader's Digest Disease Prevention Survey, we polled more than 100 doctors who specialize in preventive medicine. Among other questions, we asked them how beneficial or harmful they believe certain habits to be. Take this quiz and see how they'd rate your current lifestyle. Follow the instructions below, then turn to page 22 to learn what your score means. If your lifestyle could use some tweaking, be sure to read the 12 Steps to Total Prevention chapter to learn how to improve your odds of living disease free.

Tally Your "Angel" Habits

For each of the following healthy habits you can claim, give yourself the number of angels you see next to the statement.

Your Diet

 # OF ANGELS

1. Eat at least five total servings of fruits and vegetables a day (see "What's a Serving?" on page 320). _____

2. Have two or more daily servings of fat-free milk or low-fat yogurt. _____

3. Have two or more daily servings of 2% or full-fat milk or full-fat yogurt. _____

4. Eat fish at least twice a week. _____

5. Eat whole grain bread or another whole grain at most meals. _____

6. Eat one to three servings of soy foods a week. _____

7. Eat a clove or more of garlic on most days. _____

8. Drink a glass of wine or beer on many or most days. _____

9. Eat at least some organic foods. _____

10. Eat a small piece of dark chocolate on many or most days. _____

Your Lifestyle

	# OF ANGELS
1. Get 20 to 30 minutes of moderate aerobic exercise on most days.	😇😇😇😇😇 _____
2. Take a daily multivitamin.	😇😇 _____
3. Do strength training two or three times a week.	😇😇😇😇 _____
4. Meditate or practice another stress-relief technique regularly.	😇😇😇😇 _____
5. Always wash your hands after using the bathroom and before cooking.	😇😇😇😇😇 _____
6. Brush and floss regularly.	😇😇😇😇 _____
8. Get an annual flu shot.	😇😇😇😇 _____
9. Have your blood pressure checked regularly.	😇😇😇😇 _____
10. Have your cholesterol checked regularly.	😇😇😇 _____
11. Have sex regularly with a single partner.	😇😇😇 _____

Total "Angel" Points: _____

Tally Your "Devil" Habits

Give yourself the appropriate number of devils for all of the following habits that apply to you.

Your Diet

	# OF DEVILS
1. Regularly eat foods (chips, crackers, fried foods) that contain trans fat (hydrogenated oil).	😈😈😈 _____
2. Regularly eat canned soups, chips, and other processed foods high in sodium.	😈😈😈😈 _____
3. Use the saltshaker at the dinner table on most days.	😈😈😈 _____
4. Drink at least one 12-ounce soda every day.	😈😈😈 _____
5. Drink at least one 12-ounce diet soda every day.	😈😈 _____
6. Eat fatty red meat such as hamburgers and ribs twice a week.	😈😈😈 _____
7. Eat lean red meat such as flank steak twice a week.	😈 _____

8. Eat out (or have takeout) more than three times a week. 😈😈😈😈 ____

9. Drink three glasses of wine or beer more than twice a week. 😈😈😈 ____

10. Eat white bread or white rice at most meals. 😈😈😈 ____

11. Eat milk chocolate on most days. 😈😈 ____

12. Have a sweet dessert after every dinner. 😈😈😈 ____

Your Lifestyle

1. Smoke or chew tobacco regularly. 😈😈😈😈😈 ____

2. Smoke a few occasional cigarettes. 😈😈😈😈 ____

3. Drive without a seatbelt. 😈😈😈😈😈 ____

4. Are socially isolated. 😈😈😈😈😈 ____

5. Live with uncontrolled stress. 😈😈😈😈 ____

6. Have untreated depression. 😈😈😈 ____

7. Are 30 pounds overweight. 😈😈😈😈 ____

8. Are 10 pounds overweight (don't assign yourself points if you checked the box above). 😈😈 ____

9. Drive at 75 mph or faster. 😈😈😈😈😈 ____

10. Take aspirin, ibuprofen, or naproxen for pain nearly every day. 😈😈 ____

11. Take acetaminophen for pain nearly every day. 😈 ____

12. Get less than seven hours of sleep a night. 😈😈😈 ____

13. Talk frequently on a cell phone without a headset (not while driving). 😈 ____

Total "Devil" Points: ____

Your Score

🤤 Total "Angel" Habits _____

😈 Total "Devil" Habits _____

Total Score: _____

Subtract the devil points 😈 from the angel points 🤤 to get your score. Here's what your number means.

Over 30: Excellent. Congratulations! You're living a life that will help keep you disease free.

20 to 29: Good. Your lifestyle is quite healthy. Look for at least one more angel habit to adopt and at least one devil habit to lose.

10 to 19: Average. You're doing okay, but there's room for improvement. Look for a few more angel habits to adopt and a few devil habits to lose.

0 to 9: Worrisome. You're squeaking by with a lifestyle that's somewhat healthy but leaves a lot of room for improvement. Look back to see where you missed out on big angel points and collected too many high-ticket devil points.

-1 to -10: Dangerous. Now is the time to take your health more seriously, before you're dealing with treating disease rather than preventing it. A handful of unhealthy habits are probably dragging down your score—and chances are, you're not eating right, not exercising enough, or both. Look back to see where you can improve your score.

-11 or lower: Very dangerous. You're doing yourself a real disservice by ignoring ways to improve your health and clinging to some pretty harmful habits. But it's never too late to make changes! Even if you're a longtime smoker, quitting now will yield benefits within days. Start by making just one change (and if you smoke, quitting should be it). When you're ready, make another. Every little step counts.

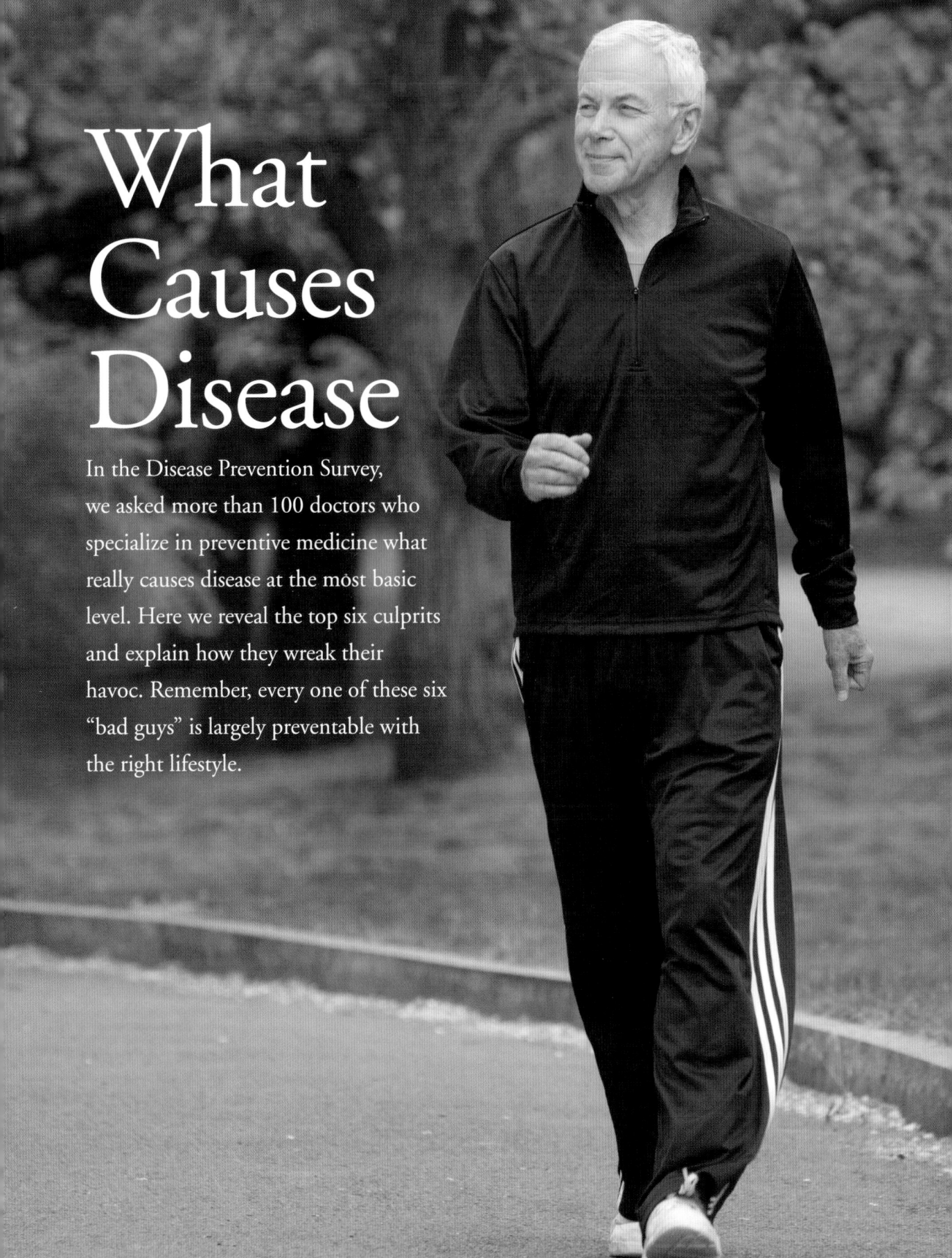

What Causes Disease

In the Disease Prevention Survey, we asked more than 100 doctors who specialize in preventive medicine what really causes disease at the most basic level. Here we reveal the top six culprits and explain how they wreak their havoc. Remember, every one of these six "bad guys" is largely preventable with the right lifestyle.

high blood pressure

what is it? Blood pressure is the force of blood against the walls of your arteries. If your arteries are healthy, they expand and contract easily with every heartbeat, keeping pressure low. But if blood vessels grow stiff, they don't expand as easily and blood pressure rises, just as a wide, lazy river becomes a raging torrent when channeled into a narrow canyon. (Stiff blood vessels are both a cause and an effect of high blood pressure.) Prehypertension begins at a reading of 120/80 mmHg; hypertension (high blood pressure) begins at 140/90 mmHg.

1 High blood pressure makes the layer of muscle inside blood vessel walls grow thicker. This narrows the arteries, raising the risk that a blood clot will completely block an artery and cause a heart attack or stroke.

LDL CHOLESTEROL

WHITE BLOOD CELL

PLAQUE BUILDUP

2 Fast-moving blood damages the delicate layer of cells that line artery walls. Damaged artery walls are magnets for white blood cells and LDL cholesterol, which accumulate and form heart-threatening plaque.

3 High blood pressure can make blood vessels in your brain grow narrow and weak, raising your risk of two kinds of stroke. A blood clot can block blood flow, causing an ischemic stroke (left), or an artery may rupture, causing a hemorrhagic stroke (right).

4 As arteries narrow, the heart works harder, and the left ventricle grows larger. But a bigger heart can't expand fully or fill completely with blood, so it becomes less efficient at pumping, raising your risk of a heart attack, sudden cardiac death, and congestive heart failure.

what causes it?
Family history, advancing age, diabetes, being male, and being African American all increase risk. So do smoking, being overweight, stress, lack of exercise, eating foods high in salt and saturated fat, and skimping on produce and dairy products. Many of these risk factors contribute to high blood pressure in part by reducing production of nitric oxide, a chemical that makes blood vessels flexible.

why is it dangerous?
It makes artery walls thicker, narrower, stiffer, and weaker, which means less blood, oxygen, and nutrients get to your organs. And blood clots are more likely to get stuck in narrowed arteries, which can trigger a heart attack, a stroke, or peripheral vascular disease. Blood vessel damage can also raise your risk of dementia, kidney failure, vision problems, and even blindness.

Top Prevention Strategies

STOP SMOKING if you haven't already.

EXERCISE to lower pressure and lose weight.

SKIP high-sodium processed foods and avoid the saltshaker.

EAT MORE fruit, vegetables, and low-fat dairy products.

intra-abdominal fat

what is it?
Fat packed deep in the abdomen, in and around your internal organs. Women with waists over 35 inches and men with waists over 40 inches are likely to have it. (For people of Asian descent, risk rises with measurements over 31.5 inches for women and 37.5 for men.) A large waist is dangerous even if your body weight is within the "healthy" range for your height. To measure your waist, wrap a tape measure snugly around your midsection at about belly-button height.

1 A high-calorie diet, lack of exercise, and chronic stress conspire to prompt your body to store dangerous fat around your liver, pancreas, and other internal organs.

2 Intra-abdominal fat pumps free fatty acids and inflammatory compounds into the portal vein, the "superhighway" that delivers blood from your lower abdomen to the liver, pancreas, and other internal organs.

what causes it?
Too many hamburgers, too much TV, and too much of all those other activities that keep you sitting down, like working and driving. In other words, a diet high in calories and a life devoid of exercise. Chronic stress plays a role, too, especially for women, since the stress hormone cortisol directs your body to store more fat in your abdomen.

3 An influx of free fatty acids causes your liver to produce more "bad" LDL cholesterol, less "good" HDL cholesterol, more blood sugar, and less adiponectin, a hormone that regulates the use of blood sugar and keeps appetite in check. The result: Your risk of heart disease and diabetes rises.

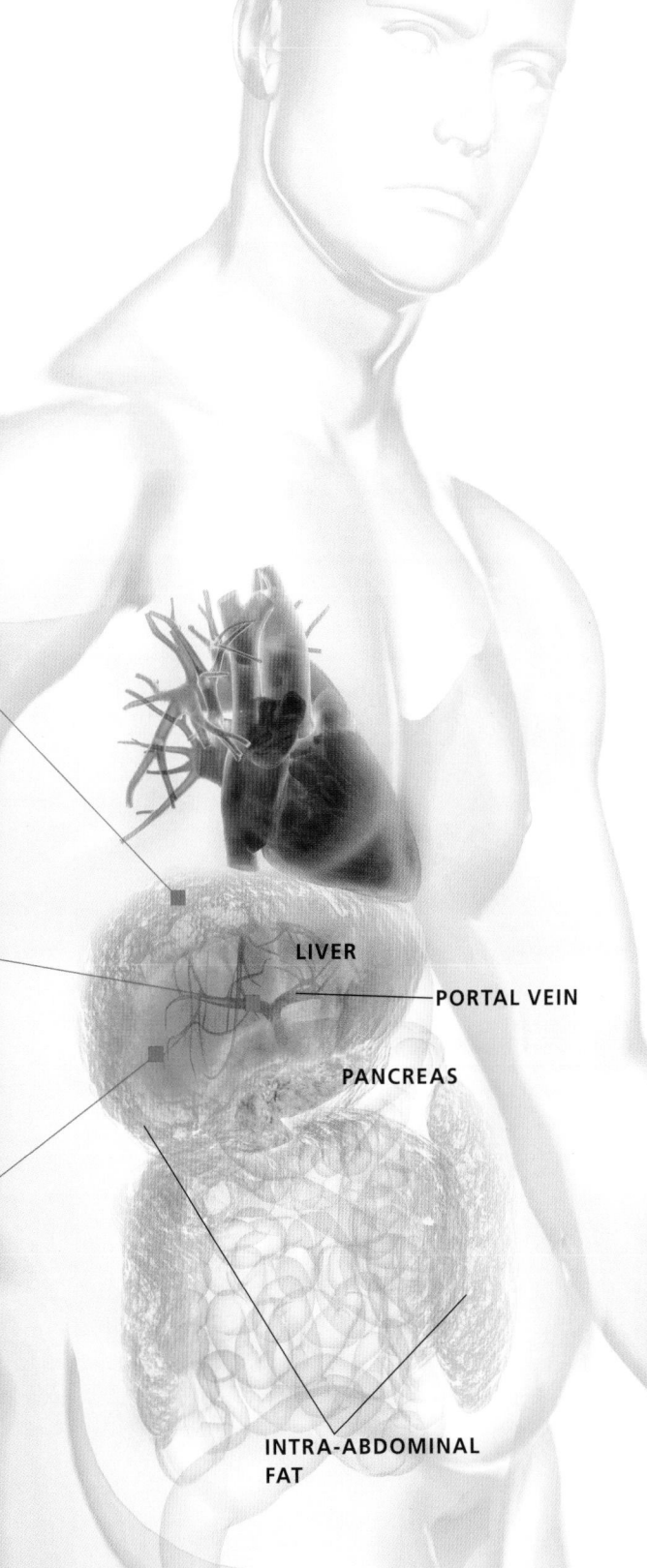

LIVER

PORTAL VEIN

PANCREAS

INTRA-ABDOMINAL
FAT

why is it dangerous?

Unlike the relatively harmless fat on your buttocks, hips, thighs, and even just below your skin at your waist, intra-abdominal fat churns out substances that raise your risk of diabetes, high blood pressure, heart attack, stroke, colon cancer, and even memory problems. These include inflammatory compounds that make blood stickier as well as free fatty acids that prompt your liver to produce more blood sugar and LDL ("bad") cholesterol.

4 The inflammatory compounds secreted by fat cells encourage the growth of plaque inside artery walls, boost blood pressure, and make blood more likely to clot—a recipe for a heart attack. They also make cells resistant to insulin, which in turn contributes to diseases from Alzheimer's to cancer.

Top Prevention Strategies

EAT MORE fruit, vegetables, and whole grains and less saturated fat.

EXERCISE most days of the week for at least 30 minutes.

FIND TIME to relax every day.

CORRECT bad snoring caused by obstructive sleep apnea.

depression

what is it? More than a passing bad mood, depression interferes with your life, your relationships, your sense of yourself, and your health. It ranges from dysthymia—low-level depression that can last for years—to major depression, which can make working, performing daily activities, and relating to your spouse, family, and friends nearly impossible. Another type is seasonal affective disorder, which occurs only during certain times of the year (usually winter).

ACTH

CORTISOL

C-REACTIVE PROTEIN

CYTOKINES

PANCREAS

FAT

1 Depression releases a hormone called ACTH that increases levels of the stress hormone cortisol in the body. Extra cortisol may be the reason people with depression have higher rates of diabetes, because it reduces production of insulin in the pancreas, letting blood sugar rise. Cortisol also prompts the body to store more abdominal fat, a risk factor for many chronic diseases.

what causes it? Often a combination of genetics, chronic stress, and difficult life experiences. Levels of the neurotransmitters serotonin, dopamine, and norepinephrine, which brain cells use to communicate with each other, may be out of balance. And areas of the brain that regulate mood, thought, sleep, appetite, and behavior may function abnormally.

SEROTONIN RETURNS TO SOURCE CELL

TOO LITTLE SEROTONIN

TOO FEW RECEPTORS

4 If you are depressed, you may have abnormally low levels of the brain chemical serotonin. The brain may not produce enough serotonin, brain cells may not have enough receptors to receive it, or it may bounce back instead of being delivered from cell to cell.

2 People with depression may have higher levels of C-reactive protein, an inflammatory compound linked with increased heart attack risk. Depression also increases the release of other inflammatory compounds, called cytokines, that fuel the growth of heart-threatening plaque in artery walls.

why is it dangerous?

Serious depression may lead to suicide. Outside of this risk, depression often coexists with diabetes, heart disease, stroke, cancer, and other major health conditions, making symptoms of these illnesses more severe and more difficult to manage. The combination can be fatal: People with diabetes and depression face a higher risk of dying from heart disease. According to new evidence, depression may even help trigger diabetes, heart disease, and osteoporosis by raising levels of inflammation and stress hormones.

3 Depression raises the risk of osteoporosis and bone fractures. Research suggests that the mood disorder triggers production of the hormone noradrenaline in bones, which reduces the body's ability to maintain healthy bone density.

Top Prevention Strategies

SEEK professional help.

EXERCISE regularly; studies show it can help prevent or lift depression.

RELIEVE STRESS every day in whatever way works best for you.

CULTIVATE a positive attitude.

CONNECT with family and friends for social support.

insulin resistance

what is it? When you eat, some of the food is turned into blood sugar (glucose), the body's main source of fuel. The pancreas responds by secreting the hormone insulin, which triggers cells throughout the body to let the glucose inside. But when cells are insulin resistant, they turn partially "deaf" to insulin's signals. The pancreas turns up the volume by churning out more and more insulin.

1 After a meal or snack, the pancreas secretes insulin to help glucose enter cells. The insulin finds its way to various cells in the body, especially muscle cells, which burn glucose for energy.

LIVER

PANCREAS

what causes it? Scientists aren't exactly sure, but genetics, advancing age, lack of exercise, and excess weight (especially intra-abdominal fat) play key roles. Diets high in saturated fat and simple carbohydrates also contribute, as do chronic infections (such as gum disease), which release inflammatory chemicals that interfere with chemical signals from insulin.

why is it dangerous?

High insulin levels can damage blood vessels and trigger the liver to produce more heart-threatening triglycerides and LDL ("bad") cholesterol and less HDL ("good") cholesterol. They also increase the risk of blood clots and prompt the body to retain more sodium, raising blood pressure. Excess insulin may even spur the growth of some cancers and contribute to Alzheimer's disease. If your pancreas can't keep pace with your body's need for extra insulin, blood sugar levels may begin to rise after years or even decades of insulin resistance—and when they do, you have diabetes.

2 Insulin binds to receptors on the cell. This triggers a series of chemical signals that allow molecules of glucose to be transported into the cell.

GLUCOSE

INSULIN

DAMAGED INSULIN RECEPTOR

NORMAL INSULIN RECEPTOR

FATTY ACIDS

4 The result: The cell can't easily absorb the glucose, and the pancreas has to churn out extra insulin. Eventually, blood sugar levels may begin to rise.

3 In insulin resistance, some insulin receptors are damaged, so the signals don't get through. Signals may also get scrambled if a cell is packed with too many fatty acids (thanks to genetics and/or excess abdominal fat). Inflammatory chemicals released by belly fat and by chronic infections can also interfere with the signals.

Top Prevention Strategies

EXERCISE on most days; exercise increases sensitivity to insulin.

CUT CALORIES and reduce the saturated fat in your diet.

LOSE just 5 to 7 percent of your body weight.

EAT MORE fruit, vegetables, and whole grains instead of refined grains and sugary treats.

bad cholesterol ratio

what is it? Your cholesterol
ratio is the proportion of "bad" LDL
cholesterol to "good" HDL cholesterol.
LDL clogs arteries, but HDL acts as a
vacuum cleaner, whisking the bad stuff
away to the liver for disposal. Optimal
LDL levels are under 100 mg/dl; optimal
HDL levels are over 40 mg/dl for men and
over 50 mg/dl for women. The lower your
LDLand the higher your HDL, the better.

LDL

HDL

OXIDIZED
LDL

1 Smoking, a diet rich in
saturated and hydrogenated
fats, overweight, and lack of
exercise lead to high levels of
LDL in the bloodstream. The
same factors, along with a lack
of "good" fats in the diet, lead
to low levels of HDL.

what causes it? A diet
high in saturated fat gives your liver too
much of the raw material it needs for
producing LDL and reduces its ability to
remove excess LDL from the bloodstream.
Eating hydrogenated fats, smoking, being
overweight, and lack of exercise can also
raise LDL and depress HDL. Skimping on
monounsaturated fats (in olive oil, nuts,
and avocados) and soluble fiber (in oatmeal, barley, beans, and pears) also hurts
your ratio.

2 Trouble starts when extra
LDL particles move out of
the bloodstream and into
artery walls. There they can
be damaged by a process
called oxidation, making them
targets for white blood cells,
which rush to the rescue.

3 HDL is your bloodstream's cleanup crew, removing LDL from circulation and returning it to the liver for elimination or reuse. HDL can even extract cholesterol from plaque in artery walls. But if levels are low, the LDL wins.

LIVER

why is it dangerous?

LDL normally moves through artery walls and into cells, where it's put to good use. But excess LDL gets "stuck" in artery walls, beginning the formation of artery-narrowing plaque. HDL can clean up this LDL mess, but if levels are low, it can't get the job done, putting you at risk for a heart attack or stroke.

PLAQUE

BLOOD CLOT

WHITE BLOOD CELL

4 The combination of LDL and white blood cells in artery walls eventually leads to the buildup of dangerous plaque. Eventually plaque can burst, leading to the formation of blood clots that can stop the flow of blood to your heart or brain.

Top Prevention Strategies

STOP SMOKING if you haven't already.

EAT LESS saturated fat and hydrogenated oils.

EAT MORE soluble fiber (from oats, barley, and beans) and good fats (from fish, nuts, olive oil, and canola oil).

DO MORE brisk walking.

ENJOY alcohol in moderation.

inflammation

STRESS

GUM DISEASE

what is it? Inflammation is a side
effect of the immune system at work. When you
have an injury or infection, immune system cells
and chemicals rush to the site to kill germs and
repair damaged tissue. You can see inflammation
in action when the skin around a cut becomes
red and swollen. Short bouts are beneficial, but
when the body is constantly barraged by inflammation—due to ongoing low-grade infections or
"injuries" from smoking and other irritants—it
ceases to help and starts to harm.

ULCER

INTRA-ABDOMINAL FAT

SMOKING

what causes it? Chronic
inflammation can be triggered by allergens,
toxins, and radiation, but also by medical
conditions such as rheumatoid arthritis,
infections such as untreated gum disease
or stomach ulcers (which are caused by a
bacterial infection), or microscopic injuries
such as damage to artery walls caused by
smoking, high blood pressure, or high cholesterol. Another culprit is intra-abdominal
fat, which secretes inflammatory chemicals.
Stress, anger, lack of exercise, and a diet
full of fast food and hydrogenated fats also
turn up inflammation.

ARTHRITIS

2 White blood cells rush to the
site of the infection or injury—
such as artery walls damaged
by oxidized cholesterol (LDL)
particles. When LDL burrows
into artery walls, the immune
cells engulf them in order to
dispose of them. But if there's
too much LDL, the white blood
cells become overstuffed,
collect in the artery wall, and
form plaque that narrows
the artery.

1 In your blood, levels of inflammatory chemicals called cytokines rise in response to smoking, bacteria, intra-abdominal fat, and other stressors to the body. Cytokines alert the body that something's wrong and set off a chain of events that causes inflammation.

why is it dangerous?

It accelerates the growth of plaque in artery walls and then makes that plaque less stable and more likely to burst open and block an artery. Chronic inflammation also contributes to insulin resistance and raises your risk of a whole host of chronic diseases, including diabetes, Alzheimer's disease, lung disease, osteoporosis, and even cancer.

3 White blood cells release more cytokines that eat away at the protective cap covering the plaque. Eventually the plaque may burst open and spill its contents into the bloodstream. A distress signal sent by white blood cells, called tissue factor, triggers a clotting response. If a blood clot blocks the artery, a heart attack or stroke can result.

WHITE BLOOD CELL

CYTOKINE

PLAQUE

INFLAMMATION

BLOOD CLOT

TISSUE FACTOR

LDL

TISSUE FACTOR

CYTOKINES

FATTY STREAK

OXIDIZED LDL

Top Prevention Strategies

STOP smoking; it inflames artery walls.

EAT MORE fatty fish, fruit, and vegetables and less fried food and hydrogenated oils.

SLEEP at least 7 or 8 hours a night.

EXERCISE moderately.

TREAT any existing infections, such as gum disease or *Helicobacter pylori*.

12 Steps to Total Prevention

When we polled preventive medicine specialists about what *really* prevents disease, their answers surprised us and challenged us to look at health in new ways. Exercising, eating fruits and vegetables, and quitting smoking are still important, as is getting necessary screening tests. But while you're having your cholesterol levels measured, you may want to measure your level of *happiness*, too. That's right—a life filled with happy interactions, devoid of chronic stress, and driven by a higher purpose emerged as the real picture of healthy living.

Step 1	Stop Smoking
Step 2	Get 30 Minutes of Light Exercise Most Days
Step 3	Eat at Least 5 Servings of Fruit and Vegetables a Day
Step 4	Get Recommended Screening Tests
Step 5	Get at Least 7 to 8 Hours of Sleep Each Night
Step 6	Take a Daily Low-Dose Aspirin
Step 7	Know Your Blood Pressure Numbers
Step 8	Have Happy Interactions with Family and Friends
Step 9	Cut Most of the Saturated Fat from Your Diet
Step 10	Get Treated for Depression
Step 11	Tame Chronic Stress
Step 12	Frequently Pray, Meditate, or Focus on a Higher Sense of Purpose

12 Steps to **Total Prevention**   37

<table>
<tr><td>Step
1</td><td>Stop Smoking</td></tr>
</table>

If you smoke, nothing else you do will offer anywhere near the benefits you'll get from quitting. It's no surprise that when our panel of preventive medicine experts ranked the habits they considered most detrimental to well-being, 99 percent put smoking first on the list, far ahead of major threats like driving without a seatbelt or being significantly overweight.

It's not news that cigarettes (as well as cigars and pipes) are lethal. Tobacco kills 5.4 million people annually thanks to lung cancer, breast cancer, heart attack, stroke, diabetes, progressive lung diseases, and hundreds of other health problems it triggers or makes worse. And we now know why it's so difficult to quit: In terms of addictive power, experts put nicotine in the same class as heroin and cocaine. So if you've tried to give up smoking and it hasn't worked, don't feel bad—and don't give up. It can take three, four, five, or more attempts before quitting works. And you don't have to go it alone; in fact, the latest research shows that using several strategies to help you quit, such as nicotine replacement and counseling, can double or even triple your chances of succeeding.

Quitting gives your health an immediate boost. Within eight hours, levels of toxic carbon monoxide gas in your bloodstream drop to normal. Within a day, your heart attack risk begins to drop. Over your first smoke-free year, your circulation will improve, your senses of taste and smell will sharpen, and you'll have fewer lung infections, cough less, and have less sinus congestion. After just a year, your odds of developing heart disease drop by half. And the payoffs mount with each smoke-free year: After 4 years, your chance of having a heart attack falls

to that of someone who's never smoked. After 10 years, your lung cancer risk drops to nearly that of a nonsmoker, and your odds for cancers of the mouth, throat, esophagus, bladder, and kidney decrease significantly, too. To help yourself quit successfully, try these strategies.

Line up help *before* your quit date. After a smoker finishes that last cigarette, a relapse can happen swiftly: Within two days, half of all new quitters light up again; by the end of the first week, two-thirds are back to smoking. Help at the right moment can be crucial, and it's easy to get. Before your quit date, set up a visit with your doctor, a cognitive behavioral therapist, or a smoking cessation support group for your first smoke-free week. Or plan to call a telephone quitline. All can offer custom-tailored help to cope with specific challenges, like what to do if you've always had a cigarette after dinner (hint: schedule an activity for that time—maybe mowing the lawn or an evening walk with a friend) or tended to smoke even more when life threw a curveball your way. In one Michigan study, 43 percent of people who used a telephone quitline were still smoke free after nine months compared to just 5 percent who didn't pick up the phone. Find a quitline in the United States, Canada, Mexico, or the European Union via the North American Quitline Consortium at www.naquitline.org.

Consider a behavioral therapy program or support group. When researchers at England's Oxford University reviewed 55 smoking cessation studies, they found that people who joined therapy groups doubled their odds of succeeding compared to those who tried to kick the habit by themselves.

Don't skimp on your nicotine replacement dose. Gum, patches, lozenges, sprays, and inhalers containing nicotine can all help you battle a nicotine addiction. All release nicotine very slowly into the bloodstream, easing symptoms of withdrawal without all the other toxins in cigarette smoke.

Studies find that the patch increases quit rates by about 7 percent compared to a placebo, the gum and inhaler by about 8 percent, and the nasal spray by 12 to 16 percent. But be sure you're getting enough. If you smoke more than 10 cigarettes a day, for example, choose a higher-dose (usually 21-milligram) patch. And if you have your first cigarette within a half hour of waking up in the morning, start the day with a 4-milligram lozenge rather than a 2-milligram dose.

If you still have cravings, using a patch plus a faster-acting product like gum, lozenges, or a spray or inhaler can further boost your chances of succeeding, say experts who reviewed hundreds of nicotine replacement studies.

Add an antidepressant. Bupropion (Zyban), prescribed as an antidepressant under the name Wellbutrin, increases your odds of quitting by 10 to 13 percent compared to going cold turkey and doubles your odds of succeeding if you're also using a nicotine patch. Experts aren't sure why it works, but they do know that it helps reduce nicotine withdrawal symptoms. And even though bupropion is an antidepressant, it helps smokers quit regardless of whether or not they're depressed. It's one of several prescription drugs available to help you stop smoking.

Schedule exercise. Exercising three times a week may work even better than a behavioral therapy program. In one study, nearly 20 percent of the exercisers were still smoke free after a year compared to 11 percent of the therapy group. They also gained less weight. Of course, counseling plus exercise is an even better idea.

<table>
<tr><td>Step
2</td><td>**Get 30 Minutes of Light
Exercise Most Days**</td></tr>
</table>

In the handful of minutes it takes to watch the depressing evening news each day, you could slash your risk of diabetes by 34 percent, of stroke by 20 percent, of a hip fracture by 41 percent, and of dying over the next few years by half—and at the same time sharpen your thinking skills, whittle your waist, and put some sparkle in your mood.

How? By exercising, of course. Our panel of experts enthusiastically ranked physical activity high on their list of health-enhancing "moves." And it couldn't be easier: They told us it takes just a half hour of light activity (a stroll, a swim, some work in the garden) most days of the week to reap its dramatic, body-wide benefits.

We'll skip the rest of that lecture because we know you've heard it 1,000 times before. The real

question about exercise and health isn't whether it works. Rather, it's why don't most of us do it?

The honest answer? We simply can't get ourselves off the couch and out the door. Maybe we're scared of the idea of exercise. More likely, inertia takes over, partly because we're so darned used to sitting on the couch and so unused to exercise. We may not even feel we have the energy to take a walk because frankly, sitting around all day makes us tired. Sound familiar?

If you've been putting it off until you feel like exercising, forget it. Waiting for the perfect wave of enthusiasm to lift you off the couch just doesn't work. Instead, make a commitment to do just 10 minutes of exercise on a certain schedule. Regular exercisers report that just getting out there—whether you feel motivated or not—creates the energy that propels your feet and buoys your mood. Just tell yourself you'll walk for 10 short minutes. Once you get started, those 10 minutes will easily turn into 20 and eventually 30.

Walking or biking is a great way to start. You'll also want to do activities that strengthen your muscles, such as working with hand weights or elastic exercise bands, doing moves like sit-ups and pushups, using the strength machines at the gym, or even working hard in your garden. You begin losing muscle mass in your thirties; as a result, your body burns fewer calories every day—making it tougher to maintain a healthy weight. A little strength training can reverse this trend and give you the strength for everyday activities like carrying heavy grocery bags as well as for fun stuff like dancing, bowling, and keeping up with the grandchildren! We recommend investing a little time and energy in learning how to do the right strength-training moves for your age and fitness level by buying a few sessions with a personal trainer or taking a class at your local gym.

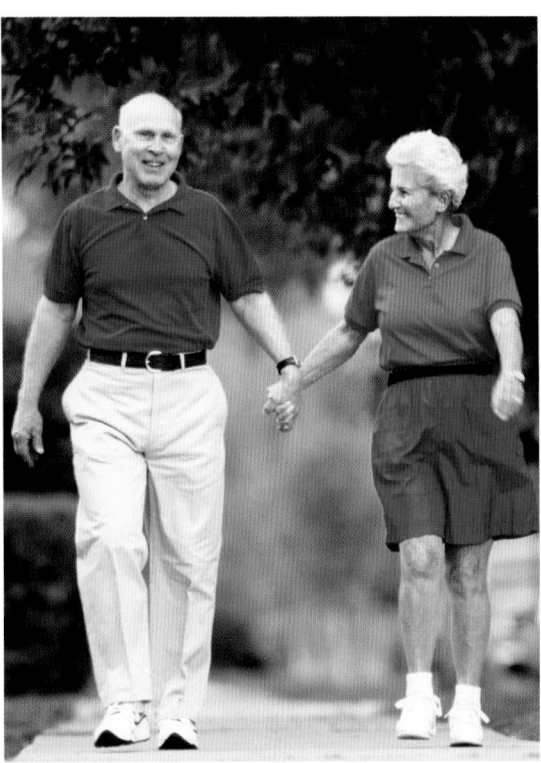

Your best exercise accessory? A mindset that helps you find a routine that works for you. Reset your attitude with these refreshing revelations.

Anything is better than nothing. No time for a 30-minute walk or a 45-minute gym workout? Then use the 5, 10, or 15 minutes you do have. Plenty of studies show that three 10-minute walks burn calories as effectively as one 30-minute jaunt and may be even better at things like keeping blood pressure lower and healthier all day. Dancing, playing energetically with the kids, hoofing it around the mall, or playing softball at the local block party can all boost cardiovascular health as well as a formal workout.

Willpower is not the answer. If you're like most people, willpower alone won't get you up every day for that 7:00 a.m. walk or pull you away from your chores for those calisthenics. Instead, set an exercise "date"—a regular walking or jogging time with a friend, a class at the gym, or even an appointment with your personal trainer. Write it in pen on your calendar.

It should be enjoyable. It's no wonder many people think they dislike exercise—how much fun is it to sit in the basement pedaling an exercise bike that's going nowhere? If you're the competitive type, take up squash, racquetball, or tennis. Are you social? Schedule walks with different friends or join a spin or water aerobics class.

Love nature? Map out some beautiful places to explore near your home. Love to garden? Plan to make the neighbors green with envy. Exercise isn't just a means to an end; it's part of your life, so it shouldn't feel like a chore.

Opportunities are everywhere. That parking spot at the back of the supermarket lot, the stairs next to the escalator, the dog with the leash in his mouth, the kid or grandkid longing for a trip to the playground—these are all golden opportunities to fit more old-fashioned, calorie-burning movement into your day. Fifty years ago, we burned about 700 more calories per day than we do today, not by running marathons but through a host of daily activities that we've engineered out of our lives, from rolling down car windows by hand to washing the dishes. It's up to you to buck the trend.

Emptier hospitals. Shorter lines at the pharmacy counter. Far fewer of the major diseases that disable and kill millions. If everyone followed the simple and delicious advice of our health experts by eating at least five servings of fruit and vegetables a day (see page 320 to remind yourself what a serving is), the results would be nothing short of miraculous.

The fact is, we humans are designed to eat these foods by the fistful every day. Our bodies are meant to be flooded with a daily deluge of amazing chemicals called antioxidants that protect cells from damage. And we need them now more than ever. Modern life triggers the production of more free radicals in our bodies than ever before—thanks to fried foods (and simply to overeating!), to more pollution, to the fact that we're living longer, and perhaps even to a thinning atmosphere.

Free radicals are atoms or groups of atoms with an odd number of electrons. They form naturally when we digest food, convert blood sugar into energy, or are exposed to sunlight or pollution. Free radicals destroy cell walls or even worse, DNA itself. The result? Increased cancer risk, cholesterol that's more likely to burrow into artery walls, and damaged cartilage that can't cushion joints properly. Your body uses the antioxidants in fruits and vegetables to neutralize free radicals before they can do harm. Shortchange yourself, and you're essentially letting rogue elements take over your body.

Fruit is simple to eat: Just grab a banana or an orange, peel, and enjoy. It also transforms meals. Think about the juicy crunch of grapes in chicken salad or the burst of sharp sweetness a few strawberries add to cereal. With a little creativity, vegetables can be just as delicious— think of ripe red tomatoes dressed with basil, zucchini fresh off the grill and dusted with a touch of sea salt, and roasted sweet potatoes with a pinch of cinnamon or nutmeg.

Putting nature's original gourmet treats on your plate may take more time than zipping through the burger-stand drive-through or tossing a frozen entrée into your microwave, but it's worth it in terms of both satisfaction and health. And thanks to a host of prewashed, precut produce available in the supermarket, you'll be surprised how easy it really can be. Try these strategies to get your fill.

Assign specific servings to each meal. For example, you might always have a small glass of orange juice plus a handful of berries or a side of melon at breakfast, start lunch with a salad (two servings of veggies), have fruit as a snack, and serve one cooked veggie and one raw veggie at dinner. That's seven servings!

Always have two colors of produce on your plate. Start breakfast with a spinach and red pepper omelet, have carrots and black beans (yes, they count as vegetables) on your lunchtime salad, and top your pasta with chopped tomatoes and steamed broccoli at dinner. It's an automatic two servings per meal and floods your body with a wide variety of antioxidants and other beneficial phytochemicals.

Double each vegetable portion you'd normally eat. This is a good approach if you're already eating several servings a day.

Load up on ready-to-use produce. Try cans of fruit in light syrup or juice, frozen plain (no sauce) vegetables, frozen berries, and presliced, pretrimmed vegetables. We also love prewashed spinach that you can microwave right in the bag.

Keep salads interesting. Plain green salads get boring, but just one new topping can make them seem new again. Try roasted sesame seeds, canned artichoke hearts, a few olives, sliced cucumbers, red peppers, hot peppers, or even a few raspberries.

new reasons to eat less

Big portions and high-fat, high-calorie processed foods are the public enemies of good health. Excess weight puts you at higher risk for heart disease and diabetes—you knew that. But a growing stack of research links obesity to an increased risk of most types of cancer, too. Our panel of experts recommends scaling back on overeating—and we agree.

Eating too much not only packs on visible pounds, it also crowds internal organs with fat that fuels the development of heart disease and diabetes. But extra calories are dangerous for a second reason: Digestion creates destructive particles called free radicals that play a role in a host of health problems, from joint pain to cancer. More food, more digestion, more free radicals. Eating just enough is a challenge in our super-size society, but it can be done.

- **Dole out single servings.** Don't put platters of food on the table or sit with an open bag of snacks.
- **Eat at home.** Women who eat out more often than five times a week consume 300 calories more each day than home diners.
- **Bulk up your meals with extra vegetables.** These add fiber, water, and heft to your meal—three qualities that make your tummy feel fuller while you're eating hundreds fewer calories. Researchers say this strategy stretches the stomach wall, activating "fullness receptors."
- **Eat only until you're 80 percent full.** This ancient Japanese custom gives your mind time to register what you've eaten. Leave the table when you still have room for a little more. Within 20 minutes, you'll realize you feel satisfied.

Get Recommended Screening Tests

Left to their own devices, invisible little health problems turn into big ones. A "touch of sugar" becomes full-blown diabetes; prehypertension becomes high blood pressure; suspicious-looking cells become cancer. Your best defense: Catch these and other silent health destroyers early, when they can most easily be reversed and even cured.

Sure, a healthy lifestyle is the best way to prevent big-league medical disasters, but trouble can brew in the healthiest of bodies. That's why our preventive medicine specialists ranked getting recommended screening tests number four on their list of "prescriptions" for a healthy life. But many of us skip these important and easy-to-get tests. Lack of time, fear of finding out that something's wrong, or the mistaken conviction that you really don't need the screenings because you're feeling fit as a fiddle can cause you to skip a test—and seriously regret it later.

See the table on the opposite page for a list of common screening tests and when to get them. And for the motivation to follow through, try out these new attitudes about the routine checks that can save your life.

Save time: Get screened when you see the doc about routine health problems. Scheduling an appointment for a sore throat, sinus infection, or other minor problem? Ask if you can get simple screening tests such as cholesterol, blood pressure, and blood sugar at the same time rather than making a separate appointment for

an annual physical. There's new evidence that annual physicals are outmoded and unnecessary; piggybacking screenings onto other visits works just fine. (Of course, you'll need a special appointment for major tests like a colonoscopy, and you'll need to go to a radiology center to get your mammogram, bone density scan, etc.)

Hate going to the doctor? Go with your spouse or a friend. Boost your odds of getting the screenings you need by seeing your family doc together for things like blood pressure checks, cholesterol and blood sugar tests, and colon cancer screenings. You can also offer to be each other's support team when it's time for specialized checks for breast and prostate cancer.

Speak up about your family history. Make sure your doctor knows your family history. If a close relative has had a stroke or heart attack or was diagnosed with cancer or diabetes, let her know.

Mention depression. Doctors should screen for depression, but they don't always. If you're feeling significantly sad or hopeless, let your doctor know. There are treatments that can help.

Ask about vaccinations. Aside from a yearly flu shot, you should get a one-time-only shingles vaccine if you're 60 or older and a one-time-only pneumonia vaccine if you're 65 or older.

Keep track. Don't wait for your doctor to tell you it's time to check your cholesterol again. Keep a record of what tests and vaccinations you've had and when in a small notebook or wherever you record birthdays and appointments.

The Tests You Need

	TEST	WHEN TO GET IT
Women	Mammogram	Yearly beginning at age 40. Once you reach 75, it's up to you and your doctor whether you should continue having mammograms.
	Pap test and pelvic exam	Yearly. If you're over 30 and have a normal Pap and a normal HPV test (which tests for the virus that causes most cervical cancers), you don't need to be tested again for 3 years. If you've had 3 normal Pap tests in a row, you can skip the next 2 or 3 years. Check with your doctor if you are over 70.
	Thyroid hormone test	Every 5 years beginning at age 35.
Men	Prostate-specific antigen (PSA) test	Yearly beginning at age 50, or 45 if you're at increased risk due to a family history of the disease or being African-American. Not everyone agrees the test is necessary; talk with your doctor.
	Digital rectal exam	Yearly beginning at age 50, or 45 if you're at increased risk due to a family history of the disease or being African-American.
Everyone	Dental exam and cleaning	Twice a year.
	Blood pressure reading	At every doctor's visit (at least once a year).
	Cholesterol test	At least every 5 years starting at age 30, or age 20 if you have a family history of heart disease or you smoke. Every 2 years in your 40s and yearly starting at age 50.
	Fasting plasma glucose (blood sugar) test	Every 3 years beginning at age 45; more often or earlier if you're overweight or at risk for diabetes.
	Skin cancer check	Every 3 years beginning at age 20; yearly beginning at age 40.
	Eye exam	At least once from ages 20–29; at least twice from ages 30–39, then every 2 to 4 years until age 65; annually thereafter.
	Hearing test	Every 10 years until age 50, then every 3 years.
	Colonoscopy	Every 10 years starting at age 50.
	Bone density scan	At least once beginning at age 65, or earlier if your doctor recommends it.

Step 5 — Get at Least 7 to 8 Hours of Sleep Each Night

Blame it on insomnia, our infatuation with caffeine, shift work, or cable TV and the Internet; whatever the cause, we've become a sleep-deprived planet. And we're paying the price with higher rates of obesity, diabetes, depression, anxiety, and even some forms of cancer—all related, in part, to lack of sleep. Our health team says it's time to turn in and snooze.

Researchers are beginning to suspect that sleep deprivation exerts its far-reaching effects on the body by disrupting levels of key hormones and proteins. These include the appetite-regulating hormones ghrelin and leptin (that's why lack of sleep contributes to weight gain); stress hormones such as cortisol that raise blood sugar and blood pressure (a reason lack of sleep makes diabetes worse); and proteins involved in chronic inflammation, a condition in which the immune system remains on high alert and that raises the risk of heart disease, stroke, cancer, and diabetes. Lack of sleep also seems to reduce levels of melatonin, a hormone that may help protect against cancer.

If you have insomnia or you're a heavy snorer and often wake up exhausted, turn to the Insomnia and Snoring chapters. But many of us are our own worst enemies when it comes to getting enough shuteye. If that's you, put these three simple strategies to work in order to get seven to eight hours of deep, refreshing sleep.

Pick your perfect bedtime, then stick with it for two weeks. Count back eight hours from the time you have to get up in the morning. This is your new, nonnegotiable lights-out time. Subtract another half hour: This is your new "get into bed" time. Subtract another half hour to find the time when you should start relaxing, getting mind and body ready for sleep. Here's an example: If you have to be up at 6:30 a.m., you'll need to start relaxing by 9:30 p.m., get into bed by 10:00, and turn out the lights by 10:30.

Turn off all electronics. A half hour before you get into bed, turn off the TV, computer, cell phone, and personal digital assistant. Politely tell anyone who calls on your home phone that you'll talk to them tomorrow (or better yet, screen your calls and return nonurgent messages later). Take a shower or bath and climb into clean, comfy pajamas. Brush your teeth, comb your hair, do a few minutes of gentle stretching or deep breathing, read a few pages, and lock up the house. Skip snacks during this time: Too often, we turn to food to fuel a burst of late-night energy.

When it's time, discipline yourself to turn out the lights. If you've trained yourself to fight back fatigue and keep on going, you may be tempted to stay up just a little later. But go ahead and turn out the light; it's time to sleep. You'll see how great you feel in the morning!

Step 6	**Take a Daily Low-Dose Aspirin**

This step applies only if your doctor says it's appropriate for you.

A tiny aspirin can battle two of our biggest killers, heart disease and stroke. Swallowing one a day can slash your odds of having a heart attack by 23 percent and a stroke by 15 percent. New research suggests it may even cut the odds for the most common form of breast cancer by 16 percent. Yet fewer than half of the people who could benefit from this inexpensive health "insurance policy" pop this potent little pill.

Aspirin guards hearts by making platelets, the special clotting cells in your bloodstream, less sticky. This means they're less likely to form a clot that can travel to your heart, causing a heart attack, or to your brain, causing a stroke. Aspirin's anticancer benefits are probably due to its anti-inflammatory effects (chronic inflammation plays a role in the development of cancer).

It sounds good—but don't take aspirin every day on your own. In some people, long-term use can provoke digestive upset and excessive bleeding, including bleeding in the brain. Doctors usually recommend daily aspirin therapy only to patients with risk factors for heart attack and stroke, such as smoking, high cholesterol, diabetes, or a family or personal history of either condition. If you're taking daily aspirin, be sure to drink alcohol only in moderation (no more than one drink a day for women and two drinks a day for men). The combination of aspirin and too much alcohol can harm your liver.

aspirin's new rules

If you take aspirin daily or are thinking about it, these smart tips can keep you safe.

- **Tell your doctor if you bleed easily** due to a clotting disorder or have asthma, stomach ulcers, or heart failure, all conditions that may prevent you from taking daily aspirin.
- **Take the dose your doctor recommends.** Some studies have found benefit from as little as 75 milligrams a day (less than the 81 milligrams in low-dose aspirin), but some doctors prefer to prescribe one regular-strength, 325-milligram tablet daily.
- **Ibuprofen interferes with aspirin's anticlotting magic, reducing its effectiveness.** If you need a single dose of ibuprofen for pain, take it two hours after taking aspirin. If you use ibuprofen regularly, talk with your doctor about strategies for getting the most from both drugs.
- **Tell your surgeon and dentist.** If you need a surgical procedure or dental work, inform your doctor about your aspirin use ahead of time to avoid problems like excessive bleeding.
- **Before you begin taking aspirin on a daily basis,** tell your doctor if you take another blood-thinning drug, like warfarin (Coumadin), or any herbs and supplements, especially vitamin E, St. John's wort, or ginkgo biloba. All can interact with aspirin and thin the blood too much.

<table>
<tr><td>Step
7</td><td>**Know Your Blood Pressure
Numbers**</td></tr>
</table>

Speaking four magic words—What's my blood pressure?—could slash your odds of a heart attack, a stroke, kidney failure, or blindness. If you don't ask, your doctor may never tell you whether you're developing high blood pressure, the killer that nearly every physician in our Disease Prevention Survey said has the greatest potential for causing chronic disease. And if you don't know your blood pressure is creeping up, you can't take steps to bring it back down, leaving the door open for years or even decades of damage to occur.

You can't feel high blood pressure. But when blood rages and bangs through your cardiovascular system, it wreaks havoc—thickening heart muscle, promoting the growth of plaque in artery walls, rupturing blood vessels in your brain, tearing others in your eyes, weakening your kidneys, and even raising your risk of dementia. Your doctor should check your pressure at every visit, but some doctors don't; if yours doesn't, ask for the check. And pay attention to the results.

Until just a few years ago, doctors thought you were in the clear if your blood pressure was below 140/90. Now we know the risk of heart disease and stroke begins to rise when BP is as low as 115/75. There's nothing "normal" about slightly high blood pressure. Being in the "prehypertensive" range—with a reading between 120/80 and 140/90—raises your risk of dying from heart disease by 58 percent, making this "little" problem more deadly than smoking!

More than one in four adults have prehypertension. Are you among them? Even if your pressure's normal now, consider this: 90 percent of us will develop high blood pressure after age 55. And don't depend on your doctor to catch rising BP early, when it's easiest to fix. Physicians often adopt a dangerous "wait and see" attitude when their patients' pressures start creeping up, studies show. It's up to you to keep tabs on your blood pressure and take any increase seriously, even if your reading is still within the healthy range.

Live a healthy blood pressure lifestyle. At breakfast, lunch, and dinner, you can choose the power foods that fight hypertension. Top eating strategy: Follow the DASH Diet, which is packed with fruits, vegetables, whole grains, and several servings of low-fat dairy foods, every day. Keep sodium low, too. Quitting smoking, treating obstructive sleep apnea, and getting regular exercise can all make big dents in elevated blood pressure, too.

Ask about medication. If lifestyle changes alone don't lower your blood pressure, medication can help. Forward-thinking doctors are beginning to prescribe BP-lowering drugs even to people in the prehypertensive category if they have other risk factors for heart disease or kidney problems, such as diabetes or kidney disease.

what your numbers mean

115/75 or lower: Ideal
Below 120/80: Healthy
120–139/80–89: Prehypertensive
140/90: High blood pressure

<table>
<tr><td>Step
8</td><td>**Have Happy Interactions
with Family and Friends**</td></tr>
</table>

You've gotta have friends…What good is sitting alone in your room?…Love makes the world go 'round. These song lyrics could be ripped from the pages of today's medical journals. A growing body of scientific research is proving that happy relationships literally change the biochemistry of your brain for the better, while loneliness raises your risk of problems like high blood pressure, depression, and even an early death. In fact, an overwhelming 79 percent of the doctors we polled said that social isolation is extremely detrimental to health. Good times with friends and family, on the other hand, pump up feelings of joy, boost immunity, lower your risk of heart trouble, and can even extend your life.

Experts are beginning to realize that we're hardwired for personal connection. Back in prehistoric times, being alone was perilous—no one was around to help fend off marauding wolves or forage for roots and berries if you were sick. Fast-forward to today: We're remarkably self-sufficient, yet our ancient responses haven't changed. When you're alone for too long (and the definition of "too long" is different for each of us), levels of the stress hormone cortisol rise, ratcheting up your odds of heart disease, high blood pressure, depression, muddled thinking, and sleep problems. One UCLA study even found that our brains register social isolation in the same way they register physical pain.

How can you get more "vitamin F" (for "friends and family")?

Reach out. Stop waiting for the perfect moment. Plenty of people you know are shy and would love it if you called with an invitation to a movie or to come over to share that fruit salad you just whipped up. Thinking that you need an elaborate plan, a perfectly clean house, or a new haircut before you can make a date just postpones happiness.

Touch. Sit closer to your spouse or romantic partner. Hold hands more often—and while you're at it, make love more often. Studies show that these physical connections buffer stress and even cut heart attack risk. Need more touch in your life? Don't overlook furry, four-legged friends. Plenty of research shows they can have profound health benefits, including reducing levels of stress hormones and calming high blood pressure.

Expand your network. Yes, old friends know us best, but relying on a small group of companions could be a setup for lonely days. Invest in your future health by reaching out to a new person this week. An easy way to begin: Strike up a conversation with someone you see often at your house of worship, in your neighborhood, at your gym, or somewhere else you go regularly. Then go a step further and ask if they'd like to join you for a cup of coffee. Chances are, they'll be delighted.

<table>
</table>

Step 9	Cut Most of the Saturated Fat from Your Diet

Steering clear of fast-food drive-throughs; custard stands; and the fatty meats, butter, and full-fat milk and cheeses at the supermarket could lower your LDL cholesterol by an impressive 10 percent. What's the big deal? Well, this drug-free drop in bad cholesterol could in turn cut your risk of having a heart attack by 20 percent. Not a bad return on a smart food investment—and that's why our panel recommends targeting saturated fat when you're ready to make some healthy dietary tweaks.

These days, experts say that getting LDL lower than ever (below 100 mg/dl for most people and as low as 70 mg/dl if you have diabetes or have had a heart attack or stroke) is a smart move. The best way to do it? Cut way back on saturated fat, the body's raw material for manufacturing LDL.

Your goal is to keep saturated fat at just 7 percent of the calories you eat. That's about 15 grams a day or 135 calories' worth if you eat about 2,000 calories a day. You can quickly see that there's little room for butter, at 7 grams of saturated fat per tablespoon; heavy cream, at 3.5 grams per tablespoon; or full-fat cheddar cheese at 6 grams per ounce (about 1 slice). Here's how to keep a lid on this dangerous fat.

Buy low-fat or fat-free milk and dairy products. Choosing fat-free over full-fat milk will save you about four grams of saturated fat per cup, and having low-fat cheese will save the same amount per slice. Hate low-fat cheese? Try soft cheeses such as goat cheese, which are naturally a little lower in saturated fat than hard cheeses. Or choose a strong-flavored cheese like Romano and grate just a bit on your food.

Skip butter entirely, and be careful what you replace it with. If you like margarine, choose a brand that's free of hydrogenated oils, which are as bad as saturated fat for your ticker. Even better: Invest in an oil mister bottle and enjoy a little olive oil on your bread instead.

Buy only the leanest beef. A three-ounce burger made from 80 percent lean ground beef has 5.1 grams of fat; one made from 90 percent ground beef has 3.5. Make your burger from extra-lean ground beef (95 percent lean), and you'll cut the saturated fat to 2.3 grams—not bad. Want to bring those numbers even lower? Avoid ground beef and go for cuts of meat like eye of round, top round, and bottom round, which come from the cow's lean back legs; skip fatty underbelly cuts like rib eye, spareribs, and brisket. A three-ounce (small!) piece of broiled top sirloin has just 1.6 grams.

Keep servings of red meat to four ounces or less per day. Cancer experts say higher amounts raise cancer risk.

Eat your chicken and turkey naked. That means no skin. Well-trimmed pork tenderloin and even well-trimmed pork chops are also good lean choices.

Be on the lookout for tropical oils. Coconut, palm, and palm kernel oil are rich in saturated fat—and they're making a comeback in some commercial baked goods like cookies and crackers. Some food makers are putting these oils back into their recipes as they remove trans fats (partially hydrogenated vegetable oils linked to higher risk of heart disease). Bottom line: If the label says "no trans fats," check the ingredients list for tropical oils and look at the Nutrition Facts label to see what the saturated fat content is.

Swap bad fat for good fat. Instead of those burgers, try fish. Instead of butter, use olive oil. Fish and olive (and canola) oil bring hefty heart benefits. And instead of doughnuts or chips, snack on nuts, which actually lower cholesterol!

can carbs keep you disease free?

Many people are cutting down on carbs to keep their weight in check. A smart idea? That depends.

Most experts agree that carbs in the form of soda and sugary fruit drinks, store-bought baked goods (like muffins), packaged snacks, and sweets make blood sugar and blood fats (such as triglycerides) soar, raising your odds for type 2 diabetes, heart disease, and even some forms of cancer.

Stock up instead on "smart carbohydrates"—whole grains like oatmeal, barley, whole grain bread, and brown rice, as well as fruits, vegetables, and beans—and you'll flood your body with powerful disease-fighting compounds. These strategies can help you replace refined carbs with more of the good stuff.

- **Say yes to breads and cereals with the word *whole* in the first ingredient.**
- **Give potatoes the night off.** White potatoes and white rice make blood sugar soar; in comparison, whole grain side dishes such as barley, quinoa, and bulgur keep it lower and steadier.
- **Have beans for supper a few nights a week.** Rinse canned beans to reduce excess sodium. Then toss 'em into soups, salads, casseroles, or pasta sauce or enjoy them with your favorite seasonings as a side dish.
- **Drink unsweetened iced tea or water.** Besides adding hundreds of waist-widening calories, soda (even one can a day!) has been linked with a higher risk of diabetes, heart disease, and overweight.

<table>
<tr><td>Step
10</td><td>**Get Treated for Depression**</td></tr>
</table>

Depression isn't a bad mood. It's a common, serious illness that puts your health in danger—so much so that our prevention experts ranked it as significantly more dangerous than having high cholesterol. It's linked with a higher risk of diabetes, heart disease, and a host of other serious health conditions. Having depression plus diabetes and heart disease (a common combination) is a deadly triple threat that increases your risk of early death by as much as 30 percent.

It's not clear why depression accompanies so many serious health problems. Some experts are beginning to suspect that stress hormones and changes in the nervous system play important roles. What is clear: Fighting depression is imperative.

The trouble is, most people with depression aren't getting the help they need. Thanks to punishing beliefs that this illness is a sign of weakness (or something you can "tough out" on your own) and to doctors who fail to recognize or treat depression, millions of people slog along on their own. If that sounds like your situation, call your doctor today and make an appointment specifically to talk about this issue and get help. No one should go through life feeling sad and

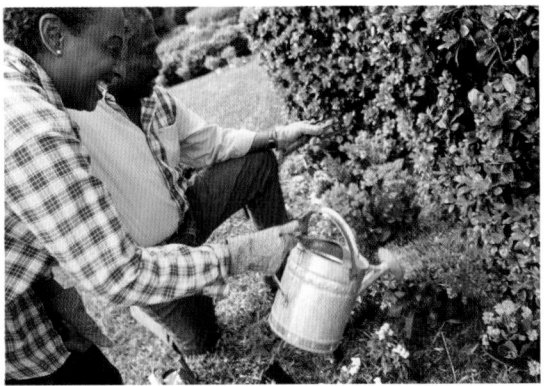

hopeless. There's just too much at stake.

We know that one of the hardest things about depression is trying to believe that you can feel better. But that belief should be your goal—and your doctor's. Mental health experts now say that feeling a bit better isn't enough. You can, and should, feel as good as you felt before the depression began. However you choose to get there, call on these three courageous qualities (and demand them of your doctor) on your journey toward feeling good again.

Be patient. Nearly 70 percent of the 3,700 people in a recent landmark study of depression treatments eventually felt as good as new. Just 37 percent got there with the first treatment (an antidepressant) they tried. The rest needed as many as four different therapies before finding the right one for them. What worked? For some, it was one antidepressant. For others, it was a combination of two drugs. For still others, cognitive therapy was the turning point. You won't know what works for you until you try—and try again.

Have high expectations. Expect to feel completely better. If you have lingering down times after giving a therapy a good try (usually 8 to 12 weeks), talk to your doctor about what else she can do to help you.

Be persistent. Plenty of people stop taking antidepressants or going to therapy as soon as they begin to feel better, but many relapse. The reason: A single episode of depression can last for 9 to 12 months. Stopping treatment early leaves you vulnerable, so stick with the one that's making your life better. If you think you're ready to go it alone, talk with your doctor about the best way to taper off a drug and how to decide whether you need to resume treatment.

Step 11 Tame Chronic Stress

The body is quite adept at dealing with short-term stress. If you need to swerve the car to avoid an accident, a burst of adrenaline will have come and gone even before your mind has time to fully process what happened. But living with chronic stress is another story altogether, one with surprising health implications. It ratchets up levels of cortisol and other stress hormones and leaves them set on "high" for days, weeks, months (or years!) on end. The result? Beyond the obvious—tension headaches, sleepless nights, disrupted digestion—researchers are finding links between this kind of stress and higher blood sugar levels, greater amounts of dangerous fat deep in the belly, and possibly even a higher risk of certain cancers. It's no wonder our panelists told us that living with uncontrolled stress is more destructive than major disease triggers such as being 30 pounds overweight or eating loads of processed food.

All of us have stress in our lives, whether it's the result of a dramatic event like divorce or a major illness or the low-level frustrations that come with a busy job, a tense home life, financial worries, or regrets about the roads not taken in life. We're not going to advise band-aid recommendations like a bubble bath, a hot cup of tea, or a good sniff of lavender; they're all very nice, but we'd rather help you get to the bottom of your stress. The best place to start? Be frank and honest with yourself about what's bothering you, then start looking for real solutions.

Admit to yourself what's really stressing you. Whatever it is, it deserves your attention and respect. Once you bring it out of the shadows and into the open, you can start dealing with it rather than letting it eat away at your insides. Don't downplay the issues that are bugging you, even if they seem commonplace. When Pace University researchers quizzed people over 50 about the biggest sources of stress in their lives, a decreasing circle of friends, slowing down physically, diminishing time left to spend with children and grandchildren, regret over earlier life choices, physical pain, memory problems, and the need to complete way too many bewildering forms (for health insurance and income taxes, for example) were issues that showed up on the list.

Once you've identified the things that are really stressing you out, write them down, leaving room beside each one to note whether it's something you can't really change and need to accept (such as that milestone birthday coming up) or something you do have some control over. If it's the latter, allow yourself some time to think, then list a few concrete steps you can take to start addressing it. Making even one small improvement can make you feel remarkably better by finally giving you a sense of control.

Ask for help where you need it. It's human nature: People are afraid to ask for help. Or they assume there's nowhere to turn, when often there are resources available. Financial planners, marriage counselors, life coaches, your doctor, or a trusted adviser from your house of worship are good resources that can help you address specific problems in your life. And friends, relatives, neighbors, or even acquaintances are usually willing to help out with small tasks if you have the courage to reach out. Maybe they could use your help with something, too.

Build, or rebuild, a social network. Loss is a theme that occurred again and again when the Pace University researchers asked people about big stresses. Their advice? Rebuild a web of caring connections through your house of worship, community groups, and volunteering (which itself makes you feel good). Don't depend on a small, close-knit circle of friends—now's the time to branch out. Scientific journals are bursting with evidence that having friends around changes the biochemistry of your brain—by pumping up feelings of joy and well-being that bolster immunity, for example—while being

lonely puts you at risk for an earlier death, high blood pressure, depression, and even accidents at home and on the road.

Learn, and practice, relaxing. Most of us aren't very aware of our bodies. If our muscles are tensed or our breathing is faster and shallower than it should be, we don't manage to notice, let alone make the connection to stress. A good solution is to find a relaxation technique you like and use it every day, regardless of how you feel that day. You can try formal meditation and mindfulness-based stress reduction (locate a class in dozens of countries around the world at www.umassmed.edu/cfm/mbsr), yoga, and breathing exercises (inhale slowly for 4 counts, pause for 1 to 2 counts, exhale for 7 to 8 counts, pause for 1 to 2 counts, and inhale again). The health benefits of relaxation include better weight control, lower blood sugar, stronger immunity, less depression, an easing of chronic pain, and even faster recovery from psoriasis.

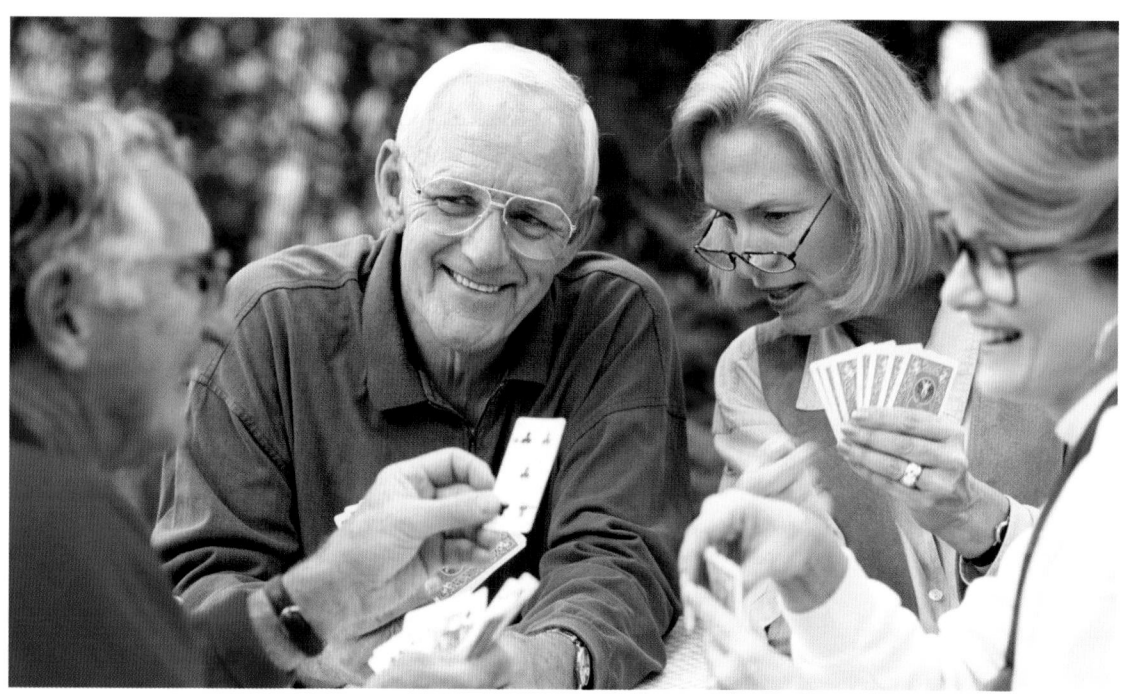

Frequently Pray, Meditate, or Focus on a Higher Sense of Purpose

Have you ever noticed that people with a deep love or passion for something outside themselves—their religion, helping others, nature, music, or art—complain less about themselves, their health, and their lives and seem more resilient when bad things happen? Perhaps they are more joyful, more thankful, or feel more at peace with the world around them. Those feelings pay off in the form of better health. The benefits are so strong, in fact, that the doctors who participated in our Disease Prevention Survey ranked praying, meditating, or embracing a higher sense of purpose as more important to disease prevention than consuming more omega-3 fatty acids or eating less sugar. And these are medical doctors!

Frankly, we were amazed at how many of the doctors we surveyed answered along the following lines when we asked what actions were important for maintaining health and preventing disease. One doctor advised our readers to "Believe in something good; practice being a loving person." Another recommended that you "Love the ones you're with (spouse, children, extended family, faith family, neighbors, co-workers, community members)." Wrote a third, "Volunteer in the community to improve the life of others less fortunate than yourself." A fourth put it this way: "Strive to achieve something bigger than yourself."

Studies show that faith, prayer, a strong core belief system, and the support of a friendly religious community can cut stress, boost immunity, improve your odds of recovering from illness, and even reduce chronic pain. Some researchers have even found that regular churchgoers tended to have lower blood pressure and higher "good" HDL cholesterol than those who didn't worship regularly.

Try these strategies to tap into your own higher sense of purpose.

Reconnect with your religion. You may already belong to a faith community or hold cherished religious or spiritual beliefs. But if you've let this dimension of life languish, it's time for a personal revival, whether you choose to attend religious services or pray on your own.

Try meditation. Doing it regularly can actually lower your blood sugar and increase your body's resistance to stress. Take a class to learn how or simply spend 10 minutes a day breathing slowly and deeply and clearing your mind by letting your thoughts flow by without dwelling on them.

Express yourself through music or art. There's no better way to free your mind of worries and keep you in the moment.

Lose yourself in nature. It's hard not to appreciate the beauty of the world when hiking through a verdant forest or strolling past a rushing stream or flowering meadow.

Give back. Volunteering is a great way to give back and restore your faith in yourself and others. If you don't want to do it formally, look for small ways to help others. Maybe older neighbors could use a hand with their lawn care, for example.

Safeguarding Your Health

Heart disease, cancer, diabetes, osteoporosis—none can stand up to the 12 Steps to Total Prevention you discovered in the previous chapter. Follow even just a few of the steps, and you're well on your way to preventing major diseases from inside your body. While you're at it, you'll also want to arm yourself against threats that lurk outside your body, from germs to toxins to tainted food, all of which can make you mildly sick, or worse. Whether you're in your home, on the road, or in the hospital, the advice in this chapter can help keep you safe and illness free.

creating a healthy home

Your house may be a haven—but a haven for what? For you and your family, or for allergens such as dust and mold, toxic gases, and waterborne threats? Experts estimate that people spend 80 to 90 percent of their time indoors, and most of that at home, so why not make your surroundings as healthy as possible? No home can ever be truly "clean," and that's okay. Just be sure to tackle any major threats lurking under your roof that could make you sick. Here are the four key steps.

1. Clear the air

HELPS PREVENT: Allergy and asthma attacks; bronchitis; lung cancer; and nervous system, developmental, and reproductive disorders (including infertility and attention deficit disorder); may even prevent death

Modern homes are sealed up tight, so you'd think they'd be practically pollution free. In fact, just the opposite is true: Indoor air is much more polluted than the air outside. Take these steps to ensure that the air you breathe isn't sabotaging your efforts to live a healthy, disease-free life.

What to Do

Wage war on dust. Dust and dust mites trigger allergy and asthma attacks, but dust itself is a "repository of pollutants," according to experts who've studied it extensively. It's a carrier of countless toxins, including pesticides, flame retardants, volatile organic compounds, or VOCs (emitted as gases by everything from paints and varnishes to cleaning products), and more. Live in a dusty house, and these contaminants enter your body every time you breathe, or eat food to which the particles have adhered. You also absorb the dust through your skin.

Battling dust doesn't necessarily mean vacuuming more often—in fact, vacuuming raises clouds of dust and other allergens, even if you use a vacuum cleaner with a fancy HEPA filter. Instead, replace carpets with hard flooring wherever possible and dust with a damp mop. (See our other tips for waging war on dust in the Allergies chapter on page 74.)

Test for radon. You can't see it, smell it, or taste it, but next to cigarettes, this radioactive gas is the leading cause of lung cancer in the world. It forms when uranium in soil breaks down, and it enters your home through cracks and holes in the foundation, which is why homes with basements tend to have the highest levels. However, any house, no matter its age or quality of construction, can have a radon problem.

Test your home for radon with either a professional testing service (check the yellow pages in your phone book) or a kit available at home centers. If levels are high, you need help from a professional radon-mitigation contractor to reduce them.

Install a carbon monoxide detector. Like radon, carbon monoxide is colorless, tasteless, and odorless—and it's fatal. It's released in fumes produced by small gas engines, stoves, generators, lanterns, and gas ranges or by burning charcoal and wood. And it kills more than 500 people a year in most countries. In addition to installing the detector, which you should test and replace every six months, here's what else you can do to prevent carbon monoxide poisoning.
- Get a qualified technician to service your heating system, water heater, and any other gas-, oil-, or coal-burning appliances each year.

- Never use a generator, charcoal grill, camp stove, or other gasoline- or charcoal-burning device inside your home, basement, or garage or near a window outside.
- Don't run a car or truck inside a garage attached to your house, even if you leave the garage door open.
- Don't burn anything in an unvented stove or fireplace.
- Never use a gas oven to heat your house.

Minimize mold. That stuffy nose, irritated throat, coughing, and wheezing? It could be a mold allergy. You may not even realize that your home has become a mold repository, but old carpets, damp basements, and even those stacks of old newspapers are likely to harbor it. Here's how to prevent mold and mold-related symptoms.

- Go to a hardware store and buy a hydrometer to measure the humidity in your home. Aim to keep indoor humidity levels between 40 and 60 percent. Use a dehumidifier in humid areas like basements, and run the air conditioner during hot, humid weather.
- Make sure that exhaust fans in your kitchen, bathroom, and laundry area are clear and vented to the outside.
- Fix any leaky roofs, windows, or pipes.
- Repair air ducts if you find a buildup of mold, dirt, or moisture inside, or if insects or rodents have taken up residence there. Keeping air filters clean and fixing leaks are the first steps—not duct cleaning, which may not even help.
- Remove mold with a bleach solution made with one cup of bleach to one gallon of water.
- Add mold inhibitors to paints before painting.
- Avoid using carpet in the bathrooms or basement.

ripping up carpeting? read this first

Wood floors are all the rage, and we recommend them to reduce allergy and asthma symptoms. But many floor finishes used in the 1950s and 1960s contain polychlorinated biphenyls (PCBs), which can retard development in fetuses and young children as well as contribute to cancer risk. As people rip up carpet in older homes and refinish floors, those chemicals are released into the air. In one study, researchers detected PCBs in the indoor air of a third of homes tested. The highest concentrations in homes and in the blood of their residents were found in homes in which the floors had just been sanded and refinished. If you're planning to refinish your floors, use a process that captures the dust so it doesn't go into the air, and make sure you and your family vacate the house during the work.

Forget the kerosene heater. It's a major source of sulfur dioxide, which is linked to respiratory illnesses like asthma and chronic obstructive pulmonary disease and even to death from these conditions.

Go green when building or remodeling. Furniture, paints, adhesives, ceiling tiles, drywall, and carpeting are major sources of VOCs such as formaldehyde. These compounds have been linked with fatigue, concentration problems, sore throats, runny noses, and even cancer. Most of these products are available in VOC-free forms; ask your contractor the next time you're redoing a room or building a new house.

2. Diagnose and treat your water

HELPS PREVENT: Diarrhea caused by bacteria in the water, miscarriage and birth defects due to pregnant women drinking water containing chlorination by-products, possible increase in cancer risk from carcinogenic pollutants, and delays in neurological development in babies and children

Simply turn on the tap and voilà—clean running water! It's a miracle, really, though we take it for granted dozens of times a day. For people who live in developed nations, enough safety standards are in place to ensure that the tap water almost certainly won't kill you. Still, your water may not be quite as pure as you'd like it to be.

What to Do

Ask for a water quality report. Even water from municipal suppliers can have more than 2,000 toxins in it, ranging from microorganisms to pesticides to radon. To find out what's in yours, ask your local water authority for a report on your water quality. If you have a private well or can't get a free report, you may have to pay for a water test by a private company. Ask for a basic test that looks for arsenic, bacteria, chlorine, copper, lead, manganese, nitrates and nitrites, and sodium. Recheck for bacteria and nitrates/

A Guide to Water Filters

All water filters are not alike. Choose the type that's right for your house after finding out what's in your water that you want to remove.

DEVICE	FORM	WHAT IT CAN DO	WHAT IT CAN'T DO
Activated carbon filter	Pitcher with filter insert, faucet attachment, countertop unit, or under-sink unit	Absorb organic contaminants that affect taste and odor; may remove chlorination by-products, cleaning solvents, and pesticides	Remove metals such as lead and copper, nitrates, bacteria, or dissolved minerals
Ion-exchange unit	Whole-house system	Remove minerals, including calcium and magnesium, that make water "hard," and fluoride; may remove radium and barium	Remove metals such as lead and copper, nitrates, and bacteria. *Note:* These units may become clogged if your water contains oxidized iron or iron bacteria.
Reverse-osmosis unit	Under-sink unit or whole-house system	Remove nitrates, sodium, and other dissolved inorganic and organic compounds as well as foul tastes, smells, or colors; may reduce levels of some pesticides, dioxins, chloroform, and petrochemicals	Remove all inorganic and organic contaminants
Distillation unit	Whole-house system	Remove nitrates, sodium, hardness, bacteria, dissolved solids, most organic compounds, heavy metals, and radionuclides	Remove some volatile organic compounds and certain pesticides. *Note:* Bacteria may recolonize on the cooling coils when the system is not activated.

nitrites (from agricultural runoff) each year and for other compounds every three years. Test for radon and VOCs every three to five years.

Choose the right filter system. No filter system is capable of removing every contaminant, off taste, and unpleasant odor from tap water. The key is choosing one designed to filter out the particular contaminants in your water. You can go with a whole-house system that cleans water where it enters your house from the public water supply or choose a point-of-entry system, like a filter that attaches to your kitchen sink or pitchers with filter inserts.

If you're worried about microscopic organisms such as cryptosporidium and giardia, common causes of intestinal infections, look for a filter with a pore size of one micron or less. (See "A Guide to Water Filters" on the previous page for more information on choosing a filter.) The stuff that's being filtered? It has to go somewhere, so wear gloves when you replace the filter.

3. Fight germs in key places

HELPS PREVENT: Viral and bacterial infections
Microbiologist and germ guru Charles Gerba, PhD, a professor at the University of Arizona, notes that "if you have the right germs in the right place and the right amount, you can get sick from anything you touch." You'll never, ever get rid of all the germs in your house—after all, bacteria are by far the most numerous organisms on Earth—so don't even imagine that you can. Instead, choose your battles strategically.

What to Do

Microwave the sponge. Your kitchen sponge is the germiest thing in your house. When researchers at the USDA tested common methods of disinfecting sponges—soaking in bleach or lemon juice, microwaving, or washing in the dishwasher—they found that microwaving for one minute zapped the most germs, followed by using the dishwasher. Save the soaking for the laundry.

Scrub the sink. After the sponge, the kitchen sink is the second most germ-laden place in your house (even worse than the toilet). Keep a spray bottle of cleaner handy and spritz the sink after each use, then wipe and rinse with hot water.

Buy a new cutting board. Older cutting boards, whether made of wood or plastic, are great hiding places for bacteria, including salmonella, thanks to all those deep knife cuts. If yours has seen better days, buy a new one and make it wood. When researchers slathered bacteria onto plastic and wooden cutting boards, they found that the bacteria snuggled deep within the pores of the wooden boards. That may sound gross, but those bugs stayed there and never reemerged, so they were harmless unless the board was scarred by a knife. The plastic boards, however, retained germs on their surface for hours. Clean your wooden cutting board in the sink with hot, soapy water and microwave it for one minute (if it will fit in the microwave) every few days to annihilate any remaining germs.

Protect your toothbrush. Store it at the opposite end of the bathroom from the toilet. When you flush, droplets containing bacteria are propelled through the air, landing on anything nearby. (It's also a good idea to put the toilet lid down before you flush.) Store your brush in an upright position after each use so the water drains away from the bristles; don't store a wet toothbrush in a closed case. And don't let the bristles of family members' brushes touch. Still worried about germs? Consider a dunk in antimicrobial mouthwash. Studies show that a 20-minute soak can eliminate germs. Don't reuse the disinfection liquid or soak more than one brush in it. If you've been sick, replace your toothbrush after you recover so you won't reinfect yourself.

Change diapers on the table. The diaper-changing table that is. If you change your granddaughter's nappy on the living room couch or floor, you'll transmit bacteria to surfaces in the room, no matter how careful you are. When you finish, wash your hands thoroughly with soap and water.

Get rid of the communal candy bowl or cookie jar. Given that only 67 percent of people who say they wash their hands actually do and that only a third of those people use soap, you can imagine what's lurking in there.

Wipe down sick surfaces. You can't go crazy disinfecting every surface in your house, but even if you did, it wouldn't make much difference. If a family member's been sick, though, it might make sense to wipe down surfaces that everyone touches all the time—doorknobs, light switches, the computer keyboard and mouse, the remote, the telephone—with disinfectant. Disinfectants don't kill all viruses (they mainly work against bacteria), but they may kill some. Experts recommend a solution of 1 part bleach to 10 parts water, which effectively kills bacteria and some viruses. Leave it on the surface for 10 to 20 seconds before wiping dry.

Wash laundry right. Yes, even laundry can make you sick. Sharing towels, for instance, is one way hepatitis B and antibiotic-resistant staph infections are spread, according to Dr. Gerba. And, he says, "If you do undergarments in one load and handkerchiefs in the next, you're blowing your nose in what was in your underwear." Make your underwear the last load, and at least once a month, run a hot cycle with bleach to clear out germs in the machine. Wash your hands after sorting laundry and before transferring wet items to the dryer. Otherwise you could transfer the bacteria on the laundry to your mouth, nose, and eyes, not to mention the clean laundry.

4. Keep your food safe

HELPS PREVENT: Diarrhea and food poisoning
Food should make you healthy, not sick. If you're careful how you handle the food you cook, you'll be much less likely to come down with diarrhea, the "stomach flu," or worse. Don't rely on your senses to judge safety—you can't see germs on food, and a food can smell okay even if it isn't.

What to Do

Thaw right. The best option is to defrost items in the fridge overnight. But if you're in a hurry, put the frozen item in a plastic bag and immerse it in cold water, changing the water every 30 minutes. Otherwise, use the microwave, but be ready to cook the food as soon as it's thawed.

Use a meat thermometer. Poultry should reach 165°F; beef roasts, at least 145°; pork and ground meat and poultry, 160°; and casseroles, 165°.

Shop in the right order. Buy nonperishables first, vegetables and fruits next, then meats and poultry, and finally, frozen food.

Take your fridge's temperature. Pick up an appliance thermometer at the hardware store and check that the fridge is at 40°F or below and the freezer at 0° or below.

Purge your pantry. Any high-acid canned foods such as tomatoes, grapefruit, and pineapple should be stored for no longer than 18 months; other canned foods can be kept for two to five years if the can is still in good shape and the label is readable. If you bought that can of peas two moves ago, it's time to say goodbye.

Wash, wash, wash. *E. coli* from spinach, salmonella from cantaloupe . . . is nothing safe? Nope, not really. Whether it's a bunch of grapes or an orange you plan to slice, rinse fresh fruits and vegetables in running tap water. Remove and toss the outer leaves of lettuce or cabbage. And don't leave cut produce at room temperature for more than an hour.

traveling disease free

It's the trip of a lifetime—a cruise to the islands, 10 days at sea, a balcony suite. But on the second day out, it hits: a dreaded norovirus, scourge of the high seas, destroyer of cruise-ship romance, death to any vacation. Or maybe you're visiting Florence for two weeks of art immersion, but you get sick on day five thanks to a virus you caught on the plane. Don't let your vacation—or even a business trip—be ruined by illness or accidents. The goal is to be disease free whether you're lounging in your living room or in the lobby of a four-star hotel. Here are the three key steps.

1. Use "plane" old common sense

HELPS PREVENT: Blood clots, respiratory illnesses, tummy troubles, flu, and dehydration
Nothing is more maddening than catching a virus on the plane ride to your vacation destination—and unfortunately, it's all too common, thanks to packed airplanes, germs that lurk on every surface you touch, and stale recirculated air (the result of airlines trying to save fuel by not allowing in as much fresh air from outside). Protect yourself with this travel-savvy advice.

What to Do

Take the first flight out in the morning. Not only is it more likely to be on time (delays haven't started building yet), reducing your stress level, but the plane will also have been recently cleaned from the previous day.

Tote a large bottle or two of water. As you've no doubt noticed, airline air is incredibly dry. That puts you at extra risk for picking up a bug, since you need moisture in your mucous membranes (your nose, throat, and eyes) to help repel viruses and bacteria. So skip the salty peanuts and pretzels (and alcohol, which is dehydrating) and drink up. Just make sure the water is bottled, whether you take it with you or get it on the plane. When the US EPA tested 158 passenger planes, it found that the drinking water in nearly 13 percent was infected with coliform bacteria, the presence of which is often used as a rough indicator of water's general cleanliness.

Stand up and walk every two hours. This helps prevent blood clots in your legs that can occur after sitting for several hours. It's easiest to get up as often as you like if you've booked an aisle seat. When you can't get up, exercise every half hour by raising your shoulders and shrugging them forward and back, dropping your chin and nodding yes and no, drawing circles with your toes, and pressing up onto the balls of your feet 10 times in a row. Don't sit with your legs crossed.

Take your own pillow and blanket. It may have been a month since the ones on the plane were cleaned. You can find inflatable pillows and travel blankets in travel stores.

Buy a pack of antibacterial wipes in the airport. Use them to wipe down your seatbelt, tray table, and armrests as well as the button that turns on the light. Take the wipes with you to the bathroom to use when opening the door and flushing the toilet.

2. Pack your suitcase right

HELPS PREVENT: Traveler's diarrhea, blisters, motion sickness, sunburn, and malaria
Sometimes it's little things like blisters or sunburn that detract from a perfect vacation. Other times it's the not-so-little things, like a bad case of traveler's diarrhea that leaves you stuck in the hotel for days. You can prevent a whole host of health problems by doing a little planning in advance.

What to Do
See your doctor two months before your trip. Ask if you'll need any vaccinations for the place you're visiting and whether malaria pills are advisable (if they are, start taking them as directed before leaving the country). If you're traveling to areas where the water quality is questionable, putting you at risk for traveler's diarrhea, also ask for a prescription for an antibiotic and fill it before you go. For example, a 200-milligram dose of rifaximin (Xifaxan), taken with the first meal you eat upon reaching your destination and followed by 200 milligrams twice a day with meals, prevents diarrhea in 72 to 77 percent of people who take it.

Take insect repellent and bug-blocking clothes. Mosquitoes aren't just annoying; the mosquitoes in certain areas of the world can transmit diseases like malaria and dengue fever. Ticks can cause tickborne encephalitis. Use an insect repellent on any exposed skin to repel mosquitoes, ticks, and fleas. Choose one that contains DEET or a newer pesticide called picaridin. Also take clothes to wear when the mosquitoes are out in force, including long-sleeved shirts, long pants, and closed shoes. If you're in really heavy mosquito territory, apply insect repellent that contains permethrin to clothing, shoes, tents, mosquito nets, and other gear (but not your skin). It keeps working even after five washings.

Screen out the sun. Whether you're skiing in the Alps or embarking on a long-awaited cruise to Mexico, keep in mind that countries near the equator and at higher elevations receive more UV rays than other parts of the globe. Plus, snow and light-colored sand reflect the sun, increasing your risk of sunburn. Even if you're not heading for the beach, slather on a high SPF sun lotion (30 is plenty) that blocks both UVA and UVB rays, and reapply it every couple of hours.

Pack flip-flops for the shower. If you plan to use the hotel pool or public showers, slip some flip-flops into your suitcase to protect your feet from athlete's foot. If you're planning to visit any rocky beaches, take aqua shoes.

Be ready for blisters. Blisters seem innocent enough, but if one becomes infected, you have a bigger problem, especially if you have diabetes. Take shoes that are already broken in, and pack a package of moleskin (sold in drugstores near the bandages) and some travel scissors. As soon as you feel a "hot spot" developing, cut a piece of moleskin large enough to cover the area and stick it on to prevent a full-blown blister.

Prevent Montezuma's revenge. You can reduce the risk of traveler's diarrhea by taking the usual precautions (such as avoiding tap water, ice, raw fruits and vegetables that you haven't peeled yourself, and so on). But also pack some Pepto-Bismol, which can even be used to prevent diarrhea; studies show it can cut your risk by 65 percent. Take two 262-milligram tablets at each meal and at bedtime. You can do this daily for up to three weeks.

Don't forget the Dramamine. Dimenhydrinate (Dramamine) and cyclizine (Marezine) work well to reduce nausea and vomiting from motion sickness. The trick is to take either drug well before you board the ship or begin a winding car ride.

Take steps against altitude sickness. This can occur if you move rapidly from sea level to more than 6,000 feet. To avoid it, move higher gradually (for instance, spend the night at 4,000 feet before continuing to your destination), slowly integrate physical activity (hint: That five-mile hike should wait a couple of days, until you're acclimated), and skip the alcohol and heavy meals. If you're prone to bad altitude sickness, talk to your doctor. There are drugs you can take ahead of time to help prevent it.

before you go

In addition to getting flu vaccine and, depending on your age and health status, pneumonia vaccine, make sure your tetanus immunization is up to date. (Hint: You need one every 10 years.) Also check which vaccinations are recommended for the areas to which you're traveling. You can search wwwn.cdc.gov/travel/contentvaccinations.aspx by your destination country. The only ones required are yellow fever vaccine for travel to certain countries in sub-Saharan Africa and tropical South America and meningococcal vaccine for travel to Saudi Arabia during the religious festival, the Hajj.

3. Keep your hands clean

HELPS PREVENT: Diarrhea, intestinal bugs, and colds and other viral illnesses

Next time you embark on a cruise, consider this: In 2007, there were 23 outbreaks of noroviruses, which cause "stomach flu," on 19 cruise ships, affecting about 3,000 passengers and crew members. Most involved person-to-person transmission, making hand washing, which studies find removes 99 percent of the virus particles, crucial. No matter where you go or what you're doing, hand washing should be your number one strategy for avoiding bugs.

What to Do

Wash with soap and hot water. Wash long and often. Plain soap and hot water are fine; you don't need an antibacterial soap. Just be sure to wash for at least 20 seconds, the time it takes to sing the happy birthday song twice at normal speed.

Load up on antibacterial hand wipes and gel sanitizers. Whenever you have access to soap and water, wash your hands—it's more effective at removing germs than antibacterial products because it physically rinses them away. Hand sanitizers aim to kill germs but don't kill all

of them. Still, for times when you can't wash your hands, alcohol-based antibacterial gels and towelettes are much better than nothing. Use a sanitizer that contains 99.5 percent ethanol, which studies find is more effective against noroviruses than any other concentration or type of alcohol-based cleaner.

Leave faucets and door handles untouched. Just think about how many people used the public bathroom in the hour or two before you did. Then consider how many of them washed their hands before leaving (far fewer than you might wish). It's not the toilet seats in these bathrooms you have to worry about; it turns out that the faucets and door handles are the germiest areas, so use a paper towel or hand wipe to turn the water on and off and to open the door when you exit.

4. Protect your physical safety

HELPS PREVENT: Accidents and injuries

You're more likely to come down with a virus or other infection on the road than to get hurt in an accident, but it can happen. According to the US Centers for Disease Control and Prevention, traffic accidents are the leading non-natural cause

protect yourself from avian flu

So far, there's no need to worry about contracting avian flu from people. It's spread from animals to people, not from person to person. But if you're traveling to a country that's had outbreaks of the disease, be sure to avoid direct contact with chickens, ducks, or geese; poultry farms; live-animal markets; and surfaces that may be contaminated with poultry feces.

of death for Americans who die in a foreign country. And let's face it, even throwing your back out trying to haul your suitcase through the airport is no fun.

What to Do

Forget about motorcycles and mopeds. Just visit a local hospital and witness all the tourists who've had vacation-ruining moped injuries. You'll be much less likely to decide to rent a scooter, no matter how cute and fun they look. Use public transportation, rent a car, or hire a driver if you're uncomfortable on strange roads. If you do rent a car, get a large one—it reduces your risk of injury if an accident does occur.

Wear your seatbelt. If the car or taxi doesn't have a working seatbelt, look for another form of transportation.

Don't cram too many into the car. Less developed countries are notorious for overfilled buses and cars. If you don't have room to sit comfortably and a seatbelt to click over you, or if the bus or van seems so top-heavy it might tip over, decline the ride.

Use rolling luggage. It saves strain on the back. And always lift with your legs, not your back.

Guard against heat exhaustion and heatstroke. Whether it's Jamaica in July or Sydney in February, the heat indexes of some countries can start your blood boiling. Drink plenty of fluids, wear light-colored lightweight clothing and a wide-brimmed hat, retire to your hotel room or anyplace with air conditioning during the hottest part of the day, slather on the sunscreen, and skip the alcohol-laced lunches.

in a germy world

Call it the revenge of the germs. Less than a century after the introduction of antibiotics, the world is facing an onslaught of super-strong bacteria—some of which are impervious to all but the most powerful of drugs—not to mention viruses that threaten to mutate and cause the next global pandemic. Short of donning a space suit, here are the two key steps you should take to protect yourself.

1. Guard against staph infections

HELPS PREVENT: Potentially deadly infection from MRSA and other staph bugs

Staph is one of the most common types of bacteria on the planet. The infections aren't always serious; often they cause only minor skin problems. But methicillin-resistant *Staphylococcus aureus* (MRSA), a common strain of staph, can be fatal because it's resistant to even the most powerful antibiotics. Some MRSA infections are relatively harmless, but in older people or those with weakened immune systems, they can cause real trouble. People at increased risk include those who've recently been in the hospital, those who live in long-term care facilities, and those who participate in contact sports.

What to Do
In Everyday Life
Wash your hands. It's a boring recommendation, but keeping your hands clean by washing with hot water and soap for at least 20 seconds is the best way to prevent MRSA. If there is a MRSA outbreak in your school or workplace, try using an antiseptic cleanser called Hibiclens. It

contains chlorhexidine, which eradicates bacteria on the skin.

Hit the showers. This is particularly important after working out. And use soap!

Cover scrapes and cuts with a bandage. Keep them covered until they heal to keep out the staph bacteria.

Practice the "ick" strategy. Meaning keep away from other people's wounds or bandages.

Be selfish. Don't share towels, razors, makeup, combs, or brushes. Even cell phones and unwashed clothing can harbor staph bacteria.

Create a barrier. Use a towel or your clothing as a barrier between your skin and any gym equipment. And wipe all equipment with an antibacterial solution or wipe before and after using it.

Play keep-away. We know you love the other guys (and gals) on the team, but try to restrain yourself from hugging, slapping, and other body-to-body contact, which can spread the bacteria.

Use the hot setting. Washing gym clothes and towels in hot water will help kill bacteria.

In the Hospital

Make like an investigator. Before you check in, ask what the hospital does to control hospital-acquired infections and about its surgical infection rates and infection-control program. If you're not happy with the responses—particularly if the person you ask bristles at providing the information—find another hospital. Many states and countries require that hospitals post their infection rates online. Check it out.

Pick the right surgeon. Ask your surgeon about her infection rate. Trust us—she'll know! You may not understand the answer, but you should get a good sense of how seriously the surgeon takes infection prevention.

Take a shower. Some authorities recommend showering or bathing with soap containing the antiseptic chlorhexidine three to five days in advance of surgery. However, recent studies suggest that using special soap isn't necessary; any will do as long as you bathe thoroughly before your operation.

Stop smoking. Give up the butts for at least four days before you're hospitalized. People who smoke have three times the risk of infection compared to nonsmokers, probably because smoking interferes with the delivery of oxygenated blood throughout the body, affecting the immune response to bacteria.

Ask about presurgery antibiotics. Studies find that giving patients antibiotics just before and/or during surgery can slash the risk of postoperative infection in half without increasing the risk of antibiotic resistance. Ask your doctor about the hospital's procedures in this regard, and gently remind her to order the antibiotics if required. Then make sure you get them when you're in pre-op.

Check your blood sugar. If you have diabetes, your risk of infection is much higher than for someone without the disease. Keep your blood sugar levels as stable as possible before entering the hospital and make sure they're checked regularly while you're there.

Remain vigilant. Insist that hospital staffers who enter your room—even your doctor—wash their hands or use alcohol-based wipes before touching you. One study found that simply increasing hand washing among intensive care unit (ICU) staff by 25 percent led to a 25 percent drop in hospital-acquired infections in the ICU. Also ask your doctor or nurse to wipe off the stethoscope before using it on you. Stethoscopes are often contaminated with MRSA.

Get the right line. A major source of MRSA infection in the hospital is a central-line catheter, a soft plastic tube surgically inserted into a large vein in your chest. It makes it easier to give you certain medications, such as those for chemotherapy. If you need a catheter, ask for one impregnated with antibiotics or coated with silver-chlorhexidine, which studies find help reduce central-line infections.

is it MRSA?

An infection usually starts out looking like a pimple or spider bite, often near a cut or scrape or on body parts such as the neck, groin, buttock, or armpit. If it becomes red, swollen, or painful or contains pus, see your doctor and ask to be tested for a staph infection.

2. Protect yourself from the flu

HELPS PREVENT: Complications, hospitalization, and even death from this virus
You may not think of the flu as deadly, but it kills tens of thousands of Americans each year (most of them elderly). And that's just the regular flu. Experts say it's only a matter of time before the big one hits—a flu pandemic reminiscent of the 1918–19 pandemic that killed about 50 million people in nearly every spot on Earth, no matter how isolated. These strategies will help protect you whether there's a flu outbreak in your neighborhood or in the world.

What to Do

Get vaccinated. The effectiveness of flu shots varies from year to year, providing anywhere from 40 to 90 percent protection against the strains of flu that are prevalent that year. But even 40 percent protection is much better than no protection. If a flu virus suddenly mutates and a pandemic strikes, you'll get at least a little boost from having had a flu shot. If you're 65 or older, also ask your doctor for a pneumococcal vaccine to protect against pneumonia.

Make sure your tetanus immunization is up to date (you need it once every 10 years). If your immune system is busy fighting off the flu, you don't want the bacteria that cause tetanus sneaking in.

Wash and wipe. Flu viruses are not like little winged insects; they don't fly from your nose to Aunt Polly's nose. They're usually spread from hand to mouth: Someone covers their mouth when they cough, gets the virus on their hands, and uses the phone. An hour later, you pick up the phone, transfer the virus to your hands, rub your eyes, and voilà—you're infected. Wash your hands as often as possible during flu outbreaks and wipe down surfaces with alcohol-based wipes or solution. You know the drill!

Dress like a surgeon. You don't need the gown, but the mask could be helpful, especially when you're on a plane full of people coughing and sneezing. Buy an N-95 face mask certified by the National Institute for Occupational Safety and Health. The masks filter out about 95 percent of particles the size of the influenza virus.

Keep your hands in your pockets. Infectious disease experts at the US Centers for Disease Control and Prevention use a greeting called the bump when they're out in the field investigating a contagious outbreak. Instead of shaking hands—which could be covered with disease-causing viruses from a sneeze or contact with virus-ridden surfaces—they politely touch elbows. Actions like this are forms of "social distancing." If you don't like the bump idea, try simply nodding and smiling.

Stay home. Next to washing your hands, the best thing you can do to protect yourself from infection is to stay home if there's a serious flu outbreak. Don't go to work or school; don't go to the movies or anywhere else you might encounter other people and their germs. Just settle in until the worst is over. This is so important that if there's a pandemic, worldwide government agencies plan to call for the shutdown of all but essential services to slow the spread of the virus.

Minimize the damage. If the flu hits, it doesn't have to be a death sentence. At the very first sign of the flu, ask your doctor for a prescription for one of the antiviral flu medicines, zanamivir (Relenza) and oseltamivir (Tamiflu). They can cut the flu short by a little over a day. Meanwhile,

take acetaminophen to bring down the fever and stay hydrated with clear liquids and tea.

Keep everything clean. If you're nursing someone who's sick, wipe down surfaces they've touched with antimicrobial solution; launder all sheets, towels, and clothing in hot water with bleach; and bathe yourself and the patient often.

is it a cold, or the flu?

Telltale signs of the flu are a fever over 101°F in adults, chills and sweating, muscle aches and pains, and serious fatigue and weakness. It's often accompanied by a lack of appetite. If your main symptoms are congestion, sneezing, a sore throat, and watery eyes, it's probably a cold.

disease prevention A to Z

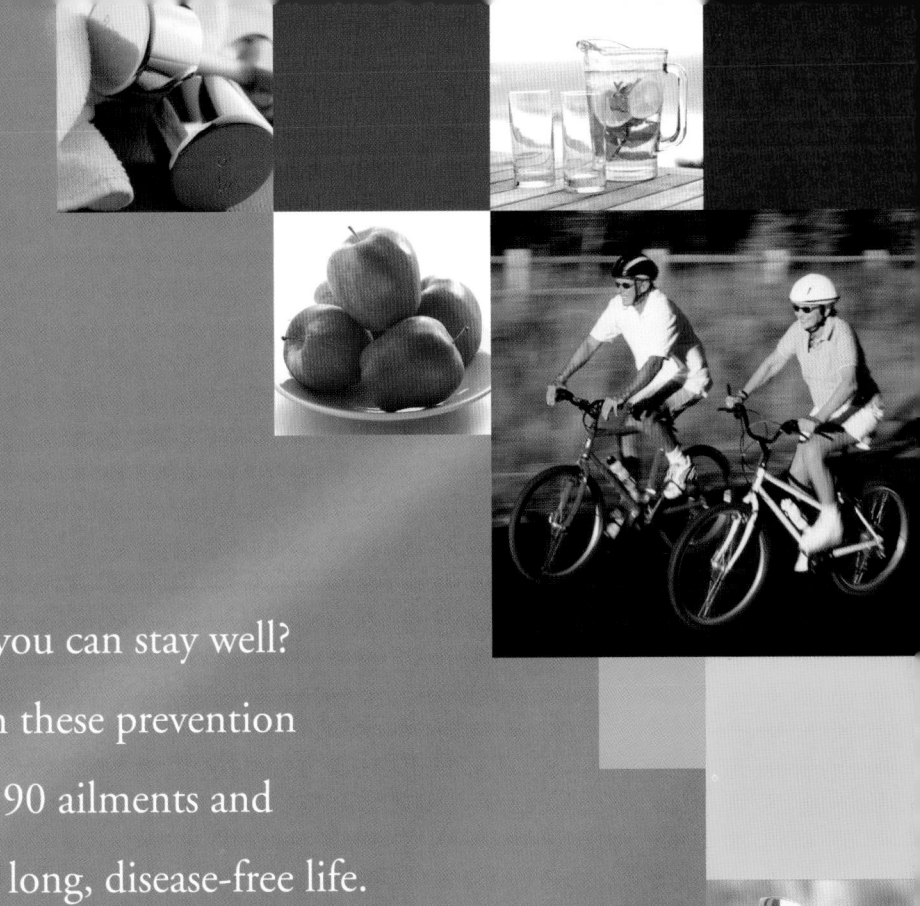

Why get sick when you can stay well?
Protect yourself with these prevention
plans for more than 90 ailments and
illnesses and enjoy a long, disease-free life.

Acne

54%

The reduction in blemishes when people with acne used a drugstore benzoyl peroxide product for four months.

Blackheads and bumps, pimples and cysts are a rite of passage for 90 percent of teenagers. But studies show that up to 54 percent of adults get acne, too. The cause? Everything from genetics to stress to hormones can initiate skin changes that clog pores, ratchet up inflammation, and give acne bacteria a cozy place to breed. If you're prone to acne, these strategies can help prevent flare-ups, whether you're 14 or 44.

Key Prevention Strategies

Open your pores with products containing salicylic acid, resorcinol, or lactic acid. These ingredients are also called alpha-hydroxy acids and beta-hydroxy acids. Available in dozens of drugstore gels and creams, they work by preventing pores from clogging by breaking down the thick, gunky mix of skin cells and excess oil that starts the whole acne cycle. Some even act as gentle chemical peels to unblock pores that are already clogged. In one State University of New York study of 30 people with acne, salicylic acid was better than benzoyl peroxide for reducing the number of pimples.

Stop bacteria with benzoyl peroxide. This inexpensive drugstore remedy is a proven bacteria stopper that fights acne's top culprit, the bacteria *Propionibacterium* acnes. Its advantage over oral antibiotics and most antibiotic creams and gels: It works even on strains of *P. acnes* that are resistant to the most widely used antibiotics for acne, such as tetracycline and erythromycin. Some experts estimate that bacteria are antibiotic resistant in at least half of all cases of acne.

In one British study of 649 people with acne, 60 percent of those who used benzoyl peroxide for 18 weeks saw significant reduction in blemishes, while only 54 percent of volunteers who got the oral antibiotics tetracycline or minocycline saw an improvement.

Benzoyl peroxide comes in several strengths; higher strengths are more likely to cause redness, irritation,

help for sensitive skin

Retinoid creams can be irritating, especially for people with sensitive skin. Here's a gentler alternative: a prescription cream containing azaleic acid (brand names are Azelex and Finacea). In one German study, an alcohol-free azeleic acid gel reduced blemishes by 70 percent after four months. Researchers also report that the cream can be just as effective as benzoyl peroxide and caused less irritation.

and even peeling. Start with a low dose and move up until you're happy with the results.

See a dermatologist for a retinoid cream. Prescription-strength creams and washes containing the vitamin A derivatives tretinoin (Retin-A), tazarotene (Tazorac), or adapalene (Differin) speed the shedding of dead skin cells so they can't clog your pores. They may also cool inflammation, easing redness and swelling. When researchers reviewed studies involving 900 people with acne, they found that tretinoin reduced the number of pimples by about 54 percent. In another study, tazarotene produced similar results. Other research suggests that retinoids may clear up 70 percent of blemishes.

Combine a pore-opening cream with an antibiotic cream. It's more effective than using an antibiotic cream alone. Your doctor can prescribe a combination cream that contains both an antibiotic and benzoyl peroxide. Another good duo: Benzoyl peroxide plus an alpha- or beta-hydroxy acid or some types of retinoids. In one Pennsylvania State University study of 517 people with severe acne, 53 percent of those who used both of these creams saw the number of blemishes cut in half after 12 weeks, compared to 35 percent of those who used benzoyl peroxide or the retinoid adapalene alone. Benzoyl peroxide can inactivate tretinoin, so don't use the two together.

Prevention Boosters

Light therapy. It works by killing bacteria and possibly reducing oil production. There are many types, including combined blue-red light therapy and pulsed-dye lasers. In one study, 85 percent of people who had four sessions of light therapy over eight weeks saw acne improve by at least 50 percent, and 20 percent of study volunteers had a 90 percent improvement. Results can last up to three months in some people.

Low-dose birth control pills. For women whose acne persists after trying many treatments, oral contraceptives could help. They can clear up skin by changing the hormone balance in your body in a way that reduces the production of oil. Research shows that the Pill can clear up 30 to 50 percent of infected, inflamed blemishes. It's recommended only for women age 35 and younger who have healthy blood pressure levels, don't smoke, and don't get migraines.

WHAT CAUSES IT Heredity and hormones. The combination causes the production of excess oil by sebaceous glands in your skin, plus a buildup of dead skin cells. Together they clog pores, creating a breeding ground for acne-causing bacteria.

SYMPTOMS TO WATCH FOR Tiny dark spots (blackheads) or small bumps (whiteheads). If clogged pores become infected or inflamed, they turn red; white pus inside may be visible. Larger bumps may signal clogs and a buildup of oil deep within pores. If these become infected, they're called cysts and can leave scars.

NEWEST THINKING Experts have said for years that foods like chocolate and french fries don't cause acne, but research suggests that diets generally high in sugar and refined carbohydrates could play a role. In a study of 43 young men with acne, those who followed a low-glycemic diet—involving foods that have a minimal impact on blood sugar levels—had 23 percent fewer blemishes after 12 weeks. Aim to get plenty of fruits and vegetables and choose whole grain products when you eat foods like rice and pasta.

Allergies

58%
The percentage of people who rated stinging nettle effective at relieving their allergy symptoms.

Have you met anyone lately who *doesn't* have allergies? Whether it's hay fever; food allergies; or allergies to dogs, cats, or cockroaches, it seems nearly everyone is sniffling and blowing these days. It's not your imagination; the incidence of allergies—including adult-onset allergies—is up in developed countries. The reasons are numerous: too much time spent indoors, higher levels of pollutants, "too clean" environments in our childhoods that led to confused immune systems. People with allergies are three times more likely to develop asthma and to have sinusitis. The following steps can help you avoid a new allergy or cut down on attacks.

Key Prevention Strategies

Wage war on dust and dust mites. Think of dust as a repository for almost every allergen you can think of: dust mites, pet dander, cockroach droppings, pesticides, and pollution blown in from outside, just for starters. Modern homes are allergen traps. You'll need to make a serious effort to reduce allergens enough to make a noticeable difference. Start with these approaches.

- **Think solid surfaces.** We're talking about hardwood, laminate, tile, and vinyl for your floors, and as much non-upholstered furniture as you can stand. Carpets and fabrics harbor dust mites and attract pet dander. They also grow mold if they get wet. One study found that the dust on walls, uncarpeted floors, and bookshelves had little impact on the overall level of dust mites in the home compared to the dust found on carpets, upholstered furniture, duvets, and mattresses and pillows.

- **"Dry steam clean" your carpets.** Vacuuming does little to remove allergens. In fact, on old carpets, it may just bring more pet dander and dust mites to the surface. But "dry steam cleaning," also known as vapor steam cleaning—not the same as regular steam cleaning—can reduce the number of dust mites for up to eight weeks. You can have it professionally done or buy a machine and do it yourself. Afterward, finish up by using a vacuum cleaner equipped with a HEPA filter.

a shot at permanent relief

The way to permanently prevent allergy attacks is to "reboot" your immune system with immunotherapy—yes, allergy shots. The shots, which you receive over a period of several months or years, contain increasingly larger doses of the substance to which you're allergic. Over time, your immune system learns to tolerate the allergen.

- **Encase your bedding.** Use hypoallergenic covers on your pillows, mattress, and box spring. They prevent dust mites from setting up house in your bed. Wash all covers in hot water (140°F) once a week and dry them in the dryer on the highest heat setting to kill dust mites. If you don't use pillow covers, choose feather pillows, which studies find harbor far fewer dust mites than synthetic pillows, probably because of the tighter weave on the covering.
- **Vacuum your mattress—top and bottom.** A Brazilian study compared dust mite bodies on the lower mattress surface (including the bed frame) and upper mattress surface and found more than three times as many dust mites on the lower surface. So flip the mattress monthly, vacuum each side, and wipe down the bed frame with hot, soapy water. For some hard-core cleaning, find out where your local used furniture stores send mattresses for sterilizing. Once it's sterile, keep it wrapped in hypoallergenic coverings.
- **Clear out clutter.** All those knick-knacks and magazine stacks are magnets for dust and mold.

If you can't part with you pet, use an air purifier. The truth is, there's scant proof that air purifiers can lessen allergy symptoms very much for most people. Buy if you buy one with a HEPA filter, use it in the bedroom, and keep your pet out of the room, you will create a friendlier environment for your respiratory system. These filters remove airborne particles, including those coated with pet dander. One study on using air filters in the bedroom found that they significantly reduced cat allergens. Another study evaluating the benefits of whole-house air cleaners fitted with HEPA filters found that they reduced levels of dog allergens 75 percent when the dog was allowed in the room and 90 percent if the dog was kept out of the room.

Rinse your nasal passages daily. Just as a rain shower rinses pollen from the air, a saline rinse washes allergens from your nasal passages. One study found that rinsing three times a day during allergy season eased congestion, sneezing, and itching and reduced the amount of antihistamines participants needed.

To make your own saline rinse, mix 1/2 teaspoon salt, 1/2 teaspoon baking soda, and 16 ounces of warm tap water. How to get it into your nose? Use an infant ear bulb syringe or a neti pot, available at health food stores and drugstores. Lean over a sink

WHAT CAUSES IT Your immune system overreacts to irritants such as dust, pollen, dander, mold, food proteins, or insect venom, releasing inflammatory chemicals that trigger allergy symptoms.

SYMPTOMS TO WATCH FOR Runny nose and itchy eyes, particularly during high-pollen seasons; sneezing; hives and/or trouble breathing after eating certain foods, such as peanuts or shellfish; red, dry, itchy skin.

NEWEST THINKING British researchers have discovered a protein called p110delta that plays a key role in triggering allergy attacks. Drugs that target it could prevent allergies, leaving existing allergy medications—which mostly reduce symptoms once the allergic reaction has occurred—in the dust.

and turn your head so your left nostril points down. Gently flush your right nostril with eight ounces of saline, which will drain out through your left nostril. When finished, gently blow your nose. Repeat with your other nostril.

Prevent attacks with stinging nettle. You may experience fewer allergy symptoms when you take this herb daily. In one study of volunteers who took 300 milligrams a day of freeze-dried nettle leaf capsules, more than half of the 69 participants said it relieved their allergy symptoms, and nearly half said it worked better than allergy medicine. Another good natural remedy to try is quercetin. Follow the directions on the label.

Prevention Boosters

Eat yogurt every day. University of California researchers found that people who ate about eight ounces of yogurt that contained live, active cultures every day had half as many days with allergy symptoms during hay fever season as people who didn't eat yogurt. The researchers aren't sure why yogurt helps, but it probably affects the immune system's response to allergens.

Eat more apples and drink more tea. Apples with the skin and green or black tea are excellent sources of quercetin. This powerful antioxidant checks the release of inflammatory chemicals from mast cells, the immune cells responsible for your run-of-the-mill allergic reaction. You'll also get quercetin from raw onions and red grapes.

Up your vitamin E intake. You'll find this vitamin in spinach, wheat germ, almonds, sunflower seeds, and sweet potatoes. A German study on the dietary habits of 1,700 adults with and without hay fever found that those who ate foods rich in vitamin E had a 30 percent lower incidence of hay fever than those who ate diets low in the vitamin.

Shut the windows. Sure, the warm spring breeze seems just the thing to freshen up your house—it's filled with pollen. Keep the windows closed and turn on the air conditioner if it's too warm.

> "Carpets and fabrics harbor dust mites and attract pet dander."

prevent allergies in your kids

Whether you're just thinking about having kids, are pregnant, or already have rug rats in the house, these measures may help reduce their risk of allergies.

During Pregnancy

1. **Follow a Mediterranean diet.** That means one rich in whole grains, fruits, vegetables, and fish, with olive oil used as the primary fat. In one study, kids whose mothers followed such a diet were 82 percent less likely to have wheezing and 45 percent less likely to have the skin rashes that predict childhood allergies.

2. **Take one grams of fish oil a day.** There is some evidence that supplementing with this anti-inflammatory fat can reduce the risk of allergies in young children. Check with your doctor first.

3. **Take a probiotic supplement.** Children whose moms take supplements of these beneficial bacteria during pregnancy—and those who received probiotics as infants—appear to be less likely to develop eczema, an itchy skin condition that's a common precursor of allergies in children.

During Childhood

1. **Feed kids plenty of fruits, veggies, and fish.** Researchers who followed nearly 500 Greek children from the time their mothers were pregnant until the kids turned 6 1/2 found that diets high in these foods significantly reduced the risk of allergies and asthma. The children who ate fruit and vegetables at least twice a day were 74 percent less likely to develop allergic rhinitis than those who ate them less often. Produce popular in Crete includes grapes, oranges, apples, tomatoes, eggplants, cucumbers, green beans, and zucchini. Eating an average of two ounces of fish daily also helped. Margarine, on the other hand, made allergies more likely, probably because hydrogenated oils trigger inflammation.

2. **Get a pet.** Some studies suggest that exposing your infant to a cat or dog during the first year can help prevent allergies to common airborne allergens like dust mites and pollen.

3. **Breastfeed for four to six months.** This is the amount of time required to reduce the risk of all allergies in your child, probably by providing important immune system support.

4. **Hold off on cereal.** Studies find that children who don't eat solid foods until they're 6 months or older are less likely to develop food allergies.

Alzheimer's Disease

60%

The difference in Alzheimer's risk between those who eat fish at least once a week and those who don't.

Alzheimer's disease was barely a dot on the horizon 50 years ago. That's because few of us lived long enough to develop it. But with life expectancies creeping into the midseventies or older, we're facing a potential epidemic of dementia. The good news is that scientists are on it; in the past decade, they've identified numerous biological and lifestyle underpinnings of Alzheimer's disease, opening the door to potential preventive strategies.

Key Prevention Strategies

Eat at least one meal of fatty fish per week. You may think of salmon as heart healthy, but it could be just as good—or even better—for your brain. Chalk up its brain benefits to omega-3 fatty acids, especially a type called DHA, which your brain is largely made of. Low levels are linked to memory and learning problems and even Alzheimer's disease.

DHA is thought to guard against the accumulation of beta amyloid proteins, the stuff responsible for the sticky brain lesions, known as plaques, that are the hallmarks of Alzheimer's disease. Fish fats also counter inflammation, which may contribute to protein buildup in the brain. When scientists added DHA to the diets of mice bred to develop Alzheimer's disease, the mice had lower levels of nasty brain plaques than mice who didn't get the DHA.

One population study suggests that eating fish once a week or more even after age 65 can reduce your risk of developing Alzheimer's by 60 percent compared to someone who eats less fish. If you don't like fish, talk to your doctor about taking one to two grams of fish oil daily.

Exercise your brain. Every time you challenge your brain to learn new information or attempt a new task (whether it's playing chess or just brushing your teeth with your nondominant hand), you create new connections between brain cells, in effect strengthening your brain.

drugs that PREVENT that DISEASE

That same daily aspirin that some people take to protect themselves from heart attacks could possibly protect them from Alzheimer's disease, too. In one study, people who took a nonsteroidal anti-inflammatory drug (NSAID) such as aspirin or ibuprofen every day for two years or more were 80 percent less likely to develop Alzheimer's than those who took an NSAID less often. Even people who took an NSAID for a month to two years reduced their risk by 17 percent. Talk to your doctor about whether it's a good idea for you to take a daily aspirin.

Research suggests that daily mental stimulation could reduce Alzheimer's risk by as much as 47 or 75 percent, depending on which study you look at. So get out those crossword puzzles, and think about learning a new language or how to play an instrument.

Walk two miles a day. At a brisk pace, this should take you no more than 30 minutes, the amount of time required to slash your risk of Alzheimer's by 50 percent, according to a Canadian study of about 10,000 people. Exercise probably has numerous benefits, including increased blood flow to the brain and increased production of a chemical called brain-derived neurotrophic factor (BDNF)—a sort of "Miracle-Gro" that encourages nerve cells in the brain to multiply and create more connections with each other.

Check the scale. If you're obese, your risk of Alzheimer's is nearly twice that of someone whose weight is normal. In fact, an analysis of several studies concluded that one in five cases of Alzheimer's disease in the United States was related to obesity. The link? For starters, carrying extra body fat—particularly around your abdomen—bumps up your risk of heart disease and diabetes, both of which make people more vulnerable to Alzheimer's. What's more, the fat itself releases inflammatory chemicals that may contribute to brain inflammation—and Alzheimer's.

Prevention Boosters

Eat your spinach. Despite what Popeye believed, it won't make your muscles strong, but it could help you maintain healthy brain function. Spinach is an excellent source of folate, a B vitamin that helps keep levels of homocysteine in check. This amino acid damages blood vessels and doubles the risk of Alzheimer's disease. Another B vitamin to look for is niacin. Studies find that a diet containing at least 17 milligrams of niacin (vitamin B_3) a day reduces the risk of Alzheimer's disease by 70 percent compared to a diet shy on niacin. You can get 14 milligrams from a 3.5-ounce serving of cooked liver, 10 milligrams from 1/2 cup of peanuts, and 13 milligrams from 3 ounces of white-meat chicken. Other great sources of B vitamins are beans and lentils, fortified grains, whole wheat breads, and nuts.

got the gene?

Researchers have identified at least 20 genes and genetic abnormalities linked to Alzheimer's disease. The best known is the ApoE gene, which affects the concentration of apolipoprotein Apo(E) in the blood. Apo(E)'s job is to help remove excess cholesterol from the blood and carry it to the liver for processing. While you can be tested for the gene, there's nothing you can do if you have it. Instead, live your life as if you do have it by following the tips in this chapter to reduce your overall risk.

Sip a glass of wine on most days. One of the best studies of dementia in the world, the Canadian Study of Health and Aging, found that drinking a glass or two of wine a day reduced the risk of Alzheimer's disease by 62 percent in women and 51 percent in all participants when men were included with the women. The benefit is probably due to something in the wine itself, since the protection afforded by wine was far greater than that from liquor or beer. Check with your doctor before increasing your alcohol intake.

Cultivate a pomegranate juice habit. The risk of developing Alzheimer's is 76 percent lower in people who drink the juice at least three times a week compared to those who drink it less than once a week, probably because of the high levels of antioxidants called flavonoids in the juice. These antioxidants neutralize free radicals, damaging molecules that attack cells and contribute to the formation of brain plaques. Pomegranate juice has already been shown to help prevent an Alzheimer's-like disease in mice.

Wear a helmet. Guard your precious noggin while biking, roller skating, or motorcycling, and avoid heading the ball during soccer matches or colliding with the head of another player during pickup football games. There's fairly good evidence that experiencing a moderate or severe head injury increases your risk of Alzheimer's disease (up to 3.5 times as much if the injury is severe).

Prevent high cholesterol. Although the theory is still controversial, population, animal, and laboratory studies suggest a link between high cholesterol levels in midlife and Alzheimer's disease. High cholesterol levels interfere with the breakdown of the amyloid precursor protein (APP), which plays a major role in the development of Alzheimer's disease. (Follow the tips on page 210 to keep your cholesterol under control.) There is also some evidence that using

check your pressure

The link between Alzheimer's disease and heart disease grows clearer every year. Now comes evidence that high blood pressure may hasten the development of Alzheimer's in people with early memory loss. Researchers following 5,092 Utah women with mild dementia for three years found that those with systolic blood pressure readings (the top number) higher than 160 mmHg declined 100 percent faster than those with normal blood pressure. Those who also had angina and/or had had a heart attack before their diagnosis declined even faster. The good news is that a study in the same group of women found that taking medication to reduce high blood pressure reduced the risk of Alzheimer's. Check your blood pressure once a week; if it's higher than 120/80, see your doctor. You may need to increase your exercise, change your diet, or take medication to bring it down to normal range.

cholesterol-lowering statin drugs may help prevent Alzheimer's, though it's too soon for doctors to start prescribing the drugs just for that reason. The link between statins and Alzheimer's prevention may actually be unrelated to the drugs' ability to lower cholesterol and may instead result from their ability to reduce inflammation.

Drink some coffee. If you enjoy a cup of coffee in the morning, don't give it up—it may be protecting your brain. According to recent research, caffeine appears to help protect the so-called blood-brain barrier from the harmful effects of high cholesterol, possibly reducing the risk of dementia. Other studies suggest that caffeine can help shore up memory in older people.

Take steps to prevent diabetes. Men who develop diabetes in midlife increase their risk of Alzheimer's disease by 150 percent, according to one study. The risk remained no matter what their blood pressure, cholesterol levels, or weight and is probably linked to low levels of insulin. Interestingly, the risk was highest in people who did not have the so-called Alzheimer's gene. (Turn to page 152 to learn how to prevent diabetes.)

Watch out for depression. A study of 486 people found that people who have experienced depression severe enough to seek medical help were 2.5 times more likely to develop Alzheimer's than those who never had severe depression. Those whose depression occurred before age 60 had a risk four times higher. One theory is that depression results in the loss of cells in two areas of the brain that also are linked to Alzheimer's disease. (Check out pages 148 for ways you can prevent depression now and in the future.)

WHAT CAUSES IT
Advancing age is the greatest risk factor, although an early form of the disease is linked to a genetic mutation. It's not clear what causes Alzheimer's, but it is associated with protein clumps, called amyloid plaques, in the brain, along with "tangles" of brain cells. It's likely that these interfere with processing in the brain.

SYMPTOMS TO WATCH FOR Memory loss, difficulty planning or completing everyday tasks, forgetting simple words or substituting unusual words in writing or speech, getting lost in familiar places; showing poor judgment (such as wearing shorts outside when it's snowing), having difficulty with abstract tasks like adding a column of numbers, putting things in unusual places, mood changes, loss of initiative.

NEWEST THINKING
People with Down syndrome all develop Alzheimer's disease by age 40. Now researchers suspect that people without the syndrome who get Alzheimer's may develop a small number of the same chromosomal abnormalities throughout their lifetimes. If true, it could one day mean new options for prevention, diagnosis, and treatment.

Anxiety

50%

The amount by which you could reduce your stress levels (which contribute to anxiety) by taking three grams of fish oil a day.

No matter the cause, chronic anxiety is bad for your health. It makes your heart beat faster than it should and even makes your blood stickier, increasing your risk of a heart attack or stroke. If you're the anxious type, do yourself a favor and try these strategies to help quiet your mind.

Key Prevention Strategies

Talk to someone. Preferably a therapist trained in cognitive behavioral therapy. In this form of talk therapy, you learn to separate worry from reality and put your fears into proper perspective. Studies find that as a treatment for anxiety disorders, it works better than medication; other research finds it can help prevent a full-blown anxiety disorder if used early on.

Stroll around the block. You know those "feel-good" hormones released during exercise? One is the neurotransmitter known as gamma aminobutyric acid, or GABA. Studies find low levels of GABA in people with some anxiety disorders, particularly panic disorder. They also find that exercise, even yoga, can increase GABA levels. How much exercise do you need? One study had 15 healthy people walk on a treadmill for 30 minutes, then gave them a drug that simulates a panic attack. Just 6 had panic attacks after exercising, compared to 12 who had them when given the drug after resting.

Breathe like a nonanxious person. Many of the symptoms of an anxiety attack are caused by hyperventilation—when you take such short breaths that you never fully release the carbon dioxide in your lungs. As the carbon dioxide builds, you don't have enough room in your lungs to bring in fresh oxygen, making you dizzy and lightheaded. Learning to breathe properly when you feel anxiety building can help stem the release of stress hormones that underlie hyperventilation.

Your best bet is to take a class in relaxation through a local

drugs that PREVENT DISEASE

If your heart races, your hands sweat, and your mouth turns dry as a desert when you have to speak in front of people, talk to your doctor about a prescription for a low dose of a beta-blocker. These medications, which include propanolol (Inderal) and metoprolol (Lopressor and Toprol-XL), block the effects of the stress hormone adrenaline, soothing the jitters of performance anxiety with no negative side effects.

hospital or wellness center. Until then, try to deliberately focus on your breathing when you feel anxious. Take one deep breath as slowly as possible (count to five as you breathe in), watching your stomach (not your chest) inflate. Hold your breath for a few counts, then let it out, again counting to five. Repeat five times.

Prevention Boosters

Rediscover your religion. A study of 718 adults found that women who had stopped attending religious services were three times more likely to have an anxiety disorder than those who still attended. The link may be related to the social interactions women get from being part of a church, synagogue, or mosque.

Supplement with kava. This herb is a member of the black pepper family. Numerous studies attest to its ability to calm anxiety. But check with your doctor before taking it; kava can interfere with how your body metabolizes certain medications and, in large amounts, could cause liver damage.

Sip some tea. As if the simple acts of brewing and sipping tea weren't calming enough, British researchers recently discovered that people who drink tea several times a day recovered faster from stressful situations designed to increase heart rate and blood pressure. The tea drinkers' blood also showed lower levels of stress hormones. Antioxidants in tea may attach to the same receptors in the brain that anti-anxiety medications target.

Swallow some brewer's yeast. Brewer's yeast is an excellent source of biotin, also called inositol or vitamin B_7. In one study, supplementing with 12 to 18 grams of inositol worked just as well as the antidepressant fluvoxamine (Luvox) for reducing the intensity and frequency of panic attacks. To prevent the attacks altogether, start taking a B vitamin supplement that contains 12 to 18 grams of biotin. Besides brewer's yeast (try sprinkling a tablespoon over cereal or yogurt), peanut butter is a good source.

Take three grams of fish oil daily. There's intriguing evidence that fish oil can help relieve depression, and now it seems it may reduce stress as well. After three months, study participants who took three grams of fish oil a day reported feeling half as stressed as those who got a placebo. Check with your doctor before taking the supplements.

WHAT CAUSES IT Just about anything in life can cause anxiety. But if your anxiety is excessive or irrational and it disrupts your life, you may have a condition known as generalized anxiety disorder.

SYMPTOMS TO WATCH FOR Restlessness, difficulty concentrating, irritability, trouble falling asleep, obsessive thoughts about something specific, racing heartbeat, shortness of breath, unusual sweating.

NEWEST THINKING In people who have experienced a traumatic situation, such as child abuse, war, or rape, intervention through counseling and other approaches can prevent an anxiety disorder.

Arthritis

30%

The reduction in arthritis risk in women who exercise for an hour a week.

Arthritis is a cruel straitjacket. If you've ever seen people hobbling on bad hips or bum knees or struggling to simply butter toast with stiff, achy fingers, you know how this disease can interfere with life. But osteoarthritis—in which the shock-absorbing cartilage between joint bones wears away—isn't inevitable. Everything from genetics to joint injuries to age-related changes in cartilage-protecting enzymes plays a role. But there's plenty of evidence that you can cut your risk significantly with the simple, proven strategies here.

Key Prevention Strategies

Lose weight. Are you carrying around a spare tire, saddlebags, or "junk in the trunk"? Here's yet one more reason to shed a few pounds: You'll put less pressure on your joints and thereby lower your risk of arthritis. Australian researchers say that osteoarthritis risk goes up 36 percent for every 11 pounds over your healthy weight range. Lose just 1 pound, on the other hand, and you'll put 4 pounds less stress on your knees. Losing 11 pounds if you're obese can cut your odds of developing arthritis over the next 10 years by a whopping 50 percent.

Losing weight benefits not only your knees but your hips, too. When Harvard Medical School researchers checked the weight and health histories of 568 women with osteoarthritis, they found that women with higher body weight were twice as likely to need hip replacement surgery.

Exercise for at least an hour a week. Arthritis has been a bit of a conundrum to doctors and scientists. Until recently, they thought that a lifetime of exercising made people more vulnerable to the disease, since studies showed a higher risk of joint problems among aging athletes. But now researchers say that joint injuries, not exercise itself, account for the difference. In fact, there's growing evidence that exercise can prevent problems by building up muscles that protect joints.

In one Australian study of middle-aged and older women, those who got 2.5 hours of exercise per week cut their odds of developing arthritic joints by about 40 percent. Exercising for just an hour a week lowered risk by about 30 percent.

Stretching exercises help, too.

Add strength training. Strengthening your muscles by using any form of so-called resistance training (using light hand weights, elastic bands, or machines at the gym or doing home exercises that use your own body weight as resistance—think knee bends) may shield joints from damage. In one study, women with stronger thigh muscles had a 55 percent lower risk of developing knee arthritis and an amazing 64 percent lower risk for arthritis of the hips than women with weaker thigh muscles.

Getting stronger helps if you already have arthritis, too. When Tufts University researchers tested a gentle, at-home strength-training program for older men and women with moderate to severe knee osteoarthritis, the results surprised and pleased study volunteers. After 16 weeks, exercisers had 36 percent less pain and 38 percent less disability. (See pages 88 for an at-home exercise routine you can try on your own.)

Experts say gentle strength training can also dampen the pain and disability of rheumatoid arthritis (RA), which occurs when the immune system attacks the tissues that protect bones. In a study from Finland, people with mild RA who followed a home strength-training program for two years saw pain decline by 67 percent and disability drop by 50 percent.

Prevention Boosters

Don't smoke. Women who smoked cigarettes raised their risk of developing RA by 30 percent in one Harvard study of 121,700 nurses. Smoking doubled the risk of the disease in another study of 30,000 women. Tobacco smoke may provoke immune system changes that lead to an attack on joints, Swedish researchers say. The good news: Women who had quit smoking had no extra risk after about 10 years.

Get more vitamin D. If you're running low on the "sunshine vitamin," your joints may be at risk. Vitamin D, produced by your skin upon exposure to the sun, may help keep the immune system healthy and protect joints from wear-and-tear damage by strengthening nearby bone, too. When researchers tracked men and women whose knees showed signs of osteoarthritis, those who took in above-average amounts of D from food and supplements were in better shape eight years later than those who didn't.

Vitamin D may protect against RA as well. When researchers at the University of Iowa followed 29,368 women ages 55 to 69 for 11 years, they found that women who got less than 200 IU of D

WHAT CAUSES IT For osteoarthritis, cartilage breakdown. Injuries, extra weight, genetics, and muscle weakness can all contribute. Over time, cartilage may wear through in spots so that bones rub against each other, creating intense pain. Rheumatoid arthritis happens when your immune system attacks the lining of your joints (the synovium), leading to intense pain, swelling, and joint deformities.

SYMPTOMS TO WATCH FOR Pain, stiffness, tenderness, and swelling in joints. Osteoarthritis most often affects the knees, hips, hands, and spine. Rheumatoid arthritis usually begins in small joints in the hands and feet, then spreads to larger joints. In addition to pain and swelling, rheumatoid arthritis can cause fever, tiredness, and weight loss.

NEWEST THINKING If you have a type of knee arthritis in which the wear and tear is harming the middle of your joint—called medial-knee arthritis—special insoles could help. Lateral-wedge insoles are thinnest at your instep and widest at the outer edge of your foot, realigning your feet and lower legs in a way that can reduce some of the twisting that wears down knee joints. Your doctor can tell you which type you have.

from food or supplements were 33 percent more likely to develop the disease.

At press time, the US Institute of Medicine recommendation was 400 IU of D per day for people ages 50 to 70 and 600 IU per day after age 70, although many experts were lobbying to have the guidelines revised upward, and some recommended 1,000 IU per day. Getting up to 2,000 IU per day is considered safe.

You'll probably need a supplement to get you there. Unless you're eating fatty fish like salmon or mackerel every day (3.5 ounces of either contains about 350 IU of D), it's awfully tough to get enough from food. (A glass of fat-free milk, another good source, has just 98 IU.) And while your body makes D from sunlight, if you can't see your shadow, the rays probably aren't strong enough. What's more, after age 50, your body simply makes less D from sunlight.

To check your vitamin D status, ask your doctor for a blood test at the end of winter, when most people's levels are lowest.

Eat colorful foods. If it's red, orange, blue, or green, chances are it's loaded with antioxidants, compounds that neutralize rogue molecules called free radicals that are thought to interfere with cartilage repair and rebuilding. Sweet, juicy mangos, peaches, oranges, and watermelon are packed with betacryptoxanthin, a tongue-twisting antioxidant and one of a pair of joint-pampering compounds that lowered the risk of arthritis by an impressive 20 to 40 percent in a University of Manchester, United Kingdom, study of 25,000 people. The other antioxidant, zeaxanthin, is found in spinach, sweet corn, peas, and orange peppers. People with the highest blood levels of both of these antioxidants cut their arthritis risk even further, by 50 percent.

Good old vitamin C is joint friendly, too. Eating plenty of strawberries, oranges, red bell peppers, and broccoli—all loaded with C—could help slow the development of knee pain if you already have osteoarthritis, say Boston University researchers. In one study, people who got the most C were three times less likely to have arthritis knee pain than people who got the least.

> "Tobacco smoke may provoke immune system changes that lead to an attack on joints."

glucosamine and chondroitin: worth It?

This dynamic duo is taken by more people with osteoarthritis than any other "joint" supplement. But a slew of recent research casts doubt on how well they work. Here's what you need to know.

What are they? Both are components of human cartilage, the smooth covering on knee bones and other joints that acts as a shock absorber. In osteoarthritis, cartilage softens, cracks, and wears out, allowing knee joints to rub together.

Glucosamine is thought to be involved in cartilage growth; supplements are derived from the shells of crabs and lobsters. Chondroitin gives cartilage its elasticity; supplements are usually derived from animal cartilage.

The claim: Proponents say that glucosamine and chondroitin relieve pain by maintaining cartilage so joint bones don't grind against each other.

The research: There's plenty of conflicting data out there. Belgian researchers recently found that glucosamine had no effect on pain or joint deterioration in people with osteoarthritis in their hips. And a large American study of 1,583 people with osteoarthritis found that this duo didn't ease joint pain any better than placebo pills. But when researchers looked at the 20 percent of study participants with moderate to severe arthritis pain, they found a benefit: 79 percent of those taking the supplements (they took 500 milligrams of glucosamine plus 400 milligrams of chondroitin three times a day) had at least a 20 percent reduction in pain, compared to 54 percent taking placebos.

What about joint protection? Other studies suggest that these supplements may help maintain "joint space"—the distance between bones. (More joint space means less grinding, less damage, and less pain.) In a Belgian study of over 300 women with osteoarthritis, those who took glucosamine for three years showed no narrowing of the space between knee bones, while those taking a placebo saw the gap grow smaller. The glucosamine group also reported a 14 percent improvement in pain and stiffness from the beginning to the end of the study, while the placebo group was a little worse by the end.

Are these supplements safe? Yes. Long-term studies have found only mild side effects such as intestinal gas and softer bowel movements.

What should I take? The Arthritis Foundation suggests this pair may be worth a try. Take a supplement containing 500 milligrams of glucosamine and 400 milligrams of chondroitin sulfate three times a day. Try it for at least six weeks (some experts recommend three months) to see if you're getting any noticeable benefit. If not, stop taking the pills.

Exercises for Arthritis Prevention

These moves strengthen key muscles in your legs and arms that act as shock absorbers for your joints, helping to protect you from developing arthritis. You'll need lightweight dumbbells (start with one-pound weights) and an exercise band. Ask your doctor if this program is right for you. If it is, start with just 10 minutes of these exercises three times a week. As you become stronger, do more repetitions, increase the weight, and switch to an exercise band that offers more resistance.

Calf Strengthener

Stand facing a chair back or table with your feet a few inches apart and hold on to the chair or table for balance. Rise onto the balls of your feet, then lower. Repeat until your calves feel tired. If this becomes easy after a few weeks, add weight: Use a small backpack with a five-pound weight in it (such as a dumbbell). To make it even harder, do the exercise (without the backpack or weight) with one foot on the floor and your other knee bent so that the foot is raised.

Quadriceps Toner

1 Sit on the floor with your left leg straight in front of you and your right leg bent. You can support your back by sitting against a wall or by putting your hands slightly behind you.

2 Keeping your abdominal muscles tight, lift your left leg off the floor. Lower and repeat until your leg feels tired. Switch legs and repeat.

Hip Flexor Builder

1 Lie on your back on the floor, bend your right knee slightly, and rest your right foot on the floor.

2 Tighten the quadriceps muscle in your left thigh, turn your leg outward slightly, and raise it as far as you can (but not above your right knee). Lower and repeat until the muscle feels tired. Switch legs and repeat.

Hamstring Builder

1 Knot an exercise band to make a medium-size loop. Stand facing a table or sturdy chair that you can use for support. Put one end of the loop under your left foot and the other around your right ankle.

2 Bend your right knee and raise your foot behind you, pulling against the resistance of the band. Don't let your back arch. Repeat until the back of your thigh feels tired, then switch sides.

Foot Builder

Spread a hand towel in front of a chair. Sit down and put one bare foot near the back edge of the towel. Keeping your heel on the towel, use your toes to gather the fabric and pull it under your foot. Keep going until you've gathered all you can. Repeat with your other foot.

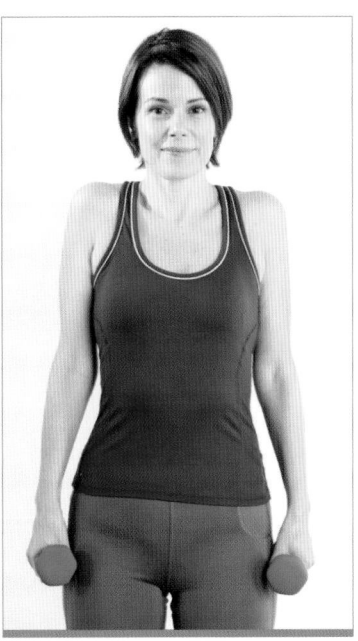

Shoulder Shrug

Stand and hold a pair of lightweight dumbbells (start with one-pound weights) at your sides. Keeping your arms straight, shrug your shoulders upward, then relax. Repeat 20 times.

Shoulder Strengthener

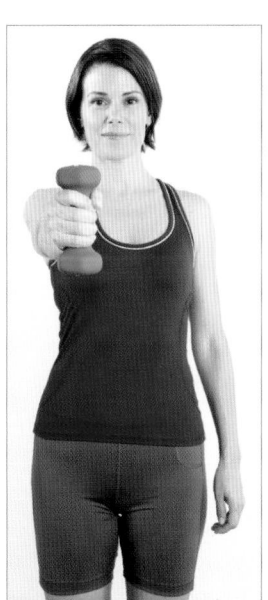

Hold a dumbbell in your right hand, with your arm down at your side. Lift the weight straight out to the side, then swing it slowly out in front of you as far as you comfortably can. Slowly swing your arm back to the side. Repeat 5 to 10 times, then switch hands.

Asthma

30%

If you have asthma, you're hardly alone; the disease is on the rise in most developed nations. Researchers think one reason is that children are rarely exposed to the germs, insects, and just plain dirt that older generations rubbed elbows with, so their immune systems never learn to react appropriately to these essentially harmless substances. Studies find that adults raised on farms are much less likely to have asthma. While it's too late to go back and relive your childhood, there's plenty you can do to prevent attacks if you already have asthma.

Key Prevention Strategies

Allergy-proof your house. More than half of all homes have at least six detectable allergens, and the remainder have at least three. And here's a real gross-out figure: More than a third of American homes have levels of mouse allergens high enough to contribute to asthma. The higher the allergen levels in your house, the more likely you or your children are to have asthma. Here are suggestions for targeting those asthma-causing mouse and cockroach allergens. (Find more tips on allergy-proofing your house in the Allergies chapter on page 74.)

Mouse allergens

- Damp-mop your floor daily. The highest levels of mouse "urinary proteins" are found on kitchen floors.
- Seal all cracks and holes in walls and doors, around window frames, and in the attic, as well as around wiring entrances to all electrical outlets and light switches and fixtures. They're perfect entry points for mice. If the cavities are too large to caulk, stuff them with mouse- and roach-repelling steel wool.
- Keep all food in sealed containers. Cardboard boxes aren't good enough; mice can easily gnaw through them.
- Use mousetraps. You can buy humane traps that keep the mouse contained until you arrive. Then you can set it free far, far away.

Cockroach allergens

- Store open boxes of food in your refrigerator, not your pantry.
- Make a natural spray with two ounces of eucalyptus or peppermint oil per gallon of water. Then spray around your

got the gene?

Because asthma and allergies tend to run in families, researchers have long suspected that certain genes make some people more susceptible. Now they're finding potential culprits. A variant in a gene called ORMDL3 seems to increase the risk of asthma in children by 60 to 70 percent.

kitchen, outside, around water pipes—anywhere you've seen roaches or suspect they may be gaining entry.

- Sprinkle a thin layer of boric acid where you've seen the insects.
- Kill them with poisoned bait (a concoction of flour, cocoa, oatmeal, boric acid, and plaster of Paris should do it). For every roach the concoction kills directly, 20 or 30 more will die from eating poisoned feces.

Check the scale. Gained a few pounds lately? Noticed your asthma is getting harder to control? It's not a coincidence. You're 66 percent more likely to have persistent asthma symptoms if you're obese than if your weight is in the normal range. Why? It may have to do with inflammatory chemicals released from fat cells.

Researchers are just beginning to study the effects of weight loss on asthma symptoms. In one small Italian study, 12 obese women with asthma who had surgery to shrink their stomachs and who lost a significant amount of weight as a result saw a 31 percent improvement in scores that measure shortness of breath and an 18 percent improvement in scores that measure the use of rescue medication compared to women who didn't have the surgery or lose weight.

Get a personalized asthma plan from your doctor. A shocking 55 percent of people with moderate to severe asthma do not have their disease under control—and these are people with health insurance and a regular healthcare provider. The result? Unnecessary emergency room visits, hospitalizations, and missed work. A major reason for uncontrolled asthma is the lack of a personalized asthma plan. These plans provide information about how and when to use daily and emergency medications and a peak flow meter to monitor lung function. They also help you know when it's time to seek emergency medical care or call your healthcare provider. Studies find that using these plans significantly reduces asthma attacks and death from asthma. The following questions can help you and your doctor develop the right plan for you.

- When should I call you?
- When should I seek emergency care?
- When is quick-relief medicine not enough?
- When, if ever, should I increase my use of inhaled steroids?
- When, if ever, should I start taking oral steroids?

WHAT CAUSES IT

A combination of genes and environment leads to an overly sensitive airway that reacts to triggers like airborne pollutants, allergens, or cold air by releasing inflammatory chemicals that lead to swelling of the bronchial tubes in the lungs, often accompanied by extra mucus production.

SYMPTOMS TO WATCH FOR Shortness of breath, coughing, chest tightness, wheezing.

NEWEST THINKING

According to Australian researchers, brief, regular exposure to ultraviolet light, found in sunlight, can suppress certain immune reactions, including those that trigger asthma symptoms—at least in mice. But wait for a UV light therapy to be developed, since too much sun exposure can cause skin cancer.

Once developed, the plan should be reviewed and updated annually and given to family members and others who might need to know what to do in the event of an emergency.

Prevention Boosters

Learn to use your inhaler properly. About one-third of people with asthma don't know how to properly use an inhaler. This lack of understanding can increase the risk of asthma attacks, hospitalization, and even death.

Use a peak flow meter. If you have trouble recognizing the early signs of worsening asthma, this small, inexpensive device can

prevent asthma in your children

Asthma prevention actually begins in the womb. Here's what you can do to reduce the risk that your child will develop asthma.

1. **Follow the right diet while pregnant.** That means one high in foods rich in vitamin E (wheat germ, sardines, egg yolks, and nuts) and zinc (red meat and shellfish). These nutrients influence lung and immune system development. At least two studies find that low levels during pregnancy can increase the risk of allergies and asthma in children. Also include fatty fish like salmon, herring, or sardines twice a week or take a daily fish-oil supplement (after checking with your doctor). Studies find that getting the healthy fats in fish and fish oil during pregnancy reduces the baby's risk of asthma, possibly by leading to healthier immune system development. Skip fish sticks, however, which can actually increase the risk of asthma in your child, perhaps because of the high levels of inflammatory trans fats some brands contain.

2. **Stop smoking.** The link between exposure to secondhand smoke in childhood and asthma is strong and undeniable.

3. **Get your kid allergy shots.** If your child has allergies, treatment with immunotherapy—either shots or under-the-tongue drops—may help protect her from developing asthma.

4. **Breastfeed for at least four months.**

5. **Hold off on solid foods.** Your child should be at least 6 months old before eating cereal or other solid foods.

6. **Skip acid-blocking meds while you're pregnant.** Researchers find that taking medications like H2 blockers such as cimetidine (Tagamet), famotidine (Pepcid), and ranitidine (Zantac) or proton-pump inhibitors such as omeprazole (Prilosec) and esomeprazole (Nexium) during pregnancy increased the risk of asthma in infants by more than 50 percent.

7. **Limit exposure to dust mites.** British researchers who followed 120 children from birth through age 8 found those who were breastfed and had limited exposure to dust mites due to the use of mattress covers and pesticides were 76 percent less likely to have asthma and 87 percent less likely to have allergies by age 8. (See page 74 for more on getting rid of dust mites.)

help. Peak flow meters measure your lung function, providing an early warning of an impending asthma attack. Using it daily and adjusting your medication based on the results can keep you attack free.

Use hypoallergenic mattress and pillow covers. One study found that these not only reduced the number of dust mites in the bed but also enabled children with asthma to cut their dose of inhaled steroids by at least 50 percent.

See an allergist. You're likely to have fewer problems controlling your asthma and less severe symptoms if your care is provided by an allergist instead of a primary care physician. You're also less likely to be hospitalized, go to the emergency room, or overuse rescue medication (a sign of uncontrolled asthma).

Serve salmon twice a week. A study of the dietary habits of 13,000 adults found that those who ate fish once a week were 30 percent less likely to have asthma than those who ate it once a month or less often and about 36 percent less likely to have asthma symptoms like wheezing. One explanation may be the anti-inflammatory benefits of fatty fish like salmon and mackerel. Asthma is first and foremost an immune system disease, in which immune cells overreact to triggers by pumping out inflammatory chemicals that narrow airways.

Stay away from traffic. Diesel exhaust (think trucks and buses) can cause serious problems for people with asthma. Just walking along busy streets can significantly reduce lung capacity and increase inflammation in people with asthma, probably because of tiny particles of dust and soot in the exhaust that are inhaled deep into the lungs and absorbed into the blood.

Take an aspirin every other day. Check with your doctor first, but if it's okay, taking a small dose (100 milligrams) of aspirin every other day could cut your risk of developing asthma by 10 percent if you're a woman who isn't obese. If you're a man, you need a higher dose (325 milligrams), but the benefits are also higher— a risk reduction of 22 percent.

"You're 66 percent more likely to have persistent asthma symptoms if you're obese."

Athlete's Foot

90%

Your odds of clearing up stubborn athlete's foot and avoiding a new infection for the next 11 months if you use a prescription antifungal cream containing butenafine.

Working out at the gym or pool is great for your whole body, from head to toe. But if you aren't taking steps to protect those toes, you may get more than you bargained for: itchy, scaly, athlete's foot. Regular folks can pick up this fungus before or after exercising (if you put your bare feet on the floor at a pool, in a shower, or in a changing room) or even at home. It's sometimes hard to knock out the fungus; preventing infection is far smarter.

Key Prevention Strategies

Keep your feet dry. Athlete's foot fungus thrives wherever there's moisture and its favorite food: keratin, a substance found in human skin. This means the insides of your sweaty shoes (and socks) are ideal breeding grounds. Change your footwear after exercise or when you come home from work, and change your socks when they're damp. Don't wear the same shoes two days in a row. When you're at home, walk around barefoot or in clean socks. In summer, wear sandals.

Store flip-flops in your pool bag and shower shoes in your gym bag. Foot protection is the best way to avoid the fungi lurking on the floors of virtually all locker rooms and public showers. These hardy little beasts thrive in damp environments, and they love to hitch a ride on bare feet: When Japanese researchers swabbed the soles of 140 people taking swimming classes at the University of Tsukuba, they found that 64 percent carried the fungus.

surprise culprit: fido

Dogs and cats can harbor hard-to-see fungal infections on their skin; you pick it up when you pet or groom them. In one study of 211 dogs, researchers found 89 fungal strains that can also infect humans—and in fact, 11 dog owners who had athlete's foot or jock itch (infection of the groin area by the same group of fungi that cause athlete's foot) were infected with the same strain carried by their pets. Look for areas of skin where fur is missing or ask your veterinarian to check your canine or kitty.

Stand on a thick towel while you're dressing in a locker room. It's nearly impossible to keep flip-flops on your feet while changing into your clothes, and socks may not offer enough protection. Researchers have found that foot fungus can easily travel between the fibers of cotton and nylon socks and attach itself to your skin; wool socks and extremely thick cotton socks do keep fungus off your feet, but you'll wind up "infecting" your shoes. A better idea:

Take an extra towel and use it only as a floor mat (then throw it in the laundry and wash it in hot water).

Wash or wipe your feet. If you forget to wear your shower shoes or flip-flops, clean your feet before putting your socks and street shoes on. Japanese researchers who study the spread of athlete's foot in public bathhouses found that washing feet with soap and water or even wiping them thoroughly (don't forget to wipe between your toes) removes a significant amount of the fungus picked up from floors.

Use an antifungal foot spray or powder to prevent repeat infections. Once your tootsies are infected with athlete's foot fungus, it's hard to get rid of it—and even tougher to stay foot-fungus free once the infection seems to clear up. The reason: The fungus hunkers down between skin layers.

If you get frequent infections, it's time to use antifungal sprays, powders, and creams. In one study of men who'd been battling on-again, off-again foot fungus, 90 percent of those who used an antifungal cream containing butenafine saw infections clear up within a week and stay away for the next 11 months. Butenafine is available in over-the-counter creams such as Lamisil Ultra. Other effective products contain terbinafine (such as Lamisil AT), tolnaftate (such as Tinactin and Altate), and miconazole (such as Micatin).

If you are prone to athlete's foot or will be spending lots of time wearing sweaty shoes or changing in locker rooms, using an antifungal product every day could help prevent infection.

Prevention Boosters

Check your family's feet. If anyone in your house has signs of athlete's foot, they could be spreading the fungus around. Take family members who seem to have athlete's foot to the doctor to rule out other causes. If it's really athlete's foot, insist that the person use antifungal sprays or foot powders until the problem is gone. Disinfect the bathtub and bathroom floor regularly, avoid sharing towels, and wash towels and sheets in hot water to kill the fungus.

WHAT CAUSES IT
The family of fungi called dermatophytes is responsible for most cases. These organisms send tendrils into the top layer of the skin, prompting increased cell production and creating thick, scaly skin.

SYMPTOMS TO WATCH FOR Burning, stinging, or itching; peeling, cracking skin between your toes or on the bottoms of your feet; extremely dry skin on the bottoms or sides of your feet; crumbling, thickened, and/or discolored nails.

NEWEST THINKING Toenail fungus? Foot experts now suspect that an ongoing nail infection can be a "reservoir" of fungus that can infect other parts of the body and that clearing it up could cut your odds of developing athlete's foot. If you have nail fungus, see your doctor; you'll need a long course of pills to clear it up.

Back Pain

50%

The amount by which you can reduce your risk of back pain through regular moderate exercise.

Exactly why is back pain the most common medical complaint in the Western world? It could be because creatures—whether human or not—were simply never meant to walk upright. This intriguing idea comes from examining the backbone of a 21-million-year-old forerunner to humans and apes. It turns out that the very evolutionary change in our spines that allowed us to walk on two limbs also made it easier for vertebrae (the bones that encase the spinal cord) to crush and strain the soft disks between them. While you can't change your heritage, you can guard yourself from the effects of this design weakness.

Key Prevention Strategies

Get yourself off the couch and out of the chair. If you're sitting around all day (which in itself is bad for the back), you're not getting exercise, the one strategy known to prevent back pain. Exercise helps keep extra weight off, strengthens abdominal and back muscles that support the spine, and increases the flow of oxygenated blood to the muscles and the vertebrae and other bones that keep your back properly aligned.

Don't worry about what kind of exercise you do; a major review of studies found that no single activity is best, nor is there any clear evidence as to how often and for how long you should work out—it may in fact vary from person to person. We always recommend that you get at least 30 minutes of moderate exercise (walking fast enough so you're slightly out of breath) at least four or five days a week.

Perfect your posture. Surprisingly, that doesn't mean sitting up straight. Scottish researchers used MRIs to evaluate three sitting postures in 22 volunteers. The participants either hunched forward, sat ramrod straight, or leaned back slightly. The researchers found the greatest risk of vertebral movement, which can lead to misaligned spinal disks, in people who sat up straight and the least in people who leaned back slightly. So find a chair that provides good back support but also allows you lean back just a bit.

mind your mattress

Tempted by a nice, fluffy, pillow-top mattress? Resist. Studies find that firm mattresses provide more support for your back, resulting in less back pain. Your mattress shouldn't be hard as a granite slab, though; choose one that's medium-firm for best results.

Here are some other posture pointers.

- **Sleep on your side or back, not your stomach.** Stomach sleeping increases the curve of your lower back, pulling it out of normal alignment.
- **Stand in front of the mirror several times a day and straighten up.** Memorize how it feels when your entire body—from your ears to your ankles—forms a straight line.
- **Check your workstation.** Even when leaning back slightly in your chair, you should be able to put both feet flat on the floor and keep your eyes level with your computer monitor without bending your neck.
- **Walk with your stomach pulled in;** don't allow your lower back to arch. Hold your head high.
- **Walk lightly.** If you literally pound the pavement, you're sending shock waves throughout your body, creating extra stress on your joints, including your pelvic and spinal joints. Have someone watch (and listen) to how you walk. If they think you walk too hard, practice walking heel-toe, heel-toe instead of landing on your whole foot. This will cushion each step and more evenly distribute your weight.

Lift like a pro. The American Academy of Orthopedic Surgeons recommends lifting like this.

- **Light objects (like a piece of paper):** Hold on to a nearby chair or table for support. Then lean over the object, slightly bend one knee, and extend the other leg behind you. Push up with your bent leg after you've picked up the object.
- **Heavy objects (grocery bag or laundry basket):** Stand in front of the object, bend at the knees, and lift with your leg muscles. Don't bend at your waist, and don't rely on arm strength alone for lifting.
- **Luggage:** Stand right next to the suitcase, bend your knees, grasp the handle, and straighten up.

Treat stress and depression. You may think depression is all in the mind, but in reality, it's often all in the back. Chronic pain like back pain can lead to depression, but it can also work the other way around, studies show. If you've lost interest in your normal activities, find yourself sleeping significantly more or less than usual, have considered hurting yourself, or have other symptoms of depression, see your doctor immediately. (Also turn to the Depression chapter for more advice.)

> "The better your spinal stability, the less likely you are to develop back pain."

Ever had a visit from your mother and suddenly found yourself flat on your back and unable to move without excruciating pain? You're not alone. At least 11 studies find a significant relationship between stress, anxiety, and back pain. We can't recommend barring your mother from your life; we can recommend learning better ways to manage stress. Here are some of our favorites.

- **Take up a repetitive hobby** like knitting, woodcarving, or crocheting.
- **Learn to meditate.** Classes are available in most communities.
- **Reframe the situation.** This means finding a more positive way to view a situation. Yes, your mother takes every opportunity to tell you what's wrong with you; isn't it wonderful to have someone who cares that much about you?
- **Volunteer.** Helping others in need puts your own issues and problems into perspective like nothing else.

Prevention Boosters

Try Pilates or PT. There's no evidence that one is better than the other for preventing future episodes of back pain. A physical therapist can develop a program of exercises for you that addresses impairments in flexibility and strength and may help you have a more active lifestyle. Pilates focuses on strengthening your core muscles—all the muscles that surround your spine and abdomen—that play a role in stabilizing your back. If you already have back problems, tell your Pilates instructor before you begin.

Work out with an exercise ball. California researchers tried an experiment on 20 sedentary office workers. Half of them exercised twice a week for 10 weeks with inflatable, oversize balls, also known as stability balls (available online and in big-box stores), which are designed to strengthen the core muscles. The other half did nothing. The people who got "on the ball" showed major improvements in spinal stability; the muscles they developed in their abs and backs acted like a thick belt around the waist to support the spine. The better your spinal stability, the less likely you are to develop back pain. The sizes of these balls vary; be sure to choose the right size for your height.

bike basics

Biking is great exercise, but hunching over the handlebars can wreak havoc on your back. Try this: Tilt the front of the bike seat down 10 to 15 degrees. It relieves pressure on your spine, in turn relieving back pain, according to a British study of 40 recreational cyclists. Also take your ride into a bike shop and ask the technician to make sure the seat is at the right height and that the frame itself is the right size. And don't let your shoulders ride up around your neck when leaning on the handlebars; try to draw your shoulders down and back.

Wear flats. When you wear high heels, you throw your body weight forward, which exaggerates the curve of the lower back, making the back muscles work overtime.

Set your alarm to get up and move. When you're sitting for a long time at the computer, in the car, or on a plane, set an alarm on your watch or cell phone to remind you to move every 20 minutes. If you can, get up and walk. If you're stuck in the car, shift your weight from one buttock to the other in a rocking movement and flex your legs to the extent you can. On long car trips, try to stop and walk around at least every hour.

Clean out your "carryall." Big purses may be great for packing it all in, but they can wreak havoc on your back, especially if you hoist them on one shoulder. They make you walk lopsided and pull your neck and shoulder—and hence your back—out of alignment. The best option is a fanny pack, which puts the weight evenly on your hips. If that's not "hip" enough for you, try a backpack or a purse slung across your body, each of which distributes the weight more evenly across your shoulders or chest. And clean the thing out! No matter what you carry, it shouldn't weigh more than 10 percent of what you do.

Use a stepstool. It will keep you from reaching too high, which could pull or strain a back muscle. If the stool has a low step, you can also place one foot on it (occasionally switching feet) to relieve your back a bit while you're washing dishes.

Counteract low kitchen counters. The typical counter height is 36 inches, which means tall people wind up leaning over when they wash dishes or prepare meals. Try putting a stool or small stepladder in front of your legs and lean the fronts of your legs against it. A study by Japanese researchers of kitchen workers and cooks found that this simple change significantly reduced lower-back strain.

Stop smoking. Smoking narrows arteries, hampering circulation and reducing the amount of oxygen-rich blood that gets to the spine and back muscles, among other areas. A lower blood supply interferes with the ability of bone and muscle to repair itself.

WHAT CAUSES IT Strained muscles or ligaments or the breakdown of the disks between the vertebrae.

SYMPTOMS TO WATCH FOR Spasms, pain that may or may not radiate down the leg, numbness in your legs, restricted function.

NEWEST THINKING You may one day be able to blame chronic back pain, in part, on your genes. Norwegian researchers believe that there is at least one genetic variant that increases susceptibility to back pain.

No-Back-Pain Daily Routine

A strong, supple back is one that's less likely to be injured. Do this series of easy exercises every day to protect yourself from nagging back pain. They strengthening and/or lengthen the back muscles, abdominal muscles (which provide support for your back), and even the hamstrings in the back of your legs, which help minimize stress on the low back. Start slowly and build up to the number of repetitions suggested.

Hamstring Stretch

1 Lie on your back, with your knees bent and feet flat on the floor. Place your hands under your left thigh.

2 Straighten your left leg until you feel a comfortable stretch. Keep your entire back on the floor. Hold for 15 seconds, then return to the starting position. Repeat 4 times on each side.

Knee-to-Chest Stretch

1 Lie on your back, with your knees bent and feet flat on the floor.

2 Using both hands, pull one knee toward your chest until you feel a comfortable stretch in your lower back. Hold for 15 seconds. Return to the starting position and repeat with other leg. Repeat 4 times on each side.

Pelvic Tilt

Lie on your back, knees bent and feet flat on the floor. Tighten your abdominal muscles and gently press your lower back into the floor. This is a small motion, mostly felt and not seen. Hold for 5 seconds. Repeat 10 times.

Back Rotation

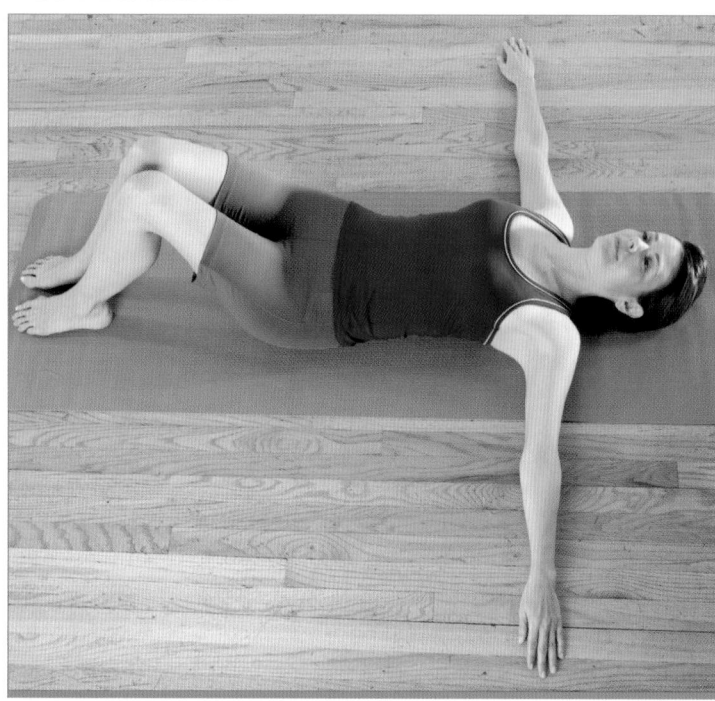

1 Lie on your back, with your knees bent, feet flat on the floor and arms out to the sides.

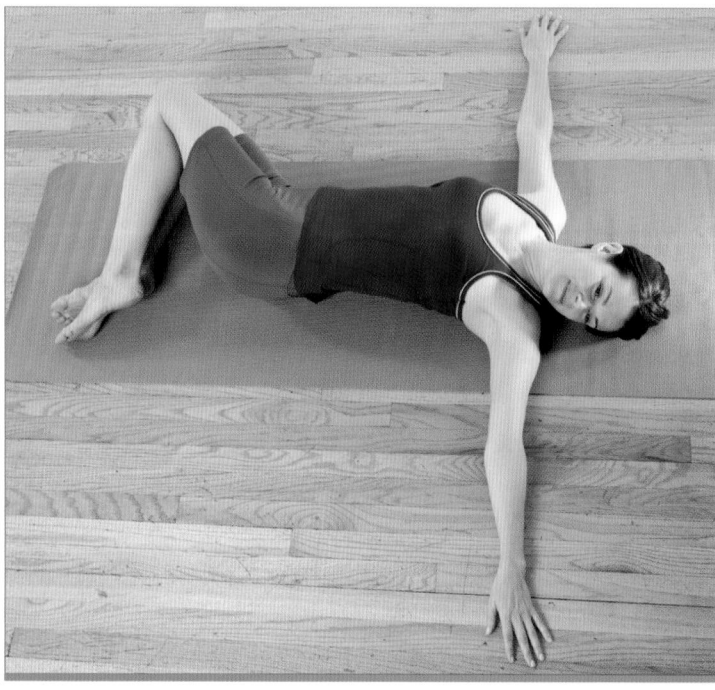

2 Keeping your shoulders on the floor, turn your head to the left and let your knees drop to the right until you feel a comfortable stretch. Hold for 15 seconds. Repeat 4 times on each side.

Back Extension

Lie facedown with a thin pillow under your stomach and a small rolled towel under your forehead. Tighten your buttocks, then lift your right hand and left leg about 4 to 8 inches off the floor. Hold for 2 seconds, then lower and repeat on the other side. Continue for 2 minutes.

Halfway Situp

1 Lie on your back with your knees bent and feet flat on the floor. Tuck your chin to your chest and stretch your arms out in front of you

2 Using your abdominal muscles, slowly curl your upper body forward, lifting one vertebra off the floor at a time, until your shoulders clear the floor. Hold for 3 seconds. Slowly lower yourself to the floor one vertebra at a time. Repeat 10 times

Hip Bridge and Roll Down

1 Lie on your back with your knees bent and your legs hip-width apart.

2 Tighten your abdominal muscles and lift your hips until your body forms a straight line from knees to shoulders. Hold for 5 seconds.

3 Slowly roll your spine back down to the starting position, touching one vertebra at a time to the floor, starting near your shoulder blades and ending with your tailbone. Repeat 10 times.

Cat Stretch

1 Get on your hands and knees on the floor.

2 Drop your head, tuck your tailbone under, and raise the middle of your back. Hold for 5 seconds. Return to the starting position.

3 Raise your head and hips and allow your back to sag toward the floor. Hold for 5 seconds. Return to the starting position. Repeat 10 times.

Belching

50%
The amount of extra air that chronic belchers swallow and release compared to people who don't burp excessively.

One dictionary definition of burping, "bringing forth wind noisily from the stomach," has a poetic ring to it. But burping is anything but poetic in real life. Experts say the occasional release of air from your stomach after a large meal is perfectly normal. Sudden, uncontrollable attacks of belching, however, are anything but. These "attacks" can be embarrassing and even painful. The good news: Most of the time, the cause is simply air that you've inadvertently swallowed. Here's how to preserve your dignity.

Key Prevention Strategies

Put your fork down between bites. Gulping your food and washing down big bites with a beverage are two surefire ways to send more air into your stomach, which is likely to resurface as a belch. Taking small bites, chewing thoroughly, and pacing your meal by putting down utensils between bites can all help because they give your body time to move trapped air into your intestines or simply absorb it. Chew especially well if you're eating a plateful of crunchy raw vegetables like broccoli, cabbage, lettuce, and cauliflower. Air becomes trapped easily between the crushed food particles and ends up in your stomach.

More mealtime tips to minimize the amount of air in your tummy include letting hot beverages cool before sipping, not using a straw, skipping carbonated drinks if they make belching worse for you, and taking a few minutes to relax before eating if you're feeling tense. Anxiety has been linked with excess air ingestion in several studies.

Keep cigarettes, gum, and hard candy out of your mouth. Chewing gum and sucking on hard candies produce extra saliva, which prompts more swallowing and sends more air into your stomach. Experts say we swallow an extra "teaspoonful" (about five milliliters) of air every time we swallow saliva. That's not much, but after several swallows, you've got a big air bubble in your stomach. And when that air is heated by your body's toasty 98.6°F temperature, the air expands by about 10 percent, creating the perfect setup for a belch. Similarly, when you smoke, you inhale air, which can return as a burp.

Conquer nervous air swallowing. Dutch researchers who compared 14 "excessive belchers" and 14 "normal burpers" came to a surprising conclusion: While both groups had the occasional "normal belch," problem belchers continually swallowed extra air and immediately let it back out. Digestion experts call this type of nervous belching eructio nervosa.

Air swallowing is often an unconscious habit. Experts suggest that approaches such as relaxation exercises, speech therapy, hypnosis, and simply holding a pencil between your teeth (you can't swallow when your jaws are separated in this position) can help keep extra air out.

Prevention Boosters

Knock out the ulcer bug. Repeated belching can be a sign of infection with the ulcer-causing bacterium *Helicobacter pylori*. This common bug can inflame the lining of your stomach and even trigger a process that burns holes in it. Along the way, it produces bloating and tummy gas. Other signs of an *H. pylori* infection or peptic ulcer include heartburn, indigestion, nausea, chest pain, weight loss, and fatigue. If you have unexplained belching, ask your doctor about a blood test or a breath test for *H. pylori*. If the results are positive, you may be treated with an antibiotic.

Fix your dentures, and clear your sinuses. Poorly fitting dentures and chronic postnasal drip can lead to excess air swallowing and excessive burping.

WHAT CAUSES IT
Swallowing air, infection with *Helicobacter pylori* (the bacterium that causes stomach ulcers).

SYMPTOMS TO WATCH FOR Expelling air from your stomach, either as a loud belch or a discreet burp.

NEWEST THINKING Up to half of all people with gastrointestinal reflux disease (GERD) belch excessively. Experts suspect that GERD sufferers may unconsciously swallow air in an attempt to burp and relieve stomach distress. If you have GERD and burp a lot, the tips recommended by experts for preventing more belching are the strategies outlined in this chapter: eat more slowly and cut back on air swallowing.

HOLDING A PENCIL BETWEEN YOUR TEETH CAN HELP KEEP EXTRA AIR OUT OF YOUR STOMACH.

Benign Prostatic Hyperplasia (BPH)

50%
The amount by which you could reduce your risk by exercising vigorously for two hours a week.

They say that as we age, our noses lengthen and our ears get bigger. Fact or fiction? Who knows. But one thing is for sure: If you're a man, your prostate gland will probably enlarge. Since the prostate surrounds part of the urethra, the tube that carries urine from your bladder to your penis, this growth could lead to annoying symptoms like having difficulty urinating or "going" too often. While nearly 80 percent of men have benign prostatic hyperplasia (BPH) by the time they turn 80, only about a third develop symptoms. Follow our advice, and you could be one of those who don't.

Key Prevention Strategies

Eat more vegetables. When researchers compared the diets of 6,000 men with BPH to 18,000 men without it, they found those who got about 10 vegetable servings a day were 21 percent less likely to have BPH. Ten servings may sound like a lot, but if you start with a veggie omelet for breakfast, snack on a dozen baby carrots with low-fat dip, and order up a large spinach salad for lunch, you're halfway there. Your best bet, the study found, is vegetables high in vitamin C and the antioxidant lutein, such as bell peppers and spinach. Also pay special attention to onions. Men who eat several portions of onions a week are far less likely to develop BPH than those who barely shed a tear over this root vegetable. Onions are high in phytoestrogens, which you'll read about next.

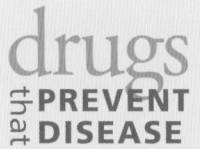

drugs that **PREVENT DISEASE**

Finasteride (Proscar) and doxazosin (Cardura) are drugs used to treat BPH. Taking the two together can also prevent early-stage BPH from advancing to the point where it causes symptoms and requires treatment, according to a major study. The combination reduced the risk of BPH progression by two-thirds compared with a placebo, while finasteride alone reduced the likelihood of surgery or other invasive therapies for BPH by 64 percent. Combining dutasteride (Avodart) and tamsulosin (Flomax) can have similar effects.

Discover flaxseed and soy. Both are sources of hormone-like plant compounds called phytoestrogens. These help guard against BPH by blocking an enzyme that converts testosterone into a different form—one that triggers prostate growth. Phytoestrogens also counteract the effects of estrogen (yes, men have estrogen, too), which also fuels prostate cell growth. Researchers think one reason men living in

Western countries have higher rates of BPH than those living in Asian countries is that they eat lower amounts of phytoestrogen-rich foods.

Flaxseed is easy to add to your diet: Buy it ground (keep it in the fridge) and sprinkle it on practically anything, from cereal to yogurt to salad. You can also add it to meatballs and baked goods.

For soy, you don't have to rely on tofu. Try snacking on soy nuts or soybeans in the pods, known as edamame (available frozen), and using soy milk in your cereal.

Burn off some calories every week. A study involving 1,000 men who were followed for nine years found that those who burned the most calories each week through physical activity were half as likely to develop BPH as those who barely moved out of the recliner. Two hours a week of swimming laps burns about 1,260 calories—putting you in the 50 percent risk-reduction zone based on this study. Other good options include running for two hours or walking for four hours a week.

Check your cholesterol levels. Here's something you probably never knew: Reproductive hormones like testosterone are largely made of cholesterol. There is some evidence that men with high levels of LDL ("bad") cholesterol are more likely to have BPH.

Prevention Boosters

Skip the doughnuts. Cutting out sugary snacks and simple carbohydrates like doughnuts, white bread, and potato chips is a good way to lose weight and also guard against high blood sugar levels. Men who are very obese (defined as a body mass index of 35 or higher) are 3.5 times more likely to develop BPH than normal-weight men. Men with high blood sugar levels are three times more likely to develop BPH than men with normal levels.

Stop at one beer. We're not suggesting you cut out alcohol altogether, but cutting back is a good idea. Men who have two or more drinks a day are one-third more likely to develop BPH than those who have less than one a month.

Reach for low-fat or nonfat options. If you're getting more than 38 percent of your calories from fat, you're not only eating a really high-fat diet, you're also about a third more likely to develop BPH than your friend down the road who is consuming fewer than 26 percent of his calories from fat.

WHAT CAUSES IT
Overgrowth of prostate tissue spurred by hormones like estrogen and testosterone. Age is the most common risk factor; 40 percent of men 60 and older have it, and 90 percent of men 80 and older do.

SYMPTOMS TO WATCH FOR Increased need to urinate, particularly at night; weaker urine stream; burning sensation during urination; problems starting to urinate.

NEWEST THINKING Men with fast-growing BPH may be more likely to develop prostate cancer, particularly if they have metabolic syndrome.

Bladder Cancer

30%

The amount your bladder cancer risk drops within four years of quitting smoking.

Most men worry about prostate cancer, but few think about bladder cancer, the second most common cancer in middle-aged and elderly men. About one in five cases occur after exposure to certain chemicals used to make dyes, paints, textiles, and other products, most of which you would have been exposed to 30 to 50 years before the cancer developed. There's not much you can do about that now, but there's a surprising amount you can do to prevent bladder cancer from other causes.

Key Prevention Strategies

Quit smoking. If you smoke, your risk of developing bladder cancer is two to four times higher than that of someone who never smoked. In fact, researchers estimate that two-thirds of all cases of bladder cancer are related to smoking. The longer you smoke and the more cigarettes you smoke, the greater your risk.

Don't try to quit on your own. Studies prove that you're more than twice as likely to be successful if you combine nicotine replacement products like gum or nasal spray with some form of organized support, like a counseling program or a telephone quit-line. (See page 38 for more advice on quitting.)

Get your water tested. If you're drinking well water, or even municipal water with high levels of arsenic, your risk of bladder cancer just went up. Arsenic levels should be less than 10 micrograms per liter. Ask your local water-treatment authority for a report on your water quality; it should indicate the amount of arsenic in your water. If you have a well, you may have to pay for a water test by a private company.

Munch on raw broccoli and cauliflower. Cruciferous veggies like broccoli, cauliflower, cabbage, kale, collards, and brussels sprouts are filled with isothiocyanates. These antioxidants inhibit enzymes that make certain chemicals in the body more likely to cause cancer. One study found that eating three or more servings a month slashed bladder cancer risk by about 40 percent compared to eating fewer servings. Cooking destroys the enzyme needed to produce isothiocyanates, reducing available amounts by 60 to 90 percent, so eat these veggies raw at least some of the time. We like crudités dipped in low-fat ranch dressing.

Prevention Boosters

Savor foods rich in selenium. This trace mineral is a powerful antioxidant linked with lower rates of several cancers, including bladder cancer. In your body, selenium comes into direct contact with bladder cells, where it is thought to prevent damage from free radicals (the unstable molecules that wreak havoc on DNA) and reduce levels of cancer-causing toxins. In one 12-year study of nearly 26,000 people, those with the lowest blood levels of selenium were more than twice as likely to develop bladder cancer compared to those with the highest levels.

Selenium is found in numerous foods, including Brazil nuts (the best source by far), whole wheat flour, pearled barley, and fish, including tuna. Most people don't need selenium supplements; check with your doctor if you want to take one.

Switch to fat-free milk and low-fat yogurt. High levels of saturated fat (found in full-fat dairy products, not to mention fatty meats and cheese) more than doubled the rate of bladder cancer in a large Spanish study. Other studies find the overall amount of fat in your diet increases your risk; follow a low-fat diet, and your risk drops.

WHAT CAUSES IT Most often, toxins coming in contact with bladder cells. Over time, they can affect the DNA in these cells, leading to cancer. These toxins can come from the food you eat and the water you drink, tobacco by-products, and environmental and occupational chemicals. Other causes include infection with certain parasites (schistosomiasis).

SYMPTOMS TO WATCH FOR Blood in the urine, pain during urination, frequent urination or feeling that you need to urinate but can't, abdominal pain.

NEWEST THINKING Surgery to remove just the tumor, followed by chemotherapy and radiation therapy, may be just as effective as removing the entire bladder for most stages of bladder cancer.

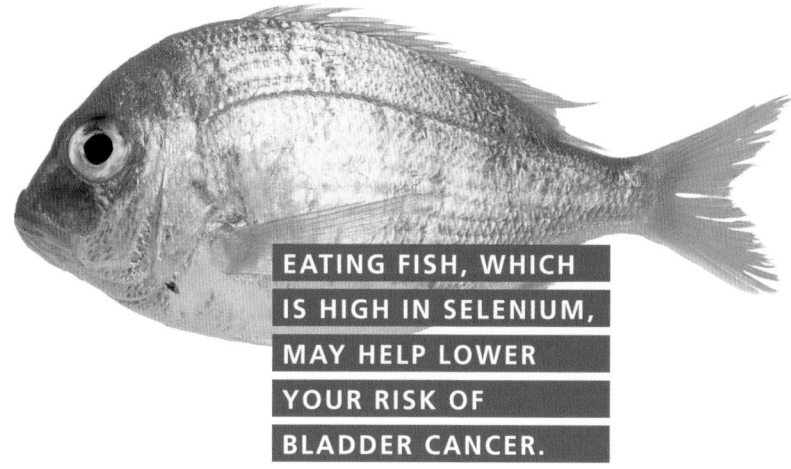

EATING FISH, WHICH IS HIGH IN SELENIUM, MAY HELP LOWER YOUR RISK OF BLADDER CANCER.

Breast Cancer

12-60%

The amount by which you can reduce your risk of breast cancer simply by taking regular walks.

Ask a woman her greatest health fear, and it's a good bet she'll say breast cancer. The bad news: It's the most common cancer in women and the second most common cause of cancer deaths in women. The good news: It's highly beatable, especially when caught early. It's also the only cancer with two drugs approved to prevent it (for women at high risk). Most women don't have to take medication to prevent breast cancer, however. Instead, follow this advice.

Key Prevention Strategies

Limit hormone replacement therapy (HRT) after menopause.
Giving breast cells extra estrogen is like pouring gasoline on a fire. It makes the cells divide faster, raising the risk that some will make a "mistake" during division, producing a cancerous cell. Your immune system can typically quash a few cancerous cells, but if you're taking estrogen, those "oops" cells could quickly overwhelm your natural defenses. One study found that undergoing HRT for just three years increased the risk of one of the most dangerous types of breast cancer fourfold.

Researchers suspect that the nearly 7 percent drop in breast cancer diagnoses between mid-2002 and mid-2003—after 20 years of increasing rates—was due to the fact that millions of women stopped taking HRT in 2002, the year a major report showed that the most commonly prescribed hormone medication increased the risk of breast cancer, heart disease, and stroke.

Researchers don't think HRT causes the cancer; instead, it enables microscopic cancers that might have faded away or remained tiny for decades to roar to life.

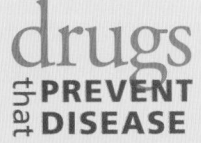

drugs ✝ PREVENT ✝ DISEASE Does the threat of breast cancer keep you up at night? Talk to your doctor. Using a simple quiz, he can determine your five-year and lifetime risk of breast cancer. If it's at least 60 percent higher than that of other women your age, you may be a candidate for chemoprevention. This means taking one of two medications—tamoxifen or raloxifene—for five years. These drugs mimic estrogen in the body, preventing the real thing from affecting breast cells. Studies find that either medication slashes breast cancer risk by a whopping 49 percent in high-risk women. If you're 35 or older, you can calculate your own risk of developing breast cancer at www.cancer.gov/bcrisktool.

Skip the molten chocolate cake.
Here's another good reason to say no to decadent desserts and padded portions: Every 11 pounds you gain after menopause bumps up your breast cancer risk by 1 percent.

The major reason: Fat cells release chemicals that can convert other hormones such as testosterone (which both men and women have) into estrogen. On the other hand, if you're postmenopausal, and you lose 11 pounds or more and keep the weight off—and you don't take hormones—your risk is 57 percent lower than that of women whose weight stays the same (and is presumably a bit higher than it should be).

Schedule that mammogram. If you want your risk of dying from the disease to be minuscule, an annual mammogram beginning at age 40 is a must. Mammograms find 80 to 90 percent of all breast cancers, most at an early stage. And studies find that 98 percent of women diagnosed with early-stage breast cancer are still alive five years after their diagnoses. Compare that to women diagnosed after the cancer has spread to their lymph nodes, whose five-year survival rate is 83 percent, and to those diagnosed when the cancer has spread to other parts of the body, whose five-year survival rate is just 26 percent. Also do monthly breast self-exams.

Prevention Boosters

Limit your drinking. A glass of wine with a great meal isn't just a pleasure, it's good for your heart. But one drink a day can very slightly increase your risk of breast cancer—probably not enough to really worry about. If you have more than one drink a day, however, you should worry. About 4 percent of breast cancers are thought to be linked to this level of alcohol intake, and the more you drink, the higher the risk. Researchers think it's because alcohol increases estrogen production.

If you decide to drink more than one serving of alcohol a day (which we don't recommend), you can hedge your bets by taking a daily supplement containing at least 400 micrograms of folic acid. This B vitamin helps repair mistakes cells make when they divide and could erase the increase in risk caused by the alcohol.

Keep moving. Whether you use the stairs instead of the elevator, take a brisk daily walk, hit the gym, or train for a 5K, regular physical activity to the tune of at least 30 minutes a day five days a week can reduce your risk of breast cancer. The reason is simple: The more physically active you are, the lower your body fat, which in turn lowers breast cancer risk. The sooner in life you start exercising, the greater your protection will be, though you'll gain benefits at any age.

WHAT CAUSES IT High circulating levels of hormones such as estrogen are the main disease drivers. After menopause, obesity and weight gain drive up hormone levels and thereby increase risk. The longer you live, the more estrogen and environmental toxins you've been exposed to and the greater your likelihood of developing the disease. That one-in-eight statistic you may have heard? That's only if you live to be 90 or older. Inherited genetic mutations account for only about 5 to 10 percent of cases.

SYMPTOMS TO WATCH FOR A lump or thickening in or near the breast or in the underarm area; tender nipples; changes in how the breast or nipple looks, including the size or shape; scaly, red, or swollen skin on the breast, nipple, or areola (the dark area surrounding the nipple); a nipple that turns inward; nipple discharge.

NEWEST THINKING Even if you carry mutations in the genes BRCA1 and BRCA2, the "breast cancer genes," your risk of developing breast cancer by age 70 is far less than once thought. Instead of the 80 percent risk often cited, new research from Memorial Sloan-Kettering Cancer Center finds a risk of between 36 and 52 percent.

Bronchitis

15%

The amount of improvement in lung function just two months after you quit smoking.

When you inhale things that don't belong in your lungs, such as tobacco smoke, viruses, bacteria, air pollutants, and chemical vapors, your bronchial tubes swell in rebellion, producing extra mucus in an attempt to isolate unwelcome intruders. As a result, you cough, wheeze, and may feel very tired. An occasional viral or bacterial attack—or exposure to lots of smoke or pollution—leads to short-lived bronchitis. Follow the advice in our chapters on colds and the flu to lower your risk. But if you have a cough most of the time for at least three months out of the year for two consecutive years, you have chronic bronchitis, usually caused by smoking. You know the solution. (You may also need medical care to assess your lung damage and determine a course of treatment.)

Key Prevention Strategies

Stop smoking. Cigarette smoking is responsible for 85 to 90 percent of cases of chronic bronchitis; experts say pipe and cigar smoking can trigger it, too. One reason: Smokers' lungs produce more mucus than those of nonsmokers. The mucus often coats airway walls in a continuous sheet, providing a place for bacteria and viruses to grow. The good news: When you quit smoking, lung improvements begin almost immediately. For many people, chronic coughing—which is a sign of all that extra mucus production—begins to subside within a month of stopping smoking.

chronic bronchitis? use a phlegm buster regularly

Over-the-counter and prescription drugs known as mucolytics thin the phlegm in your lungs so it's more liquid and easier to cough up, allowing you to clear your lungs and breathe more easily. Active ingredients include guaifenesin (available in dozens of brand-name tablets and liquids, including Mucinex and Robitussin) and acetylcysteine (Mucomyst). When researchers from the University of Auckland in New Zealand reviewed studies of 7,335 people with chronic bronchitis, they found that those who took mucolytics reduced the odds of having a bronchitis flare-up by 20 percent.

Avoid secondhand smoke. Cigarette smoke irritates lung tissue, triggering inflammation and raising your odds of lung infections. In a German study, chronic exposure to secondhand smoke at work raised the odds of developing chronic bronchitis by 90 percent. Exposure every day of the week—for example, in people who live with a smoker—tripled the risk.

Wash your hands frequently and carry an alcohol-based hand sanitizer. Scrubbing up five times a day with soap and water slashed the number of upper respiratory infections among Navy recruits by 45 percent in one two-year study conducted by the Naval Health Research Center in San Diego. Stash hand sanitizer gel in your purse, your car, your gym bag, and your briefcase for times when you can't get to a sink. Studies show that a sanitizer containing 60 percent ethyl alcohol can kill most bacteria and viruses.

Prevention Boosters

Wear a respirator at work if the air is dirty. Exposure to dust, fumes, chemical vapors, and gases on the job causes about 15 percent of cases of chronic bronchitis. In one Stanford University study of 517 nonsmokers, those who were exposed to dirty air on the job were twice as likely to have recurring lung infections or chronic bronchitis. If you already have chronic bronchitis, exposure to dust, fumes, chemical vapors, and gases at work can raise your risk of flare-ups. Poor ventilation, closed-in work areas, and heat boost your odds of developing bronchitis.

Get a flu shot every year and a pneumococcal vaccine at least once. Acute bronchitis and flare-ups of chronic bronchitis are often the result of the flu. An annual flu immunization can cut your risk of bronchitis, and a pneumonia vaccination offers similar protection. If you have chronic bronchitis, you're at higher risk of getting the flu or pneumonia and also at higher risk of getting sicker or even dying from these respiratory infections. In one study from Taiwan, the death rates for chronic bronchitis fell steadily after the government began providing free flu vaccines to people at high risk.

Use your woodstove and fireplace less often. Smoke from fireplaces and wood-burning stoves has been linked with higher rates of lung infections and chronic bronchitis in children and adults. If you use a woodstove for heat, be sure it is well sealed and burns efficiently (generally, stoves manufactured after 1992 are more efficient and release less smoke and fewer fine particles into the air). If you burn wood in a fireplace or stove for enjoyment, consider doing so less often to give your lungs a break. Have the chimney cleaned and maintained regularly to make sure the fumes are venting properly.

WHAT CAUSES IT Viruses and bacteria, often after a cold, the flu, or a sinus infection, that inflame the breathing tubes in your lungs. You can also develop bronchitis from breathing in cigarette smoke, polluted air, or household cleaners or from inhaling tiny amounts of stomach acid into your lungs if you have gastroesophageal reflux disease (GERD).

SYMPTOMS TO WATCH FOR A cough that brings up yellowish, gray, or green mucus; chest soreness or tightness or a tickling feeling when you breathe; infections, chills, and a low fever; tiredness; wheezing; sore throat; sinus congestion.

NEWEST THINKING A healthy diet can protect your lungs from bronchitis. In a recent study of 2,100 high school students, researchers from the Harvard School of Public Health found that those who ate the most fruits and vegetables, fish, nuts, and whole grains had the lowest risk of symptoms of chronic bronchitis.

Bursitis and Tendinitis

up to 90%

One rheumatologist's estimate of the cases that can be prevented by increasing exercise gradually and doing aerobics and stretching and strengthening exercises regularly.

Variety is good for both mind and body. What your body may not like is performing the same movements—say, swinging a golf club or tennis racket or throwing a bowling ball—over and over again, which sometimes ends in tendinitis. It's caused by inflammation of a tendon, a tough band of tissue that connects bones to muscles. Unfortunately, tendons lose some of their elasticity with age, making the condition more likely. Overuse of a joint can also cause bursitis, or inflammation of the fluid-filled sacs that cushion pressure points where muscles and tendons move across bone. (You can even get a form of tendinitis by leaning on your elbows too much!) Protect yourself with these steps.

Key Prevention Strategies

Revamp your exercise routine. Overuse or misuse of joints and muscles causes the majority of tendinitis and bursitis cases. Don't quit exercising! Instead, follow these tips for injury-free movement.

- **Book a session or two with a personal trainer** to evaluate your regular workout and identify movements that may be putting unnecessary strain on your joints and tendons.
- **Start slowly.** Just as it takes a few minutes for the water in your shower to warm up, it takes a few minutes for your muscles and joints to warm up when you start working out.
- **Be consistent.** That means exercising several times a week, not just once or twice a month. It also means you shouldn't throw yourself into a competitive basketball game if you haven't played or exercised in a while. Increase exercise by no more than 5 to 10 percent each week, in terms of either time spent or weight lifted.
- **Switch activities throughout the week.** For instance, if you work out with weights twice a week, spend one day on leg exercises and one day on upper-body exercises. If you run three times a week, bike on the other days. If you garden intensively one day, water the lawn or take a walk the next.
- **Rest.** Give yourself at least one day off each week. And if you

help for "housemaid's knee"

If you kneel a lot on the job, while cleaning, or when gardening, you're at risk of developing this condition, officially known as repatellar bursitis. Investing in a thick pair of knee pads, available at home improvement and hardware stores, can save you from the pain.

feel any joint soreness after a workout, ice the joint to ward off inflammation.

Stretch and strengthen. Range-of-motion exercises and weight-bearing exercises designed to strengthen muscles can reduce strain on joints, helping to prevent overuse injuries. For best results, book a few sessions with a personal trainer or physical therapist to identify the best exercises for you based on the activities you do most.

Cut your calories. As with many conditions related to the joints, being overweight increases the pressure on joints, bones, and tendons, increasing the risk of injury.

Prevention Boosters

Use insoles or orthotics if you need them. A major cause of Achilles tendinitis, an injury to the tendon that attaches the calf muscle to the heel bone, is hyperpronation of the foot—a fancy term that simply means your ankles roll in. When you shop for sneakers, do it at an athletic shoe store, not a department store, and ask the salesperson to help you find a shoe with the support you need.

If your pronation is bad, you may want to see a podiatrist to be fitted for custom orthotics, or start with a basic pair of shoe inserts from the drugstore and see if they help. In addition, wear the right shoes for the sport you're playing. For instance, if you play basketball, wear high-top sneakers.

Pay attention to pain. If your joint feels sore, take some ibuprofen or ice it. Both can relieve inflammation, possibly preventing long-term damage.

Use a band or brace where you need it. Supports for elbows and knees help reinforce and protect tendons during activities. There are many different types available, so check with your doctor or physical therapist about which one to choose.

WHAT CAUSES IT Aging, repetitive movements, biomechanical problems with joints.

SYMPTOMS TO WATCH FOR Pain and tenderness near a joint that gets worse with movement. The skin over the area may become red or warm to the touch. Your doctor (you may need to see a specialist) can tell whether it's bursitis or tendinitis based on where the problem occurs.

NEWEST THINKING A minimally invasive procedure using ultrasound can reduce pain from rotator cuff tendinitis and restore mobility. The procedure, called ultrasound-guided percutaneous (through the skin) therapy, uses ultrasound to guide the injection of saline solution into the shoulder and break up calcium deposits in the tendon. The doctor then removes the calcium remnants with a syringe.

Canker Sores

64%

Potential drop in your odds for repeat canker sores if you switch to a toothpaste that does not contain sodium lauryl sulfate.

Ouch! Somewhere in your mouth or along your gums, a tiny white sore is sending strong signals of pain, making it difficult to eat and maybe even to talk. It's a canker sore, a mysterious malady triggered by everything from food to toothpaste ingredients and sharp-edged potato chips to stress. Researchers aren't sure what causes these sores, known to doctors as aphthous ulcers. We know they can hurt. These strategies can keep them at bay.

Key Prevention Strategies

Use toothpaste that does not contain sodium lauryl sulfate (SLS). This ingredient can irritate the delicate lining of the mouth and trigger canker sores in some people. In a Norwegian study of 10 people who got recurring canker sores, switching to an SLS-free toothpaste cut their rate of new sores by nearly two-thirds.

But don't skimp on dental hygiene. Brushing and flossing twice a day can keep your mouth free of tiny food bits and bacteria that can irritate the lining of your mouth and kick-start a new canker sore. Scrub gently to avoid activating a new sore.

Swish with an antibacterial mouthwash. Rinses containing triclosan, chlorhexidine (available by prescription), and other antibacterial ingredients have significantly reduced the number of canker sores in people who get these painful mouth ulcers over and over again, several studies show. These may work because they wash away debris from hard-to-reach spots, because they prevent the flare-up of tiny infections which could trigger a canker sore, or by helping to prevent infection if you do get a sore.

the gluten connection

An estimated 1 in 20 people who get regular canker sores have celiac disease, an intolerance to the gluten protein found in wheat and some other grains. But don't give up wheat yet. If you think you may have celiac disease, talk to your doctor about testing and treatment. Other symptoms of gluten intolerance include diarrhea, abdominal pain, weight loss, fatigue, and gas pain.

Avoid these food culprits. Some canker sores are caused by a food or food additive. Citrus fruits, tomatoes, eggplant, tea, and cola drinks all triggered mouth ulcers in one study from Turkey, presumably because these foods irritated the lining of the mouth. Benzoic acid (a food preservative), cinnamon, milk, coffee, chocolate, potatoes, cheese, walnuts, and figs are said to be other culprits.

Say no thanks to spicy foods, which can also irritate sensitive mouth tissue. And skip sharp-edged edibles such as pretzels and chips.

Before you banish all these foods from your diet, look for connections between foods you've eaten recently and the onset of a new canker sore. Experts recommend eliminating a suspect for a few weeks, taking note of whether you get fewer sores, and then introducing the food again to see if it triggers a sore.

Ask about levamisole. This prescription-only pill stimulates the immune system in ways that can help prevent canker sores. In four studies of people who got frequent sores, the number of repeat attacks was cut in half for 43 percent of volunteers who took the drug. Some experts consider this the safest and most effective medication for preventing mouth ulcers.

Prevention Booster

Be calm. Stress is a classic instigator of mouth ulcers. In one study of people with canker sores, 16 percent said that extreme stress triggered outbreaks. Experts think stress may be a factor in up to 60 percent of first-time canker sore episodes. Irish researchers have found higher levels of the stress hormone cortisol in the saliva of people who get the sores, too. Try exercise, warm baths, deep breathing, or anything else that helps you relax.

Take a vitamin B$_{12}$ supplement. When Israeli researchers gave 15 people with recurring canker sores either an injection of B$_{12}$ or a daily B$_{12}$ tablet, canker sores dropped from an average of 10 per month to about 1 every three months. Several studies have found low levels of B$_{12}$ in people who get canker sores regularly. People in the study took 1,000 micrograms of B$_{12}$ daily, but talk to your doctor before taking that much. (Some experts recommend a more conservative 100 micrograms per day.) Top food sources include fortified cereals, meat, fish, and poultry.

Clear up other nutritional deficiencies. About one in five people with recurring canker sores have a nutritional deficiency. Some need more vitamin B$_{12}$. Others are low in other B vitamins, zinc, or folic acid or have iron-deficiency anemia. Correcting low iron could cut your odds for more canker sores by 71 percent, studies show. We don't recommend that you take extra iron on your own; for some people, it can be harmful. Ask your doctor whether you need a blood test to check for deficiencies.

WHAT CAUSES IT No one knows. Experts suspect that canker sores are caused by several factors, including tiny immune system attacks on healthy mouth tissue, allergic reactions, low levels of B vitamins and iron, injury and irritation of the lining of the mouth, additives in foods and toothpaste, menstrual cycle hormone changes in women, and stress.

SYMPTOMS TO WATCH FOR Small round sores under your tongue, inside your cheeks or lips, or at the base of your gums. Most are less than 1/3 inch in diameter, but some canker sores can be large and can take up to a month to heal.

NEWEST THINKING Some children get recurring mouth ulcers along with a fever and sore throat on a regular basis between ages 3 and 10. This newly recognized condition, called periodic fever, aphthous-stomatitis, pharyngitis, and adenitis (PFAPA) syndrome, returns like clockwork every few weeks or months. No one's sure what causes it, and there's no recognized treatment, though new research from Children's Hospital Boston suggests that removing the tonsils of a child with PFAPA can stop future attacks.

Carpal Tunnel Syndrome

49%

The percentage of people whose carpal tunnel symptoms improved after they wore a wrist splint at night.

You know that saying, "Hard work never hurt anyone"? Well, it's not always true. If your job (or your life) involves typing on a computer all day, cutting meat, using sign language, or any other repetitive task involving your wrists and hands, you could be in danger of developing carpal tunnel syndrome. Hobbies like knitting, sewing, guitar playing, and woodcarving also put you at risk. The condition is caused by inflamed tendons or ligaments in the wrist that put pressure on a nerve running through the base of your palm. It's marked by numbness, tingling, and pain in the hand and fingers. If it gets bad, you may even have trouble picking up your coffee cup. Prevent the pain with these suggestions.

Key Prevention Strategies

Embrace proper ergonomics. Good posture can help you avoid carpal tunnel syndrome. That means sitting up straight and not letting your shoulders roll forward (which puts pressure on nerves in the back and arms), and not rounding your lower back or thrusting your chin forward—all common postural mistakes we make at the computer that squeeze the muscles in the neck. That in turn can affect muscles and nerves in your hands, wrists, and fingers. It's also important to keep your wrists relatively straight—not bend them up or down. If you're sitting at a keyboard, follow the advice in "Type Smart," on page 124.

Warm up, and take breaks. Flex your fingers up and down 10 times whenever you've been away from your workstation or haven't been using your hands for more than 5 minutes. It's also important to give your wrists a rest. Take a 30-second break every 20 minutes, and schedule a 5-minute stretching

when carpal tunnel is a symptom

Studies find much higher rates of carpal tunnel syndrome in people with rheumatoid arthritis, hypothyroidism, type 1 diabetes, fibromyalgia, and certain other conditions. In fact, some experts think that carpal tunnel syndrome may actually be the first symptom of these diseases. Other conditions that can cause it include multiple myeloma, non-Hodgkin's lymphoma, and acromegaly, a disease in which the bones grow very long. If you have any of these diseases or conditions, managing them with lifestyle changes and medical treatments may reduce your risk of carpal tunnel or improve it if you already have it. Pregnancy and menopause also increase the risk, suggesting that hormones may play a role.

break every hour (keep a full water jug at your workstation; drinking throughout the day will force you to take breaks to hit the bathroom!).

Vary your tasks. If you just spent two hours typing, switch to drafting an outline using a pen and paper (the fatter the pen, the better), meet with co-workers, or read a hard copy report.

Use a wrist splint. Wearing a splint that keeps your wrist in a neutral position can help prevent the kind of damage that turns into carpal tunnel syndrome. In one study, 63 people with early signs of carpal tunnel wore custom-fitted wrist-hand splints nightly for six weeks. After six weeks, about half reported that their symptoms improved, with scores on a test measuring pain severity dropping from an average of 7.24 to 4.43. Even if you don't wear the splint every night, slip it on when you feel the first painful twinges.

Perform gentle stretching. Try the exercises starting on page 125. They tone and stretch muscles and ligaments in your hands and wrists to help guard against injury.

Prevention Boosters

Use the right tools. Product designers have caught onto our need for more ergonomically correct tools, whether hammers, screwdrivers, or can openers. Toss your old tools and kitchen implements and restock with tools that distribute the force of your grip across the muscle between the base of your thumb and your little finger, not the center of your hand. If you use tools that vibrate (like a motorized saw or knife), add shock absorbers to reduce vibration or wrap the vibrating part in a towel.

Check your risk of metabolic syndrome. This condition is marked by three of the following factors: low HDL ("good") cholesterol, a waist measurement greater than 35 inches (for women) or 40 inches (for men), high blood pressure, high triglycerides, and insulin resistance. When researchers studied 107 people, they found that 75 percent of those with metabolic syndrome also had carpal tunnel. The more severe the metabolic syndrome symptoms, the more severe the carpal tunnel. Metabolic syndrome also increases your risk of diabetes, and studies find that people who have diabetes are much more likely to have carpal tunnel

WHAT CAUSES IT Repetitive hand movements, particularly if you have to pinch or grip something while your wrist is bent. This inflames the nine tendons in the carpal tunnel, a narrow passageway that runs from the forearm through the wrist. These tendons enable you to flex your fingers. When they become inflamed, they put pressure on the median nerve, which also runs through the tunnel and supplies feeling to several fingers.

SYMPTOMS TO WATCH FOR Pain, numbness, and tingling in the affected hand and/or fingers, especially the thumb and index and middle fingers. The pain and numbness may be worse at night; sometimes it's bad enough to wake you up. You may find you have trouble holding objects tightly and have weakness in your thumb.

NEWEST THINKING Perhaps we need to stop pinning the blame for carpal tunnel syndrome on work. One study found that people who used a keyboard for four or more hours a day were significantly *less* likely to have carpal tunnel than those who used it for an hour a day or less. Other risk factors include rheumatoid arthritis, hyporthyroidism, type 1 diabetes, and non-Hodgkin's lymphoma. Pregnancy and menopause also increase risk.

than those who don't have diabetes. (The tips on page 152 for preventing diabetes and on page 206 for preventing high blood pressure can help you avoid metabolic syndrome.)

Get treated for depression. A British study found that 14 percent of adults with carpal tunnel syndrome had symptoms of major depression, while 22 percent had depression or some other psychological condition, such as an anxiety disorder. (You can find tips on preventing depression on page 148; for treatment, talk to your doctor.)

Drop a few pounds. If you're overweight, your risk of carpal tunnel syndrome is twice that of someone of normal weight.

Do the downward dog. Oddly enough, yoga may help protect your wrists. First, it can help you manage stress, which may contribute to carpal tunnel syndrome. It can also strengthen your wrist grip. In one study, people who participated in twice-weekly yoga sessions for eight weeks saw their grip strength increase by 25 mm/Hg, and pain in the carpal tunnel region of the wrist dropped by nearly half on a scale that measures pain.

Bump up your Bs. Vitamin B_6 is essential to healthy nerves. While the vitamin has primarily been studied for relieving the pain of carpal tunnel, it's worth increasing your intake from food (yellowfin tuna, cod, and roasted chicken or turkey breast are among the best sources) or supplements (aim for 200 milligrams daily) to help prevent it as well.

type smart

Practice smart ergonomics at work, and you'll be less likely to ever suffer from carpal tunnel syndrome.

- **Adjust your chair** so you can sit with your back against the chair back, your shoulders relaxed, your elbows along the sides of your body, your wrists straight, and both feet flat on the floor or propped on a footrest.
- **Keep materials used for typing at eye level** so you don't have to drop or twist your neck.
- **Change the setting on your keyboard** (usually found in the software that came with the keyboard) so you can gently tap the keys instead of having to pound them.
- **Keep your wrists flat while typing.** A wrist rest under the keyboard can help, but don't rest your wrists on it while typing.
- **Make sure the surface supporting the keyboard is at least 30 inches wide** to accommodate both the keyboard and mouse. Don't put the mouse on a higher or lower level than the keyboard.
- **The keyboard should be between 28 and 30 inches off the floor.** If you can type with your elbows bent at a 90-degree angle, it's at the right height. Pull it close to your body to maintain that 90-degree angle.
- **Use a computer table.** This furniture piece is thinner than a regular desk, allowing plenty of thigh clearance.
- **Place the monitor directly in front of you**, with the top of the screen at eye level or below. You should be looking down slightly as you type.

Exercises for Hands and Wrists

Repetitive wrist and hand motions can lead to painful carpal tunnel syndrome. Taking regularly scheduled breaks to do these exercises may help prevent the condition. Perform each one before you begin work, once an hour while you're doing a repetitive task such as typing, and at the end of the day before you go home. Hold each move for 5 seconds. When you're done, repeat the routine 10 times, then stand with your arms relaxed by your sides for 10 seconds.

Fist Flex

1 Hold your arms straight in front of you, then make fists with your hands and squeeze tightly.

2 Keeping your hands in fists, bend your wrists down at a 90-degree angle.

3 Straighten your wrists and let your relaxed fingers hang down.

Wrist Flex

Hold your right arm out in front of you. With your left hand, gently pull back your fingers until you feel a stretch in the bottom of your forearm. Ultimately your wrist should be bent at a 90-degree angle so your fingers point straight up. Repeat with the left arm.

Muscle Strengthener

1 Place a rubber band around your slightly separated fingertips.

2 Slowly spread your fingers, then close them, keeping a steady resistance against the rubber band. Repeat 10 times.

Forearm Stretch

1 Press your right hand against a wall, with your fingers open. Press your palm into the wall.

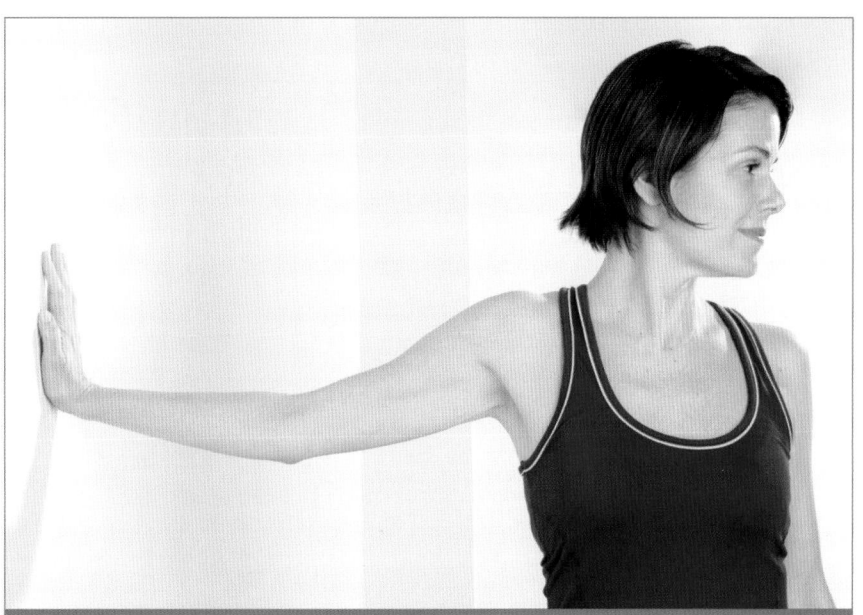

2 Slowly bring the tip of your right shoulder blade forward, turning your head to the left, until you feel a stretch in your arm.

Cataracts

66%
The potential drop in your risk of cataracts if you shield your eyes by wearing a broad-brimmed hat and sunglasses.

When the normally clear lenses in your eyes grow cloudy, you've got cataracts. Vision blurs, driving at night can become difficult due to headlight glare, and colors grow muted. French impressionist painter Claude Monet had cataracts and was forced to choose colors for his famous outdoor scenes by reading the labels on tubes of paint. "Reds had begun to look muddy," he lamented. "My painting was getting more and more darkened." Cataract surgery can replace clouded lenses with artificial ones, but you may not need it if you take these steps now to prevent cataracts.

Key Prevention Strategies

Enjoy a spinach salad with hard-boiled eggs, mandarin oranges, and almonds at lunch. Getting plenty of the antioxidants lutein and zeaxanthin as well as vitamin E—all present in this yummy salad—cut cataract risk 16 percent in a Harvard School of Public Health study of over 23,000 women. Other studies show that getting plenty of vitamin C is also protective.

Your body stores lutein and zeaxanthin in high concentrations in the lenses of your eyes, where they seem to work like sunglasses to filter out harmful ultraviolet rays. Antioxidants, including C and E, also seem to protect proteins in the lens from damage by destructive oxygen molecules called free radicals.

Eating just five servings of fruit and vegetables a day plus two servings of nuts is enough to provide your body with plenty of these important nutrients. Top sources of lutein and zeaxanthin include dark green vegetables like kale, collard greens, turnip greens, spinach, broccoli, and zucchini, as well as eggs and corn. For E, turn to almonds, hazelnuts, peanuts, and whole grains. For C, choose citrus fruits, red bell peppers, and strawberries.

Keep your blood sugar low and steady. Diabetes raised cataract risk 80 percent in one study of 6,000 people. Experts suspect that high blood sugar damages proteins in the lens of your eye. Even high-normal blood sugar and prediabetes increase your odds: In a British study, people with a prediabetic condition called impaired fasting glucose had double the normal risk. If you have diabetes, work with your doctor to keep blood sugar under control. If you're at risk, follow all the steps in Diabetes chapter to keep your blood sugar low and healthy.

Wear sunglasses and a broad-brimmed hat. When scientists checked the eyes of nearly 900 Chesapeake Bay fishermen, they found that those who spent the most time in the sun were three times more likely to have cataracts than those who spent the least. But wearing sunglasses plus a brimmed hat reduced the risk by two-thirds. Experts suspect that solar radiation alters proteins in the eye's lens, causing it to cloud.

Inexpensive sunglasses can be just as good as high-priced types. Just look for a label or tag that says the lenses protect against 99 percent of UVB and 95 percent of UVA rays—or say "UV absorption up to 400 nm"—and you're covered.

Stop smoking. Puffing cigarettes doubles your risk for cloudy lenses. Quit, and your risk begins to drop, say Swedish researchers who tracked the health of 34,595 women. Light smokers (who smoked 6 to 10 cigarettes a day) completely erased their added risk 10 years after quitting; heavier smokers (over 10 daily cigarettes) who quit needed 20 years to reduce their risk to that of nonsmokers.

Prevention Boosters

Lose weight. Carrying extra pounds can raise your risk for cataracts by as much as 36 percent, says a Harvard study of 133,000 women and men. The reason? If you're overweight you're more likely to have blood sugar problems (even if you're not diabetic). You may also have high blood pressure or high triglycerides. Other research suggests that these factors can raise risk by about 80 percent.

If you use steroid medications, get an eye exam soon. Oral steroids increase cataract risk; in one study of 2,446 people taking steroid pills to treat conditions such as rheumatoid arthritis, asthma, chronic obstructive pulmonary disease, lupus, and inflammatory bowel disease, those who took 10 milligrams of steroids per day for a year raised their cataract risk 68 percent. By 18 months, risk increase rose to 82 percent. At higher doses, inhaled steroids may also raise risk, according to British researchers. Steroid creams and steroid eyedrops may also push your odds higher. If you're using steroids long term, make an appointment for an eye exam and ask your opthalmologist how often you need repeat checks.

WHAT CAUSES IT Sunlight, smoking, a low-antioxidant diet, high blood sugar, and other factors seem to deactivate compounds, called alpha-crystallins, that normally prevent proteins in the eye's lens from clumping. Clumped proteins make the lens cloudy, distorting or even blocking the passage of light.

SYMPTOMS TO WATCH FOR Cloudy or blurry vision; glare or a halo around lights; poor night vision; double vision; colors that look faded; frequent prescription changes in your glasses or contact lenses.

NEWEST THINKING Cholesterol-lowering statin drugs pack a surprising vision bonus. In a study of 6,000 people, published in the *Journal of the American Medical Association*, those who took statins cut their risk for cataracts by 60 percent. Researchers suspect that statins act as antioxidants, protecting proteins in the lens from damage.

Cervical Cancer

70%

The percentage of cervical cancers that could be prevented with the Gardasil vaccine.

If you think that medical research moves at a glacial pace, you haven't been paying attention to advances in cervical cancer. As recently as 20 years ago, we didn't even know what caused it. Now we know it's caused by the human papillomavirus (HPV)—and we have a vaccine to prevent infection with that virus. Someday, maybe in your lifetime, cervical cancer will have gone the way of polio, diphtheria, and other viral illnesses vanquished with vaccines.

Key Prevention Strategies

Get vaccinated. We prevent tetanus, whooping cough, meningitis, and numerous other illnesses with vaccines; now, for the first time, we can prevent cancer with a series of three shots. The Gardasil vaccine prevents infection with four HPV viruses that cause about 70 percent of all cervical cancers. Ideally, women should be vaccinated before they become sexually active, which is why Gardasil is recommended for girls as young as 11 (it is licensed for girls as young as 9). In reality, any woman can get the vaccine as long as she is not pregnant, but there is no evidence of a benefit in women who have already been infected with HPV.

Have regular Pap smears. Cervical cancer is one of the few cancers that can be prevented with regular screenings. Pap smears, in which the doctor scrapes a few cells from your cervix for examination under a microscope, can pick up very early cellular changes that may eventually turn into cancer. Burning, cutting, or freezing off those cells can prevent the cancer. In fact, Pap screenings are the primary reason cervical cancer rates have plummeted 70 percent since the 1950s.

Get your first Pap when you turn 21 or within three years of becoming sexually active, then annually until you turn 30 if your healthcare professional uses the regular Pap test, or every two years if she uses the more sensitive liquid-based Pap (Thinprep). After you turn 30 and have had three normal Paps in a row, you can get a Pap every two to three years. Another option is to get screened every three years with either the conventional or liquid-based Pap plus an HPV test, which directly tests for the presence of the virus (something a Pap doesn't do). Once you turn 70 and have had three consecutive normal Paps and no abnormal Paps in the past 10 years, you can stop screenings.

Prevention Boosters

Choose a nonhormonal contraceptive. If you're worried about cervical cancer, avoid birth control pills that combine estrogen with progestin. They're actually classified by the International Agency for Research on Cancer as a cause of cervical cancer. A review of 24 international studies found that the longer you use this form of contraception, the greater your risk. Using birth control pills for 10 years beginning around age 20 to 30 nearly doubles your risk of cervical cancer. As soon as you stop using them, your risk drops; after 10 years, it's the same as that of a woman who never used contraceptives. The risk seems to be linked to the fact that women who use birth control pills are more likely to be infected with HPV, possibly because they have more sexual partners than women who use other forms of birth control.

Settle on one partner. The more sexual partners you have, the more likely you are to become infected with HPV.

Watch your stress levels. Being infected with HPV doesn't automatically mean you'll develop cervical cancer; many women, especially those under 30, can shake off the virus as easily as they shake off dozens of other viruses they encounter on a daily basis. But daily stress—from having a difficult boss, problems with your kids or spouse, or money worries—can impair your ability to fight off all viruses, including HPV, increasing your risk of long-term infection that could lead to cervical cancer.

WHAT CAUSES IT The primary cause is the human papillomavirus (HPV), which is spread via sexual contact.

SYMPTOMS TO WATCH FOR There are no symptoms with early cervical cancer. In later stages, the most common symptoms are abnormal vaginal bleeding (not during your period) or discharge. In the very late stages, it may cause pelvic pain.

NEWEST THINKING An interaction between cigarette smoking and HPV may increase the risk of cervical cancer. Carcinogens in cigarette smoke are thought to enable the virus to stick around longer and replicate, making the cervix more vulnerable to cellular changes that can lead to cancer.

Chronic Obstructive Pulmonary Disease

50%

The drop in your risk of COPD if you follow a Mediterranean diet full of fruit, vegetables, beans, olive oil, and fish.

Although it sounds rare and obscure, chronic obstructive pulmonary disease (COPD) is shockingly common. When a team of researchers scanned the lungs of over 9,000 people around the world, they found that 1 in 10 had moderate to severe COPD. In some nations, it's the fourth leading cause of death, right behind heart disease, cancer, and stroke. Smoking causes 85 to 90 percent of COPD cases. It weakens the tiny tubes and air sacs in your lungs so that they can't force out stale air, leaving little room for your next fresh, oxygen-rich inhalation. COPD makes you cough, wheeze, and feel oh, so tired; it also raises your risk of lung infections and life-threatening lung damage. People who have it usually have chronic bronchitis, emphysema, bronchial asthma, or some combination of these. Your first line of defense: Protect your lungs from tobacco smoke as well as dust and fumes on the job.

stop a COPD flare-up before it starts

If you've been diagnosed with COPD, these strategies can help you avoid flare-ups that can land you in the hospital and further damage your lungs.

- **Get a yearly flu vaccination.** Viral and bacterial infections can make breathing problems worse. This vaccine can cut the risk of influenza among people with COPD by up to 81 percent.
- **Get a pneumonia vaccination at least once.** COPD raises your risk of life-threatening forms of pneumonia.
- **Use an over-the-counter mucus thinner.** Medicines like Mucinex dilute mucus and make it easier to cough up. It can cut flare-ups by 20 percent.
- **Use an inhaler with one or two medications.** A long-acting bronchodilator or an inhaled corticosteroid can each cut flare-ups by 20 percent. Combining the two cuts your odds by 25 percent.
- **Follow a progressive exercise routine.** Work with your doctor or a pulmonary rehabilitation program. A half hour of exercise most days of the week can ease breathlessness significantly.

Key Prevention Strategies

Stop smoking. Smoking cigarettes, cigars, and pipes causes an estimated 85 percent of COPD cases. Over a lifetime, half of all smokers will develop this debilitating lung disease. Quitting is the most effective way for smokers to reduce their risk. We'll be honest: If you already have COPD, quitting won't reverse lung damage that's already been done, but experts say it's still crucial. By kicking the habit, you can cut future declines in lung function by half.

Refuse to be a passive smoker. Secondhand smoke is packed with chemicals and particles that irritate your lungs. Living with a smoker raises your own odds of developing COPD by 55 percent. Working in a smoky environment (such as a bar) raised risk 36 percent in one study. Insist on smoke-free air in your home and car.

Steer clear of fumes, vapors, and dust on the job. University of California, San Francisco, researchers concluded that workplace exposures to bad air double COPD risk. If your job involves breathing in dust, fumes, or vapors, wear a respirator.

Eat like a Sicilian fisherman. Pile your plate with fruit, vegetables, beans, and fish; use olive oil in place of butter; and enjoy a glass of wine with your dinner. This Mediterranean-style way of eating cut the risk of COPD in half in one major study. (Processed foods, red meats, and refined sugars raised risk.) Antioxidants in the Mediterranean menu may protect cells from damage, while compounds in fish and olive oil help cool chronic inflammation, which also plays a role in lung destruction.

Prevention Boosters

Get a spirometry test. Millions of people have undiagnosed COPD and are missing out on treatments and strategies that could literally save their lives. If you're a smoker or show any signs of COPD, ask your doctor about this simple test that measures how much air you can expel from your lungs and how fast.

Say no thanks to cured meats. In one study, people who ate cured meats such as bacon, sausage, lunchmeats, and cured ham 14 or more times per month were 93 percent more likely to develop COPD than those who never ate them. Nitrites used as preservatives and color fixatives in these meats may raise levels of cell-damaging particles called reactive nitrogen species in the bloodstream.

WHAT CAUSES IT Most of the time, cigarette and cigar smoke, secondhand smoke, pollution, and fumes damage bronchial tubes and air sacs in the lungs. In rare cases, a genetic disorder called alpha-1-antitrypsin deficiency causes airway damage that leads to COPD.

SYMPTOMS TO WATCH FOR A cough that won't go away; coughing up mucus on a regular basis; shortness of breath, especially when you're physically active; wheezing; a feeling of tightness in your chest; frequent bronchitis, sinus infections, and/or colds.

NEWEST THINKING Research from Cardiff University in the United Kingdom found that people with COPD have arteries that are about 25 percent stiffer than the arteries of people without the disease, raising their risk of heart disease and high blood pressure. They were also nine times more likely to have osteoporosis. Experts suspect that the lung damage that causes COPD puts the immune system on high alert; this in turn speeds the development of plaque in artery walls and may weaken bones.

Colds

30%

The amount by which you can cut colds if you use a saline nasal spray every day.

Avoiding even a single nasty cold is worth far more than you'd pay in a year for hand soap, the only ingredient (along with water) you'll need to slash sniffling, sneezing sick days by 45 percent. Along with sound sleep and good nutrition, hand washing is your best defense against cold viruses, which can survive for up to seven days on light switches, ATMs, doorknobs, and other surfaces—and for at least three hours on unwashed hands. Should some of those viruses make it inside your nose, mouth, or eyes, a strong immune system is your best defense.

Key Prevention Strategies

Wash your hands frequently with soap and water. Do this even if your hands don't look or feel dirty. Scrubbing five times a day with soap and water slashed the number of upper respiratory infections among Navy recruits by 45 percent in one two-year US study. A brisk, 10-second scrub rinses away 99 percent of viruses. This cuts your odds of infection substantially, but not completely; a single viral particle can start a cold! For best results, wet your hands, lather vigorously for a full 20 seconds, rinse, and dry with a clean paper towel. Use the towel to turn off the tap, too. Any soap will do—washing works by scrubbing viruses off your skin, not by killing them (and antibacterial soaps don't kill viruses anyway).

Walk five days a week. Regular exercise invigorates your immune system's natural killer cells and virus-killing antibodies. University of South Carolina researchers found that adults who exercised moderately to vigorously at least four times a week had 25 percent fewer colds over one year than those who moved less. A brisk 40-minute walk five

the new cold fighters

Echinacea may be the top-selling herbal supplement in the United States and Europe, but its cold-battling prowess remains controversial. The latest: An authoritative German review of 16 clinical trials concluded that it doesn't prevent colds (though other research says it does). A worse bet: vitamin C. A definitive analysis of 29 well-designed studies involving over 11,700 people concluded that C has no power to prevent a cold. Instead, try one of these.

Andrographis. In one well-designed study, volunteers who took two 100-milligram tablets a day for three months had half as many colds as volunteers who got placebos.

Probiotics. These beneficial bacteria seem to increase production of immune cells where you need them most to fight colds: in the tissues lining your respiratory system. Capsules containing the bacteria *Lactobacillus gasseri*, *Bifidobacterium longum*, and *B. bifidum* MF shortened colds by an average of two days in volunteers who took them daily for three months.

days a week should do it; in another study, this much exercise cut in half the number of days volunteers had cold symptoms. But don't overdo it: Working out for an hour and a half or more could reduce immunity.

Use a saline nasal spray daily. Moist nasal passages are less receptive to cold viruses than dry ones. In one 20-week study of military recruits, those who used a saline nasal spray every day had 30 percent fewer colds and 42 percent fewer days with runny noses or congestion. Key times to spritz: In winter, when heated indoor air is dry, and during airplane flights.

Prevention Boosters

Tame the stress monster. In a year-long Spanish study of 1,149 university professors and staff, sniffles were twice as likely among people who felt the most stressed or reported experiencing the most stressful events compared to those with the least. And once you catch a cold, stress can make symptoms worse.

Season or supplement with garlic. This ancient remedy may help by boosting the activity of your immune system's virus-killing T cells. When 146 women and men took either a garlic capsule or a placebo pill daily during cold season, the garlic group caught 24 colds, while the placebo group got 65. Researchers at England's Garlic Centre say that garlic takers who did get sick recovered in just 1.5 days, while the placebo group had the sniffles for an average of 5 days. (Other research is less positive about garlic.) If you love garlic, use it liberally. Remember to "chop, then stop"— let chopped or crushed garlic sit for 10 minutes before using to maximize levels of its most active component.

Use alcohol-based hand sanitizers when you can't get to a sink. These gels and sprays kill bacteria and some viruses, but don't put all your eggs in this basket. Studies show that brands containing 60 percent ethanol alcohol are powerless against rhinoviruses (which cause colds). Some researchers report that a 70 percent ethanol sanitizer can be effective.

Hop into a sauna twice a week. In an Austrian study, people who did this twice a week for six months had half as many colds as those who didn't use the sauna. The link may be air temperature—at over 80°F, sauna air is too hot for cold viruses to survive.

WHAT CAUSES IT At least 250 viruses—and possibly hundreds more. The sheer number has made it impossible so far for scientists to develop an effective vaccine. But time's on your side: The human body develops some resistance to each cold virus it encounters, which is one reason we get fewer sniffles as we age.

SYMPTOMS TO WATCH FOR Sore throat, stuffy and/or runny nose, sneezing, coughing, and even a mild fever. It may be the flu if you have chills, body aches, significant fatigue, and/or a higher fever.

NEWEST THINKING Perhaps your mom was right: Being cold can up your risk of catching a cold, at least according to one study. People exposed to a chill were three times more likely to develop cold symptoms than those who stayed cozy and warm, according to a study of 180 people from the Common Cold Centre in Wales. The cold-cold connection: Being chilly constricts blood vessels in the nose, reducing the supply of nutrients to infection-fighting white blood cells. This may allow dormant infections to roar to life.

Colorectal Cancer

50%

The amount of risk reduction achieved by getting 15 minutes of sun exposure a day.

Imagine our surprise when a slew of clinical study reviews found that high-fiber diets didn't protect against colon cancer as much as we thought. Twenty-five years of advice down the proverbial drain. But the news isn't all bad. Although colorectal cancer is the third most common cancer worldwide and the fourth leading cause of cancer deaths, it's also the most preventable cancer in the world after lung cancer. There are numerous lifestyle and medical steps you can take to protect yourself against this cancer, many of which, as you might imagine, still involve your diet.

Key Prevention Strategies

Get screened. Colorectal cancer is one of only two cancers that can be completely prevented through screening. Having a colonoscopy means taking a day off from work and letting a doctor snake a tube with a tiny camera through the entire four or five feet of your colon to search for potentially dangerous polyps in the colon's nooks and crannies. It sounds worse than it is. For one thing, you're sedated; for another, even the night-before prep to clean out your colon has gotten a tad easier with the introduction of pills instead of chalky liquid. The actual procedure takes about 30 minutes or less.

If the doctor sees anything suspicious, he can be snip it out and biopsy it while you're still sedated. In this way, colonoscopies prevent about 80 percent of all colorectal cancers. Most medical groups recommend having a colonoscopy every 10 years starting at age 50, or more often (and earlier) if you have a family history of the disease or a history of colon polyps.

Get out there and exercise. An analysis of 19 studies found that men who are physically active reduce their risk of colon cancer about 21 percent; for women, the benefit of brisk walking, heavy-duty gardening, biking, swimming, etc. is greater, yielding a 30 percent risk reduction.

should you go "virtual"?

Many doctors agree that virtual colonoscopy, which involves lying on a table and passing painlessly through a CT or MRI scanner to have detailed 3-D images of your colon taken and examined, isn't "ready yet" as a tool to replace traditional colonoscopy. It doesn't excuse you from the pretest bowel-cleansing ritual that no one enjoys. And if the test finds a polyp, you'll need to follow up with a traditional colonoscopy—and repeat the bowel cleansing—to have the polyp removed. If you decide to get virtual colonoscopy, be sure you go to a doctor who's very experienced with the procedure; otherwise, the results may not be as reliable as they should be.

Cut back on red meat. Here's a simple equation: The less red meat you eat, the lower your risk of colorectal cancer. Eating 18 ounces a week (the amount in two large hamburgers) increases your risk by about 30 percent; every 1.5 ounces after that increases your risk by another 15 percent, according to the American Institute for Cancer Research. (Just for comparison's sake, most people in Western countries eat an average of 36 ounces of red meat a week.)

There are several possible reasons for the link. First, people who eat a lot of meat tend to eat fewer health-protective fruits and vegetables. But a diet rich in fatty red meat also contributes to "oxidative stress"; in other words, it creates harmful free radicals in the body that can damage cells, DNA, and other microscopic components of your digestive tract. Some of those interactions are as dangerous as those caused by radiation! That's why high consumption of fruits and vegetables is so important; they contain valuable antioxidants that help stem that oxidative damage. So if you must toss a steak on the grill, make it no larger than your hand and grill some peppers, onions, and pineapple to go with it.

Skip the cold cuts. Eating about two ounces of processed meat (about two slices of bologna) a day could increase your risk of colorectal cancer by 50 percent compared to people who eat no processed meat. The culprit may be n-nitroso compounds (NOCs), the result of nitrates used to preserve meat.

Go heavy on fish. When you put colon cancer cells in a dish with fish oil or feed fish oil to animals, the number of colorectal tumors drops, along with the overall risk of colorectal cancer. We're not quite sure what goes on in humans, but it appears that people who eat fish once or twice a week reduce their risk by about 12 percent compared to those who eat it less; each additional serving reduces the risk by another 4 percent. The link between fish and colorectal cancer prevention may be due to the high levels of selenium and vitamin D in fish, both of which are also prized as colorectal cancer preventives.

Limit yourself to one alcoholic beverage a day. That's 4 ounces of wine, 12 ounces of beer, or 1.5 ounces of liquor. As your body breaks down alcohol, cancer-causing acetaldehyde forms. Alcohol also appears to make cells more permeable to other cancer-causing compounds. An analysis of more than 4,600 cases of colorectal cancer among 475,000 participants found that those who drank

> "Colorectal cancer is one of only two cancers that can be completely prevented through screening."

more than 45 grams of alcohol a day (about four beers) increased their risk of colorectal cancer by 41 percent. The risk increased 16 percent in those who consumed 30 to 44 grams a day. One beer contains 12.8 grams of alcohol, 4 ounces of wine contains 10.9 grams, and 1.5 ounces of 80-proof liquor contains 14 grams.

Prevention Boosters

Eat your beans. Beans, lentils, and peas are excellent sources of folate, a B vitamin also known as folic acid. According to a Harvard study of nearly 89,000 women, those with a family history of colon cancer who consumed more than 400 micrograms of folate each day lowered their risk by more than 52 percent compared to women who consumed 200 micrograms a day. You can get almost 300 micrograms by eating one cup of chickpeas or cooked spinach, another great source. If you take a multivitamin, you may already be getting enough folate.

Season with garlic. About six cloves of garlic a week, whether raw or cooked, can help reduce your risk of colorectal cancer by as much as 31 percent, according to one University of North Carolina analysis of many studies. The benefit probably comes from allicin compounds in garlic that prevent colorectal tumors from forming, possibly by forcing aberrant cells to commit the equivalent of cellular suicide.

Drink a glass of fat-free milk every day. Just eight ounces a day reduces women's risk of colorectal cancer by 16 percent and men's risk by 10 percent, according to an analysis of studies by researchers at

If you're already taking aspirin or another nonsteroidal anti-inflammatory drug (NSAID) such as celecoxib (Celebrex), you may enjoy a happy side benefit: a lower risk of colon cancer. When women take at least 325 milligrams of regular aspirin twice a week for at least 10 years, their risk of colon cancer plummets by a third compared to women who take aspirin less often. And in a study of people who had already had precancerous polyps removed, those who were taking 400 milligrams of celecoxib a day were one-third less likely to have the growths return within three years. Unfortunately, it's too soon to recommend taking drugs like these solely to prevent colon cancer, as they can have unwanted side effects.

Statins, the drugs prescribed to lower cholesterol, may also lower the risk of colon cancer. A study involving 4,000 people found that taking these drugs for at least five years cut the risk of colon cancer nearly in half. But as with aspirin and NSAIDs, statins have side effects, and doctors aren't ready to prescribe them unless you need them to regulate your cholesterol.

All these medications have one thing in common: They reduce inflammation, which can contribute to cancer development. But they likely work in other ways as well. Researchers around the globe are now studying their mechanisms to try to figure out a way to create a drug with all the cancer-preventing benefits and none of the negatives.

Brigham and Women's Hospital and Harvard Medical School. Every two additional glasses drops the risk another 12 percent. Why? It may be the vitamin D that's added to milk, or its calcium (high calcium consumption is also linked to lower rates of colon cancer). Milk also contains the fatty acid conjugated linoleic acid and the protein lactoferrin, both of which help prevent colon cancer in animals.

Use olive oil, not butter, as your fat of choice. Animal fats like butter are associated with an increased risk of colorectal cancer, probably because diets high in fat lead to increased levels of bile acids in the colon to break down that fat. These bile acids can be converted to cancer-causing compounds. This is another reason to get your protein from sources like fish, soy, or legumes rather than fatty red meat.

Drop a few pounds. Being overweight considerably increases your risk of cancer, including colorectal cancer. An analysis of numerous studies found that men's risk jumped 37 percent if they were overweight or obese; women's risk inched up 7 percent. Researchers think the higher levels of hormones like insulin, leptin, and insulin-like growth factor in overweight people are to blame. All provide fuel for cancer cells.

Get 15 minutes of sunscreen-free sunshine a day. It's your best source of vitamin D, one of the most important vitamins when it comes to preventing colorectal cancer. An analysis of five studies found that getting at least 2,000 IU a day from diet, sunlight, or supplementation could cut the risk of colorectal cancer in half. How? By detoxifying a dangerous form of bile.

During the winter months, get your D from your diet or a supplement. Three ounces of cooked salmon or mackerel contains about 350 IU, three ounces of tuna has about 200 IU, and a cup of fat-free milk fortified with vitamin D provides about 100 IU. If you supplement, aim for 800 IU daily.

WHAT CAUSES IT Aging, genetic abnormalities, diseases like inflammatory bowel disease.

SYMPTOMS TO WATCH FOR Blood in your stools; narrowing of stools; a change in bowel habits, including diarrhea or constipation for more than a couple of weeks; cramps, gas, or pain; abdominal pain with a bowel movement; feeling that your bowel doesn't empty completely; weakness or fatigue; unexplained weight loss.

NEWEST THINKING A simple blood test could provide a warning about precancerous colorectal growths. The test, currently under investigation, detects chemical markers of colon cancer that make their way into the bloodstream.

Congestive Heart Failure

30%

The reduction in heart failure risk if you eat whole grain cereal for breakfast every day.

Heart failure is one of the fastest-growing heart conditions in the world, thanks to everything from the obesity epidemic and rising rates of high blood pressure to the fact that more people are surviving heart attacks and facing life with damaged tickers. When your heart is too weak or too stiff to pump enough blood to the organs and tissues in your body, your lungs can fill with fluid, your kidneys can fail, and you become very, very tired. The condition kills 80 percent of men and 65 percent of women within six years of a diagnosis. Here's how you can avoid it.

Key Prevention Strategies

Exercise and follow a heart-healthy diet. If you think heart failure happens only to other people, consider this statistic: Your odds of developing it after age 45 are one in five. The biggest contributors are high blood pressure and heart attacks. Your best move right now: Put down this book and go for a brisk walk. At your next meal, load your plate with fruits, vegetables, and whole grains. Small changes can make a big difference. Simply eating a whole grain breakfast cereal every morning lowers your risk by 30 percent.

If you already have heart disease or high blood pressure, talk to your doctor or experts at a cardiac rehabilitation program about what kind and amount of exercise is right for you.

Maintain a healthy weight. Every 5 to 10 pounds you gain—whatever it takes to raise your body mass index (BMI) one point—increases a woman's risk for heart failure by 7 percent and a man's by 5 percent, say researchers with the landmark Framingham Heart Study. Being obese, with a BMI of 30 or higher, doubles your odds. Extra pounds hurt your heart by raising your risk of high blood pressure and diabetes. They also put a strain on your heart that can damage muscle.

step on the scale—and check your socks

If you have any health conditions that put you at increased risk of heart failure, stay alert for early signs. Watch unusual weight changes: An increase of three pounds in a day or five pounds in a week could mean you're retaining fluid because your heart is losing its ability to effectively pump blood. Another sign: Swollen ankles or calves that make your socks feel tight.

Tame high blood pressure. Ninety percent of people who have heart failure had high blood pressure first. When your pressure is high, your heart has to pump harder to force blood through the miles of blood vessels in your body. Over time, this can make the chambers of your heart grow "muscle-bound," a condition called left ventricular hypertrophy that interferes with the heart's pumping ability. A 10-point drop in systolic blood pressure (the top number) can cut your risk of heart failure by 50 percent, say researchers from McMaster University in Montreal, Canada.

If you need medication, ask about a diuretic. Studies show these drugs cut heart failure risk more than other, more expensive drugs such as alpha-blockers and calcium channel blockers.

Ask about ACE inhibitors after a heart attack. About one in four men and half of all women who survive a heart attack will be disabled by heart failure within six years. Drugs called ACE inhibitors reduce that likelihood. In one study, an ACE inhibitor called ramipril (Altace) cut heart failure risk by 23 percent in 9,000 high-risk women and men, many of whom had had heart attacks. These drugs ease the strain on the heart by relaxing blood vessel walls and lowering blood pressure.

Prevention Boosters

Gain good blood sugar control if you have diabetes. If you have type 2 diabetes, your risk of heart failure is five times higher than normal if you're a woman and nearly four times higher than normal if you're a man. Since people with diabetes often have coronary artery disease or high blood pressure or have even had silent heart attacks, your doctor may prescribe medications to help guard your ticker. But don't overlook the power of blood sugar control. In one study, people with diabetes who kept their blood sugar within a healthy range were half as likely to develop heart failure as those whose blood sugar remained high.

Make broiled or baked fish your automatic order when you eat out. Harvard Medical School researchers who tracked the health of 4,738 adults found that those who ate broiled or baked tuna or other fish once or twice a week cut their risk of congestive heart failure by 20 percent. More is better: Those who had fish five times a week cut their risk by 32 percent. *Note:* Fried fish did not protect against this heart problem.

WHAT CAUSES IT Damage or death of heart muscle due to narrowed arteries or a heart attack; high blood pressure, which makes heart muscle grow large and stiff; malfunctioning heart valves (due to a birth defect, infection, or heart disease); heart-rhythm problems.

SYMPTOMS TO WATCH FOR Breathlessness; coughing and wheezing; swollen feet, ankles, legs, or abdomen; fatigue; lack of appetite; nausea; confusion and memory loss; rapid heartbeat.

NEWEST THINKING Depression can make heart muscle stiffer, raising the risk of heart failure. University of Maryland School of Medicine scientists found that depression raised levels of chronic inflammation in the body, which stimulated the production of collagen, a protein that can stiffen heart muscle.

Constipation

68%

The drop in your risk of constipation if you eat a high-fiber diet and exercise most days of the week.

Sometimes it's the little things that "block" us from feeling our very best, and constipation is one of them. Normal bowel movements range from a prodigious three a day to a spartan three per week, so don't assume you're constipated unless you're having the symptoms described on the next page. If you can't seem to "go" when you need to, chances are good that you're not eating enough fiber or drinking enough fluids. Anxiety, medications, and conditions like pregnancy and diabetes also contribute.

Key Prevention Strategies

Increase the fiber in your diet. Getting at least 20 grams of fiber a day could cut your risk of constipation by 46 percent, say Harvard School of Public Health researchers who tracked more than 60,000 women. Those who ate less than 7 grams a day had the highest constipation rates. Fiber helps by making your stools bulkier and heavier, which allows tiny hairs along the inner walls of the intestines to whisk them toward the finish line with greater ease. Fiber may even make your bowels move faster.

You can get to 20 grams by starting the day with oatmeal or high-fiber cold cereal (top with berries and a sprinkling of wheat germ or flaxseed for even more fiber), having your sandwich on whole grain bread, eating a serving of barley or brown rice at dinner, and consuming plenty of fruits and veggies (including beans) throughout the day. Keep at it—it may take a few weeks to see an improvement.

Drink plenty of water. If you've just started a higher-fiber diet or have been following one and feel constipated, put down this book and drink a glass of water. If you're taking a fiber supplement, water is even more important. When researchers gave 117 people with chronic constipation a fiber supplement, the group that was also told to drink two liters (about 8.5 cups) of water a day saw more improvement than those who drank half that amount.

biofeedback for stubborn constipation

One in three people with chronic constipation get little relief from standard approaches, say University of Iowa researchers. In a little-recognized, lifelong constipation problem called dyssynergic defecation, the muscle contractions that should move stools along are weak and uncoordinated, and it's hard to sense when there's stool ready to exit the bowels. The fix? In one study, a biofeedback technique that involves using a pencil-thin rectal probe and artificial "practice stools" helped 80 percent of people with this problem learn to push at the right time and overcome constipation.

Take a walk. When middle-aged Dutch men and women with chronic constipation took a brisk 30-minute walk every day, researchers found that they didn't have to strain as much during bowel movements and had fewer hard stools. Food also passed more quickly through their intestinal tracts. As a result, the number with constipation dropped by a third. And in a Harvard School of Public Health study of 62,036 women, those who got some kind of physical activity every day were 44 percent less likely to be constipated than women who were active less than once a week.

While you're at it, stack the deck by eating more fiber. These two strategies seem to do more together to prevent constipation than either one can alone: In the study, active women who also ate a high-fiber diet were 68 percent less likely to be constipated than inactive women who ate a low-fiber diet.

Prevention Boosters

Munch a few dried plums or sip some prune juice. Research has confirmed something many of us have experienced firsthand: There's something in prunes that gets the bowels moving. Studies show that it stimulates contractions of the intestinal wall and seems to make bowel movements wetter, which can make elimination easier. In one Boston University study, prunes stimulated the bowels more than any other food tested.

Change your prescription. Experts estimate that prescription and over-the-counter drugs and remedies are responsible for up to 40 percent of constipation problems. If you take any of the medications on this list and are having trouble with regularity, ask your doctor if you can switch to another drug: antacids containing aluminum or calcium, antidepressants, antihistamines, calcium channel blockers, diuretics, iron supplements, opioids, and pseudoephedrine (found in many cold medicines).

Sit on "the throne" a half hour after eating. The gastrocolic reflex—a wave of muscle activity along the intestines that leads to a bowel movement—usually happens within a half hour after a meal. Digestion experts often recommend that people prone to constipation make it a point to spend some time on the toilet after meals as a form of "bowel retraining"—getting your body on a schedule that can lead to better regularity. If nothing happens, don't linger—sitting for a long time won't help.

WHAT CAUSES IT Slow movement of waste material along the intestinal tract due to a lack of fiber and fluids, aging, lack of a regular bathroom routine, or taking medications or having a health condition (such as diabetes) that slows bowel speed.

SYMPTOMS TO WATCH FOR Bloating, abdominal discomfort, having two or fewer bowel movements per week with hard stools, straining and pushing when you have a bowel movement, feeling that your bowel movement was incomplete.

NEWEST THINKING People with chronic constipation are twice as likely to have frequent headaches as people with regular bowel movements, report researchers from the Norwegian University of Science and Technology. The more frequent the headaches, the worse the constipation. Experts aren't sure why the two are connected, but they warn that prescription painkillers such as morphine, codeine, and oxycodone could make constipation worse.

Coronary Artery Disease

80%

The number of cases that could be prevented through lifestyle changes such as getting more exercise and eating more fruits, vegetables, and fish.

You don't just wake up one day with heart disease; the stage is set decades in advance. As early as your teens or even your preteens, habits like getting too little exercise and eating too much of the wrong fats begin to pad artery walls with plaque. Fast-forward 20, 30, or 40 years, and you may have chest pain as narrowed arteries can't deliver enough blood to heart muscle—or worse, a heart attack. While genes play a role, your heart's fate is mostly in your hands. Even if your arteries are less than squeaky clean today, changing your ways can change your future.

Key Prevention Strategies

Walk for 30 minutes five times a week. Our advice: Keep some walking shoes in sight at all times. Getting out for a walk at a moderate clip—a pace brisk enough to quicken your breathing a little—five days a week can cut heart disease risk in half, according to one large study of middle-aged and older women. Researchers looking at men found that those who rarely if ever exercised were three times more likely to die from heart disease than men who exercised at least five days a week.

Exercise helps your heart in many ways. It raises HDL ("good") cholesterol, lowers LDL ("bad") cholesterol and triglycerides, puts a damper on high blood pressure and heart-threatening inflammation, and can even improve the circulation of antioxidants that protect the cells of the heart and the cells lining blood vessels from injury.

One study really demonstrates the heart-friendly powers of exercise. Researchers looked at 101 men who had surgery to open blocked arteries in their hearts. Half of them received stents to keep the arteries open. The other half didn't; instead they rode exercise bikes for 20 minutes a day to achieve the same effect. The result? The bike riders had fewer heart attacks, strokes, and serious chest pain. A good reason to invest in an exercise bike!

Quit smoking. Cigarette smoking doubles, triples, or even quadruples your risk of developing heart disease; once you have the disease, smoking doubles your risk of sudden cardiac death.

Tobacco smoke damages arteries, giving plaque an easier foothold. Nicotine constricts blood vessels. And the carbon monoxide in cigarette smoke displaces oxygen in the bloodstream, forcing your heart to pump harder to deliver oxygen to cells.

Quit, and you'll begin to lower your risk almost immediately. Within two years after your last cigarette, risk drops by more than 30 percent, and it drops to normal within 10 to 14 years. (Turn to page 38 for the best strategies for kicking the habit.)

Eat more fish. Want to get dinner on the table fast and also protect yourself from heart attacks? Serve fish. You'll eat fewer calories than you would if steak were on your plate, and you'll not only avoid the "bad" saturated fats that raise cholesterol levels but also get "good" fats that keep your ticker happy. In one study of nearly 85,000 women, those who ate fish a mere one to three times a month cut their risk of developing coronary heart disease by 21 percent; eating fish five times a week or more lowered it by 34 percent. Fish fat helps prevent blood clots and inflammation of the arteries, and it protects against irregular heart rhythms that can lead to heart attacks.

Aim to eat at least two servings (8 to 12 ounces total) of fatty fish such as salmon, mackerel, halibut, or canned light tuna a week. Don't worry too much if your salmon is farmed or wild; unless you're pregnant, the benefits of eating it outweigh any risks.

Consider fish-oil capsules. The American Heart Association recommends getting 1 gram of DHA plus EPA a day from fish or fish-oil capsules for people who already have coronary artery disease and up to 4 grams of DHA plus EPA a day (under a doctor's care only) if you have high triglycerides (studies show this can lower triglycerides by up to 30 percent). In one study, people who got 1.5 grams of these omega-3 fatty acids a day from fish-oil capsules saw plaque regress after two years.

Even if you don't have heart disease, ask your doctor about taking one gram of fish oil daily as a preventive measure. Vegetarians can look for omega-3 capsules that provide DHA from algae instead of fish.

Eat nuts and heart-healthy oils. Walnuts, canola oil, ground flaxseed (keep it in the refrigerator), tofu, and soybeans are all good sources of alpha linolenic acid (ALA), a type of omega-3 fatty acid that your body converts into DHA and EPA.

"Getting out for a walk five days a week can cut heart disease risk in half."

These foods are not a replacement for fish and fish oil—your body gets only a small amount of DHA and EPA from them—but they're a good add-on.

Eat foods that "Offer Best Protection." It's a mnemonic device for remembering foods richest in soluble fiber—oatmeal and oranges; beans, barley, and berries; and pears and peas. Soluble fiber forms a gel in your intestines that actually reduces the absorption of the fat you eat, which in turn lowers cholesterol. In one study that followed 9,776 women and men for 19 years, those who got about six grams of soluble fiber a day (about the amount in a bowl of oatmeal, 1/2 cup of barley, and a pear) had a 15 a percent lower risk of heart disease than those who got less than a gram a day.

Choose smarter carbs. The key here is whole grains. Studies show that people who eat more of them (think 100 percent whole grain bread, whole grain breakfast cereal, and whole grains such as brown rice and bulgur) are less likely to have heart disease, whereas people who eat a lot of refined grains (think white bread; white rice; and snack foods like crackers, cookies, and doughnuts) have more heart attacks. Chalk up the difference largely to the effects of refined grains on insulin; generally speaking, they raise insulin more than whole grains do, and high insulin levels have a domino effect that raises heart disease risk. A diet that keeps insulin low also helps lower levels of potentially harmful blood fats called triglycerides.

Go low salt. A recent Harvard Medical School study shows that cutting back on salt cuts your risk of heart disease by 25 percent, even if you don't have high blood pressure yet. Taking the saltshaker off your table is just the first step. Infinitely more important is fervently avoiding most processed foods, from which we get 70 to 80 percent of the salt we eat. That means everything from lunchmeats and canned soups to microwave meals and salad dressings. Make your own or look for low-sodium versions.

Ask your doctor about wine. Drinking any form of alcohol in moderation (up to one drink a day for women or two for men) can lower your risk of heart disease as much as 30 percent by improving cholesterol ratios and helping to prevent blood clots. But if your triglycerides are high, drink wine only in moderation or not at all. While some studies suggest that just one glass a day may lower triglycerides, this strategy doesn't work for everyone.

The American Heart Association suggests cutting out alcohol entirely if your triglycerides are high. (If you have trouble keeping your drinking in check, do the same. Drinking to the point of drunkenness even once a month increases heart attack risk.)

Lower your blood pressure. High blood pressure stresses your heart, making it grow thicker and stiffer. The extra pressure damages artery walls, speeding up the accumulation of plaque. It can also mute your sensitivity to chest pain so you don't notice warning signs of heart disease and could even suffer a "silent" heart attack, say Montreal Heart Institute researchers who studied 900 people with hypertension. Lowering blood pressure can cut heart disease risk by up to 30 percent, studies show.

Watch your cholesterol levels. If you don't know your cholesterol levels—LDL, HDL, and total cholesterol—go to your doctor for a blood test. Check them again every five years, or more often if they're out of whack. While many people who have heart attacks don't have high cholesterol, having high cholesterol does increase the risk. If your ratios are less than ideal, take steps to bring them into range (see the High Cholesterol chapter).

Prevention Boosters

Brush and floss regularly. The cheapest heart protection tools of all? A toothbrush and dental floss. When used daily (brush at least twice and floss once), they can cut your risk of gum disease, which recent studies suggest doubles your odds for heart disease. The link? Inflammation caused by bacteria. People with severe gum disease have four times higher levels of bacterial by-products, called endotoxins, in their bloodstream than people with healthy gums. Battling these toxins involves an immune system response that triggers inflammation, and chronic inflammation contributes to the formation of plaque in artery walls.

Have a sweet, dark treat. An ounce of dark chocolate a day—that's just a small piece, mind you—helps arteries stay flexible and can help nudge your blood pressure lower, studies show. But it has to be the dark stuff.

Avoid secondhand smoke. Breathing in the smelly smoke from someone else's cigarettes raises your own risk of developing heart disease by 25 to 30 percent.

WHAT CAUSES IT Damage to the inner layers of arteries in your heart due to high blood pressure, smoking, and high blood sugar. As your heart tries to heal itself, fatty plaque accumulates in artery walls, especially if you have high levels of "bad" LDL cholesterol. This buildup narrows arteries and can lead to the formation of heart-threatening blood clots. Infections like gum disease and excess belly fat fuel the process by releasing inflammatory compounds into the bloodstream that spur the growth of plaque.

SYMPTOMS TO WATCH FOR Chest pain, or angina, which occurs when the heart muscle can't get enough oxygen-rich blood. Angina can feel like pressure or squeezing in your chest, but you may also feel it in your back, jaw, shoulders, neck, or arms. It usually gets worse during activity and improves when you stop.

NEWEST THINKING Marital stress can harm the heart. In a University of Utah study of 150 couples, those who deployed angry, mean-spirited verbal grenades during a six-minute conversation about a sore subject had more atherosclerosis (caused by severe plaque buildup). Husbands had a 30 percent higher risk of atherosclerosis when either spouse was dominant or controlling; wives' risk rose by 30 percent when either partner was hostile.

Depression

61%
The amount by which learning to problem solve could reduce your risk of depression.

When we asked more than 100 doctors which health conditions are most likely to cause chronic disease, depression ranked surprisingly high—not far below high blood pressure. Depression is linked with a higher risk of nearly every major health issue, from diabetes to heart disease, and is the leading cause of physical disability in the world. And it's hardly the type of thing you just "snap out of." The best way to beat depression is to prevent it in the first place or, barring that, prevent a recurrence (up to 60 percent of people who have had one major depressive episode go on to have another). Here's what the research finds helpful.

Key Prevention Strategies

Learn to solve problems. Often, depression starts with a challenge in your life that you just don't know how to cope with. Finding ways to manage the issues you're facing now can help you avoid depression down the line. Think of it as preventive maintenance for your mind.

One study looked at older adults who were just diagnosed with macular degeneration, a leading cause of vision loss. Those who were taught to solve many of the problems they would encounter as their sight failed were 61 percent less likely to be depressed two months after their diagnoses than those who didn't receive such coaching. They were also less likely to have to given up an activity they enjoyed—the very types of activities that help prevent depression.

Learning to solve problems can be as simple as sitting down with paper and pen, listing the issues that are making you unhappy, and identifying three concrete steps you can take to make things better. Other options include brainstorming solutions with friends or family or scheduling a few sessions with a therapist trained in cognitive behavioral therapy.

drugs that PREVENT DISEASE

If you've had at least two episodes of major depression, or you have a chronic illness such as diabetes, heart disease, or cancer, talk to your doctor about continuing your antidepressant medication for longer than the recommended six months after the depression recedes. A review of several studies found that about 60 percent of people are at risk of having another depressive episode within a year of stopping treatment, but just 10 to 30 percent of people who continue antidepressants will have a recurrence. Another study found that people with a form of depression called seasonal affective disorder (SAD), which occurs in fall and winter, can prevent an episode by starting antidepressants early in the season, while they still feel well.

View the glass as half full. Numerous studies find that optimistic people are less likely to develop depression than pessimistic people. In fact, in one study of 71 older adults, researchers found that people who expected that bad things would happen in the coming month experienced more depressive symptoms at the end of the month than those who didn't have negative expectations, regardless of what actually happened.

Not everyone is a born optimist, but anyone can work on adopting a more positive attitude. Being an optimist begins with the belief that bad events are temporary and changeable. For instance, rather than complaining about a bad boss and assuming nothing will change, an optimist would identify opportunities for growth elsewhere in the company, update his résumé, and apply for a new—possibly better—job. It also involves looking on the bright side. If a pessimist were diagnosed with breast cancer, she might immediately assume she's going to become sick from chemotherapy, lose her hair, and eventually die from the disease. An optimist might count herself lucky that women today are much less likely to die from breast cancer and that new treatments relegate many of the negative effects of chemotherapy to the past.

See a therapist once a month. If you've ever been diagnosed with major depression, a once-a-month psychotherapy session may be all that's required to prevent a recurrence. Researchers randomly assigned 99 previously depressed women to interpersonal psychotherapy (a short-term form of counseling that focuses on resolving issues related to grief, role transitions, or problems interacting with others) weekly, twice a month, or once a month for two years or until they had another depressive episode. The result? Just 26 percent of the women who completed the maintenance phase saw their depression recur (versus an average 60 percent recurrence rate), no matter how often they had therapy.

Stay connected. Join a bowling league, a sewing club, or a committee at your child's school or your church—anything to bring you into regular contact with others and enhance your social network. Such connections, researchers find, do a great job of inoculating you against depression.

Prevention Boosters
Seek treatment for anxiety. If you find that you're worrying beyond reason, obsessing over events in your life, or pathologically

> "Anyone can work on adopting a more positive attitude."

afraid of certain things like going outside or being around other people, you may have an anxiety disorder and thus an increased risk of depression. The more severe your anxiety, the more likely you are to become depressed. Researchers think the anxiety disorder may alter the way the brain releases and takes up serotonin, a chemical important to mood. Or the anxiety may change your normal interactions and lifestyle so much that it triggers depression. Regardless, your best option is to seek out a therapist trained in cognitive behavioral therapy, which studies find is the best way to treat most anxiety disorders.

Lace up your sneakers. Countless studies underscore the emotional boost that exercise provides and its ability to help relieve symptoms of depression. But a pile of research also suggests that people who get regular exercise are less likely to become depressed in the first place. A recent British study showed that at least in middle-aged men, more intense exercise (think running or playing soccer or basketball) was most effective. But in another study of older adults with arthritis, simply taking aerobics classes led to fewer depression symptoms. It may be key to get your heart rate up; slow walking or weight lifting probably won't do the trick.

10 instant mood boosters

Snapping at the kids, your spouse, or the clerk at the convenience store? Feeling out of sorts or just sad for no reason? Here are 10 quick ways to raise your spirits.

1. **Call a friend and gab about nothing.** It's an instant stress buster!
2. **Take a walk in the sunshine.** Sunlight has proven mood-boosting powers, as does exercise.
3. **Meet someone for coffee.** Good conversation coupled with an energy burst from the caffeine. What could be better?
4. **Give thanks for something.** You'll remember how much you have to be grateful for and stop dwelling on your problems for a minute.
5. **Plant some geraniums.** The physical activity of planting and the bright colors of the flowers will raise your spirits in no time.
6. **Bake a loaf of bread (even an instant mix works!).** Nothing says contentment like the scent of freshly baked bread filling the house.
7. **Clean out a closet.** You'll get an instant sense of accomplishment. Donate the extra clothes and get the added mood benefit of helping someone else.
8. **Soak in a hot bath.** Light some candles (try lavender or vanilla scents, which studies find can relieve anxiety and boost mood), scan a trashy magazine, or just drift for 20 minutes. What was bothering you again?
9. **Pet a puppy.** Actually, even a full-grown dog will work. Studies find that petting animals reduces stress and boosts mood.
10. **Enjoy a small piece of dark chocolate.** It contains compounds that influence levels of serotonin, a feel-good brain chemical.

Broil some salmon for dinner. Can twice-weekly meals of salmon, mackerel, or tuna help keep depression at bay? It's entirely possible. Fatty fish like these are excellent sources of omega-3 fatty acids. In countries where people consume a lot of these healthy fats, depression rates tend to be low. In fact, women who dine on "fin food" often have half the risk of developing depression than those who don't eat fish often. If you don't eat fish, ask your doctor about taking a daily fish-oil supplement containing at least two grams of omega-3 fatty acids.

While you're at it, cut back on corn, safflower, and sunflower oils as well as processed foods such as chips and cookies. These are high in omega-6 fatty acids, which counteract the beneficial effects of omega-3's.

Get a good night's sleep. Researchers used to think that insomnia was a symptom of depression. Now they're finding that it typically precedes depression, with up to 50 percent of people with insomnia that lasts two weeks or longer later developing a major depressive episode. Of course, the insomnia may be a sign of an underlying problem in your life that may lead to depression, but good evidence shows that poor sleep by itself can lead to symptoms of depression. (See the Insomnia chapter for tips.)

Make your cereal whole grain. Just 3/4 cup of whole grain cereal contains about 800 micrograms of folate, a B vitamin in which many people who are depressed are deficient. Studies find that men who get 234 micrograms of folate for every 1,000 calories they eat are half as likely to become depressed as men who get 119 micrograms. Other great sources of folate include lentils (358 micrograms in 1 cup of cooked lentils), chickpeas (282 micrograms in a cup), and spinach (263 micrograms in 1 cup of frozen cooked spinach).

WHAT CAUSES IT Usually a mix of factors that results in an imbalance in mood-regulating chemicals called neurotransmitters (such as serotonin and dopamine). These factors may include a genetic predisposition, a single traumatic event, and stress, particularly the kind of stress that comes from feeling a loss of control over your life. Other triggers include specific situations, like the death of a loved one.

SYMPTOMS TO WATCH FOR Changes in your sleeping and/or eating habits; loss of pleasure in things that you used to enjoy; thoughts of hurting yourself; lack of interest in sex; feeling hopeless or worthless; crying for no apparent reason; trouble concentrating and making decisions; irritability or restlessness; feeling fatigued or weak; unexplained physical problems, such as back pain or headaches.

NEWEST THINKING People who have had depression are more likely to develop Alzheimer's disease than those who were never depressed. Researchers don't know yet whether the depression contributes to the development of Alzheimer's or whether something else is at work to cause both the depression and the Alzheimer's.

Diabetes

58%

The drop in your odds
of developing type 2
diabetes if you lose just
7 percent of your
body weight

It doesn't take a rocket scientist to figure out why so many people are developing diabetes. Genes do play a role, but the less exercise you get and the more you weigh, the greater your risk. If you aren't part of the "diabetes epidemic" yet, congratulations. But there's a shadow epidemic of prediabetes—elevated blood sugar that's not yet high enough to trigger alarms—that you should worry about now. Doctors don't look for prediabetes often enough (a fasting blood test can give a pretty good indication if you have it), but now's the time to prevent it from turning into diabetes.

Key Prevention Strategies

Drop just a few pounds. Excess weight is the number one reason adults and kids are at higher risk for type 2 diabetes now than ever before. Gaining weight can pack excess fat around internal organs at your midsection—especially if you're stressed out on a regular basis (stress hormones can send extra fat to the belly). New research shows that this dangerous abdominal fat sends out chemical signals that desensitize cells throughout your body to insulin, the hormone that persuades cells to absorb blood sugar. Insulin resistance is the first step on the path to type 2 diabetes.

The good news: In a landmark clinical trial that followed 3,234 people with prediabetes for three years, those who lost just 7 percent of their body weight (10.5 pounds if you now weigh 170) lowered their diabetes risk by 58 percent. In fact, weight loss worked better than insulin-sensitizing diabetes drugs at cutting the odds of diabetes!

A brisk cardio workout three to five times a week can melt belly fat better than dieting, say Syracuse University researchers. Brisk walking for 30 minutes daily also works.

Aim for five to nine servings of fruit and vegetables every day, plus three servings of whole grains. Following a low-glycemic diet packed with produce and whole grains—and cutting back on white bread, white rice, foods like pancakes and bagels made with white flour, and sweets—helps keeps blood sugar low and steady. Research shows it also cools chronic low-grade inflammation in the body, which interferes with the action of insulin and the absorption of blood sugar by cells.

In a recent study of 486 women, Harvard School of Public Health researchers found that those who ate the most fruit were 34 percent less likely to have metabolic syndrome, a cluster of risk factors, including insulin resistance, that predispose a person to diabetes. Women who ate the most vegetables cut their risk of metabolic syndrome by 30 percent. Meanwhile, German researchers who followed 25,067 women and men for seven years recently found that those who got the most fiber from whole grains were 27 percent less likely to develop diabetes than those who got the least.

Give up "liquid candy." Start quenching your thirst with water, club soda (with a spritz of lemon or lime), unsweetened tea, or fat-free milk instead of soda, fruit punch, or sweetened iced tea drinks.

A single daily serving of soda raised the risk of metabolic syndrome (described above) by a staggering 44 percent in a headline-grabbing study from Boston University School of Medicine. The reason? Experts have many theories. It could simply be all those extra calories in soda and other sugary drinks or in the high-fat, high-calorie foods we tend to pair them with (think french fries and pizza). Experts are also finding that drinking even a single soda a day is associated with being overweight—perhaps because the calories in beverages don't register in our brains, so we don't compensate for them by eating less food.

Yet another possible culprit: high-fructose corn syrup. It's essentially table sugar in liquid form, except that for technical chemistry reasons, some experts believe it's more likely to lead to insulin resistance.

For a healthier thirst quencher, drop several teabags (black, green,

10 great low-glycemic snacks

Low-glycemic foods are those that have only a minimal or moderate effect on blood sugar. Studies show that people who eat more of these foods and fewer high-glycemic foods are less likely to develop insulin resistance, a core problem underlying type 2 diabetes. Low-glycemic foods are often rich in fiber, protein, or fat, though it's not smart to eat fatty foods just for the sake of your blood sugar unless those fats are "good" (unsaturated) fats.

1. **An apple with the skin**
2. **Whole wheat crackers with peanut butter**
3. **Baby carrots dipped in low-fat sour cream**
4. **A small handful of walnuts or almonds**
5. **Low-fat yogurt sprinkled with fresh fruit or bran cereal**
6. **A toasted whole wheat pita with bean dip**
7. **Soybeans with a little salt**
8. **Air-popped popcorn**
9. **Dried apricots (no more than 1/3 cup)**
10. **A hard-boiled egg**

or herbal) into a plastic pitcher filled with water and refrigerate overnight, then enjoy. And don't discount a glass of fat-free milk. The calcium, vitamin D, and other minerals in dairy foods may be the reason that getting at least one serving of low-fat or fat-free milk (or yogurt or cheese) a day lowered metabolic syndrome risk by up to 62 percent in a British study.

Turn off the TV and go for a walk. Exercise helps protect against diabetes by transporting blood sugar into fuel-hungry muscle cells and making cells more sensitive to insulin. A Harvard study of 40,000 women found that 30 minutes a day of brisk walking, plus a TV limit of 10 hours per week, cut diabetes risk by 43 percent. Bored by walking? Spend Friday night at the local YMCA recreational swim, take up bowling, gather the kids or grandkids for a nature hike, or just put on some music and dance.

Eat less fast food. Does drive-through dining lead to diabetes? Consider this: When University of Minnesota researchers tracked the eating habits and health of 9,514 people ages 45 to 64 for up to 10 years, they discovered that those who ate two servings of red meat (like hamburger patties) a week were 26 percent more likely to wind up with metabolic syndrome. A daily helping of french fries or other fried foods raised it another 10 to 25 percent. These foods are high in saturated and trans fats, which have been linked to diabetes.

Trade burgers and butter for fish and olive oil. Each bite of that burger and each smear of that butter is full of saturated fat. This stuff not only clogs arteries, it also increases insulin resistance, which jet-propels you down the path to genuine diabetes. These fats also trigger inflammation, which is toxic to cells, including those that handle blood sugar. Fish and olive oil have the exact opposite effects and could actually lower your diabetes risk. The same goes for nuts (even peanuts!) and canola oil.

Of course, you don't want to overdo even these good fats, which are high in calories. Cutting total fat intake as well as saturated fat helped participants in the Diabetes

get out the tape measure

Women whose waists measure 35 inches or more and men whose midsections measure 40 inches or more are more likely to have fat deep in their abdomens, which can triple the risk of diabetes. While you're probably overweight if your waist is big, researchers report that they're seeing more people at a normal weight who also have big waists, so don't think it's enough to simply watch the numbers on the scale.

Prevention Program study slash their diabetes risk. Participants limited saturated fat to 7 percent of total calories a day, about the amount in two ounces of cheese plus one pat of butter if you eat 2,000 calories a day.

Prevention Boosters

Eat breakfast. In one study, people who ate breakfast were 35 to 50 percent less likely to be overweight or have insulin resistance than breakfast skippers. What's going on? An overnight fast puts your body into "starvation mode." If you don't eat breakfast, your liver churns out stored glucose to keep your blood sugar levels up. At the same time, skipping breakfast flips biochemical switches that reduce the body's response to insulin. And it raises levels of an appetite-stimulating hormone called ghrelin so you want to eat more all day long. Do this often enough, and you gain weight, say scientists from Children's Hospital Boston.

What's for breakfast? Certainly not a bagel (too many carbs) or a store-bought muffin (too many calories and hydrogenated oils). Instead, pour yourself a bowl of high-fiber cereal with fat-free milk and throw some berries on top for good measure. One University of Toronto study of people with prediabetes found that high-fiber cereals made their cells "listen" better to insulin than lower-fiber fare. Yogurt with fresh berries is also a good choice.

If you're depressed, get help. If you're depressed, you're much less likely to exercise and eat well. But the health dangers don't end there. Stanford University scientists think that depression itself alters body chemistry in profound ways that spell trouble for anyone at risk for diabetes. Rates of insulin resistance were 23 percent higher among depressed women than among women who weren't depressed, regardless of body weight, exercise habits, or age. (See the Depression chapter for prevention advice.)

Get better sleep. A chronic lack of sleep leads to weight gain and reduces your body's sensitivity to insulin. In one Yale School of Medicine study of 1,709 men, those who averaged five to six hours of slumber per night doubled their risk of diabetes. Studies of women have found similar results.

WHAT CAUSES IT Genetics definitely play a role, but it usually takes extra pounds and a sedentary lifestyle to develop type 2 diabetes. Excess body fat (especially visceral fat deep in the belly) and inactivity conspire to make cells stop obeying signals from insulin to absorb blood sugar. Your body compensates by pumping out more insulin, but if it can't keep pace, you've got high blood sugar.

SYMPTOMS TO WATCH FOR Often, there are none. You can have type 2 diabetes for years without noticing anything's amiss. But as it progresses, symptoms include thirst, frequent urination, intense hunger, weight loss, tiredness, blurry vision, sores that are slow to heal, and more frequent bladder and vaginal infections for women.

NEWEST THINKING Think diet soda is safe? Think again. Sipping just one can of diet soda per day raised the risk of metabolic syndrome by 34 percent in one recent study and 48 percent in another. Experts aren't sure why.

Diarrhea

59%

When you're sprinting for the bathroom, diarrhea seems more like an uncomfortable inconvenience than one of Mother Nature's most ingeniously simple health-protection strategies. It's designed to flush out invaders as quickly as possible, but it can have serious consequences such as dehydration and loss of electrolytes—sodium, calcium, potassium, magnesium, and other important minerals. You can sidestep the bouts of diarrhea most of us get four times a year by tackling the bugs, the drugs, and the ingredients that trigger it. If your problem is irritable bowel syndrome, see the advice in that chapter.

Key Prevention Strategies

Wash your hands frequently. It's the best defense against the viral and bacterial infections that cause most diarrhea, say researchers who reviewed 14 studies of hand washing and diarrhea risk. Their conclusion: Scrubbing up can cut risk by at least 30 percent. Wash for 20 seconds, the amount of time it takes to warble the happy birthday song twice. Any soap will do; washing works by rubbing and rinsing viruses and bacteria off your skin. What about antibacterial soaps? Save your pennies. University of Michigan researchers who analyzed 18 studies of these germ killers found that plain soap was just as effective at preventing diarrhea.

Rub on an alcohol-based hand sanitizer when you can't wash. Using one regularly in addition to regular hand washing cut the risk of diarrhea and vomiting by an impressive 59 percent in a Children's Hospital Boston study of nearly 300 households. Families in the study all had at least one child age 5 or younger enrolled in daycare, where the germs that cause gastrointestinal illnesses sometimes run rampant.

prevent traveler's diarrhea

Planning a trip to an out-of-the-way foreign locale? Be prepared. Your odds of developing traveler's diarrhea in a developing country are one in three. These infections are usually bacterial and can lay you up for three to five days—waylaying your plans to explore museums, ruins, markets, and other exotic wonders. Experts say that observing the five "Ps" can cut your odds dramatically.

- **Take Pepto-Bismol** four times a day. Take two 262-milligram tablets at each meal and at bedtime. Studies show it can cut your risk by 65 percent. You can do this daily for up to three weeks.
- **Peelable, packaged, purified, or piping-hot food** is safest. Stick with bottled water (tie a ribbon on the tap in your hotel bathroom to remind you not to fill up a glass and sip it!); skip ice cubes in drinks (even alcoholic ones); and avoid salads and other raw vegetables, fruit you can't peel, mayonnaise, pastry icing, unpasteurized dairy products, and undercooked shellfish.

Participants kept sanitizer gel in the bathroom and kitchen and near diaper-changing tables and rubbed it on their hands after using the toilet, before preparing food, and after changing diapers.

Practice good food safety. Food poisoning—from undercooked meats, edibles left sitting out too long, and food contaminated by contact with cutlery and cutting boards used with raw meats—causes millions of cases of mild to severe diarrhea every year. Just a few of the rules: Don't let other foods touch raw poultry or other raw meats; don't put cooked meats, fish, or poultry back on the plate that held the raw product; wash cutting boards and knives in hot, soapy water after using them for raw meats (wash the sink, too); wash your hands frequently during and after handling raw meat; don't eat or serve food that's been out of the refrigerator, off the stove, or out of the oven for more than two hours; and if food looks or smells bad, throw it out. Use a meat thermometer to be sure meats are heated to the proper internal temperature to kill bacteria. Examples include T-bone steaks, 145°F; hamburgers, 160°F; hot dogs, 165°F; and chicken breasts, 170°F.

Prevention Boosters

Cut back on sugar-free and low-carb treats. Many "sugar-free" and low-carb chewing gums, hard candies, chocolates, cookies, cake mixes, and even pancake syrups are sweetened with sugar alcohols such as sorbitol and mannitol. Your body can't absorb most of the sugars (and calories) in these sweeteners, making them seem like the perfect choice for dieters. But the unabsorbed sugars draw water into your intestines and encourage the growth of bacteria, leading to bloating, gas, and sometimes severe diarrhea.

Eat more "good bacteria." Antibiotics can trigger diarrhea by slaying beneficial bacteria in your intestinal tract. Studies show that getting more of these good guys by eating yogurt with live, active cultures or taking a probiotic supplement can help. When British researchers checked on 135 people taking antibiotics, those who also drank a yogurt drink every day cut their risk of loose bowels by 21 percent compared to those who got a placebo drink without beneficial bacteria. The yogurt drink contained the bacteria strains *Lactobacillus casei*, *L. bulgaricus*, and *Streptococcus thermophilus*, commonly found in commercial yogurts and in probiotic supplements available at health food stores or drugstores.

WHAT CAUSES IT Bacteria, viruses, parasites, antibiotics, sugar-free foods, stress.

SYMPTOMS TO WATCH FOR Frequent, loose, fluid-filled stools, perhaps accompanied by abdominal pain, cramps, and bloating.

NEWEST THINKING Love turtles, snakes, or lizards? If you keep a reptile as a pet or can't resist touching or picking one up at a pet store, petting zoo, or a friend's house, be sure to scrub up afterward. Reptiles are responsible for 6 percent of salmonella infections, which cause bloody diarrhea, fever, and vomiting. The infections can be so severe that they require hospitalization and are sometimes deadly. Many reptiles are carriers of the bacteria that cause the infection.

Diverticular Disease

Years of constipation, straining during bowel movements, and eating a low-fiber diet can take an invisible toll on the walls of your intestinal tract. Hard stools and repeated high-pressure "pushing" can create tiny, pea-size pouches that balloon outward. These sacs, called diverticula, can number in the hundreds—and usually cause no trouble at all. But if stool gets trapped in a pouch, the sac can become inflamed and even infected, and you have diverticulitis, which can cause intense abdominal pain, fever, nausea, and constipation or diarrhea. You're even at risk for intestinal blockages or tears and for bleeding if a blood vessel near a pouch bursts. You can cut your odds of developing these troublesome pouches—and of having problems with existing ones—with these strategies.

Key Prevention Strategies

Eat more fiber. Packing about 30 grams of fiber into your diet each day could cut your risk of developing diverticulitis by 47 percent, say Harvard School of Public Health researchers who tracked the health and diets of nearly 44,000 men for four years. And if you've already had a painful episode, boosting the fiber in your meals could help prevent a repeat attack. In one British study of people who had been hospitalized once for diverticulitis, 90 percent of those who switched to a high-fiber diet were symptom free and stayed that way when researchers checked up on them seven years later.

Provided you drink plenty of fluids along with the fiber you eat, fiber protects intestinal walls by making stools soft and fluffy, which makes them easier to pass, and by decreasing tension within the walls. Researchers now suspect that it also promotes a healthier environment in the intestines by providing a haven for beneficial bacteria and by maintaining the layer of protective mucus that lines the inner walls. This healthy "inner landscape" seems to prevent the immune system from overreacting and causing inflammation in diverticula.

If you're planning to increase your fiber intake, go slowly. Add a few higher-fiber foods to your diet each week over the course of a month or two so you and your body grow accustomed to the changes. And be sure to drink several large glasses of water a day to avoid discomfort.

Add a fiber supplement. Can't get 30 grams of fiber from food every day? Experts say it's okay to use a fiber supplement to close the gap. (Avoid supplements during flare-ups of diverticulitis, though. They can cause discomfort.)

Snack on fruit instead of chips, cookies, and fries. Eating french fries, cookies, or a small bag of chips five or six times a week raised the risk of diverticular disease by as much as 69 percent in one study of 48,000 men. In contrast, those who snacked regularly on peaches, blueberries, apricots, apples, or oranges lowered their risk by as much as 80 percent. Avoid any fruits that give you diarrhea.

Have chicken or fish instead of fatty or processed red meat. Greek researchers have found that a diet loaded with red meat can raise your odds for diverticulitis a whopping 50 times higher than a vegetarian diet can. Eating even a medium (four- to six-ounce) serving of beef, pork, or lamb five or six nights a week tripled the risk of diverticular disease in the Harvard study mentioned earlier. Having a weekly hot dog raised the odds by 86 percent; a serving of processed meat (such as lunchmeat or ham) five or six times a week nearly doubled the risk. In contrast, fish and chicken eaters barely increased their risk at all.

Some experts speculate that red meat may prompt bacteria in your colon to produce substances that weaken the intestinal wall, so it's easier for pouches to form.

Don't worry about coffee or tea. In the past, people at risk for diverticulitis have been warned to avoid these popular drinks. But newer research suggests that they actually have little effect on diverticulitis. (Of course, if a food or beverage makes your symptoms worse, you should give it up.)

Foods That Fight Diverticular Disease

Fruits, vegetables, and whole grains packed with a type of insoluble fiber called cellulose seem to have a special talent for protecting intestinal walls from damage that leads to problems, researchers report. These foods pack the most.

FOOD	SERVING	TOTAL FIBER	CELLULOSE
Dried beans (legumes)	1/2 cup	6.7 grams	2.8 grams
Peas	1/2 cup	4.4 grams	2.1 grams
Tomato sauce	1/2 cup	4.2 grams	2.0 grams
Potato, with skin	1 medium	4.2 grams	1.6 grams
Apple	1 medium	3.7 grams	1.0 grams
Carrots	1/2 cup	2.6 grams	1.0 grams
Whole grain cereal	1 cup	6.0 grams	0.7 grams
Banana	1 medium	2.7 grams	0.5 grams
Whole grain bread	1 slice	1.1 grams	0.3 grams
Orange	1 medium	3.0 grams	0.3 grams

Get moving. Perhaps because it can prompt stools to move more swiftly through the intestinal tract, physical activity lowered the risk of diverticular disease by as much as 48 percent in one study. People who jogged got the most benefit, but any kind of exercise may help, experts say, especially if you also eat a high-fiber diet.

Schedule time in the bathroom. Straining to have a bowel movement puts extra pressure on the intestinal walls, setting the stage for the formation of pouches. If you're prone to constipation, be sure to take advantage of a key, after-meal opportunity for a bowel movement. During the half hour or so after eating, your gastrointestinal system makes room for the new food by moving everything else farther down the line. This wave of muscle activity, called the gastrocolic reflex, often results in a bowel movement if you let it by spending a few minutes in the bathroom about 30 minutes after a meal.

Ask about your medications. Ask your doctor if constipation is a common side effect of any prescription or over-the-counter medicine you're taking. Culprits include antacids that contain aluminum or calcium, antidepressants, antihistamines, calcium channel blockers, diuretics, iron supplements, opioid painkillers, and pseudoephedrine (found in many cold medicines). You may be able to substitute a different drug.

Prevention Boosters

Consume more good fats. Getting plenty of omega-3 fatty acids from fish, flaxseed (which also acts as a laxative) and flaxseed oil, walnuts, or fish-oil capsules may nudge down levels of inflammation in your colon—a big plus because inflammation can trigger serious diverticulitis symptoms. Taking one gram of fish oil once or twice a day could help, say digestive disease experts from the University of Maryland. Check with your doctor before starting fish-oil supplements.

Add a probiotic. Diverticular disease can decimate beneficial bacteria in the gut. These "good guy" bacteria, available in supplements known as probiotics, play a role in the speedy movement of stools, in protecting the lining of intestinal walls, and even in reducing inflammation. Studies from Italy and Germany are beginning to suggest that bolstering their levels may cut the risk of repeat attacks of diverticulitis. Look for *Lactobacillus acidophilus, L. plantarum, Saccharomyces boulardii*, and bifidobacteria. Many probiotic products include a combination of these.

If you've had an attack of diverticulitis, probiotic supplements alone may not be enough to prevent a repeat. Be sure to see your doctor and follow her advice about medication and lifestyle steps you can take.

Lose weight. Traditionally, diverticular disease has been a problem for people over age 50, brought on by decades of low-fiber eating and constipation. But that may be changing. Thanks to the obesity epidemic, doctors are beginning to notice that people as young as 20 have the thin-walled, bulging pouches along their intestines. Yet another good reason to keep your weight in check.

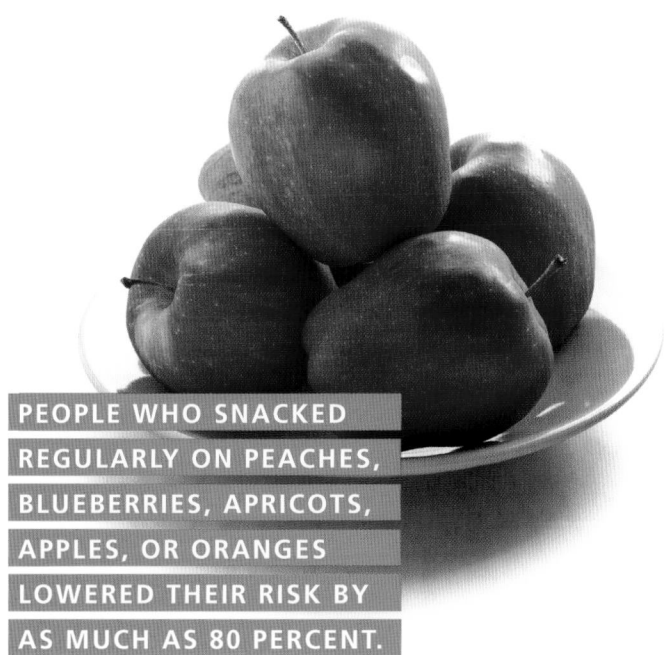

PEOPLE WHO SNACKED REGULARLY ON PEACHES, BLUEBERRIES, APRICOTS, APPLES, OR ORANGES LOWERED THEIR RISK BY AS MUCH AS 80 PERCENT.

WHAT CAUSES IT

Increased intestinal wall tension from hard stools plus straining to have a bowel movement can make tiny sections of the wall bulge outward. If these pouches become infected or inflamed, you may experience pain, bleeding, or even perforations in the intestinal wall.

SYMPTOMS TO WATCH FOR

You may have severe, sharp pain in your abdomen (often on the lower left side) or milder pain that lasts for several days and may occasionally get worse. Other symptoms include fever, nausea, bouts of diarrhea or constipation, and bloating. If you have severe pain or bleeding, call your doctor immediately.

NEWEST THINKING

Nuts, seeds, and popcorn are okay. In the past, doctors have told people with diverticular disease to avoid these nuggets, fearing that they could get stuck in the intestinal pouches. But when researchers tracked more than 47,000 men for 18 years, they found that those who ate these healthy, high-fiber foods had no extra risk of problems. In fact, those who ate popcorn twice a week had a 28 percent lower risk of flare-ups than those who indulged less than once a month, possibly because popcorn is a good source of fiber.

Dry Eyes

68%

The reduction in your risk of having dry eyes if you eat foods high in omega-3 fatty acids five or six times a week.

Tears aren't just for sadness and joy. They are your eyes' first line of defense against infection and damage from dust and airborne debris. Each time you blink, a new layer of this moisture—a beautifully balanced blend of water, fat, and mucus—rolls across the surface of your eyes. Or at least it should. If tears evaporate too quickly (thanks to age-related changes in tear production) or aren't renewed often enough (because you're staring at the TV or computer for far too long), your eyes begin to dry out. These steps can keep your peepers comfortably moist.

Key Prevention Strategies

Remind yourself to blink. Your "blink rate" drops from a normal 17 to 22 blinks per minute to as few as 4 when you're doing anything that requires intense visual focus. In one study, people playing computer games blinked just once every 2 to 3 minutes! Keeping your eyes wide open allows the protective film of tears to evaporate. To protect your eyes, remember to blink whenever you turn a page in your book or check your rear-view mirror while driving (which should be several times each minute). If you're working at a computer, try the 20-20 rule: Give your eyes a 20-second rest every 20 minutes. Look out a window or at something across the room and be sure to blink.

Lower your computer monitor. Shifting your eyes upward to read the top lines on your screen could double your odds for dry eyes. The reason: Looking up exposes more of the surface of your eyes to the air. (This is one reason computer use dries out eyes more than reading a book does—when you read, you tend to look down, which partially closes your eyes.) Raise your chair or lower your monitor so you can see the top third of the screen while looking straight ahead.

medical help for dry eyes

If self-care steps aren't enough to keep your eyes moist, see your eye doctor. He may suggest one of these treatments.

Restasis for "better" tears: These prescription eye-drops boost the production of tears for about 15 percent of the people who try them, studies show. The drops seem to trigger tear production by soothing inflammation on the surface of the eyes.

Punctal plugs for more tears: These tiny silicone stoppers, installed in your doctor's office, close off your eyes' drain holes for tears. Some doctors use temporary plugs first so you can see if they'll help. They are usually recommended for people with moderate to severe dry eyes who aren't helped by other treatments.

Eat "good" fats. When researchers from Brigham and Women's Hospital in Boston checked the diets and eye health of nearly 32,500 women, they found that those who ate the most good fats had the lowest risk of dry eyes. In fact, those who ate tuna or tuna salad sandwiches at least five or six times a week were 68 percent less likely to have dry orbs than those who had less than one weekly serving of tuna or other rich sources of omega-3 fatty acids. Choose "light" tuna if you go this route; it's far lower in mercury than albacore. And to avoid eating too much of even this tuna, aim to get your omega-3's from a variety of sources, including salmon, halibut, sardines, and herring as well as flaxseed, flaxseed oil, canola oil, soybeans, pumpkin seeds, and walnuts.

Eye experts think fish-oil or flaxseed-oil capsules may also promote eye health, but they're still debating the best dosage. Follow the package directions on one of the dry eye–prevention supplements available in drugstores, such as TheraTears Nutrition, or take fish-oil capsules with a total of one gram of DHA and EPA per day. It may take up to three months to notice a difference.

Stop smoking. When University of Wisconsin Medical School in Madison researchers checked the lifestyle habits and eye health of several thousand people, they found that current smokers had an 82 percent higher risk of dry eyes than nonsmokers.

Prevention Boosters

Take care of rosacea, blepharitis, and eyelid problems. All can cause dry eyes. People with rosacea have a 50 percent chance of developing ocular rosacea, which can cause dry eyes, frequent sties, and the feeling that there's something in your eyes. Tell your eye doctor that you have rosacea and ask about a check for this type, too. The doctor can also help treat blepharitis, or inflammation of the eyelids, as well as eyelids that curl outward or inward with age. Both conditions can change the way you blink so tears aren't spread across your entire eye.

Use artificial tears. Keep artificial tears, also called lubricating drops, on hand for times when you'll be in air-conditioned or heated buildings or in a car, airplane, desert, or any other place with extremely dry air. Eye experts recommend choosing preservative-free drops if you'll be using them more than four to six times a day for more than two or three days; otherwise, your eyes may become sensitized to preservatives and become inflamed.

WHAT CAUSES IT
Aging; for women, hormonal changes at menopause; eye problems that interfere with blinking or tear production; medications such as antihistamines, diuretics, sleeping pills, birth control pills, and tricyclic antidepressants; exposure to dry air; medical conditions such as diabetes, rheumatoid arthritis, lupus, scleroderma, and Sjögren's syndrome.

SYMPTOMS TO WATCH FOR A stinging, burning, or scratchy sensation in your eyes; sensitivity to light, wind, and/ or smoke; stringy mucus in or around your eyes; blurry vision at the end of the day or after focusing intently on a close-range task.

NEWEST THINKING
Before having LASIK surgery, have a dry-eye checkup. A hefty 50 percent of people who opt for laser surgery to improve their vision wind up with dry eyes for at least a few months after surgery—and 10 percent develop ongoing, severe problems. If your eyes are dry, ask your doctor about starting treatment with artificial tears, prescription eyedrops such as Restasis, and/or tear duct plugs before surgery.

Eczema

Could itchy skin be worse than a life-threatening health condition like diabetes or high blood pressure? When scientists asked 92 adults with severe eczema about the quality of their daily lives, they reported that having one of those serious medical problems might be easier than dealing with itchy, bumpy, scaly skin all the time. Half said they would trade up to two hours a day of their lives for normal skin, and 74 vowed they'd spend over $1,000 for a cure. But eczema eruptions don't have to rule your life. These strategies can help you avoid flare-ups and outsmart the "itch, scratch, itch" cycle that can make skin worse when you do have one.

Key Prevention Strategies

Avoid hidden triggers. Many everyday things can rub hypersensitive skin the wrong way. Among them: perfumes and dyes in laundry and personal care products, dust, cigarette smoke, walking barefoot in sand (or letting it rub the creases of your legs or arms at the beach), and chlorine or bromine left on the skin after swimming in a pool or soaking in a hot tub. Avoid them or get them off your skin as soon as possible. Sunburn is another trigger.

Bathe less often. Long, hot baths or showers can take the natural oils out of the skin, making it drier and more easily irritated. While some experts recommend a long soak in a tepid tub to soothe skin, many others say it's better to go a day or two between showers or baths. When you do wash up, keep it short and use warm—not hot—water. Use a mild soap that's not too drying; avoid antibacterial or deodorant soaps, which may strip more moisture from your skin. In fact, use soap only where you really need it: on your face, underarms, genitals, hands, and feet. Try using just water everywhere else. When you're done, pat yourself dry, then slather on moisturizer.

Keep your skin super-moist. If you have eczema, you know firsthand how dry, itchy, and sensitive your skin is, and that dryness makes itching and rashes even worse. That's why it's important to apply a thick layer of moisturizer once or twice a day to seal the water in the top layer of skin. Keeping your skin moist may mean you'll need less steroid cream to control rashes. In a Spanish study of 173 kids with eczema, those who were slathered daily with moisturizers needed 42 percent less high-potency steroid cream.

Be sure to apply moisturizer generously. In one German study of 30 adults with eczema, those who applied the amount their doctors recommended saw their itching, dryness, and skin crusting improve about 20 percent more than those who skimped. If you're using moisturizer and a steroid cream, apply the steroid first.

Keep a steroid cream handy just in case. Steroid creams, ointments, gels, and lotions can't cure eczema. But when it flares, they're the best choice for controlling it. The catch: Overuse (more than four continuous weeks) can lead to thinning of the skin, reduced bone density in adults, and growth problems in kids—but these side effects are rare. In fact, some researchers say fear of steroid creams can have worse side effects than the creams themselves. In one British study of 200 people with eczema, 73 percent admitted to being worried about using a steroid cream, and 24 percent admitted to skimping on or skipping the treatment as a result. But studies show that smart use brings relief, usually without problems.

If you're worried about stronger creams recommended by your doctor, remember that they're safe and very effective when used as directed. When British researchers followed 174 kids and teens with mild to moderate eczema for 18 weeks, they found that when treating flare-ups, three days of a high-dose cream worked as well as seven days of a low-dose cream. Both groups had the same number of itch-free days and neither showed signs of skin thinning.

Get tested for allergies. Pet dander, pollen, and dust mites can all trigger eczema flare-ups. In fact, one Scandinavian study of 45 people with eczema found that everyone with severe skin problems was allergic to at least one of these airborne troublemakers. But before you give the cat away, get an allergy test. It makes sense to know who (or what) the enemy is before you launch an all-out battle.

sunlight, a tanning bed, or the doctor's sunlamp?

Answer: the sunlamp. Stubborn, severe eczema that isn't healed by creams or even steroid pills may respond to exposure to ultraviolet (UV) light. In one study of 73 people with moderate to severe eczema, those who got twice-weekly "narrow-band UVB" treatments with sunlamps for 12 weeks saw a 28 percent reduction in itching, oozing, and crusting of their skin rashes. In contrast, those who were exposed to regular sunlight saw a 1.3 percent improvement. See a dermatologist about UV therapy—and don't go to a tanning salon unless the doctor recommends it; the potential benefit has to be balanced against the risk of skin cancer.

Experts have conflicting opinions about the effectiveness of strategies for avoiding allergens at home (such as removing carpets, keeping pets out of the bedroom, and covering mattresses and pillows with allergen-proof covers). While some recommend it, studies tend to show that these steps often don't reduce eczema flare-ups, simply because it's tough to keep the air completely allergen free. What can help: Allergy shots. In one German study of 89 people with eczema who were allergic to dust mites, those who got immunotherapy had an easier time keeping their eczema under control than those who didn't have the shots.

Consider food allergies. Allergies to milk, wheat, and other foods may sometimes cause flare-ups in kids with eczema. While food allergies are usually rare among adults with eczema, don't rule them out. In one Danish study, 25 percent of adults with severe eczema were allergic to at least one food. Before you start cutting whole food groups out of your diet on your own, though, talk to an allergist, a dietitian, or a naturopath about the best way to test yourself. Often this involves keeping a detailed food diary, removing one suspect food from your diet for several weeks, and then eating it again to see what happens.

cut your baby's odds for eczema

Most eczema begins in early childhood. Now it appears that what Mom eats during pregnancy can lower her child's risk of the condition. Scientists from the University of Aberdeen in the United Kingdom tracked moms' eating habits as well as allergies and asthma in 1,212 kids from birth to age 5 and found that the babies of women who ate fish once a week or more often during pregnancy were significantly less likely to develop eczema. They also concluded that a woman's diet during gestation may have a bigger impact on a child's risk of developing eczema than the child's own diet in the first few years of life. Fish is a rich source of inflammation-soothing omega-3 fatty acids, but scientists aren't yet sure how this healthy food may bolster protection in a child. For toddlers who are eating solid foods and can have dairy products, adding probiotic-rich foods such as yogurt with live, active cultures may help, too.

Try an immunomodulator cream for severe eczema. If moisturizers and steroid creams don't control outbreaks, an immunomodulator cream could help. Tacrolimus (Protopic) and pimecrolimus (Elidel) reduce eczema symptoms by 50 percent or more, say British researchers who reviewed 31 well-designed studies. The verdict: A 0.1 percent tacrolimus cream may be your best bet. It was about 42 percent more effective than pimecrolimus.

Tacrolimus ointment and pimecrolimus cream don't have the skin thinning and other side effects of steroid creams, so they are often used for sensitive areas like the face or body folds. They can also be used for long-term control of eczema. Talk to your doctor about the "black box" cautions on these drugs, which warn of increased risk of skin cancer and lymphoma. Major medical organizations say that the evidence for a connection is extremely weak and that these well-intentioned warnings may keep people from getting the eczema relief they need.

Prevention Boosters

Soothe your emotions. Several studies have linked stress and anxiety with eczema outbreaks. If anger, frustration, or stress seems to trigger a rash, consider adding a little "emotional therapy" to your skin care routine. Studies show that relaxation therapy, cognitive behavioral therapy (find a therapist trained in it), and biofeedback can all help. For best results, ask your dermatologist for a reference to a psychologist or program specifically for people with skin conditions.

Dress for comfort. Rough, scratchy fabrics and clothing that's too tight can irritate sensitive skin. Instead, choose smooth cotton weaves and knits to avoid irritation and allow skin to breathe. Avoid itchy wool and synthetic fabrics that trap sweat.

Wash all new clothes before you wear them to remove irritating chemicals used to make them look smooth and wrinkle free in the store. If you suspect that your laundry detergent or fabric softener is irritating your skin, switch to products without perfumes or dyes and rinse clothes twice in the washing machine.

Keep your home's temperature and humidity levels comfortable. Too much humidity in the air can make you sweat; too little can leave skin parched and flaky. Both situations can prompt an eczema flare-up. Keep your home's humidity level comfortable by using an air conditioner in summer and a humidifier in winter if your heating system dries out the air too much. Research suggests that big temperature swings can also trigger flare-ups, so keep the temperature on an even keel.

Keep using your medications. A recent study showed that patients' use of medication recommended for eczema dropped by 60 percent within three days of starting treatment—maybe because their skin improved quickly or because they were afraid of side effects. Let your doctor know if you have any concerns about the treatment and how often you really use the medication so he can plan the treatment that's best for you.

WHAT CAUSES IT
Experts are still trying to identify the culprits behind eczema. While the causes aren't fully understood, allergies, dry skin, and low levels of a skin-protecting protein may play roles.

SYMPTOMS TO WATCH FOR Small, itchy bumps that may leak fluid when scratched; dry, itchy, red to brownish-gray skin patches or areas of thick, scaly skin, especially on the hands, feet, arms, neck, face, and chest and behind the knees.

NEWEST THINKING
While many experts have traditionally believed that allergies trigger eczema, there's evidence that a genetic quirk that makes skin fragile could be behind many eczema cases. Researchers in Ireland and Scotland have found a lack of filaggrin, a compound that normally makes the skin's outer layer watertight, in up to half of adults and kids with eczema. The result: The skin dries out, and particles of dust, pollen—virtually anything— from the outside can creep in, causing irritation. While experts continue investigating this intriguing clue, researchers say it underscores the importance of protecting eczema-prone skin by slathering on moisturizers.

Emphysema

27%

The reduction in your risk of emphysema if you eat several servings of fruit a day.

Like old or broken party balloons, the millions of air sacs in your lungs just don't work properly if they've been damaged by tobacco smoke or environmental pollutants. The result: emphysema. You feel tired and short of breath because the air sacs can no longer force stale air out of your lungs. Protecting your airways from cigarette smoke—yours and other people's—is a top priority for prevention. Here's how that and other proven strategies can keep you breathing easy.

Key Prevention Strategies

Quit smoking. About 90 percent of people with emphysema are smokers. If you smoke, your chances of developing emphysema are one in four. Cigarette smoke paralyzes the tiny hairs, or cilia, that normally sweep germs and irritating chemicals and particles out of your airways. Instead, irritants invade the millions of air sacs in your lungs and ultimately destroy them. Cigar and pipe smokers are also at risk, as are marijuana smokers. In one Australian study, researchers found that habitual marijuana smokers showed signs of lung damage years sooner than cigarette smokers. Other studies suggest that a single joint is as destructive as 2 1/2 to 5 cigarettes.

Quit, and the risk of future damage drops. Nine months after your last cigarette, the cilia will be functioning normally again. And while quitting will not reverse existing damage, it will slow the progression of the disease.

Avoid secondhand smoke. Breathing in other people's smoke on a regular basis—at home, on the job, or out with friends—can damage healthy lungs and raise the risk of emphysema attacks if you already have this condition. When researchers at Children's Hospital of

stop an emphysema flare-up before it starts

If you already have emphysema, try this trifecta of strategies to help you avoid wheezing episodes.

Exercise: Getting regular exercise and building endurance can prevent a flare-up. Ask your doctor about rehab programs for people with chronic lung problems in your area.

A cold-air face mask: This protects your lungs from wintry air that can constrict your airways, while letting air in comfortably for breathing. Buy one in a drugstore or medical supply store.

A yearly flu vaccination and a pneumonia vaccination every five years: They won't help you avoid emphysema flare-ups, but studies show that these shots reduce death rates from the flu and pneumonia in people with emphysema and other lung problems.

Philadelphia scanned the lungs of 61 adults, they found that 35 percent of those who were exposed to secondhand smoke regularly showed early signs of lung damage.

Bad air at work? Ask for a respirator. Chemical fumes as well as dust from grain, cotton, wood, or mining products can raise your emphysema risk whether or not you smoke. A face mask fitted with special air filters could save your lungs.

Keep the air at home clean. If you already have emphysema, you can cut your risk of an attack by avoiding fumes from paint as well as perfumes and the smell of burning candles and incense. Even cooking odors can make you cough or wheeze. Keep the humidity in your home between 40 and 50 percent (you can buy a device that measures humidity at the hardware store) and check air filters on your furnace and air conditioning systems regularly—as often as monthly—and clean or change them when they look dirty so the air stays irritant free.

Prevention Boosters

Skip bacon, hot dogs, and other cured meats, especially if you smoke. Eating cured meats at least once a day raised smokers' risk of emphysema and other progressive lung problems 2.64 times higher than that of those who ate these foods only a few times a year, according to a Harvard School of Public Health study of nearly 43,000 men. Nitrites in these meats generate cell-damaging particles called free radicals in the body. People with higher levels of free radicals are more susceptible to lung damage.

Eat more fiber. Getting about 27 grams of fiber a day translated into a 15 percent drop in risk for emphysema and other lung problems compared to eating just 9.5 grams a day, according to a study of nearly 12,000 people. People who got a lot of their fiber from fruit cut their risk further—by 27 percent. The reason? Fiber may simply be a marker for a diet that includes more fruits and vegetables. It's possible that the real protectors are the antioxidants in produce, which protect lungs from damage caused by free radicals.

WHAT CAUSES IT
Smoking and chronic exposure to fumes and dust. Occasionally, genes play a role.

SYMPTOMS TO WATCH FOR A chronic cough that may produce sputum or phlegm; fatigue; in later stages, you may have loss of appetite and weight loss.

NEWEST THINKING
A new twist on standard breathing exercises makes exhaling even easier for people with emphysema. University of Michigan researchers have found that people with emphysema who learn to play the harmonica improve their breathing significantly—and the longer and stronger your exhalations, the better your version of "Yankee Doodle" will sound!

Erectile Dysfunction

70%

The amount by which you can reduce your risk if you stay physically active in middle age and beyond.

Before 1998, you rarely heard anyone utter the words *erectile dysfunction* or *impotence.* Then came a diamond-shaped blue pill called Viagra, and suddenly everything changed. The ability to have and maintain an erection was on the evening news, peppering comics' riffs, and requiring that your 8-year-old leave the room or be distracted during certain commercials. Although there are now three medications approved to treat it, simple lifestyle changes could prevent it for good.

Key Prevention Strategies

Eat like the Greeks. Do you think the ancient Greeks and Romans depicted in all those statues had problems in the bedroom? If they didn't, they may have had their diets to thank. The Mediterranean diet is rich in healthy monounsaturated fats from foods like olive oil. It's also loaded with fruit, vegetables, nuts, legumes, whole grains, and fish and is relatively low in red meat. When Italian researchers compared 100 men with erectile dysfunction (ED) to 100 men without it, they found that those whose diets most closely matched a Mediterranean diet were significantly less likely to be impotent. The reason, researchers speculate, is probably the anti-inflammatory effect of the diet. Inflammation contributes to plaque buildup, narrowing blood vessels, and narrowed vessels mean less blood gets through to the penis, making an erection less likely.

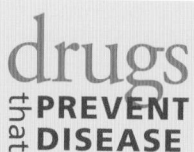

drugs that PREVENT DISEASE

Although drugs like sildenafil (Viagra) are designed to be used on an as-needed basis, preliminary studies suggest that taking them every night for a year could actually prevent impotence once you stop using the drug. German researchers had 112 impotent men take either 50 milligrams of Viagra every night or 50 or 100 milligrams as needed for a year. After six months with no treatment, 58.3 percent of the men who took nightly Viagra had normal erections without any medication, compared to only 8.2 percent of those who used the drug as needed. One drug, tadalafil (Cialis), is already approved for daily use.

Take up a new sport (or rediscover an old one). Exercise isn't just good for your muscles; it's also good for your erections. Men who become more physically active in middle age slash their risk of impotence by 70 percent compared with men who stay on the couch. In fact, physical activity—no matter what kind—reduced the risk of impotence even more than quitting smoking, losing weight, or drinking less booze.

Stop smoking. If the idea of protecting your heart and lungs isn't enough to make you stop smoking, maybe the threat of sexual embarrassment is. One study of 7,684 Chinese men found that smoking probably accounted for about one in five cases of ED. The more you smoke, the more likely you are to have problems. The study found that smoking just 20 cigarettes a day increased the risk by 60 percent compared to not smoking at all. The reason? Smoking constricts blood vessels and contributes to the buildup of plaque, both of which reduce blood flow—and you know what that means. Smoking also reduces levels of nitric oxide, a chemical compound that keeps blood vessels, including those in the penis, dilated. Even one day without a cigarette can improve erections.

Prevention Boosters

Maintain normal blood sugar levels. Half of all men with diabetes have erection problems—twice the rate of men without the disease. (See page 152 for tips on preventing diabetes.)

Pop a pill. You have three choices: sildenafil (Viagra), tadalafil (Cialis), and vardenafil (Levitra). All work by increasing levels of nitric oxide, the chemical that helps dilate blood vessels in the penis and keep them dilated so you can have and maintain an erection. The major difference between the three is how long they take to begin working. Levitra works the fastest, with one study finding it began working in as few as 10 minutes and remained effective for up to 12 hours. However, if you're away for a romantic weekend, consider Cialis: Studies find that one dose continues working for up to 36 hours. It's also approved in some countries (including the US) for daily use.

WHAT CAUSES IT
Anything that affects the health of blood vessels—heart disease, diabetes, high blood pressure, or smoking—can affect a man's ability to have an erection. Stress and relationship problems are other causes.

SYMPTOMS TO WATCH FOR Inability to have or maintain an erection.

NEWEST THINKING
Men with impotence have a greater risk of developing Parkinson's disease. Researchers evaluating the medical records of 32,616 medical professionals found those with a history of ED were nearly three times more likely to develop Parkinson's than those who didn't have erection problems. The link seems to be related to damage in the autonomic nervous system, which regulates functions like breathing and digestion. Identifying the underlying reasons for the link could theoretically lead to ways to prevent Parkinson's.

EVEN ONE DAY WITHOUT A CIGARETTE CAN IMPROVE ERECTIONS.

Fatigue

65%

The best way to characterize fatigue is by saying what it's not: energy. When you're fatigued, you may not need to sleep, but you sure don't feel like doing much else. Your brain feels like cotton, your muscles like lead. Fatigue can be the result of a condition like depression, cancer, diabetes, fibromyalgia, or congestive heart failure, but about one in four people experience fatigue that's not related to any medical problem.

Key Prevention Strategies

Get a good night's sleep. It's the most obvious way to keep your natural energy up. If you're tossing and turning, waking up in the middle of the night, or waking up too early, see the Insomnia entry on page 228. If you snore, also read the Snoring entry on page 292. Obstructive sleep apnea, which is associated with severe snoring, is a common cause of daytime tiredness.

Hit the walking trail. As few as 10 minutes of brisk walking helps power up energy levels more effectively—and for much longer—than eating a candy bar. Just 20 minutes of strolling three times a week can increase energy levels by 20 percent and reduce fatigue by 65 percent.

Eat a high-fiber breakfast. One study found that people who started their mornings with a high-fiber meal were more alert throughout the morning, probably because these meals take longer to digest than, say, a bowl of cornflakes or a doughnut, so blood sugar levels remain steadier. It also helps to include some protein with breakfast—and every other meal.

Good breakfast options, then, are whole grain toast with a slice of cheese or a teaspoon of peanut butter and a piece of fruit, a bowl of high-fiber cereal (aim for at least five grams of fiber a serving) with milk, or a bowl of oatmeal sprinkled with ground flaxseed. For an afternoon snack, instead of a candy bar or pretzels from the vending machine, choose almonds, trail mix, or whole grain crackers with peanut butter.

Get your blood tested. Common causes of fatigue that a blood test can reveal are low iron levels (you don't have to be anemic to be low on iron) and hypothyroidism, which occurs when the thyroid gland doesn't make enough thyroid hormone. Both are common in women and often go undetected. One US study found that about 16 percent of women had low iron levels.

Prevention Boosters

Tip your head up to the sun. Bright light—whether from the sun or a full-spectrum fluorescent light designed to mimic the sun's rays—pumps up alertness levels like a shot of adrenaline. You don't have to sunbathe; in one Japanese study, women who sat near a sunny window for 30 minutes reported feeling more alert than when they sat in a darkened room for the same time period. Sunlight boosts activity in brain regions associated with alertness and dampens levels of the "sleep hormone" melatonin.

Sip mini coffees. Too much caffeine can backfire by keeping you up at night, but sipping just two ounces of coffee every hour from about 10 a.m. to 2 p.m. boosts alertness levels, thanks to caffeine's ability to block a sleep-inducing brain chemical called adenosine.

Use the power of peppermint. If you need a quick pick-me-up, the smell of peppermint may do the trick. Purchase peppermint essential oil from a natural foods store and rub a drop between your hands once every hour, or place a few drops on a tissue and breathe in the scent.

Find a new hobby. Boredom and loneliness are twin contributors to depression, which is a major cause of fatigue. Join a book group, a bowling league, a knitting club—anything that gets you out of the house, helps you meet new people, and gives you something interesting to do.

WHAT CAUSES IT
The most common reason for fatigue is lack of sleep, but it can also be a side effect of illness, cancer treatment, or medical conditions like fibromyalgia, chronic fatigue syndrome, diabetes, lupus, multiple sclerosis, low iron levels, or hypothyroidism. Depression and boredom may also contribute. Certain medications, either prescription or over-the-counter, can have the side effect of causing fatigue as well.

SYMPTOMS TO WATCH FOR Lack of energy, inability to concentrate.

NEWEST THINKING
In women with breast cancer, fatigue from chemotherapy can last up to six months or more after the treatment ends. But a recent review of studies shows that good old exercise is effective at relieving even cancer-related fatigue.

Flatulence

45%

The percentage of people who had no gas after taking Beano when eating a bowl of bean chili.

Flatulence is hardly a "disease." In fact, everyone passes gas from 14 to 23 times a day (women emit as much as men), though most of the time, it's odorless. But that knowledge doesn't make an ill-timed release any less embarrassing. If odoriferous emissions are causing your social life to suffer, follow this advice right away.

Key Prevention Strategies

Go easy on beans and windy vegetables. Dried beans are oh, so good for you, helping to fend off any number of health problems. But gas is sometimes the tradeoff. The culprit is an indigestible sugar called raffinose, also found in cabbage, brussels sprouts, broccoli, and asparagus. Humans lack an enzyme needed to break down raffinose, so beneficial bacteria in the intestinal tract do the work of munching on this sugar. The bacteria emit gas, and within a few hours, you do the same. Experts from the University of Michigan say that by gradually increasing the amount of beans and other gas producers in your diet, you can minimize this stinky side effect.

Banish bean gas. Draining and thoroughly rinsing canned beans before use gets rid of some of the gas-causing raffinose. If you're cooking dried beans, be sure to soak them first. Add 1/8 teaspoon of baking soda to the soaking water to leach out more raffinose, and be sure to rinse soaked beans well. Never cook beans in their rinse water; it's full of raffinose.

Add Beano. Sprinkling a few drops of Beano on your first bite of beans or gassy vegetables (or taking a tablet before eating) could significantly reduce the gas you produce after a

is gas trying to tell you something?

Sometimes intestinal gas is a sign of a food intolerance or digestive condition. Among the most common:

Lactose intolerance: If you have gas and abdominal pain after eating dairy products or drinking milk, you may lack the enzyme lactase, needed to break down the sugar, called lactose, in these foods. A simple breath test can diagnose this problem. The solution: lactase supplements, lactase drops to add to milk, and lactose-reduced dairy products.

Gluten intolerance: If your body can't digest gluten, a protein found in wheat and some other grains, you may experience gas, bloating, weight loss, oily and foul-smelling stools, and other symptoms. The only solution is to avoid gluten, but see your doctor first for a diagnosis.

Irritable bowel syndrome (IBS): If you emit normal amounts of gas but feel extremely bloated on a regular basis and have bouts of diarrhea and/or constipation, you may have IBS. Dietary changes, stress reduction, and medications may help.

meal. Beano, sold in drugstores, contains an enzyme that breaks down the sugars in beans.

Check your reaction to these major gas producers. Other foods contain tough-to-digest sugars that often become food for gassy bacteria in your gut. Everyone reacts differently, so don't write off a nutritious fruit or veggie unless you're sure it's causing a reaction. Prime culprits include foods high in the sugar fructose, such as dates, grapes, apples, and pears, as well as foods that contain sorbitol, such as apples, pears, peaches, and plums.

Prevention Boosters

Order water instead of seltzer. All those bubbles in seltzer and soft drinks contain gas, and you swallow a lot of it when you sip a carbonated drink. Switching from the fizzy stuff to the "still" stuff helps. (Beer and champagne lovers, that includes you.)

Have rice instead. Starchy side dishes such as potatoes, noodles made from wheat flour (that's most pasta), and corn produce gas when they're digested in your large intestine. Rice won't—it's just about the only starch that is completely absorbed in the small intestine, making it a more comfortable choice if you're bothered by gas.

Skip the low-carb sweets. Many "sugar-free" and low-carb chewing gums, hard candies, chocolates, cookies, cake mixes, and even pancake syrups are sweetened with sugar alcohols such as sorbitol and mannitol. When bacteria in your intestinal tract break them down, the result can be rumbles and embarrassing emissions.

Switch antacids. Using baking soda or an antacid containing sodium bicarbonate to ease heartburn and acid indigestion could backfire, loudly. Experts caution that while it's busy neutralizing stomach acid, it produces plenty of carbon dioxide—some of which may exit through your intestinal tract. As little as 1/2 teaspoon of baking soda could produce enough gas to fuel a hard-to-hide eruption. Look for another type of antacid, such as one that contains calcium carbonate, which neutralizes acid, or ask your doctor about H_2 blockers, which reduce acid production.

Season beans to chase gas away. Researchers from India report that adding garlic and ginger (either fresh or dried) to beans while they cook can reduce gas when you eat them.

Flu

81%

The drop in your risk if you take an antiviral drug as soon as someone in your household shows signs of the flu.

Like poker, bingo, and the slot machines in Las Vegas, the flu is a gamble. Your odds of catching it range from 5 to 20 percent each winter, depending on the virulence of the virus circulating in your community. That sounds low, but once you've suffered through a miserable case of the flu, you'll be motivated to tilt those odds a little more in your favor. Start by doing all you can to keep your immunity strong: Eat a healthy diet and get plenty of sleep and physical activity. Beyond that, these flu stoppers can stack the deck in your favor.

Key Prevention Strategies

Get the flu vaccine. The flu isn't just miserable; it can be dangerous, especially in older folks. In a 10-year study of thousands of older people, having a flu shot cut the risk of being hospitalized with flu-like illnesses by 27 percent and reduced the risk of dying from the flu by 48 percent.

This is not a perfect vaccine; it works better some years than others. At best, it protects against 70 to 90 percent of the flu viruses being passed around. At worst, it may provide only 40 to 50 percent immunity. But those are still far better odds than with no flu shot.

Definitely get one if you're over 50, if you have a medical condition that lowers your immunity or affects your lung function, or if you live in a household with anyone on that list (to protect yourself *and* them).

Hate shots? Consider the inhaled vaccine FluMist. In the United States, it's approved for people ages 2 to 49. It can cut your risk for the flu by 30 to 57 percent. It's not recommended for kids with asthma, pregnant women, or anyone with a suppressed immune system.

vaccine busters and boosters

The flu vaccine works by introducing a tiny dose of several flu viruses into your body (if you get a shot, the viruses are dead; if you get an inhaled vaccine, they're live but weakened, so you can't get sick). Your body then produces antibodies, which will be ready to fight if you're exposed to the real thing. The more antibodies, the better the protection. These factors can affect the vaccine's effectiveness.

Stress: Feeling stressed out 8 to 10 days after your shot could suppress your immune response to the vaccine by 12 to 17 percent.

A fever: If you're running a fever on the day of your shot, reschedule. Fever is a sign that your immune system is already fighting an infection; don't ask it to multitask.

Sleep: Getting several good nights' sleep before your flu shot could boost your antibody production by 50 percent.

Tai chi or qigong: University of Illinois researchers found that people who performed one of these two activities for one hour three times a week for 20 weeks produced significantly more antibodies after getting a flu shot.

Take an antiviral drug as soon as someone in your home gets the flu. People who took the prescription drug oseltamivir (Tamiflu) or zanamivir (Relenza) after someone in their household caught the flu significantly reduced their risk of getting it themselves in one major study. Among people who took oseltamivir, 81 percent didn't get sick; among those who took zanamivir, 75 percent stayed well. People who got a placebo were five to seven times more likely to develop flu symptoms than those who took the antiviral drugs. The only potential downside: An upset stomach.

Wash your hands often. The flu virus can survive for hours on hard surfaces like metal, glass, and plastic—and even on cloth, paper, and tissues. Your best defense is washing your hands, the more often the better. Lather vigorously for at least 20 seconds to get rid of all the germs. Choose hand washing over antibacterial hand wipes and gels when you have the option; relying on rubs and wipes could allow bugs to build up on your hands if you use them many times in a row without washing.

Carry the right alcohol-based hand sanitizer. Viruses are hard to kill; even some alcohol-based hand sanitizers won't kill them if the alcohol concentration isn't high enough. (Hand washing doesn't kill viruses; it simply washes them away. That's why you don't need antibacterial soap.) Buy a sanitizer that contains 60 to 95 percent ethyl alcohol. Rub the gel or foam on all sides of your hands, then rub your hands together vigorously until they're dry.

Prevention Boosters

Sneeze smarter. Virus-killing tissues are no substitute for hand washing, but they could cut the number of virus particles on your kids' hands and may even reduce the number lurking on surfaces in your home. Also, teach your kids to sneeze into the crook of their elbow, not their hand.

Move your exercise routine indoors. In a small Canadian study, people who exercised most days of the week for three months had fewer flu symptoms and higher levels of flu-fighting immunoglobulin A in their bloodstreams compared to people who didn't exercise. We know that exercising can be a challenge when the weather's cold and roads are slick. How about popping in an exercise DVD, doing old-fashioned calisthenics like sit-ups and jumping jacks, or clearing off that stair-stepper?

WHAT CAUSES IT
Dozens of strains of the influenza virus. These viruses are extremely infectious because they're always mutating. This means that even though you develop antibodies to the flu if you're infected, your immune system won't recognize and fight off a new strain.

SYMPTOMS TO WATCH FOR A sudden, high fever; severe headache; aches and pains; fatigue; chest discomfort; coughing; sometimes a sore throat, stuffy nose, and sneezing.

NEWEST THINKING
To avoid flu over the holidays, don't fly. In 2002, the flu season started several weeks later than usual and peaked in March instead of January or February. Harvard University researchers suspect the cause was the 27 percent drop in air travel after the terrorist attacks of September 11. Exposure to airport crowds and germs on airplane surfaces plus hours spent in close quarters can increase your risk of catching the flu bug.

Food Poisoning

97%
The number of cases of food-borne illness that could be avoided if home cooks and consumers followed safe food-handling rules.

Most of the foods we eat naturally contain tiny amounts of bacteria and viruses that are harmless for most of us. But if foods are poorly handled or improperly cooked, these germs can grow to threatening levels, making your tummy mildly unhappy or making you desperately sick. Don't rely on the "sniff" test to tell if a food is okay; while you can smell rotten food, you can't smell bacteria. In fact, food safety experts say the most dangerous disease-causing bugs don't alter the look, smell, or taste of food. Instead of using your senses, practice safe shopping, cooking, and storage. And use good judgment when eating away from home (for more on traveler's diarrhea, see the Diarrhea entry on page 156).

Key Prevention Strategies

Separate meat, chicken, and seafood from the rest of your groceries. Put them in plastic bags to contain any juices. Pack them into separate bags at the checkout, too. At home, use containers or sealable plastic bags to store raw meats, poultry, and seafood in the refrigerator to make certain the juices can't escape.

Buy perishables last and refrigerate them fast. Store meats on the bottom shelf so juices can't drip on other foods. Freeze poultry and ground meat that won't be used within one or two days; freeze other meats within four or five days.

Don't defrost on the kitchen counter. Germs can grow quickly on fish, chicken, turkey, and other meats left at room temperature even while defrosting. Use these techniques instead.

- **Plan ahead and defrost in the fridge.** Put the frozen item in a zipper-lock bag or wrap well to contain juices. Place the package on a plate or in a bowl in the refrigerator until defrosted.
- **Use the microwave.** Set your microwave to "defrost" or use a low power setting (such as 50 percent) so the thinner edges of the meat won't cook while the middle thaws. Cook immediately.
- **Dunk in cold water.** Seal food in a zipper-lock bag and place in a large bowl of cold water, or under cold running water, until just thawed. Cook immediately.

Marinate safely. Keep marinating foods in the refrigerator. Don't use the marinade from raw seafood, poultry, or meat during cooking or on cooked food unless you've brought it to a full boil first to kill any bacteria. Toss the rest after use.

Wash up before you cook and again as needed. Scrub your hands vigorously with soap and water for 10 to 15 seconds immediately before handling food. Dry with a clean paper towel or kitchen towel. Wash your hands after handling raw foods and again before eating. Surveys show that 25 percent of cooks do not wash their hands after handling raw meat and fish, and 66 percent don't wash up after handling raw eggs.

Guard against cross-contamination. Keep raw meat, poultry, seafood, and their juices away from ready-to-eat foods. Do not reuse knives, utensils, cutting boards, or other kitchen equipment that's been exposed to raw meats before washing it thoroughly. Serve the food on a clean plate, platter, or cutting board—don't reuse one that held raw food.

Clean up carefully. When Utah State University researchers watched 100 home cooks prepare meals, they found that just 29 percent cleaned counters and refrigerator doors adequately after contact with raw meat. An antibacterial cleaning product or a solution of one teaspoon bleach to one quart hot water will do the trick; dry with a clean paper towel.

Cook it through. Kansas State University research reveals that color isn't a good indicator that meat or poultry is fully cooked; ground beef may look fully browned when the internal temperature is just 130°F—far from the 160°F needed to kill disease-causing bacteria. To add to the confusion, some lean ground beef and some poultry may look pink even after it's reached a safe temperature. To get it right, use a food thermometer. You can also buy disposable "pop-up" thermometers

leftover 411

Leftovers are a blessing the next day—but make sure they're safe.

Refrigerate or freeze foods promptly. Discard perishable food left at room temperature longer than two hours, or one hour in temperatures above 90°F.

Divide and conquer. Split large amounts of leftovers into small shallow containers for quick cooling in the refrigerator. Remove the stuffing from poultry and other meats immediately and refrigerate it in a separate container.

In doubt? Throw it out. If you suspect food may have been sitting out for too long, don't take any chances. Toss it.

to use in roasts or poultry, but experts suggest double-checking internal temperature with a conventional food thermometer for extra safety. Wash the probe end in warm sudsy water and dry with a paper towel after use.

For seafood, look for these signs that it's done. Fish flesh should be completely opaque and flake easily with a fork. Cook lobsters or crabs until the shells turn red; their flesh—and that of shrimp—should be pearly and opaque. Cook clams, mussels, or oysters until the shells open; don't eat any that stay shut.

Keep hot foods hot and cold foods cold. If food won't be served and eaten immediately—such as at a picnic, party, or buffet—keep hot food at or above 140°F in chafing dishes, a preheated steam table, warming trays, and/or slow cookers. To keep cold foods at or below 40°F, put food in containers on ice.

Keep your refrigerator cold. One in three refrigerators are set too warm to keep foods cold and safe, researchers say. Be sure yours is set at 40°F or lower and the freezer at 0°F. To make sure your fridge is cold enough, buy a refrigerator thermometer. And don't overload the fridge—air needs to circulate in order to chill food fast.

Keep fresh produce safe. From baby spinach to melons and raspberries to onions, fresh fruits and vegetables are now the source of three times more food poisoning cases than beef and almost twice as many as poultry, reports the US Center for Science in the Public Interest. Despite TV and newspaper headlines about outbreaks, most produce is still safe, experts say. These strategies can keep it even safer.

- Buy fresh-cut produce like half a watermelon or bagged salad greens only if they're refrigerated or surrounded by ice.
- Store perishable produce (like strawberries, lettuce, herbs, and mushrooms), pre-cut produce, and peeled produce in the refrigerator.

when is it done?

Cook until food reaches these recommended internal temperatures.

Ground poultry: 165°F

Whole chicken, duck, goose, turkey, or dark meat: 180°F

Poultry breast: 170°F

Poultry stuffing: 165°F

Ground beef, lamb, pork, or veal: 160°F

Medium-rare beef: 145°F

Medium beef or pork: 160°F

Well-done beef or pork: 170°F

Fresh ham: 160°F

Fully cooked ham: heat to 140°F

All leftovers: heat to 165°F

- Wash fruits and vegetables under running water before eating, cutting, or cooking, even if you're going to peel them. Use a clean vegetable brush on the rinds of melons and squash. Don't use dish detergent or hand soap—it can leave a residue that could make you feel sick. Dry with a clean paper towel when possible; there's evidence that this removes more germs. Experts say there's no proof that special produce cleaners remove any more germs than does washing with water and drying with a clean paper towel.
- Remove the outer leaves of head vegetables like cabbage and lettuce.
- Skip all raw sprouts, such as alfalfa, bean, broccoli, and radish sprouts, even if you've grown them at home. Their warm, moist growing conditions encourage growth of dangerous bacteria.
- Choose pasteurized juice and cider instead of unpasteurized types (or boil unpasteurized cider for five minutes before drinking).

Prevention Boosters

Keep meats hot without overcooking. Once meat reaches the right internal temperature on the grill, keep it hot if you aren't going to serve it right away by moving it to the side of the grill, away from the flames or coals. If you've cooked foods in the oven or on the stove, you can keep meats hot in a 200°F oven until you serve them.

Keep the fridge clean. Clean up food spills promptly with a solution of baking soda and water. If meat juices leak, use a weak solution of one teaspoon bleach in one quart of warm water to kill any germs, then wipe with baking soda and water to remove the bleach.

If you're transporting food to a picnic or party, use a cooler. Use enough ice or ice packs to keep foods at 40°F or below. Keep coolers out of the sun and try to keep the lid shut as much as possible. Put meats and other foods in separate coolers.

WHAT CAUSES IT
Bacteria such as *Campylobacter jejuni, Escherichia coli, Giardi intestinalis, Listeria monocytogenes, Salmonella*, and *Staphylococcus aureus*, as well as viruses such as norovirus, *Vibrio vulnificus*, and *V. parahaemolyticus*.

SYMPTOMS TO WATCH FOR Abdominal cramps, diarrhea, and vomiting 12 to 24 hours after eating tainted food. You may also have a headache, fever, and chills. If vomiting and diarrhea continue for more than two days or you have signs of dehydration, call your doctor. Young children, older people, and those with lowered immunity need prompt medical care if food poisoning strikes.

NEWEST THINKING
Should you rewash triple-washed salad greens? Some experts say yes. While studies show that triple-washed greens sold in sealed bags are safe, some food safety experts say rewashing can't hurt. Food-borne illnesses traced to salad greens have risen 39 percent in the past decade. The truth is, you can't always remove all germs from leafy greens; researchers say they're sometimes inside the leaves or cling tightly to them. But washing helps.

Gallstones

30%
The drop in your risk if you eat magnesium-rich foods like nuts, fish, and spinach every day.

Gallstones are like pearls—very, very painful pearls. Built from layers of cholesterol or calcium salts, they grow slowly and silently in your gallbladder or bile ducts the way a pearl grows inside an oyster. While most gallstones never cause a problem, some trigger exquisitely painful attacks and ultimately have to be treated with surgery or medications. Fortunately, there's plenty you can do to lower your chances of developing these painful "rocks" and to prevent their return if you've had them.

Key Prevention Strategies

Aim for a healthy weight and a trim waist. Being overweight or obese more than triples your odds for gallstones. Carrying extra pounds around your middle is especially dangerous: In a Harvard School of Public Health study of more than 42,000 women, those whose waistlines measured 36 inches or more were twice as likely to have gallstones that required surgery compared to women whose waists measured less than 26 inches. If you're not within your healthy weight range now, losing extra pounds slowly and steadily is the best way to protect yourself. Don't crash diet; losing more than 3 pounds a week raises gallstone risk, while losing 1 to 1.5 pounds a week doesn't seem to.

foods that fight gallstones

A diet rich in magnesium can lower gallstone risk by 30 percent, according to a University of Kentucky study. Men with the lowest risk got an average of 454 milligrams a day from supplements plus foods. A standard multivitamin has about 100 milligrams. These 10 foods deliver a big dose of magnesium.

Almonds	1/4 cup	98 mg
Black beans, cooked	1 cup	120 mg
Brown rice, cooked	1 cup	84 mg
Flaxseed, ground	2 Tbsp	70 mg
Halibut, cooked	4 oz	121 mg
Pinto beans, cooked	1 cup	94 mg
Pumpkin seeds	1/4 cup	184 mg
Salmon, cooked	4 oz	138 mg
Spinach, cooked	1 cup	155 mg

Don't yo-yo diet. The more weight you gain and lose repeatedly, the higher your risk of gallstones becomes. Researchers at the University of Kentucky Medical Center found that men who lost and regained as few as 5 to 9 pounds in five years had a 21 percent higher risk of gallstones compared to those who maintained the same weight. Men whose weight fluctuated by 10 to 19 pounds raised their odds by 38 percent. Weight-cycling 20 pounds or more increased risk by 78 percent.

Why is yo-yoing so risky? While dieting, you may not be eating enough fat to keep your gallbladder active; this may allow cholesterol to sit long enough to begin forming stones. Meanwhile, when you regain weight, you may develop insulin resistance because most of the pounds you put back on after a diet are body fat (not muscle), and body fat increases the risk of this condition. Changes in body chemistry that lead to insulin resistance also increase gallstone risk, the researchers say.

Lace up your roller skates. Or go for a jog, or join the gym. Getting two to three hours of physical activity per week can lower your risk of gallstones by 20 percent.

Focus on good fats. A low-fat diet isn't necessary; in fact, cutting out too much fat could cause problems. Eating regular meals that contain a little fat helps prevent gallstones by prompting the gallbladder to empty, pumping bile acids into your digestive system to help digest your meal. But the type of fat you eat *does* matter: In studies from Denmark and France, people who ate more saturated fat (found in fatty meats, ice cream, and cheese) were more likely to develop gallstones. Getting more of your fat from olive and canola oils, nuts, and fatty fish is a better idea.

Cut back on sugar and add fiber. Eating 40 grams of sugar a day, the amount in eight teaspoons of sugar or a serving of sweetened breakfast cereal plus a couple of cookies after lunch, doubles gallstone risk, according to University of Kentucky researchers. The reason? Experts think that it's an increase in cholesterol in the bloodstream, which is triggered by the surge of insulin that happens when blood sugar rises. Eat a high-fiber diet, on the other hand, and you'll protect against gallstones by whisking cholesterol (found in bile acids) out of your body.

Prevention Boosters

Enjoy coffee. A cup or two of java in the morning could slash your risk of gallstones by 40 percent, say researchers who tracked the gallbladder health of more than 46,000 men for a decade. Components in coffee stimulate the release of bile acids and lower levels of stone-forming cholesterol in bile fluid.

Toast to your gallbladder's health. One drink a day can lower gallstone risk by 27 percent. Alcohol may help by raising "good" HDL cholesterol, which whisks "bad" LDL (found in gallstones) out of your body. Beer, wine, and hard liquor were equally protective.

WHAT CAUSES IT
An imbalance of the "ingredients" in bile acids, the digestive juices that break down dietary fat, or incomplete emptying of your gallbladder. Either problem can allow cholesterol particles from bile acids to group together, forming stones.

SYMPTOMS TO WATCH FOR Indigestion, which may be worse after you eat a high-fat meal. Also gas; bloating; sudden, steady pain in your right upper abdomen; nausea; and vomiting.

NEWEST THINKING
Research suggests that people of European ancestry have a 10 percent chance of having a gene variation that increases gallstone risk. Carrying the gene doubles or even triples the risk by causing the liver to pump extra cholesterol (a major component of gallstones) into the gallbladder. But experts say that eating well and exercising can prevent gallstones from ever causing trouble.

Glaucoma

Glaucoma is a sneaky thief. It slowly destroys the delicate fibers of the optic nerve, making it impossible for your eyes to tell your brain what they're seeing. The result: You can't see anymore. The damage usually begins decades before you realize something's wrong, as pressure within your eyes builds and begins erasing peripheral vision. Untreated, it leaves you with tunnel vision—and then darkness. Regular vision checks can find dangerously high eye pressure early. Prescription eyedrops and surgery can bring it under control to help save your sight.

Key Prevention Strategies

Show up for your eye checks. Everyone should have comprehensive eye exams every two to four years beginning at age 40 and every one to two years after 65. Your eye doctor will dilate your pupils to look for signs of optic nerve damage, measure pressure levels in your eyes, and check the thickness of your cornea (a thin cornea is associated with higher glaucoma risk). You should also have a visual field test to check for tiny blind spots in your vision.

Know your risk. While anyone can develop glaucoma, your risk is significantly higher if other people in your family have it, if you're over age 60 (especially for Mexican-Americans), or if you're African-American and over age 40. Compared to Caucasians, African-Americans are 5 times more likely to develop glaucoma and 15 times more likely to become blind due to glaucoma between the ages of 45 and 64. Diabetes, high blood pressure, nearsightedness, severe eye injuries, and long-term use of steroid medications may also increase your risk.

If you're at increased risk, catching problems early should be a top priority. You may need more frequent eye exams as recommended by your doctor.

the coffee controversy

Glaucoma specialists don't all agree, but several studies suggest that a serious coffee habit could raise eye pressure and your risk of optic nerve damage. Harvard researchers found that downing five cups a day increased glaucoma risk by 61 percent in a long-term study of more than 76,000 women. Meanwhile, Australian researchers who studied the eye health of more than 3,600 people found that the more coffee they drank, the higher their eye pressure. Some studies suggest that caffeine's the culprit, but in other research, tea and caffeinated sodas seemed to have little effect—but coffee did.

If your doctor prescribes eyedrops, use them. If the pressure inside your eyes is elevated, using pressure-lowering eyedrops every day could save your vision. In a landmark study of 1,686 people with high eye pressure but no signs of optic nerve damage, those who used drops cut their risk of damage over the next five years in half. If eyedrops don't work, or if your optic nerve loss is progressing despite the use of drops, your doctor may suggest surgery to help lower your eye pressure.

Control diabetes. Having type 2 diabetes raises your risk of developing glaucoma by 70 percent, say Harvard School of Public Health researchers. Experts suspect that diabetes may somehow raise eye pressure or make the optic nerve more vulnerable to damage. If you have diabetes, keep your blood sugar under control and be sure to have your eyes checked once a year for glaucoma and other diabetes-related vision problems.

Prevention Boosters

Move it! It's no substitute for eye exams and eyedrops, but physical activity is a great "add-on" strategy for lowering glaucoma risk. Studies show that doing exercise that raises your heart rate (such as walking, swimming, or even vigorous work around the house) for about 20 minutes can lower your eye pressure by four points immediately afterward. Exercising four times a week can keep your pressure lower throughout the day. (If you use eyedrops, keep using them unless your doctor says otherwise.) Avoid moves that involve lowering your head below heart level (such as headstands, the downward-facing dog position in yoga, or any exercises that keep you bent over); these can raise pressure in the eye.

Quit smoking. When Greek researchers reviewed seven glaucoma studies, they found that smokers were 37 percent more likely to develop glaucoma than nonsmokers. Not all studies have found an association, but if you've been told you're at risk for glaucoma or already have it, it's just another good reason to kick this habit.

Relax and refresh. There's some evidence that emotional stress raises fluid pressure inside the eyes and that relaxation techniques can reverse that trend. In one German study of people with glaucoma, those who did guided imagery exercises to relax reduced their eye pressure significantly. Again, it's no substitute for drops if you need them, but it could help.

WHAT CAUSES IT
Untreated elevation of intraocular pressure. Pressure can build if your eyes' drainage system doesn't work efficiently. Some people with apparently normal pressure also develop glaucoma.

SYMPTOMS TO WATCH FOR Usually, none. In advanced glaucoma, you will develop tunnel vision. A less common form of glaucoma, called acute angle-closure glaucoma, causes very sudden blurred vision, halos around lights, red eyes, severe eye pain, and nausea and vomiting, all due to a rapid, dramatic increase in eye pressure. It's a medical emergency.

NEWEST THINKING
Glaucoma is a warning sign of heart trouble. When Stony Brook University researchers followed the health of 4,092 Barbados residents for five years, they found that those with glaucoma were 38 percent more likely to have fatal heart disease. The connection could be underlying health problems that lead to both. If you have glaucoma, keep tabs on your blood pressure and cholesterol levels, too.

Prevent **Glaucoma** 185

Gout

40%

The reduction in your gout risk if you lose just 10 pounds.

In Victorian times, gout afflicted only wealthy types who feasted heartily and drank heavily. Today it's an egalitarian epidemic, visiting excruciating joint pain on a growing number of men and women, thanks to the world's obesity epidemic—and to the fact that more people are eating foods, drinking beverages, and taking medications that raise levels of uric acid in the bloodstream. Too much leads to the development of agony-causing crystals that congregate in joints. Here's how to avoid them and to sidestep another attack if you already have gout.

Key Prevention Strategies

Maintain a healthy weight. Gaining 30 pounds could more than double your risk of developing gout, report researchers from Massachusetts General Hospital in Boston. Losing just 10 pounds lowered the odds by 40 percent.

Sweat a little. In a California study of 228 men, those who were leaner *and* fitter were less likely to develop gout than men who could claim only one of those healthy attributes. In the study, men who ran about four miles a day lowered their risk by 50 percent, but doing any form of aerobic exercise—such as brisk walking, swimming, or biking—for any amount of time will help some.

Choose chicken and beans instead of a steady diet of red meat or seafood. A daily serving of red meat raised the likelihood of developing gout by 45 percent in a study of 228 men conducted by researchers from the Lawrence Berkeley National Laboratory in California. Meanwhile, guys who ate the most seafood (including fatty fish) increased their risk by 51 percent in another study. Why? Purines, found in foods (game and organ meats and seafood including anchovies, sardines, and scallops have especially high levels) and in our body tissues. When purines break down, blood levels of uric acid rise.

Best protein for your plate? Try chicken or beans, and limit meat and seafood to three to four ounces just a few times a week. (If you don't have problems with gout, keep eating fish.)

Have a daily bowl of bing cherries. Cherries are an age-old folk remedy for gout. Now science reveals why it works. When 10 volunteers breakfasted on 45 red, ripe bing cherries for two days, researchers at the University of California, Davis, discovered that levels of uric acid in their blood fell by an impressive 30 points.

Eat a banana with breakfast and strawberries in the afternoon.
Eating two servings of fruit a day cut gout risk by 50 percent compared to eating less than a half serving a day, say researchers from the Berkeley National Laboratory. Fruit may simply be a sign of an overall healthy diet, or the fiber may help prevent gout. If you already have gout, however, it may be smart to avoid fruits that are highest in fructose, such as pears, apples, dates, grapes, and watermelon.

Ask for a different hypertension drug. Studies suggest that blood pressure–lowering diuretics can push gout risk 3.5 times higher than normal. Older, "thiazide" diuretics may raise risk most. If you're bothered by gout and take one of these drugs, ask your doctor about an alternative medication.

Drink wine instead of beer. A little alcohol may protect your heart, but it also raises gout risk. In one study, men who drank two or more 12-ounce beers a day increased their odds 2.6 times more than those who abstained. But two small glasses of wine did not raise risk. Beer contains higher levels of purines than most wines.

Skip sweetened soft drinks. Sweetened sodas, bottled iced teas, and fruit punches raise gout risk just as much as alcohol does. It's the fructose that seems to increase uric acid levels. Diet drinks seem safe.

Prevention Boosters

Indulge your coffee habit. Sipping four or five small cups of coffee a day cut gout risk by 40 percent compared to rarely downing java, according to a California study of 228 men. Decaffeinated coffee lowered risk, too, but tea had no effect, leading researchers to speculate that a strong antioxidant in coffee called chlorogenic acid is the ingredient at work.

Sip low-fat milk and spoon up some yogurt. Two servings of dairy a day can lower gout risk by about 45 percent—as long as it's low fat, researchers report. Proteins in dairy called casein and lactalbumin may protect against this painful problem by promoting the excretion of uric acid in your urine.

WHAT CAUSES IT
High blood levels of uric acid, which crystallizes in joints, causing inflammation and pain. Certain foods and beverages raise uric acid levels, and some medications may make it more difficult for your body to excrete it.

SYMPTOMS TO WATCH FOR Sudden, severe pain; redness and tenderness in joints. It often begins in a big toe or knee.

NEWEST THINKING
People with gout have a 20 percent higher risk for a heart attack than people who don't have gout, say University of Pittsburgh School of Medicine researchers. The connection may be inflammation: Gout can trigger ongoing inflammation in the body, and inflammatory compounds may also trigger blood clots that can lead to a heart attack. If you have gout, be extra vigilant about your cholesterol, blood pressure, and blood sugar to help protect your heart. People with gout also have an increased risk of kidney failure.

Gum Disease

38%

The reduction in the risk of bleeding gums after two weeks of brushing your tongue and teeth and flossing twice a day.

Having teeth fall out because you don't brush or floss enough is bad enough, but gum disease can affect more than just your mouth. Heart disease, diabetes, pneumonia, and chronic obstructive pulmonary disease are all linked to gum disease, probably because of the low-level inflammation created as bacteria from your gums travel throughout your bloodstream. What better reasons to protect your smile?

Key Prevention Strategies

Floss frequently. We're not sure why people hate to floss. It takes less than a minute, there are all those nifty flossing tools, and it's one of the best ways to prevent bad breath. Here are a few tips to make flossing easier.

- **Buy nonshredding monofilament floss.** The only thing worse than food stuck between your teeth is floss stuck between your teeth.
- **Keep floss everywhere.** At your desk, in your purse, in the bathroom (of course).
- **Buy minty floss.** The fresh taste in your mouth is a bonus.
- **Use a battery-operated flosser.** A 10-week study found that these automated flossers got rid of considerably more plaque on molars, premolars, and hard-to-reach back teeth than regular floss.
- **Ask for a demonstration.** Although the process may seem obvious, there is a right and wrong way to floss. Ask your dentist or dental hygienist for a demonstration.

Rinse with an antibacterial mouthwash daily. If you absolutely won't floss, try rinsing with a mouthwash containing antimicrobial chlorhexidine or cetylpyridinium chloride. A study in 156 healthy volunteers found those who brushed *and* used either mouthwash had lower scores on a test that measures plaque levels than those who brushed and flossed or those who only brushed.

Try a battery-powered toothbrush. After six months of brushing—but not flossing—with an automatic toothbrush, people who already had gum disease showed significantly less plaque in the morning and immediately after brushing than those using a regular toothbrush.

Put out the smokes. Not only is cigarette smoking a major risk factor for gum disease, but even exposure to secondhand smoke can increase your risk by up to 70 percent.

Prevention Boosters

Watch your blood sugar. If you have diabetes, your risk of gum disease is already higher than it is for someone who doesn't have diabetes. But if your diabetes isn't well controlled, you're really in the danger zone. Researchers find that people with poorly controlled diabetes have more inflammatory chemicals like cytokines in their gums, which contribute to gum disease.

Suck an orange a day. When researchers evaluated the link between diet and gum disease in 12,400 adults, they found that those who didn't get the recommended daily amount of vitamin C (50 milligrams, or about the amount in one orange) were nearly 20 percent more likely to have gum disease than those who got more vitamin C. Centuries ago, sailors at sea sucked on limes to prevent bleeding gums, but all citrus fruits and many brightly colored vegetables, such as red peppers, are rich in C.

Get a milk mustache. People who get less than 500 milligrams of calcium a day (one cup of milk has about 300 milligrams) are nearly twice as likely to have gum disease as those who get at least three servings a day of calcium-rich foods (a serving is one cup of milk or yogurt, six sardines, or five figs). Calcium helps build density in the bone that supports the teeth, enabling it to withstand the bacterial attack from plaque.

Don't overdose on alcohol. Researchers have found a direct correlation between the amount of alcohol people drink and their risk of gum disease. Ten drinks a week increased the risk 10 percent, 20 drinks increased it 20 percent, and so on. Heavy drinking may influence gum disease by affecting the immune system's ability to fight infection, interfering with blood clotting, and leading to vitamin and protein deficiencies that impair healing.

Talk to your doctor if one of your medications dries out your mouth. Dozens of drugs, including some antidepressants and cold remedies, contain ingredients that dry up saliva production. Saliva helps clean teeth and hinders the growth of bacteria, so if your mouth is like a desert, you're courting gum disease.

WHAT CAUSES IT
Bacteria in plaque (a sticky, colorless film that forms on teeth) inflames gums. Over time, the inflammation can spread beneath the gumline.

SYMPTOMS TO WATCH FOR Gums that become reddish, swell, or bleed easily; later, you may have loose teeth, bad breath, and visibly receding gums.

NEWEST THINKING
New research suggests that obesity and gum disease may be related. When you're very overweight, fat cells release inflammatory chemicals that can contribute to numerous diseases, including gum disease.

Headaches

50%

The decrease in the number and severity of headaches if you exercise for 30 minutes most days of the week.

On a pain scale ranging from ouch! to my head's about to explode!!! most headaches are manageable. But none are convenient. Whether you get a tension headache once in a while or experience fiercely excruciating "cluster" headaches, the best headache is the one you don't get at all. Experts say most headaches can be avoided with these steps. (If you get migraines, see page 254.)

Key Prevention Strategies

Stick to your schedule. Sleeping in on weekends and postponing that first cup of tea or coffee could trigger a weekend headache—just when you were looking forward to a relaxing morning and a fun Saturday. One survey conducted by the National Headache Foundation found that 79 percent of headache sufferers have pain in the brain if they sleep longer than eight hours. And if you're used to that 7 a.m. cup of coffee, delaying your morning caffeine hit could make blood vessels clench, leaving you with a pounding noggin.

Show up for breakfast, lunch, and dinner. If you get "hunger headaches," the culprit could be low blood sugar. Keeping your blood sugar on an even keel with healthy meals could help. Try to include whole grains, fruit and vegetables, and protein to keep levels steadier for longer. Avoid loading up on white rice, white bagels, white potatoes, and high-sugar snacks and desserts, which make blood sugar spike and then dip again.

Move your muscles. Getting a half hour of exercise most days of the week can cut headache pain and frequency by an impressive 50 percent, research shows. Physical activity fights headaches two ways: It boosts feel-good brain chemicals called endorphins and eases stress.

Melt tension away every day. You don't have to meditate—any kind of relaxation that eases your stress could help you escape from frequent tension headaches. Italian office workers who took brief relaxation breaks every two to three hours cut

drugs that PREVENT DISEASE

Cluster headaches are excruciating and can be a daily problem for weeks, months, or years on end. The most popular prevention drug, verapamil, is effective but has risks. In one study of 30 people, 12 of 15 participants who got the drug had fewer attacks in just two weeks. But other research shows that it significantly raises the risk of irregular heart rhythm. If you try this medication, be sure your heart is monitored regularly by your doctor.

their monthly headaches by 41 percent, report researchers from the University of Turin. And when Ohio University researchers tracked 203 adults with chronic daily tension headaches, 35 percent of those who got five sessions of stress management advice saw headache frequency fall by more than 50 percent. Ask your doctor for a referral for mindfulness-based stress reduction training, given at many hospitals and community centers. Meanwhile, try walks outside or a few minutes of slow, deep breathing on a regular basis.

Don't let your computer hurt your head. Reposition your chair, desk, and computer screen so you can sit up straight with your feet on the floor. The center of your monitor should be just below your gaze when you look straight ahead. Make sure your eyeglass prescription is current (if you need a new pair, spring for the anti-glare coating). Finally, get up and take frequent breaks from the screen.

Quit your pain reliever. If you take medicine for head pain more than 15 times each month, you may have "medication overuse headaches" or "rebound headaches." These happen when your painkiller wears off and blood vessels swell. Pain returns, you take something to relieve it, and the cycle begins again.

Studies show that rebound headaches can happen with over-the-counter remedies like ibuprofen and aspirin and with stronger prescription drugs for headaches and migraines, such as opioids, triptans, and ergots. The best remedy: Quit your pain reliever. Yes, it'll hurt. But once the rebound effect wears off, your doctor will be able to treat the underlying cause of your headaches.

Prevention Boosters

Stay hydrated. That nagging pain could be your brain's way of asking for a glass of water. Mild headaches can be a sign of mild dehydration, so drink up.

Let go of tension in your jaw, face, shoulders, and/or neck. It's easy to unconsciously clench muscles in these areas when you're tense, boosting your odds for a headache. Studies confirm that this is a frequent cause of chronic tension headaches. So stop right now and "listen" to the muscles in these areas; if they're tight, take a few deep, slow breaths and imagine the stress flowing out until you feel the muscles relaxing. Repeat several times a day.

WHAT CAUSES IT
No one's quite sure what causes tension headaches, but researchers now suspect that fluctuating levels of serotonin, feel-good endorphins, and other brain chemicals play an important role. Anemia, anxiety, arthritis of the neck or spine, depression, menopause, muscle tension, severe high blood pressure, and sinus infections can cause headaches. So can prescription and over-the-counter drugs, including oral contraceptives, some antihistamines and decongestants, and therapeutic hormones for women.

SYMPTOMS TO WATCH FOR Head pain, of course, as well as trouble sleeping, tiredness, irritability, loss of appetite, and difficulty concentrating. If you have cluster headaches, you will have intense pain plus teary, swollen eyes; a stuffy nose; and sweaty skin.

NEWEST THINKING
Chronic headaches and depression are linked. In a study, one in four women and men with chronic headaches also had major depression, report researchers from the University of Tsukuba in Japan. The researchers suggest that if you have had chronic headaches for longer than six months, see your doctor for an evaluation for depression. You deserve to feel better!

Hearing Loss

189%
The amount by which you could reduce your risk if you quit smoking.

"What?" Many older folks find themselves saying this a lot, and their spouses may cringe as they turn the TV volume up and up. Hearing does tend to worsen with age, partially due to conditions such as high blood pressure and diabetes, not to mention smoking and years and years of noise. But thanks to rock bands, leaf blowers, and electronic kids' toys, noise-related hearing loss is now turning up in younger adults and in children as young as 6. Keep your hearing sharp and clear with these strategies.

Key Prevention Strategies

Protect yourself against diabetes, heart disease, and high blood pressure. All can increase the risk of age-related hearing loss, probably by impeding blood flow to the inner ear. Find tips for preventing them in their respective entries.

Use the lawnmower test. If something sounds as loud as a lawnmower (90 decibels), it's too loud. You need to cover your ears with earmuffs or at least use drugstore earplugs. Here's another way to gauge whether your chores or hobbies are hurting your hearing. Before heading out to mow the lawn or go to the shooting range, turn on the television and set the volume on low. Notice how well you hear what's said. After your outing, try the test again. If you don't hear as well, you're experiencing some temporary hearing loss. With continued exposure, it could become permanent.

Turn down the volume on your MP3 player. When you're plugged into your MP3 player, you may not realize how loud the sound really is. When in doubt, turn down the volume. If you keep the volume control no higher than 50 percent of max, you can listen as long as you want. But if you're used to turning up the sound loud enough so that someone standing next to you could identify the song, limit yourself to 5 minutes if you're using an iPod with earbuds that sit inside your ear and 18 minutes if you use earphones that rest on top of your ears. Any longer, found researchers, and you're putting your hearing at risk.

Quit smoking. Add hearing to the list of body functions damaged by cigarette smoke. After analyzing eight major studies, researchers concluded that smoking increases your risk of hearing loss by 33 to

got the gene?

While most hearing loss results from noise, everyone's hearing reacts differently. Two people exposed to the same noise level could experience it differently in each ear, even at different times of the day. That makes researchers suspect there's some genetic component to hearing loss. Another clue to your risk may come from your blood type. In one study, researchers found noise-induced hearing loss much more common among people with blood group O. The bottom line: If your parents or grandparents wore hearing aids, or you have type O blood, you may have a higher risk of noise-related hearing loss, so be extra careful about prevention.

189 percent. It reduces the flow of blood and oxygen to your inner ear, weakening those all-important hair cells that transmit sound to your brain.

Get plenty of B vitamins. A growing body of evidence suggests that people with low levels of the B vitamins folic acid and B_{12} tend to have poorer hearing. When Dutch researchers gave 728 older men and women 800 micrograms of folic acid or a placebo daily for three years, those who got the vitamin had less hearing loss than those who got the placebo. In another study, researchers injected 20 young volunteers daily with either a placebo or vitamin B_{12} for seven days, then exposed each group to a loud noise. The vitamin group's hearing recovered better from the noise than the placebo group's did.

B vitamins reduce levels of the amino acid homocysteine, which damages blood vessels. Clear out the homocysteine, and you improve blood flow, leading to healthier inner ear hair cells. That's important, given that loud noises can slash blood flow to the cochlea, or inner ear, by up to 70 percent. Good sources of B vitamins include leafy green vegetables, lentils, beans, clams (for B_{12}), and fortified cereals.

Prevention Boosters

Hop on a bike or take a jog or walk. After biking twice a week for 30 minutes a day over two months, 17 moderately fit young adults suffered less hearing loss after a loud noise than before they started biking. It was as if the exercise "inoculated" them against noise-related hearing loss. The link? Researchers suspect it's related to the bikers' stronger hearts. The stronger the heart and the better the circulation (which exercise improves), the more oxygenated blood gets to those fragile inner ear hair cells, helping them resist noise-related damage.

Sauté some Swiss chard. It's packed with magnesium, which studies find can help prevent hearing-related damage. When researchers had 20 men drink juice containing 122 milligrams of magnesium or a placebo for 10 days, then exposed them to a white noise designed to exhaust the cochlear hair cells, they found the men recovered more hearing more rapidly after the magnesium-laced juice than after the placebo drink. Researchers think it's because magnesium helps cells use energy better, the kind of energy you need to repair noise-induced damage. Oat bran, barley, spinach, and pumpkin seeds are also good sources.

WHAT CAUSES IT
Noise damages minuscule hair cells in your inner ear that transmit sounds to your brain. When these cells die, they can't be replaced. You're born with about 16,000 hair cells, and you can lose between one-third and one-half of them before you notice yourself saying "what?" a lot.

SYMPTOMS TO WATCH FOR Ringing in the ears, dizziness, difficulty perceiving and differentiating consonants, feeling that words often "run together," inability to hear high-pitched sounds like a ringing phone or a crying baby.

NEWEST THINKING
One reason noise damages ears may be because it stimulates the production of free radicals, dangerous molecules that can damage cells. Antioxidants in your body neutralize free radicals, but if you're exposed to too much noise, those antioxidants can't keep up. In animals, antioxidants like n-acetyl-l-cysteine and acetyl-l-carnitine reduce the risk of that damage.

Heartburn and GERD

50%

The reduction in your risk of acid reflux if you add more fiber to your diet.

A muscular valve at the bottom of your esophagus normally keeps corrosive digestive juices where they belong—in your stomach. But if you have heartburn, this valve sneaks open at inopportune times, like after a big meal, letting acid go where it doesn't belong and causing pain that can be mild or so bad you may think it's a heart attack. Over time, heartburn becomes gastroesophageal reflux disease (GERD), a more serious condition that may raise your risk of esophageal cancer. Take it seriously—and try these strategies to discourage acid backwash.

Key Prevention Strategies

Put on a few pounds since high school? Slim down. Shedding 27 pounds cut reflux episodes 40 percent in one study reviewed by researchers from Stanford University. Why it helps: Losing weight may lower pressure at the valve that keeps stomach acid put, known as the lower esophageal sphincter (LES). It also reduces the body's output of acidic digestive enzymes.

Catch the early-bird special. When Japanese researchers tracked the bedtimes and GERD symptoms of 441 women and men, they found that those who went to bed within three hours of finishing dinner were 7.5 times more likely to have acid indigestion than those who turned in four or more hours later. If you go to bed at 10:30, aim to finish dinner no later than 6:30.

Prop up the head of your bed. Raising the head of your bed about 11 inches with bricks or wood blocks could cut reflux episodes dramatically and make the ones you do have shorter.

Recline on your left side. In one study, people who slept on their left sides had only half as much reflux as right-side sleepers. Due to the location of your stomach and esophagus, lying on your right side puts more pressure on the LES.

Take the pepperoni pizza test. There's plenty of controversy about which food demons trigger heartburn. The truth is, what bothers you may be no problem at all for the guy in the next booth at the pizza parlor. (He, on the other hand, may be in agony after downing a few chocolate-covered after-dinner mints.)

194   Disease Prevention **A to Z**

When researchers from Stanford University reviewed more than 100 studies of lifestyle remedies for acid reflux, they found that avoiding chocolate, mint, spices, grease, and late-night noshing doesn't help most people. But plenty of other research, and the experience of digestive disease specialists, suggests that for some people, these are exactly the things they should avoid.

The take-home lesson? Figure out what your personal trigger foods are, then steer clear of them. Possibilities include citrus fruits; chocolate; coffee and tea; alcohol; fatty and fried foods; garlic and onions; mint flavorings; spicy foods; and tomato-based foods such as spaghetti sauce, salsa, chili, and pizza.

Avoid sleeping pills. According to a large health survey, people who took benzodiazepines such as diazepam (Valium), alprazolam (Xanax), and triazolam (Halcion) in order to fall asleep were 50 percent more likely to have GERD at night than those who didn't take the drugs. Other research has shown that these drugs loosen the LES, lowering your chances of a comfortable night's sleep.

Stop smoking. A Swedish study of more than 43,300 people found that long-time smokers had a 70 percent higher risk of heartburn and GERD than nonsmokers. Smoking raises risk four ways: It may make you cough more, which puts pressure on the LES; it can weaken the LES; it reduces production of saliva, which normally neutralizes stomach acids that find their way into your esophagus; and it boosts production of corrosive digestive acids.

Prevention Boosters

Pop that gum. No antacid on hand? Head off heartburn with a stuck of chewing gum. A small British study found that chomping on gum for 30 minutes after a big fatty meal doubled saliva production and saliva swallowing; researchers estimate that 10 extra swallows could cool mild heartburn by pushing acids back where they belong. Other research shows that gum chewing neutralizes the acids in stomach backwash for up to three hours after a meal.

when to call the doctor

Chronic or severe heartburn can be a sign of more serious reflux disease or other digestive problems. Call your doctor if you have heartburn for more than two weeks or if it is making you wheeze or giving you a sore throat; preventing you from sleeping; interfering with daytime activities; causing pain in your neck, chest, or back; creating discomfort or difficulty when you swallow; making you vomit or have black stools (from digested blood); or causing weight loss.

Take a relaxation break. Science has yet to uncover the link between stress and acid indigestion, but plenty of heartburn sufferers know it exists: In one survey conducted by the National Heartburn Alliance, 58 percent of people who had frequent heartburn said hectic lifestyles made their pain worse. Stress may prompt you to smoke more, drink more alcohol, eat the foods that trigger acid backwash, or simply feel discomfort more intensely. Pay attention to your own stress levels, and when they get too high, look for ways to relax, such as deep breathing.

drugs that PREVENT DISEASE

If you already have GERD, acid-stopping drugs known as H_2 blockers and proton-pump inhibitors (PPIs) can help you accomplish two important health goals: halting the searing pain of heartburn and healing damaged tissue in your esophagus. (Note that there is also non-acid reflux that does not respond to PPIs.)

H_2 blockers: Drugs such as nizatidine (Axid), cimetidine (Tagamet), ranitidine (Zantac), and famotidine (Pepcid) reduce acid levels in your stomach. Your doctor may suggest over-the-counter H_2 blockers for two weeks to relieve symptoms or prescription-strength forms for long-term relief. Studies show that H_2 blockers work best for people with mild to moderate reflux problems but are less effective if your esophagus is inflamed or has already been damaged by exposure to stomach acids. If you know which foods or situations make heartburn flare up, taking an H_2 blocker in advance may help you avoid discomfort better than taking an antacid afterward.

Proton-pump inhibitors: Drugs such as rabeprazole (Aciphex), esomeprazole (Nexium), lansoprazole (Prevacid), omeprazole (Prilosec), and pantoprazole (Protonix) work by blocking production of about 90 percent of stomach acids. Doctors often prescribe PPIs if H_2 blockers don't bring relief or if you have severe heartburn or esophageal damage. In one study of people with GERD, 78 percent of those who took a PPI saw damaged esophageal tissue heal in four to eight weeks. After about eight weeks, your doctor should check to see if your esophagus is healing and may cut back on your dosage.

Control asthma. Three out of four people with asthma also have acid reflux. The connection? Coughing and difficulty exhaling may trigger the backwash of stomach acid into the esophagus. Asthma drugs that widen airways in the lungs may also relax the LES. Keeping your asthma under control can help, but if you still have acid reflux, tell your doctor.

Keep blood sugar within a healthy range. Over time, the high blood sugar levels that come with type 1 and type 2 diabetes can damage nerves throughout your body, including those that regulate the emptying of your stomach. If food sits in your stomach, it can be regurgitated more readily into your esophagus. Some studies suggest that better blood sugar control can help, but it's still important to use the other lifestyle strategies mentioned here.

Ask if any of your pills are culprits. Many prescription and over-the-counter drugs and supplements can keep the LES from staying tightly shut. These include some antibiotics, antidepressants, calcium channel blockers, opioid pain relievers like codeine and hydrocodone, osteoporosis drugs, sedatives, and tranquilizers as well as over-the-counter pain relievers and supplements such as iron, potassium, and vitamin C. If you have heartburn or GERD, ask your doctor if any of these could be contributing to your discomfort and whether you should switch to another drug or remedy.

Up your fiber intake. People who ate high-fiber breads (think whole grain) had half the risk of GERD compared to people who ate low-fiber breads (think white) in one large Scandinavian study. Fiber may help by soaking up excess nitric oxide, a compound that relaxes muscles in the digestive system. When researchers at the Houston Veterans Affairs Medical Center scanned the esophaguses of 164 people, they found that those who ate more fruits, veggies, whole grains, and beans were 20 percent less likely to have signs of erosion of delicate esophageal tissue caused by reflux. At higher risk: people who took in more fat, protein, and calories.

Skip the cola. When researchers from the University of Arizona College of Medicine polled more than 15,000 people about their lifestyle habits and history of GERD, they found that those who drank more than one carbonated, caffeinated drink per day were 24 percent more likely to have sleep-disturbing nighttime reflux than those who drank less soda. Many bubbly drinks have a high acid level, which may explain the connection, they say.

Add acupuncture if your prescription drug isn't working. When 30 people with persistent heartburn received either a double dose of proton-pump inhibitors or twice-weekly acupuncture plus their regular dose for four weeks, the acupuncture group enjoyed a significant decrease in GERD symptoms. The group that simply got more drugs didn't see much improvement at all, report University of Arizona researchers.

WHAT CAUSES IT
Weakening or relaxation of the lower esophageal sphincter, the muscular valve at the bottom of your esophagus. Normally, the LES keeps digestive juices and food in your stomach. But smoking, alcohol, lying down too soon after a meal, some foods, and some medications can weaken or partially open the LES, allowing stomach acids to backwash into your esophagus.

SYMPTOMS TO WATCH FOR
A burning pain in your throat or chest, under your breastbone. It may become worse after a meal, at night, or when you lie down. Less obvious symptoms include a persistent cough and chronic laryngitis.

NEWEST THINKING
New research shows that nearly 40 percent of heartburn/GERD sufferers who use an acid-stopping PPI drug once a day still get heartburn symptoms two to four times a week. Many wind up popping antacids, which can stop pain but may not protect the esophagus from damage. If you're taking medication for heartburn or GERD and are still in pain, ask your doctor about upgrading your treatment plan.

Heavy Periods

50%

The amount you can reduce menstrual bleeding by taking the prescription drug tranexamic acid.

Every woman has the occasional day when a heavy period overflows her protection. But when the bleeding becomes so heavy that you can't leave the house without worrying or continues for seven or more days, you have more than just a period; you have menorrhagia, the medical term for excessive or prolonged menstrual bleeding. Prevent the flood—or at least reduce it significantly—with these recommendations. Remember that bleeding sometimes becomes heavier as menopause approaches; that problem will resolve itself.

Key Prevention Strategies

Ask your doctor about a prescription drug. Tranexamic acid (Cyklokapron) is the most effective medical treatment available for preventing heavy bleeding. It is an antifibrinolytic, which means it prevents blood clots from disintegrating. It also stimulates clot formation. More clots mean less bleeding. Studies find the drug can reduce heavy menstrual bleeding by as much as 50 percent.

Try Advil or another NSAID. Over-the-counter painkillers like ibuprofen (Advil, Motrin) and naproxen (Aleve) and the prescription drug diclofenac (Cataflam)—all known as nonsteroidal anti-inflammatory drugs, or NSAIDs—can help prevent heavy menstrual bleeding by reducing levels of prostaglandins, hormone-like chemicals that interfere with blood clotting. Mefenamic acid (Ponstel), a prescription NSAID, may be less likely to irritate the stomach and reduces bleeding by 22 to 46 percent. Avoid aspirin, which may increase bleeding.

Consider birth control pills or an IUD. Because oral contraceptives thin the lining of your uterus, there is less lining to shed and less bleeding. Studies find that birth control pills can reduce menstrual bleeding by up to 60 percent. Taking continuous birth control pills, which skip the week of placebo pills that trigger a period, often prevent menstruation altogether and can significantly reduce heavy bleeding even if your periods continue.

A hormone-releasing IUD is another option. The IUD Mirena releases a progestin hormone called levonorgestrel. Progestins help prevent heavy bleeding by reducing the growth of the uterine lining. Numerous studies find that Mirena works as well as surgery for controlling heavy menstrual bleeding. It may even stop your periods altogether.

Prevention Boosters

Try chasteberry. *Vitex agnus castus,* better known as chasteberry, is an herb often used to treat reproductive issues in women. Studies find that as little as 15 drops of a tincture of extract can significantly reduce the number of days of heavy bleeding, though it may take several months before you see a benefit.

Get tested for a bleeding disorder. Blood clotting disorders such as von Willebrand's disease often underlie heavy menstrual bleeding, yet many doctors don't think to check for them. Women who have had heavy periods since they were young girls are most likely to have bleeding problems. If you have a clotting disorder, regular injections or infusions of missing clotting factors could make your heavy periods a thing of the past.

STUDIES FIND THAT BIRTH CONTROL PILLS CAN REDUCE MENSTRUAL BLEEDING.

Hemorrhoids

750%

The amount your risk of hemorrhoids could drop if you eat breakfast every day.

Hemorrhoids are one more indignity of middle age, not to mention pregnancy. Over-the-counter treatments can help some people, but if the problem gets bad, you may need more serious help. In fact, hemorrhoids, marked by swollen and inflamed veins around the lower rectum, form a large portion of any colorectal surgeon's workload. They're also probably much more common than we know, since many people are understandably too embarrassed to admit they have them. Avoid the surgeon's scalpel and the pain and itching with these suggestions.

Key Prevention Strategies

Don't strain! If you have to bear down to have a bowel movement, something's wrong. And if you've been sitting on the toilet for more than five minutes, you've been there too long. Stop. The straining is the primary cause of the hemorrhoids, and the time spent on the toilet doesn't guarantee success. Instead, give up and try again an hour later.

Soften your stool. The reason you're straining is probably constipation. Keep things moving along by heeding the following advice.

Focus on fiber. When we asked a leading gastroenterologist what he recommends to his patients to prevent hemorrhoids, he answered with one word: flaxseed. It's one of the best sources of fiber you'll find, with nearly three grams in one tablespoon. Add a couple of teaspoons of ground flaxseed to muffin or pancake batter and sprinkle it over yogurt or oatmeal. Add the ground seeds to salads for added crunch, to spaghetti sauce for added bulk, and even to your evening bowl of ice cream. Fiber acts like a sponge in your intestinal

stop the burning

Once you have hemorrhoids, it's even more difficult to go to the bathroom; you're afraid something might burst, not to mention the burning. Try these suggestions.

- **Instead of dry, scratchy toilet paper,** use moist towelettes to wipe your bottom.

- **Use over-the-counter hemorrhoid cream or pads.** They usually contain topical anti-inflammatories to decrease inflammation and anesthetics to reduce pain.

- **Try a sitz bath.** Sit in about six inches of warm water for about 20 minutes. Or you can hold a washcloth soaked in warm water over the sore area. Do this several times a day.

- **Sit on a doughnut.** You can find these rubber circles, which keep the pressure off your bottom, at medical supply stores.

tract, soaking up liquid and creating bulkier stools that are easier to move out of your body.

Get out of the chair. A good way to get your bowels moving is to get yourself moving with regular exercise. It can be biking, swimming, walking, tennis—anything that gets the blood flowing. One study of 43 people with constipation found that those who walked every day for 30 minutes and did 11 minutes a day of weight-based exercises at home improved their rankings by nearly 35 percent on a scale designed to evaluate constipation.

Drink up. A major reason people get constipated and have a hard time moving their bowels is that their stools don't absorb enough water. Often it's because they're not drinking enough fluids, so carry a water bottle with you and make sure you refill it at least six times a day.

Go on a schedule. Believe it or not, there's actually an ideal time for a bowel movement: about 30 minutes after you wake up, just after a cup of hot coffee or tea, and about 30 to 60 minutes after meals. So plan for some bathroom time, even if nothing happens. What you're doing is training your bowels to "let go" at the same time every day.

Prevention Boosters

Change your position. Modern toilets work against you when it comes to hemorrhoids, since they require you to sit instead of squat; squatting facilitates bowel movements. To get around this, try propping your feet on a small footstool and pulling your knees toward you.

Load up on berries. Not only will the extra fiber help with constipation, but these fruits are also high in flavonoids, natural plant compounds that help reduce inflammation and strengthen blood vessel walls. In some countries, prescription medications containing highly purified flavonoids are used to treat hemorrhoids. In studies, the drugs significantly reduced the risk of bleeding, pain, and itching and also lowered the risk of recurrence by 47 percent. Ask your doctor about taking one, or simply plan to eat 3/4 cup of your favorite berries every day.

WHAT CAUSES IT
Pregnancy, in which hemorrhoids occur because of changing hormones and abdominal pressure; straining during bowel movements due to constipation; obesity; sitting for prolonged periods.

SYMPTOMS TO WATCH FOR Bright red blood covering the stool, on toilet paper, or in the toilet bowl. An internal hemorrhoid may protrude through the anus outside the body, becoming irritated and painful. Other symptoms include painful swelling or a hard lump around the anus.

NEWEST THINKING
To treat bad hemorrhoids, instead of surgery or cutting off the blood supply to hemorrhoids with a tight band, doctors can now zap them with infrared light to cut off the blood flow. No blood flow, no hemorrhoid.

Hepatitis

80-95%

How much you'll reduce your risk of hepatitis B by being vaccinated.

Hepatitis means inflammation of the liver. There are five types of viral hepatitis: A, B, C, D, and E. The three you need to worry about most are A, B, and C. The viruses all head for the liver. If they gain a toehold, they infiltrate liver cells and turn them into virus-producing factories. Sometimes hepatitis heals on its own; other times, it can last a lifetime. Cirrhosis, liver failure, and liver cancer may result from years of infection. These steps can protect you.

Key Prevention Strategies

Get vaccinated. The number one way to prevent hepatitis A, B, and D is with a vaccine. Unfortunately, there are no vaccines yet for hepatitis C and E, though researchers are working on them.

- **Hepatitis A vaccine:** Recommended for all children between 12 and 23 months, travelers to countries where the virus is prevalent (for a complete list, visit www.cdc.gov/ncidod/ diseases/hepatitis/b/country_listing.htm), homosexual men, users of IV and injectable drugs, people with blood disorders like hemophilia that often require transfusions, those with chronic liver disease, and those who work with the virus in laboratory settings. The vaccine requires two doses given 6 to 12 months apart in children and 6 to 18 months apart in adults. Studies suggest it could last up to 25 years or more.

- **Hepatitis B vaccine:** Recommended for all infants and anyone who works in the healthcare field. If you're under 19 and have never been vaccinated, do it now. The vaccine is also recommended for homosexual men, heterosexual people who have had a sexually transmitted disease or more than one partner in the previous six months, and those traveling to areas of the world with high rates of infection (for a list, see the Web site above). It's typically given in three doses over six months, though a few studies find that a shorter dosing schedule is also effective— maybe more effective. In one study, participants who received the second dose two weeks after the first showed protective antibody levels much higher than in those receiving the vaccine according to the traditional schedule. The protection lasts for

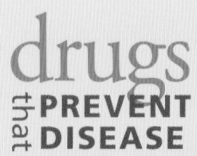

drugs that **PREVENT DISEASE**

If you think you've been exposed to the hepatitis A virus, see your doctor as soon as possible. He may give you a shot of immune globulin, which contains antibodies that destroy the virus. The sooner you receive the shot after being exposed to the virus—ideally, within two weeks—the more likely it will work.

at least 15 years but in most cases is believed to be lifelong. However, if you're over age 40 or obese, have kidney failure, are on dialysis, or have a suppressed immune system, it's not quite as effective. This vaccine also protects against hepatitis D.

- **Combined vaccine:** Three combination vaccines protect against both hepatitis A and B. Two of them are for infants and young children; the third is for adults. The vaccine is given either three times in six months or three times in 30 days, followed by a fourth at one year.

Prevention Boosters

Wash up. Not everyone hits the sink on the way out of the bathroom. Shake that person's hand, touch a doorknob he touched, and then touch your mouth, eyes, or nose, and you could be on your way to a hepatitis A infection. Especially if you're traveling to a country where hepatitis A is prevalent, wash with soap and water whenever you can, and for times when you can't, carry hand wipes. Always wash up after using the toilet or changing a diaper and before preparing food.

Use condoms. Safer sex is one of the best ways to prevent transmission of the hepatitis B virus.

Stay away from injected drugs. We're talking here about recreational drugs, not insulin. The most common cause of infection with hepatitis B and C viruses is use of injectable drugs, often beginning in adolescence or early adulthood.

Get your own razor. Using razors, toothbrushes, or any other personal item that could have come in contact with an infected person's blood can lead to hepatitis B or C infection.

Choose your tattoo parlor carefully. It's possible, though unlikely, that you'll get more than you bargained for when you get a tattoo, in the form of hepatitis C. If you must have that little flower permanently engraved on your ankle, make sure the tattoo parlor you choose is licensed (check with your state and local health departments), looks clean and tidy, and uses an autoclave to sterilize all equipment. The artist should remove the needles and tubes from a sealed package and wear gloves while working.

WHAT CAUSES IT

Hepatitis A and E: Ingesting food or water contaminated by stool from an infected person or through some other contact with an infected person's stool, such as during diaper changing or shaking hands with someone who didn't wash after using the bathroom.

Hepatitis B and D: Unprotected sexual contact with an infected person, sharing needles or drugs, or getting stuck by an infected needle. These viruses can also be passed from mother to infant during childbirth.

Hepatitis C: Exposure to infected blood products or sharing needles. It can also be passed from mother to infant during childbirth.

SYMPTOMS TO WATCH FOR
Infection may initially go unnoticed or feel like a mild case of the flu. With serious infection, you may experience jaundice, fatigue, abdominal pain, loss of appetite, nausea, diarrhea, fever, and dark urine. Hepatitis B infection may also cause skin rashes, joint pain, and arthritis.

NEWEST THINKING
People infected with hepatitis B should be started on treatment as early as possible, even before they show signs of liver damage. Doing so may help prevent the damage.

Herpes

75%

The percentage of genital herpes outbreaks that can be prevented if you take an antiviral drug daily.

Herpes—whether it's cold sores on your lips or blisters on your genitals—is painful in many ways. The blisters sting and burn for days. And while an attack is under way, herpes is embarrassing *and* risky because it's so contagious. Once you've been infected, this virus lives in your skin cells or nerve cells, dormant until it's reactivated by stress; sun exposure; trauma; surgery; illness; or, infrequently, menstrual cycles. These strategies can keep it under control and help you stay safe.

Key Prevention Strategies

Not infected? Practice safe sex—and safe kissing. If your partner has herpes blisters around the mouth or genitals, avoid skin-to-skin contact. An estimated 60 percent of adults harbor the herpesvirus—and at least one in five never have symptoms but could be contagious anyway. The reason: Tiny viral particles can migrate to the skin's surface without causing an outbreak. This is known as viral shedding, and it's dangerous because it makes it possible to pass the virus around even when no one can see it. That's why it's so important to practice safe sex. This includes using a condom during intercourse, though condoms won't always prevent spread of the virus simply because they don't cover all the areas that are infected or could become infected. The surest way to avoid genital herpes is to abstain from sexual contact or to stay in a mutually monogamous relationship with a partner who has been tested (testing for herpes antibodies is available) and is known to be uninfected.

Keep antiviral drugs on hand. These prescription pills can short-circuit a cold sore and dramatically reduce genital herpes outbreaks and viral shedding. The drugs are valacyclovir (Valtrex), acyclovir (Zovirax), and famciclovir (Famvir). In one international study of 384 women and men with genital herpes, 71 percent of those who took Valtrex every day for six months had no more outbreaks, compared to just 43 percent of those who took a placebo. Daily use can also reduce viral shedding by 94 percent, helping to keep partners infection free.

In cold sore studies, antivirals healed outbreaks in 3 days, compared to 4.3 days for placebo pills, and reduced the number of blisters by 50 percent. You can take these in advance to prevent cold sores, too, such as when you'll be outdoors in bright sunlight all day. Your doctor will tell you what dosing schedule to use.

What about antiviral creams? The truth is, many doctors don't even recommend them anymore. In some studies, they've proven no more effective than a placebo cream for clearing up blisters. And they're expensive. Having a supply of antiviral pills on hand, and even carrying some in your purse or briefcase for sudden outbreaks away from home, is a much better herpes-control strategy.

Always wear sunscreen. The sun's ultraviolet rays may reactivate the herpesvirus. In one National Institutes of Health study of 38 people prone to cold sores, 71 percent developed blisters after exposure to UV rays. The number dropped to 0 when they all wore lip balm with sunblock.

Prevention Boosters

Breathe in…breathe out…release the tension. In one survey of nearly 500 Canadian doctors, dentists, and pharmacists, 60 percent said their patients and customers complained that emotional upheaval was sure to bring on unwanted blisters. The fix: your favorite stress reduction technique. In one study, men who made time for daily relaxation had lower levels of antibodies associated with herpes.

Eat well, sleep well. Experts aren't sure why, but letting yourself become rundown increases blister risk, perhaps due to stress, lowered immunity, or both. When your life is tense, make an extra effort to turn in earlier, to order the salad at the fast-food drive-through—simply to pamper yourself so you don't feel worn out.

WHAT CAUSES IT
The herpes simplex virus. Type 1 usually causes oral herpes and type 2, genital herpes. But either type can show up in either area.

SYMPTOMS TO WATCH FOR Open sores or small, painful blisters surrounded by swollen, painful skin. Often there's pain or tingling for a day or two before the blisters appear. They typically occur around the lips or on the genitals, but they can also show up in your nose, mouth, or eyes; on your chin or fingers; or on your buttocks or the upper part of your inner thighs. Outbreaks may be accompanied by flu-like symptoms.

NEWEST THINKING
Your doctor's not talking—or you're not listening. A Canadian survey found that 75 percent of people with herpes say they were never told about antiviral drugs that can control this virus, but doctors say they're telling 60 percent of their patients about them. If you haven't heard, ask.

High Blood Pressure

If avoiding a single health problem could cut your odds of having a stroke by 30 percent, reduce your chances for a heart attack by 23 percent, and slash your risk of heart failure and dementia by half, wouldn't you drop everything and start right now? You'll reap these huge health dividends—and more—by making small changes that keep your blood pressure at a healthy level. After age 55, your odds of developing high blood pressure jump to 90 percent—unless you take action. If your numbers are already creeping over 120/80, don't wait for your doctor to get on your case.

Key Prevention Strategies

Drop those extra pounds now. Carrying extra weight, especially around your waist, raises your odds for high blood pressure by a whopping 60 percent. The reason: Belly fat pumps inflammatory compounds into your bloodstream, where they stiffen artery walls. Stiff arteries mean higher blood pressure. Excess fat can also interfere with your kidneys' ability to filter pressure-raising sodium out of your bloodstream.

Being overweight seems to be the cause of half of all cases of high blood pressure, researchers say. Losing a modest amount can protect you from this silent killer. When researchers followed 1,191 overweight women and men with high-normal blood pressure for more than two years, 65 percent of those who lost 10 pounds and kept it off nudged their blood pressure down to healthy levels.

Start sooner rather than later. Researchers suspect that over time, chemicals churned out by body fat can make artery stiffness hard to reverse.

Slash the sodium. A little sodium—a component of salt—is essential for human survival; too much is a problem. When sodium levels in your blood rise, your body pumps more water into your bloodstream to dilute it. The outcome: Your blood volume grows, and the speed of the blood pumping through your body increases. Too much sodium, research suggests, can also stiffen arteries, further raising blood pressure.

If you make just one dietary change to protect your pressure, eat less sodium. In a Duke University study of people with high blood pressure, 71 percent of those who cut back on salt but made no other menu changes brought their numbers down to normal. If your pressure is optimal, health experts recommend getting less than 2,400 milligrams of sodium a day—that's less than a teaspoon of salt. If your pressure is beginning to rise, aim for no more than 1,500 milligrams. Most of us eat nearly twice that much. And don't believe the hype that only an unlucky few are "salt sensitive"; chances are good that you are if your blood pressure has crept up even a little over the years.

When you cook, add salt at the end (if at all); long cooking dulls salt's flavor, so you're more likely to add more at the table.

Let produce lower your pressure. A low-fat diet packed with fruit and vegetables can work blood pressure–pampering magic. In one remarkable study, people with high blood pressure who followed a low-fat diet rich in fruits, veggies, and low-fat dairy products for just eight weeks lowered their systolic pressure (the top number) by 11.4 points and their diastolic pressure (the bottom number) by 5.5 points—an improvement on par with the effect of some blood pressure drugs. Blood pressure began to fall after just two weeks. Other studies show that eating this way every day can lower your odds of developing high blood pressure in the first place.

The miracle ingredients in produce? Calcium, magnesium, and potassium. These three minerals help lower pressure in several ways; for example, potassium helps the body excrete excess sodium, while calcium and magnesium work together to keep artery walls flexible.

The developers of the highly effective blood pressure–control eating plan called the DASH (Dietary Approaches to Stop Hypertension) Diet recommend four to five servings each of fruit and vegetables every day. To get the most of the miracle minerals, choose these top sources.

- **Potassium:** Baked potato with skin, tomato sauce, lima beans, orange juice, cooked spinach, winter squash, bananas, raisins, prune juice.
- **Calcium:** Dairy foods have the most, but cooked spinach, turnip greens, and broccoli are also good sources.

is your diet saltier than you think?

Most people eat double or even triple the amount of salt recommended by blood pressure experts. You could be one of them if you answer yes to one or more of these questions.

1. Do you often use prepared foods, such as frozen dinners, packaged or canned goods (including soups and vegetables), processed meats, cheeses, or bottled salad dressings?

2. Do you often eat salty snack foods, such as potato chips, salted nuts, cheese snacks, or pretzels?

3. Do you often eat in restaurants or fast-food places?

4. Do you often salt your food during cooking and/or at the table?

- **Magnesium:** Bulgur, oat bran, barley, beans (black, navy, pinto), okra, cooked spinach, plantain, pumpkin seeds.

Have milk or dairy foods two or three times a day. How about a slice of low-fat Swiss cheese on your sandwich? A smoothie whipped up with fat-free yogurt and fresh, juicy strawberries? Even homemade cocoa with fat-free milk, unsweetened cocoa, and a teaspoon of sugar (or artificial sweetener)? Developers of the DASH Diet say these treats are more than delicious; they're an essential part of a strategy to keep blood pressure healthy. Dairy foods are a top source of calcium, which helps prevent artery walls from stiffening. Stick with low-fat or fat-free versions to keep the saturated fat in your diet low. If you absolutely hate dairy products, get 600 to 900 milligrams of calcium a day in supplement form.

Keep walking shoes in your car, at your desk, and by the front door. A half hour of brisk walking three to five days a week can keep your blood pressure 5 to 6 points lower than if you didn't exercise. No time? No problem. When British researchers checked the blood pressures of 106 government workers on a walking program, they found that those who got their exercise in short bursts enjoyed the same blood pressure–lowering benefits as colleagues who preferred one longer exercise session a day.

Other research suggests that exercising in short bursts is actually better: In one study, people who used this strategy saw their numbers stay lower, longer during the day compared to people who got all their activity in one "dose."

Kick the habit. Irish researchers have found that puffing on a single cigarette makes arteries less elastic, allowing blood pressure to rise even if you're young, slim, and fit. Smoking 15 cigarettes a day raises your risk of high blood pressure by 11 percent; smoking 25 cigarettes raises it 21 percent.

Snorers, ask your bedmate this question. "Do I seem to stop breathing, then catch my breath, during the night?" If the answer is yes, or if you wake up tired despite a full night of rest, you may have obstructive sleep apnea, which makes your high blood pressure risk up to seven times higher than normal, report Pennsylvania State University researchers. Mild sleep apnea raised risk 2.5 times, and even snoring, without apnea, doubled it.

Disturbed sleep raises levels of artery-tightening stress hormones in your body. (See the Snoring entry on page 292 for solutions.)

Prevention Boosters

Reach for coffee instead of cola. Drinking just one diet cola a day raised the risk of high blood pressure by 5 percent, and a four-cans-a-day habit increased the odds by 19 percent in a landmark Harvard School of Public Health study. Risks were even higher for women who drank regular colas. Experts can't explain the association but suggest that coffee might be a better alternative; women who sipped java every day had no added risk for hypertension. While coffee triggers a temporary rise in blood pressure, it doesn't persist in people who drink it regularly.

Spend some time at "om." Regularly practicing meditation, yoga, or another relaxation technique can help pressure-proof your blood vessels. When University of Kansas scientists analyzed 107 studies of the effect of meditation on blood pressure, they concluded that it produces significant drops (one of the studies found a 10-point drop in systolic pressure and a 6-point drop in diastolic pressure). When Yale University School of Medicine researchers tested the blood pressure of 33 people taking a yoga class that met three times a week, they found improvements after just six weeks. Average blood pressure fell from 130/79 to 125/74. Tai chi has also been shown to be effective.

Sip some beet juice. That juicing machine gathering dust in your pantry could help keep your blood pressure in tiptop shape. British researchers report that drinking two cups of beet juice a day can lower your blood pressure by 8 to 10 points, fast. Volunteers who sipped two cups a day saw their pressure drop significantly after three hours and stay lower for up to a day. Emerging research suggests that nitrates in beets (and in green leafy vegetables) keep the whisper-thin lining of your arteries (called the endothelium) supple.

Have a bite of dark chocolate after dinner. That's right, just one bite! When people with slightly high blood pressure ate 30 calories' worth of dark chocolate (about the amount in one Hershey's Kiss) each night after dinner for 18 weeks, their blood pressure fell by 2 to 3 points. Artery-friendly compounds called flavonols may be responsible for the improvement. Dark chocolate is also a good source of magnesium.

WHAT CAUSES IT
Stiff arteries and excess salt play a role. Eating too much salt prompts your body to pump extra water into your bloodstream in an effort to dilute high sodium levels. Meanwhile, everything from smoking to being overweight to eating a diet low in produce, dairy, and whole grains can stiffen arteries, leaving them unable to flex, stretch, and make room for fast-moving blood.

SYMPTOMS TO WATCH FOR Usually, none. To keep tabs on your pressure, have it checked at least every two years and ask your doctor for your reading. If it's 120/80 or higher, it's time to take action—even if your doctor doesn't suggest it first. Studies show that many physicians aren't aggressive enough about putting a lid on pressure that's inching higher, especially in people over age 60.

NEWEST THINKING
There's nothing normal about "high-normal" blood pressure. Until recently, experts thought blood pressure readings between 120/80 and 140/90 were perfectly healthy. Now those levels are considered "prehypertensive" or "high normal"—and they can raise your risk of dying from heart disease by 58 percent, making this "little" problem more deadly than smoking.

High Cholesterol

17%

The amount you can lower "bad" cholesterol if you have two servings of soluble fiber (such as oatmeal and barley) every day.

Poor cholesterol—it's doomed to be misunderstood. The fact is, cholesterol is necessary to make cell membranes and even hormones. Your body produces cholesterol. Your diet also contributes, but it's not so much the cholesterol you eat as the *saturated fat* in your diet that raises your levels. Even more confusing, some cholesterol is "bad" (LDL attacks arteries and contributes to plaque buildup), while some is "good" (HDL escorts the bad stuff out of the body). Only about half of people who have heart attacks have high cholesterol, but it's still important to keep your levels healthy. For every 1-point drop in LDL, heart attack risk falls by 2 percent; every 1-point rise in HDL reduces your risk of a fatal heart attack by 3 percent.

Key Prevention Strategies

Eat less saturated fat. Yes, this is the stuff in burgers, steaks, butter, cheese, and ice cream. If you want to avoid a heart attack, you'll want to switch to skinless chicken breasts, fish, olive or canola oil, and low-fat frozen yogurt. Experts estimate that for every 2 percent decrease in calories from saturated fat—about what you'd get if you had baby carrots instead of an ounce of regular potato chips or drank two cups of fat-free milk instead of two cups of 1 percent milk—you would lower your LDL by 1 point. Keeping your daily intake of saturated fat to less than 7 percent of your daily calories—that's about one tablespoon of butter or one slice of cheddar cheese plus 1/2 cup of ice cream if you eat 1,800 calories a day—can lower your LDL by 9 to 11 percent.

cholesterol targets

Total cholesterol: Under 200 mg/dl.

LDL ("bad" cholesterol): Officially, under 160 if you have no heart disease risks, below 130 if you have some risks, under 100 if you have high risk, and below 70 if you have diabetes or have had a heart attack or stroke. But we think everyone should aim for a level under 100.

HDL ("good" cholesterol): Over 50 for women and over 40 for men.

Triglycerides: Like cholesterol, these blood fats are dangerous to the heart. Ideal levels are below 150 mg/dl.

Get the word *hydrogenated* off your menu. Read the back of a bag of chips or a box of cookies, crackers, or baked goods, and you're all too likely to see "partially hydrogenated" oil on the list. These oils, also known as trans fats, extend the shelf life of a product, but they can shorten *your* shelf life by raising LDL and triglycerides, reducing HDL, and increasing your odds of having a heart attack. In one study of 50 men with healthy cholesterol levels, eating trans fats for five weeks raised LDL 5 percent and lowered HDL a heart-damaging 11 percent.

Food served in restaurants and at fast-food chains—especially fried food—can also be high in trans fats; many eateries have promised to change the oil in their deep fryers, but not all have followed through. Even if they have, fried food is still generally too high in fat and calories to eat safely except on rare occasions.

Stop smoking. Smoking depresses levels of good cholesterol by 7 to 20 percent and at the same time can raise your bad cholesterol 70 percent, according to one analysis of several studies. It also unleashes toxic chemicals that make LDL more dangerous to arteries. Quit, and you'll see benefits fast: Levels of heart-protecting HDL bounce back within a month or two.

Eat oatmeal, barley, and/or beans every day. These three foods are packed with a type of soluble fiber called beta-glucan. It acts like a sponge, trapping cholesterol-rich bile acids in your intestines so they can be eliminated before they can raise your cholesterol. Whole grains such as whole wheat bread and brown rice, which are rich in *in*soluble fiber, just can't do that trick. In one study of 36 overweight guys, those who ate two large servings of foods rich in soluble fiber a day lowered their LDL by 17 percent. Here are three great ways to get more into your diet.

- Enjoy grated apples over oatmeal at breakfast; in one review of 10 studies, people who started the day with a big bowl of oats had LDL levels 7 points lower than those who didn't have oats.
- Cook up quick-cooking barley in just 10 minutes and serve it instead of rice. In a study from the USDA's Beltsville Human Nutrition Research Center, 25 people with slightly high cholesterol who ate barley daily for several weeks slashed their LDL by up to 17 percent.
- Enjoy beans as a main dish in chili or soup, as a side dish at lunch or dinner, or sprinkled on salads. In a University of Colorado study of

the green heart-friendly fruit

If you haven't yet discovered the rich, creamy flavor of avocados, it's time. Slice one up and enjoy a few pieces as a snack, add them to salads, or use them in sandwiches or on chili instead of cheese. In a study from Mexico's Instituto Mexicano del Seguro Social, women and men who ate one avocado a day for a week saw total cholesterol drop by 17 percent. "Bad" LDL cholesterol fell, and "good" HDL rose. The reason? Avocados are incredibly rich in heart-healthy monounsaturated fat and contain respectable levels of beta-sitosterol, the same stuff found in some cholesterol-lowering margarines.

17 people, those who ate 1/2 cup of canned pinto beans a day cut their bad cholesterol levels by 8 percent.

Snack on nuts. It seems backward, since nuts are fatty, but they really are good for your cholesterol, thanks in part to the cholesterol-lowering monounsaturated fats they contain. Choosing almonds instead of a doughnut, chips, or pretzels for your afternoon snack every day could cut "bad" cholesterol by nearly 10 percent. A bonus: Vitamin E in the almond's "meat" plus flavonoids in its papery skin protect LDL from oxidation, the first step in the development of artery-clogging plaque.

Want to raise your HDL at the same time? Choose walnuts. Bad cholesterol fell 10 percent and good cholesterol rose 18 percent when 58 women and men in one study snacked on about 14 walnut halves a day for six months.

Nuts are high in calories, so be smart about portions. A 0.5-ounce, 90-calorie serving is about 12 almonds, 8 whole cashews, 8 pecans, 26 pistachios, or 7 walnut halves. Double that for a 180-calorie serving. One great portion-control trick: Stash 22 almonds in a metal breath-mint box and munch them instead of a candy bar at work.

Feast on fruit, double your vegetables. Filling up on produce by aiming for nine servings of fruit and vegetables a day can reduce your LDL by as much as 7 percent. Researchers aren't sure why, but it could be because of soluble fiber, which blocks the reabsorption of cholesterol found in the bile acids (digestive juices) that make their way into your intestines. This effectively lowers your LDL levels. Apples, pears, and prunes are all good sources of soluble fiber. Or it could be even simpler: People who eat more produce probably eat fewer fatty meats, snacks, and desserts.

mind over cholesterol?

Stress can raise levels of "bad" LDL cholesterol— and relaxation exercises such as yoga and tai chi can lower them, studies suggest. In one study of 113 people with heart disease, researchers from India report that those who added regular yoga sessions to a healthy diet lowered their LDL by 26 percent after one year. If yoga doesn't appeal to you, relax regularly in any way that's soothing.

Get moving to boost good cholesterol. Recently, doctors have discovered that having high levels of good cholesterol is every bit as important as having low levels of the bad stuff. Unfortunately, there aren't a lot of effective ways to increase your HDL— but exercise is one of them! Aerobic exercise, whether it's walking, swimming, biking, or even working hard in your garden, can raise HDL by 5 to 10 percent. If you're also following a healthy diet, adding exercise can nudge LDL down 3 to 16 points, other studies suggest. A recent Japanese study of 1,400 people found that those who got 40 minutes of brisk walking four times a week raised their HDL by about 2 points—enough to lower heart disease risk by about 6 percent. For raising HDL, longer workouts are better than several short ones.

Prevention Boosters

Women: Lift one glass. Men: Have up to two. Studies suggest that people who drink alcohol in moderation (one drink per day for women and up to two for men) get a double cholesterol benefit. In one study, a glass a day lowered LDL nearly 8 points. Drinking moderately also increases HDL; in one Dutch study, HDL rose by a respectable 7 percent.

Trim your personal fat zones. Losing about 6 percent of your body weight (about 11 pounds if you now weight 180) could lower your LDL by 12 percent and raise your HDL by 18 percent, researchers say. The best pounds-off strategy for making your cholesterol numbers healthier? A moderate-fat diet with lots of fruit, vegetables, and unsaturated fat from fish, nuts, and olive and canola oils. Skip extremely low fat diets. While research shows that they can make plaque in arteries shrink, they're impossibly difficult for most people to follow. And plenty of studies show that a moderate-fat diet not only protects your ticker well but is also much more pleasurable.

Nudge your LDL lower with sterols and stanols. These natural compounds, found in many cholesterol-lowering fortified foods like margarines and orange juice, block the absorption of some cholesterol in your intestines. In one study, people with normal cholesterol levels who used margarines fortified with sterols and stanols saw their bad cholesterol decrease 7 to 11 percent after three months. Experts recommend getting up to two grams of sterols and stanols a day, about the amount in 2 1/2 tablespoons of fortified margarine or two eight-ounce glasses of fortified orange juice. Eat an extra serving of red, yellow, or orange fruit or vegetables a day if you use these cholesterol-lowering products; they can reduce absorption of heart-friendly compounds called carotenoids from the foods you eat.

WHAT CAUSES IT
For most people, a high-fat diet plus a sedentary lifestyle combine to raise levels of "bad" LDL and decrease "good" HDL. Cholesterol levels also rise with age. Your genes play a role, too: A few people inherit a genetic mutation that raises total cholesterol sky-high (over 600 mg/dl).

SYMPTOMS TO WATCH FOR Usually none. If you have inherited familial hypercholesterolemia, you may develop small, bumpy cholesterol deposits on your elbows, knees, and buttocks. If you have them, have your cholesterol checked right away; diet and exercise can help, but it's likely you'll need medications to bring levels down to normal.

NEWEST THINKING
Don't worry (too much) about cholesterol in food. Studies show that for most people, foods like whole eggs and even shrimp won't raise bad cholesterol. Harvard researchers have found, for example, that eating up to seven eggs a week doesn't raise LDL levels. And despite the fact that 12 large shrimp deliver 200 milligrams of cholesterol, a Rockefeller University study found that people who ate shrimp did raise their LDL slightly, but their cholesterol ratios improved because HDL rose even higher and triglycerides fell.

Hip Fractures

19%

The amount you can cut your fracture risk by taking a daily calcium/ vitamin D supplement.

The most common reason for hip fractures? Falling, particularly if you're 65 or older. In fact, about 1 percent of all falls in older people result in hip fractures. The injury means more than time lost to healing or surgery; it also increases the risk of dying during the following year by 20 to 36 percent, partly because it sends many older people to nursing homes, where they may experience a downward spiral. There are two main ways to prevent hip fractures: prevent falls, and maintain your bone density so that if you *do* fall, you wind up with a bruised—not broken—hip.

Key Prevention Strategies

Take a daily calcium and vitamin D supplement. Aim for a total of 1,200 milligrams of calcium (taken in two doses) and a minimum of 1,000 IU of vitamin D. (Anyone with darker skin and/or living in northern climates needs 2,000 IU of vitamin D a day.) The combination throws a one-two punch at the bone-thinning disease osteoporosis, which turns solid bones into Swiss cheese. One analysis of eight studies found that supplementing with the two nutrients reduced the risk of hip fractures by 19 percent. Surprisingly, vitamin D may even help prevent falls. One large study found that women with low blood levels of D were 77 percent more likely to fall than women with normal levels.

Circle the block 15 times. Weak legs can increase your risk of falling fourfold. Bolster your leg strength with that most basic yet effective exercise: walking. Aim for at least 30 minutes a day on most days. To further protect yourself, throw in a few lunges and squats. Another good exercise for improving balance and leg strength is tai chi. Studies find it effective for improving balance, strengthening legs, and reducing the risk of falls.

Get your vision checked. You're 2.5 times more likely to fall if you have vision problems than if you don't. That means getting glasses, increasing your prescription strength, or having your cataracts removed could prevent a broken hip.

Ask your doctor to review your meds. Certain drugs, including tranquilizers, some antidepressants, anti-arrhythmia drugs, digoxin (used to treat congestive heart failure), and diuretics significantly increase the risk of a fall. Regardless of what you're taking, if you take three or more medications, you're also more likely to fall than someone who takes fewer. Never stop taking a prescription drug without talking to your doctor, though.

Hire a professional organizer. Ask for help in decluttering your house, focusing not only on surfaces but on the floor as well. Throw rugs, floor plants or decorations, and end tables filled with pictures and knickknacks can all trip you up. You can find an organizer in your area by visiting the National Association of Professional Organizers Web site at www.napo.net.

Prevention Boosters

Install bright bulbs. No matter how good your eyesight is, if it's too dark to clearly see obstacles in your way, you're heading for a fall. Make sure all reading lamps have at least 60-watt bulbs but preferably 75 watts; put 100-watt bulbs in all overhead fixtures and turn on the lights when you enter a room.

Check your mood. Are you depressed? If you are, get to the doctor now for treatment. Depression doubles your risk of falling. Researchers don't know why, but it could be related to paying less attention, drinking more alcohol, eating less food, or even side effects of the medication (although few antidepressants cause dizziness these days). Turn to page 148 for prevention tips.

Sip water all day. Although the old target of drinking eight glasses of water a day has gone by the wayside, staying hydrated is still important, particularly as you age. One reason is that it becomes harder to recognize thirst as you get older; also, many older people don't want to drink too much because they're afraid they might not make it to the bathroom in time. (If that's your worry, see page 220.) Dehydration contributes to low blood pressure and dizziness, which, of course, contributes to falls. A good strategy is to keep a water bottle with you and make it a point to empty it by the time you go to the bathroom.

Strap on some hip pads. These devices, sold at medical supply stores, are worn over the hips but under clothing. An analysis of 11 studies found they could reduce the risk of hip fractures in nursing-home patients by 23 percent.

WHAT CAUSES IT
Ninety-five percent of hip fractures are due to falls. Fractures are most common in older people because they are more likely to have lower bone density, making their bones more likely to break.

SYMPTOMS TO WATCH FOR Dizziness and problems with your vision are warnings that a fall may be in your future. While osteoporosis has few symptoms, any fracture after age 50 is a warning sign that you may have a bone density issue. If you do fracture your hip, you'll have pain and be unable to walk.

NEWEST THINKING
An infusion of zoledronic acid (Zometa), a drug used to treat bone loss in cancer patients, within 90 days after surgery to fix a hip fracture could reduce the risk of new fractures by 35 percent in the following two years and cut the risk of death by nearly 30 percent.

Balance Exercises

One of the best ways to prevent falls—and therefore hip fractures—is by improving your balance and strengthening the muscles in your legs and around your hips. The following exercises are designed to do just that.

Start out by holding onto a sturdy chair or table. As you get stronger and your balance improves, hold on more loosely and then with just one finger; finally, don't hold on at all.

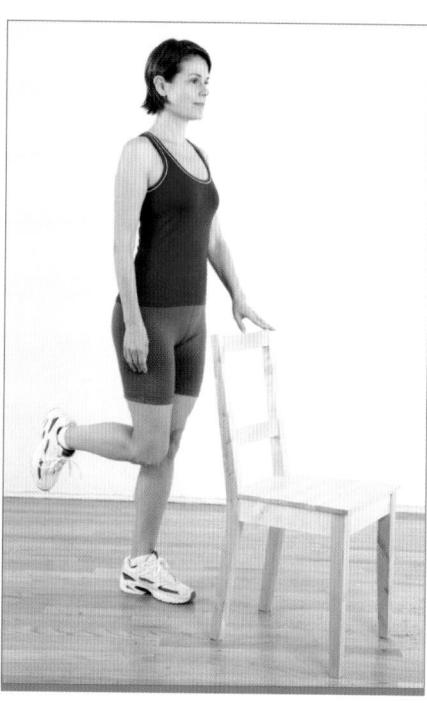

Knee Bend

1 Stand straight with one hand on a table or chair back for balance.

2 Bend your right leg at the knee, bringing your foot as far up behind you as possible. Hold for 5 seconds, then lower your foot and repeat with your left leg. Repeat 10 times on each side.

Heel Raise

1 Stand straight with one hand on a table or chair back for balance.

2 Rise on the balls of your feet as high as possible. Hold for 5 seconds, then lower your heels to the floor. Repeat 15 times. Rest for a minute, then repeat another 15 times.

Hip Stretch

1 Stand sideways behind a chair, with one hand holding onto the back for balance.

2 Slowly raise one knee toward your chest while keeping your waist and hips straight. Hold for 5 seconds, then slowly lower your leg and repeat with the other leg. Repeat 10 times on each side.

Hip Strengthener

1 Stand 12 to 18 inches away from a table or behind a chair. Lean forward and hold onto the table or chair with both hands.

2 Slowly lift one leg back and up without bending the knee. Hold for 5 seconds, then slowly lower your leg and repeat with the other leg. Repeat 10 times on both sides.

Side Leg Raise

1 Stand straight and hold onto a table or chair back for support.

2 Keeping your back straight, slowly raise one leg to the side as far as you can. Hold for 5 seconds, then slowly lower your leg and repeat with the other leg. Repeat 10 times on each side.

Hot Flashes

90%

The amount by which supplemental estrogen therapy can reduce hot flashes.

It begins as warmth in your chest, then slowly rises into your neck and face like mercury rising in a thermometer. A few minutes later, you're chilled and shivering. It's not a fever but a hot flash, something 80 percent of women experience as they move through the menopausal transition. Most women aren't too bothered by them, but for some, hot flashes and their nocturnal cousins, night sweats, can make life miserable. Here's how to keep hot flashes to a minimum.

Key Prevention Strategies

Take hormone replacement therapy (HRT). Nothing works as well as supplemental estrogen to cool hot flashes, with studies finding it reduces episodes by up to 90 percent. The key is to take the lowest possible dose for the shortest possible time. Although a major study found higher rates of breast cancer, heart disease, and stroke in women who took an estrogen-plus-progestin drug (progestin is included with estrogen therapy to lower the risk of uterine cancer) and higher rates of stroke in women who took an estrogen-only drug, major medical organizations say it's safe to use HRT short term (a year or two) to get you through the worst of the menopausal transition. The risks of any health problems are even lower if you're under 60.

Take a soy supplement. Make it one that contains isoflavone aglycones, phytoestrogens found in soy products. A study of 190 menopausal women who received either a placebo or 40 or 60 milligrams a day of a supplement containing these compounds for 12 weeks had about half as many hot flashes by the study's end, while the placebo group had about 39 percent fewer hot flashes. In another study, women who took an extract containing 40 milligrams of isoflavones every day for 10 months reported that the severity of their hot flashes dropped by 70 percent, compared to a 34 percent drop in the placebo group. Don't overdo it with soy, however; large amounts could slightly increase your risk of breast cancer. If you've already had an estrogen-dependent form of breast cancer, skip the soy.

Try antidepressants. No, not for depression, but to prevent hot flashes. Researchers trying to find nonestrogen options to relieve hot flashes in women with breast cancer stumbled onto the cooling benefits of certain antidepressants prescribed in lower-than-normal doses. These include venlafaxine (Effexor), fluoxetine (Prozac), and paroxetine (Paxil). Studies find they can reduce the number of hot flashes by up to 63 percent compared to a placebo.

Prevention Boosters

Drop a dress size. Researchers used to think that having a bit of extra padding would actually reduce hot flashes because hormones in body fat called androgens are converted to estrogen, which helps prevent hot flashes. It turns out they were wrong. A study of women ages 47 to 59 found that those with the highest percentages of body fat were about 27 percent more likely to have hot flashes than those with lower percentages. Ideally, aim for body fat levels below 33 percent (but above 5 percent). There are devices you can buy to measure your body fat percentage; your gym may have one. Your doctor can also perform a more accurate test. In this study, the average body fat percentage was 37.9.

While losing weight will certainly reduce your overall body fat, strength training is your best option for converting fat into muscle (and losing the aforementioned dress size, even if your weight remains the same). Consider a couple of sessions with a personal trainer to get you started.

See a homeopath. Homeopathy is a controversial treatment option, and very few studies have been done on its effects on hot flashes. One study, however, had 99 physicians in eight countries prescribe homeopathic medicines to 438 women with hot flashes. The most prescribed medicines were Lachesis, Belladonna, Sepia, Sulphur, and Sanguinaria. Ninety percent of the women said their symptoms either disappeared or were not nearly as severe. Find a practitioner trained in homeopathy rather than trying to treat yourself.

Consider vitamin E. Studies on its benefits for preventing hot flashes are mixed, but one recent study in which 51 women received either 400 IU of vitamin E or a placebo found that those taking vitamin E had about two fewer hot flashes a day compared to when they took a placebo, and the flashes they did have were less severe. High doses may increase the risk of stroke, so be sure to talk with your doctor before supplementing with vitamin E, and don't take more than 400 IU.

WHAT CAUSES IT
Fluctuating levels of estrogen and progesterone. These fluctuations affect the temperature control system in the brain so it overreacts to tiny changes in temperature by dilating blood vessels in a mistaken attempt to cool you down.

SYMPTOMS TO WATCH FOR A feeling of warmth, flushing, heavy perspiration. When hot flashes occur at night, they can disrupt sleep and leave you lying in a muddle of wet sheets.

NEWEST THINKING
Ultra-low doses of estrogen, as little as 25 percent of previously used conventional doses, can still significantly improve a woman's hot flashes.

Incontinence

81%

The term "overactive bladder" may have been dreamed up by marketing gurus at some pharmaceutical company, but the reality is that up to 25 percent of women and 5 percent of men under 65—and much higher numbers of those who are older—experience some form of urinary incontinence at some point. It's embarrassing, smelly, and one of the major reasons older people end up in nursing homes. Follow these recommendations to stay dry.

Key Prevention Strategies

Do Kegel exercises every day. These exercises strengthen the pelvic floor muscles, which help control the release of urine. The stronger the muscles are, the less likely you are to have an accident. In fact, Kegels are even better than medication at improving existing incontinence. They are particularly effective in pregnant women and in men who have undergone surgery for prostate cancer.

You can do them anytime, anywhere because no one knows you're doing them. First, figure out which muscles to target by stopping in midstream when you're urinating. The muscles you use to do this are your pelvic floor muscles. To perform Kegels, squeeze those muscles and hold for a count of 10. Relax, then repeat. Perform at least three sets of 10 contractions a day.

Eat smaller portions. You'll lose weight, which studies find is one of the most effective ways, next to pelvic floor exercises, to prevent incontinence. Always dole out appropriate-size portions onto your dinner plate and leave the platter on the stove or elsewhere in the kitchen—not on the dinner table, where you'll be tempted to go for seconds. Another trick: Use the smallest dinner plates you own. The plate will be fuller, so it will look like you're eating more.

Put your bladder on a schedule. Doctors think one reason for incontinence is that some people tend to go too often. This can reduce the amount your bladder can hold and teaches your bladder muscles to send "must go" signals even when your bladder is barely half full. If you find yourself going every hour or two, try bladder training. Numerous studies find that this approach, which strengthens bladder muscles, improves incontinence, so there's good reason to think it could help prevent it in the first place.

One way to train your bladder is to start out by going to the bathroom every hour whether you have to or not. The next day, go every hour and a half. Continue to increase the time between bathroom visits by 30 minutes a day until you're going about every few hours, or whatever timeframe works best for you to prevent incontinence. Also, make sure you empty your bladder after each meal.

Prevention Boosters

Avoid caffeine. If you're a tea drinker, you're more likely to develop incontinence, according to a large Norwegian study. It may or may not be due to the caffeine; researchers suspect that tea contains other chemicals that contribute to incontinence, although they don't yet know what they are. There *is* a link between caffeine and incontinence if you drink more than four cups a day.

Avoid a hysterectomy. Studies suggest that women who have hysterectomies, the most common gynecological surgeries in the world, are twice as likely to later require surgery for urinary incontinence than women who don't have them. Many hysterectomies are medically unnecessary; if your doctor recommends one, ask about other options and get a second opinion.

WHAT CAUSES IT
There are numerous causes, ranging from urinary tract infections to pregnancy to being overweight. Over time, particularly after menopause in women, bladder muscles can thin and weaken. In men, removing the prostate can lead to incontinence. And in both men and women, weak pelvic floor muscles often play a role.

SYMPTOMS TO WATCH FOR Releasing small amounts of urine when you laugh, sneeze, cough, or otherwise exert yourself and/or a sudden urge to urinate that you may or may not be able to control until you get to the bathroom.

NEWEST THINKING
An injection of botulinum A (Botox) into the bladder muscle can improve incontinence even in people who haven't responded to medication or other treatments.

WEIGHT LOSS IS ONE OF THE MOST EFFECTIVE WAYS TO PREVENT INCONTINENCE.

Infertility

25%

The increase in fertility that women can achieve by taking 750 milligrams of vitamin C a day.

Within a year of trying, 92 percent of healthy couples will find themselves pregnant. The other 6 percent, however, face the possibility that they will never become pregnant without medical help for one or both partners. Don't automatically blame the female half of the couple; the cause of infertility is just as likely to lie with men as with women. Our advice for reducing the risk of infertility includes options for both of you.

Key Prevention Strategies

Start trying to conceive early. The odds of getting pregnant plummet with age. In men, the drop usually begins in the early forties thanks to sperm that, like men themselves, tend to move slower with age. Women are most fertile between 19 and 26, when they have a one-in-two chance of getting pregnant if they have sex when they're most fertile (typically, two days after ovulating). A woman age 35 to 39 has only about a one-third chance of getting pregnant during that time, and less if her partner is at least five years older.

Maintain a healthy weight. In women, obesity plays havoc with reproductive hormones, more than doubling the risk of infertility and increasing by tenfold the likelihood that it will take longer than usual to get pregnant. In men, a 20-pound weight gain increases the risk of infertility by about 10 percent. If you decide to lose weight by dieting, consider a high-protein, low-carbohydrate approach, which several studies suggest works best to return reproductive hormones to normal levels.

boxers or briefs?

As it turns out, it probably doesn't matter. For a long time, experts advised men to switch to boxers since briefs, which are tighter, trap more heat in the area. This heat was thought to cause a drop in sperm count. But recent studies discount this theory. Researchers measured scrotal temperatures among 97 men who wore either boxers or briefs and found that those who wore boxers were just as heated as those who wore briefs.

Quit smoking. Men, did you ever consider that your smoking habit lessens your chances of getting your wife pregnant? It does. Smoking creates free radicals, molecules that damage healthy cells. Having too many free radicals, also triggered by a poor diet, affects how many sperm you make and how fast they swim.

Prevention Boosters

Chill out. It's not clear whether stress contributes to infertility or vice versa, but studies find that infertile women who seek help from assisted reproductive techniques like in vitro fertilization (IVF) have much higher levels of stress hormones than women who aren't infertile. Studies also find higher levels of stress hormones in women with disturbances in their menstrual cycles that could affect fertility, such as endometriosis. One study also found lower rates of pregnancy associated with higher stress levels in couples undergoing IVF.

Switch from wine to water. Women trying to become pregnant shouldn't wait until they conceive to go on the wagon. One study of healthy women who were not alcoholics found that those who imbibed more than three drinks a day had disrupted menstrual cycles and temporary infertility.

Consider some supplements. A German study of 7,900 women found that taking a daily multivitamin for a month before trying to get pregnant increased women's fertility rate by 5 percent compared to taking a placebo containing trace elements.

Studies also find improved fertility in men and women who take vitamin C supplements. In men, supplementing daily with 200 to 1,000 milligrams of C increases sperm production. Buy a vitamin C supplement that contains flavonoids; the two together work better than either alone to reduce oxidative damage to sperm. In women, the dose required to boost fertility was 750 milligrams a day. Don't take more than 500 milligrams at once, however; your body can't absorb more than that.

Men should also consider selenium and vitamin E, both strong antioxidants. A study of 54 infertile men found that those who supplemented daily with 400 IU of vitamin E and 225 micrograms of selenium for three months had healthier and faster sperm. Talk with your doctor before taking either of these supplements.

Get regular screenings. Women who are sexually active but aren't in committed relationships should be screened at least annually for sexually transmitted infections (STIs). They can cause pelvic inflammatory disease, in which bacteria move up through the cervix into the uterus and fallopian tubes, creating scarring that can prevent a normal pregnancy. In addition to STIs, men should be checked regularly for inflammation of the prostate gland. All can damage sperm.

WHAT CAUSES IT

In women, common causes include problems with ovulation, such as polycystic ovary syndrome (PCOS), blocked fallopian tubes, and endometriosis, in which uterine tissue grows outside the uterus. In men, the most common causes are slow sperm, low sperm count, and malformed sperm.

SYMPTOMS TO WATCH FOR

If you are under 35 and have been trying to get pregnant for a year or more with no success, or if you're 35 or older and have been trying for at least six months, you should see a doctor. Also see a doctor if you or your partner has any known fertility issues (such as previous cancer treatment, endometriosis, blocked fallopian tubes, etc.) or other reproductive problems (uterine fibroids or ovarian cysts in women or testicular problems in men).

NEWEST THINKING

Chlamydia reproduces inside the early bundle of cells that forms after conception and replicates, which hinders the cells' production of estrogen and progesterone, hormones needed to keep the embryo growing. This can lead to early miscarriage.

Inflammatory Bowel Disease

66%

The drop in your risk if you load your plate with produce, whole grains, fish, and nuts—and stay away from meats and sweets.

Inflammatory bowel disease (IBD) encompasses two painful and sometimes life-threatening conditions: ulcerative colitis and Crohn's disease. Both trigger ongoing inflammation of the intestinal system, leading to pain, sometimes-debilitating diarrhea, and infections. For many, surgery to remove parts of the intestines brings relief. While most IBD begins in young adulthood, experts have noticed an upswing among people in their fifties and sixties. If you don't have IBD, the strategies here can lower your odds, which is especially important if close family members have this disease. If you do have it, these steps can help you avoid relapses and sidestep complications.

Key Prevention Strategies

Stop smoking. Smoking cigarettes tripled the risk of Crohn's disease in one Scandinavian study of 317 sets of twins. If you already have Crohn's, continuing to smoke raises your odds for relapses and needing bowel surgery or aggressive drug treatment. The reason? Experts suspect that smoking strangles blood flow to your intestines or somehow puts your immune system on high alert, making the intestinal walls extra sensitive. Oddly, smoking seems to slightly reduce the number of flare-ups for people with ulcerative colitis—but that's no reason to light up! Smoking's just too hazardous for your health in many other ways.

Eat more vegetables, fruits, olive oil, fish, grains, and nuts. At the same time, have less red meat and fatty foods (like french fries and nachos with cheese). Canadian researchers who studied 400 children found that those who ate diets packed with produce; whole grains; and good fats from fish, nuts, and olive oil cut their IBD risk by two-thirds compared to those whose diets included more meats, saturated fats, and sweets. Eating the "bad" diet raised risk nearly five times higher than normal, report the researchers from the University of Montreal.

When the scientists looked more closely, they found that the most protective dietary components were fiber (think fruit, vegetables, and whole grains) and omega-3 fatty acids. You'll find those in fish, walnuts, flaxseed, canola oil, and, if you don't eat some source of good fats every day, in fish-oil capsules.

Kick the sugar habit. Many people are addicted to sugar and don't even realize how much they're consuming. Instead of a cookie or candy bar in the afternoon or cake for dessert, have fresh fruit instead. While eating more fruit cut the risk of IBD in several studies, eating more desserts and refined sugar tripled the odds of developing Crohn's disease and ulcerative colitis. In one study, people who developed Crohn's reported eating twice as much refined sugar in the months and years before their diagnoses as people without this painful condition.

Use pain relievers sparingly. Aspirin and other nonsteroidal anti-inflammatory pain relievers like ibuprofen and naproxen can all raise the risk for a relapse of IBD, probably because they can damage the lining of the upper intestinal tract. In one study, 28 percent of people with IBD taking these drugs had a relapse within nine days. If you have IBD plus arthritis or another chronic pain condition (or just need relief for a big headache), talk with your doctor about your options. There's some evidence that acetaminophen and the prescription pain reliever celecoxib (Celebrex) don't trigger relapses.

Cut back on red meat and processed meats. When researchers at the University of Newcastle in England followed 191 people with ulcerative colitis for one year, they found that those who ate red meat (like roast beef, hamburgers, and steaks) and processed meats (such as sausage and hot dogs) the most often were five times more likely to have painful relapses than those who ate very little of these foods.

Go easy on the alcohol. In the same British study, people who drank the most alcohol were four times more likely to have relapses of ulcerative colitis compared to those who drank little, if any, beer, wine, or spirits.

Skip cola drinks and chocolate. When researchers from the Netherlands checked on the eating habits and relapse rates of 688 people with IBD and 616 people without it, they discovered that these two dietary splurges were big troublemakers. Drinking cola and nibbling on chocolate doubled the risk of both ulcerative colitis and Crohn's disease.

got the gene?

Having a parent or sibling with Crohn's disease raises your own risk 6 times higher than normal; having a close family member with ulcerative colitis raises your risk 2.5 times. Scientists have begun to identify the genes behind IBD, and they hope their discoveries will yield new treatments. One promising lead: In a study of nearly 2,000 people, Yale researchers have uncovered a genetic variation that appears to play an important role in raising risk. Those with an "unhealthy" version of a gene called IL23R were two to four times more likely to develop IBD than those with a "healthy" variant. This gene helps regulate inflammation, the core problem in IBD.

Prevention Boosters

Snack on yogurt. Your intestines are home to millions of bacteria. Some of them are there to help digest the food you eat and keep your bowels healthy. But different bacteria—the "bad guys"—may contribute to or even cause IBD problems. Having enough beneficial bacteria in your body keeps the troublesome types in check. You can make sure you have enough by eating yogurt that contains active cultures or by taking a probiotic ("good" bacteria) supplement.

When researchers at the University of Alberta in Canada gave a probiotic supplement to 34 people with mild to moderate ulcerative colitis, 53 percent felt completely better after eight weeks, and 24 percent felt somewhat better. The supplement, called VSL, contained eight species of lactobacillus bacteria, a type also found in yogurt with live, active cultures. In another Canadian study, researchers found that when people with ulcerative colitis and Crohn's disease ate yogurt every day for a month, blood tests showed that inflammation levels in their intestinal tracts were reduced. Some studies suggest that probiotics are more helpful for preventing relapses of ulcerative colitis and less helpful for Crohn's.

Take a break. Stress doesn't cause IBD, but it may make it worse. Some studies suggest that stress increases levels of inflammation in the intestines and that the inflammation persists even when your stress levels subside. It makes sense to find time to unwind on a regular basis, in whatever way works for you—time in the garden, yoga, a hot bath, a good book, or breathing deeply as you let tension flow out of your body.

Drink lots of water. If you already have IBD, you're at risk for dehydration due to frequent and severe diarrhea, which flushes excess fluid from your body. Be sure to drink

have IBD? protect your bones

As many as 60 percent of people with IBD may have low bone density, raising the risk of osteoporosis and bone fractures. The reason: Long-term use of glucocorticoid drugs (such as prednisone and cortisone) that keep a lid on intestinal inflammation can also interfere with your body's ability to maintain healthy bones. And if you have severe IBD or have had surgery to remove part of your intestines, your body may not absorb enough calcium and vitamin D, nutrients essential for strong bones. It's smart to take in 1,000 milligrams of calcium a day (1,200 a day after age 50). You'll get there with three servings of low-fat dairy foods a day or a mix of dairy plus calcium supplements (don't take more than 600 milligrams with a meal, since your body can't absorb more than that at once). And get at least 400 to 800 IU of vitamin D daily, too, to help your body absorb and use all that calcium. Weight-bearing exercise such as walking also helps. Talk with your doctor about whether you need a bone density test or are a candidate for bone-strengthening osteoporosis medications.

plenty of fluids every day; some experts recommend 0.5 ounce for each pound of body weight. If you weigh 160 pounds, that's 80 ounces—or ten 8-ounce glasses of water or other fluids a day. And watch for signs of dehydration such as dry mouth, extreme thirst, or weakness.

Avoid dietary irritants. Normally we're cheerleaders for foods like whole wheat bread, fruits, vegetables, and nuts. But if you have Crohn's disease that isn't improving, cutting back could give your intestinal tract the break it needs. Avoid berries (because of the seeds), whole grain breads and cereals, potatoes with skin, nuts and seeds, raw fruits and vegetables, and tough cuts of meat. Do this under your doctor's care; he may want you to add back some of the foods once the inflammation subsides.

For ulcerative colitis, consider soluble fiber. Soluble fiber forms a protective gel in your intestinal tract and releases compounds that soothe inflammation and promote healing of the intestinal wall. Ask your doctor if you should eat a daily serving of foods such as barley, oatmeal, pears, and beans, or if you should try a fiber supplement with ingredients like methylcellulose (Citrucel) or psyllium (Metamucil).

Watch your reaction to dairy. An estimated 35 percent of people with Crohn's disease and 12 to 20 percent of those with ulcerative colitis lack the digestive enzyme that breaks down the sugars in milk. If milk, ice cream, and cheese cause discomfort, switch to milk with added lactase and take lactase tablets before eating dairy foods. Yogurt with live, active cultures is usually safe.

WHAT CAUSES IT

Inflammation of the intestines. Experts don't know what triggers it but suspect that genetics and an immune system response—perhaps to "bad" bacteria in the intestinal tract, or perhaps to nothing at all—are responsible.

SYMPTOMS TO WATCH FOR

Diarrhea, which can range from slightly loose stools to dozens of liquid bowel movements per day; abdominal pain and cramps; blood in the stool; lack of appetite; weight loss. You may also have fatigue, night sweats, and/or fever.

NEWEST THINKING

Doctors aren't screening enough people with IBD for colon cancer. If you have Crohn's disease or ulcerative colitis, your risk of developing colon cancer is up to five times higher than normal. Experts recommend early checks for this cancer, with a colonoscopy 8 to 10 years after you first have IBD symptoms.

BE SURE TO DRINK PLENTY OF FLUIDS EVERY DAY.

Prevent **Inflammatory Bowel Disease** 227

Insomnia

50%

The amount you could reduce the risk by practicing techniques like progressive muscle relaxation when you get into bed.

Having a hard time falling asleep may seem like no big deal when compared to, say, having heart disease. But in fact, insomnia raises the risk of depression, makes you more sensitive to pain, compromises concentration and memory, and significantly increases the risk of accidents while driving. There's even evidence that poor sleep wreaks havoc with the hormones that control appetite and metabolism and may be partly responsible for the current obesity epidemic. To prevent insomnia and guarantee a good night's sleep, follow this advice.

Key Prevention Strategies

Stick to a regular sleep schedule. That means going to bed at the same time every night and waking up at the same time in the morning, even on weekends. Think of it as training your body to fall asleep when it should.

Create the perfect sleeping environment. If you have bills stacked on the nightstand or piles of laundry waiting to be washed or folded, your bedroom is hardly an oasis for sleep. Clear the clutter and move the bills to another room. Also banish the TV and computer from the bedroom, which should be used only for sleeping and intimate time with your partner. Don't read in it, eat in it, or work in it. Don't even talk on the phone in it. This way, as soon as you enter the room at night, your body knows it's time for sleep.

If your windows let in too much light, it may also help to invest in room-darkening shades. And keep the room cool, which helps induce sleep.

Limit your time in bed. The harder you try to fall asleep, the less likely you will. If you haven't fallen asleep in 15 minutes, get out of bed and move to another room. Do something quiet, like reading or needlepoint, until you feel sleepy enough to nod off, then go back to bed. Continue this pattern until you finally fall asleep.

Walk outside. Exercise can improve sleep, and doing it outside in bright sunlight can have an even greater effect by ensuring that your body clock is properly set. In one study, people who got 30 minutes a day of bright light therapy with full-spectrum lamps that mimic sunlight (available online and in lighting stores) increased their total sleep time by 44 minutes.

Hit the gym or take a jog. One of the best ways to get a good night's sleep is to exercise. Studies find that in athletes, just one day without exercise leads to worse sleep and increases the time they need to fall asleep. Most researchers think that exercise reduces insomnia in part by raising body temperature. If you exercise vigorously enough to raise your temperature in the late afternoon, it will fall around bedtime—and decreased body temperature naturally triggers sleep. Exercise also helps by lowering stress hormones. Most people with insomnia have high levels of these hormones, or they release them with very little provocation. Exercise initially increases the hormones, but a few hours later, seeking to return to balance, your body sends out signals to reduce them. That's why you shouldn't exercise in the evening; try to end your workout at least six hours before bedtime.

Prevention Boosters

Talk to a therapist. A form of therapy called cognitive behavioral therapy (CBT) can help with insomnia by teaching you techniques to overcome it—and your anxiety about it. For instance, after a few sleepless nights, many people begin to stress about their ability to *ever* fall asleep, starting what becomes a self-perpetuating cycle. They also underestimate how much sleep they actually get and overestimate how much time they

10 soothing ways to fall asleep

1. **Sip a cup of chamomile tea before bed.** There's a reason it's called "Sleepy Time" tea.

2. **Cover your eyes.** You can find eye masks in the drugstore. They work wonders for banishing even the tiniest glow of a nightlight.

3. **Cool down your bedroom.** Open the windows, turn on a ceiling fan, or run the air conditioner. Reducing your body temperature signals your brain to release the sleep hormone melatonin.

4. **Read a book of poetry.** The cadences of the lines and the images the words invoke can be much more calming than a novel. Better yet, listen to poetry on tape or CD—it's almost like hearing a bedtime story.

5. **Make a list.** Before you get into bed, make a list of everything that's on your mind. Then you don't have to lie awake worrying about it.

6. **Listen to white noise.** Turn on a loud fan, tune the radio to a station with static, or buy a white-noise machine.

7. **Spray lavender scent on your pillow and sheets.** Lavender is known for its calming effects.

8. **Try progressive muscle relaxation.** Starting with your feet and working up to your eyes, tense and relax one group of muscles at a time. This forces every muscle in your body to relax.

9. **Sleep in your underwear.** You'll feel cooler and sleep better.

10. **Wear earplugs.** They can come in particularly handy if you sleep with someone who snores (or a dog).

spend lying awake. CBT helps put things into perspective by teaching you more about insomnia and how to address it.

Skip the martini. While alcohol may help you fall asleep, you're likely to wake up again as the effects wear off and find yourself unable to fall back to sleep. If you want a drink, have it in the late afternoon or early evening.

Stay away from cigarettes. Nicotine is a central nervous system stimulant, which means it keeps you awake. Even just being around cigarette smoke within a couple of hours of bedtime could interfere with your ability to fall asleep or stay asleep.

Check your medications. Numerous drugs, particularly some prescribed for attention deficit disorder, high blood pressure, asthma, underactive thyroid, depression, and neurological problems like Parkinson's disease, can keep you up at night. If you're having trouble drifting off or staying asleep, ask your doctor whether one of your medications may be to blame and what you can do about it.

Get treated for allergies. Sneezing your head off because of pollen and other seasonal allergens may be more than annoying: It may keep you up at night. French researchers found that 41.6 percent of people with seasonal allergies said they had trouble falling asleep compared with just 18.3 percent of those who didn't have allergies. The worse the allergies, the longer it took people to fall asleep, and the more sleeping pills they took.

Swallow a pill. To prevent occasional insomnia, over-the-counter or prescription sleeping pills can help and, if you use them only for the short term, probably won't hurt. Over-the-counter sleeping aids contain an antihistamine, either alone or together with a painkiller. They can leave you with a sleep "hangover" the next day, however. A better option is one of the newer prescription sleep aids, such as eszopiclone (Lunesta), zaleplon (Sonata), zolpidem (Ambien), or ramelteon (Rozerem). The first three are sedatives. They work similarly and carry a risk of similar side effects, including performing activities while you're asleep, like eating or even driving. Rozerem works differently, helping reset your circadian rhythm by mimicking the sleep hormone melatonin. It has a much lower risk of next-day sleepiness or performing activities while asleep.

Turn on some music. Soothing music really does work to send you off into dreamland. A study by Taiwanese researchers compared the effects of soft music on sleep in 63 people who had trouble sleeping. Half listened to 45 minutes of music when they went to bed; half listened to nothing. The result? Those who listened to music slept better and longer, took less time to fall asleep, and functioned better the next day. Overall, sleep quality improved 45 percent in the music group compared to the control group. Plus, the group's sleep quality improved more with each week of music.

Take a short nap. Long naps will only keep you up at night, but short naps could make a positive difference. A very small Japanese study found that a 30-minute nap after lunch followed by some stretching and flexibility exercises in the early evening significantly improved sleep quality and reduced the amount of time it took to fall asleep.

Join a tai chi class. When researchers assigned 118 older adults to either a tai chi or another low-impact exercise class for three hourly sessions a week over 24 weeks, they found that people taking tai chi improved significantly more than the control group in quality of sleep, the time it took to fall asleep, and the total time spent asleep. In fact, the tai chi participants fell asleep an average of 18 minutes faster than those in the other group and slept nearly an hour longer per night. The study authors theorize that tai chi helps in part by enhancing overall well-being through relaxation and diaphragmatic breathing.

SOOTHING MUSIC REALLY DOES WORK TO SEND YOU OFF INTO DREAMLAND.

WHAT CAUSES IT
Anyone can have trouble falling asleep during a stressful time. Other causes include chronic pain, depression, and anxiety disorders. You can also "train" yourself to have insomnia by worrying so much about whether you'll fall asleep that you stress out when you hit the bed. Watch out for daytime sleepiness and snoring; the two together are often a sign of sleep apnea, which contributes to numerous medical conditions.

SYMPTOMS TO WATCH FOR An inability to fall asleep or stay asleep, or waking up too early in the morning. Trouble falling asleep may be related to anxiety, whereas waking up too early could be related to depression.

NEWEST THINKING
Treating the insomnia that exists alongside medical or mental health conditions not only relieves the insomnia but can actually improve the coexisting condition. However, most doctors still treat only the coexisting condition, believing that once it improves, so will the insomnia.

Irritable Bowel Syndrome

75%

The improvement in pain and cramps when people with IBS took the antibiotic rifaximin for 10 days.

Irritable bowel syndrome (IBS) is a frustrating mystery. Experts say that this digestive problem's pain, cramps, diarrhea, and constipation seem to be the result of bowels that move too quickly or too slowly and nerves that become exquisitely sensitive to the slightest pressure after you eat a meal. These solutions work, but be patient—you may have to try a combination of several before finding a prevention plan that works for you.

Key Prevention Strategies

Pinpoint trouble foods. Many people with IBS know from experience which foods trigger trouble. Common problem foods include alcohol, chocolate, caffeinated beverages, dairy products, and sugar-free sweeteners such as sorbitol and mannitol. People who have problems with gas and bloating may be bothered by beans, broccoli, cabbage, and cauliflower, too. For others, high-fat foods can cause intestinal pain.

When researchers at St. Georges Hospital Medical School in London tested the blood of 132 people with IBS and 42 healthy people who had been exposed to 16 common foods, people in the IBS group had higher levels of an antibody called IgG4 (associated with food intolerances) in response to beef, lamb, pork, soybeans, and wheat—leading the scientists to say that if you have IBS, pay careful attention to how you feel in the hours after eating these foods. Here's how to pinpoint your trouble foods.

Step 1: Track your symptoms. Write down the date, the type of symptoms you're having, how long they last, what you ate (and how much) during the preceding day or two, any medications you took, and what you were doing just before your discomfort began. After 14 days, look for patterns.

Step 2: Eliminate one suspected trigger food at a time. In another British study, people who eliminated problem foods saw symptoms improve by 26 percent. Cutting out one food at a time will give you a clearer picture of what helps and what doesn't.

Investigate antibiotics. Digestive disease researchers are beginning to suspect that an overgrowth of bacteria in the upper intestines—

a place where few bacteria should be living—may explain many of IBS's confusing and hard-to-treat symptoms. In one study, University of Southern California researchers found evidence that 84 percent of study volunteers with IBS had an overgrowth of bacteria in the small intestine. Those who took antibiotics to wipe out these unwanted guests saw IBS symptoms improve by 75 percent. (Other studies found a lower, 36 percent improvement rate.)

Some doctors use a 10-day course of rifaximin (Xifaxan), an antibiotic that stays in the intestines (it's not absorbed into the bloodstream). Others use a broad-spectrum antibiotic. Experts say people with IBS may need to repeat treatment every two to three months.

Try a little fiber. Until recently, digestive disease experts heartily recommended higher-fiber diets for people with IBS. Conventional wisdom said that soluble fiber—the type found in beans, pears, barley, and some fiber supplements—could firm up the stools of people with diarrhea, while soluble *and* insoluble fiber (the type found in whole wheat bread and many vegetables) would speed up bowels slowed by constipation. Sometimes it works. In one University of Pittsburgh study of 81 people with IBS, 26 percent reported less abdominal pain and bloating when they switched to a diet with more than 25 grams of fiber per day. But other studies show that fiber's no miracle fix: It makes pain worse for some people and has little effect for others.

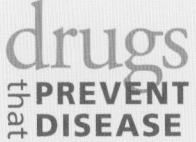 **drugs that PREVENT DISEASE**

A wide variety of drugs can help prevent and control the most difficult IBS symptoms, from constipation and diarrhea to pain and cramps.

Antidepressants, even if you aren't depressed: Antidepressants can block pain signals traveling between your intestines and your brain and can even help your bowel movements become more normal. In one study, people with IBS who took citalopram (Celexa) reported that abdominal pain and bloating improved significantly in just a few days. Which one's best for you? Expect pain and cramp relief with any of them. Constipation seems to improve more with selective serotonin-reuptake inhibitors (SSRIs) such as Celexa, escitalopram (Lexapro), paroxetine (Paxil), sertraline (Zoloft), and fluoxetine (Prozac). Diarrhea seems to ease more with tricyclic antidepressants such as amitriptyline (Elavil), imipramine (Tofranil), desipramine (Norpramin), and nortriptyline (Pamelor).

Antispasmodic drugs for pain and cramping: These medications include Levsin (hyoscyamine) and Bentyl (dicyclomine). They work by relaxing the walls of the intestines. You may have to try several to find one that's best for you.

Diarrhea medications: The over-the-counter diarrhea medication loperamide (Imodium) works for many people. For severe diarrhea, your doctor may prescribe a potent drug called alosetron (Lotronex). It works, but you must be monitored carefully while using it since it blocks blood flow to the colon in about 1 in 500 people who use it.

Mild laxatives for constipation: Plain old milk of magnesia is often effective for constipation. If it doesn't help, see your doctor. If your constipation is severe, he may suggest medications that can help prevent future problems, such as polyethylene glycol (Miralax), a milder version of the laxative once given to people to clean out their intestines before a colonoscopy.

If you'd like to give it a try, go slowly. Swap one low-fiber food for a higher-fiber one a day (replace white bread with whole wheat, for example) for a week and monitor how you feel. If all's well, make another swap. Be sure to drink plenty of water so the fiber won't cause constipation.

Relax—from the tips of your toes to the top of your head.
Progressive muscle relaxation eases stress, which in turn seems to reduce IBS pain sensitivity. In one small study from the State University of New York at Albany, people with IBS who practiced this technique daily for a month were five times more likely to experience improvement in pain and cramping than those who didn't use the technique. How to do it: Sit or lie down in a comfortable place. Shut your eyes, breathe deeply, and imagine stress flowing out of your muscles. Beginning with your feet, tense each muscle group tightly, then let the tension go so the muscles feel more relaxed than when you started. Move on to your calves, upper legs, and all the way up to your neck, face, and head.

Prevention Boosters

Lace up your tennis shoes. Exercise eased gastrointestinal symptoms in one large University of Washington study. The researchers weren't looking specifically at IBS, but there's plenty of other proof that being physically active can help by relaxing your bowels. Intestinal activity often quiets during exercise, during which your body shunts more blood to your legs and arms. It also relieves stress and boosts mood, making pain easier to cope with.

Peppermint-oil capsules for spasms. This minty remedy relaxes muscles in your gastrointestinal tract. In one well-designed study of 57 people with IBS, 75 percent of those who took peppermint-oil capsules saw symptoms improve by 50 percent or more after four weeks, compared to 38 percent who took a placebo. Study volunteers took two capsules twice a day. Use enteric-coated capsules so the oil is released in your intestines, not your stomach.

Hypnotherapy. In one British study, people with IBS who tried five sessions of hypnotherapy had less pain and diarrhea after three months than study volunteers who didn't have therapy. Benefits faded over time; after a year, the hypnosis group needed less medication to control IBS, but their symptoms were about the same as the nonhypnosis group. In another study, people who got

12 sessions over three months were still feeling better five years later. Ask your doctor for a referral to a licensed practitioner trained in hypnotherapy and familiar with "gut-directed" hypnotherapy, a technique that teaches you how to ease your own symptoms.

Soothe with yoga. In one study from India, men with IBS had equal reductions in diarrhea after two months of daily yoga or two months of daily doses of the over-the-counter drug loperamide (Imodium). Yoga seemed to soothe overactive nerves that stimulate bowel activity, reported researchers from the All India Institute of Medical Sciences in New Delhi. Meanwhile, a Canadian study of teenagers with IBS found that doing yoga routines as instructed in a video daily for a month eased anxiety.

Talk with a cognitive behavioral therapist. This practical type of counseling is aimed at helping you perceive and respond to every-day problems in new ways and to find solutions that really work. You may also work on relaxation skills. Some studies find a benefit for IBS, while others don't. Still others have found that it works for a little while, but then the effects wear off. It may be worth a try if you find that coping with IBS is overwhelming or if you just can't do all the things you want or need to do in your life. It seems to work best as an add-on therapy along with medications.

Try biofeedback. If you're bothered by constipation, learning how to properly use your abdominal muscles during a bowel movement could improve results—and make you feel better. In an Australian study, 25 women with IBS used biofeedback to help them as a doctor and nurse gave them "advanced training" in the proper way to push out stools without straining. (They practiced with small water balloons, not the real thing!) This type of biofeedback uses a probe inserted in the rectum to measure pressure exerted on stools. The result: 75 percent reported that things had improved. Other types of biofeedback can help people with IBS learn to control stress, too.

Send in the "good" bacteria. Probiotics—as supplements or in yogurt with active cultures—may help IBS symptoms by raising levels of healthy bacteria in your intestinal tract. In one study, 44 people with IBS took a supplement containing lactobacillus and bifidobacteria (also found in yogurts containing live, active cultures) for a week. Symptoms like pain, spasms, constipation, and diarrhea improved by 50 percent.

WHAT CAUSES IT
The root cause of IBS remains a mystery. Experts suspect that an overgrowth of bacteria, a gastrointestinal infection, or other factors make muscles in the intestinal wall move too quickly or too slowly; in addition, nerves in the intestines seem to become oversensitive.

SYMPTOMS TO WATCH FOR Abdominal pain and cramping, bloating, flatulence, diarrhea or constipation (or alternating bouts of both), mucus in your stools.

NEWEST THINKING
Slow down and rest when you have a stomach bug. There's new evidence that trying to "tough out" a gastrointestinal infection raises your risk of developing IBS afterward. When researchers at the University of Southampton in England contacted 620 people with past gastrointestinal infections, they found that those who had pushed themselves hard (for example, they kept working until they collapsed in bed) during their illnesses were more likely to develop IBS than those who took it easy.

Jet Lag

60 minutes

How much earlier you should hit the pillow each night for three nights before traveling eastward if you want to help prevent jet lag.

If you've ever taken an overnight flight to Europe and spent the following day in a stupor, you know the effects of jet lag. Even flying through just two time zones—especially if you're traveling east—is enough to mess with your body clock so that you can't fall asleep or wake up at the "right" time, leaving you bleary-eyed and exhausted. Chronic jet lag experienced by airline personnel and frequent business travelers even plays havoc with women's menstrual cycles and can increase the risk of cancer, heart disease, and peptic ulcers. The next time you travel by plane, take these steps to keep jet lag from ruining your trip.

Key Prevention Strategies

Sleep on the plane. This works only if you sleep when it's nighttime at your destination—for instance, if you're flying from New York on an overnight trip to London or Paris. Use earplugs and eye shades to block out light and sound. You can also try taking three milligrams of melatonin, which some studies suggest may help you fall asleep.

Turn on the lights. If you're exhausted when you arrive, it's temping to nap, even if it's morning. Resist the urge! Instead, go for a walk and try to get at least three hours of sunlight to help your body adjust more quickly to the new time zone.

Reset your body clock before your trip. The idea is to start shifting your bedtime and wakeup time to more closely resemble the schedule you'll be on at your destination. If you're traveling east through several time zones, go to sleep one hour earlier each night for three days before your trip—and get up an hour earlier, too. When you wake up, try to expose yourself to bright light for several hours. While sunlight is best, a full-spectrum light or light box can also work. You can buy them online or ask your doctor for a prescription; your health insurance company may pay for it. Some jet lag experts recommend combining this strategy with taking 0.5 milligram of melatonin in the afternoon to increase the hormonal signals that tell your body it's time for bed, so you can fall asleep earlier.

If you're flying west across several times zones, *delay* your sleep by an hour a night. If you're traveling through eight or more time zones, go to bed two hours earlier each night.

Prevention Boosters

Use sleeping pills when you arrive. One study of travelers who traveled five to nine time zones eastward found that those who took 10 milligrams of zolpidem (Ambien) for three or four nights once they arrived slept better and longer than those who didn't take the medication. Studies also find that taking 2 to 3 milligrams of melatonin on your first night in your new destination and for up to four days after arrival can improve sleep and reduce jet lag symptoms. You might also consider ramelteon (Rozerem). Although it hasn't yet been evaluated for jet lag, it works to enhance the effects of melatonin in the body, so researchers think it could be a good option. Take only one type of sleep aid at a time.

Drink a little coffee in the morning. It sounds simple, but caffeine is one of the best ways to improve your energy and concentration after flying across time zones. Don't drink too much, or it may affect your sleep that night.

SUNLIGHT HELPS YOUR BODY ADJUST MORE QUICKLY TO THE NEW TIME ZONE.

Jock Itch

90%

Your chances of staying free of jock itch if you clear up an existing infection with an antifungal cream.

Could there be a less convenient place to develop an itchy rash? "Jock itch" might as well be called "athlete's groin," because it's caused by the same fungus that causes athlete's foot. And just as with that embarrassing itchy foot condition, you don't have to be an athlete to get it. Sweaty workouts, mowing the lawn, and even failing to dry off well after a shower all cause the moist conditions that let this fungus, which is naturally present on skin, thrive. These steps can keep it from taking over.

Key Prevention Strategies

Stay clean and dry. Take a shower or bath every day. After a workout, change out of sweaty clothes (including underwear) and shower as soon as you can. Carefully dry your genital area, buttocks, and inner thighs with a clean towel. Leaving skin damp gives fungus a foothold, not only because moisture encourages the fungus to multiply but also because sweat and water dilute your natural oils, which contain fungus-fighting compounds.

Wear boxers, not briefs. Snug underwear traps moisture, so go loose with boxers and roomy shorts or pants. Choose smooth, breathable fabrics such as cotton and wool instead of synthetics. Avoid scratchy material that irritates your skin; fungus thrives on broken skin.

Wash shorts, underwear, and athletic supporters after each use. They're not just a smelly turnoff; they may also carry fungus. Remember, they've gotten sweaty, and chances are they've also hit the germy locker room floor at some point. Get them out of your gym bag right away when you get home;

can your feet give you jock itch?

Yes. The same fungus that causes athlete's foot is responsible for many cases of jock itch, too. If these little nasties are living on your feet, they can hitch a ride to your nether regions.

At the gym or pool: Wear sandals on the pool deck and in the shower or steam room and put a thick towel on the locker room floor when changing clothes.

At home: If family members have athlete's foot, you're at risk, too. Keep the tub extra-clean and be sure they use antifungal creams to clear up the problem.

After a shower: Dry yourself from head to toe. We mean that literally—start with your head and dry your feet last. That way, if there's fungus on your feet, you won't transfer the infection to your groin. If you have or suspect you have jock itch, consider using a hair dryer on the coolest setting to dry your privates instead of using the towel.

Wherever you dress: Start with your socks. You can transfer the fungus to your underwear while getting dressed if you pull your undies over your bare feet.

fungus can breed in the bag's damp, dark interior. In fact, if your bag is wet, spray it with disinfectant spray, dry with a paper towel, and let it air out in the sun for extra protection.

Dust yourself with an antifungal powder. Using an antifungal powder such as Cruex, Desenex, or Zeasorb in skin folds at your groin can help discourage itchy fungal growth and keep you dry. Using them proactively during hot weather and when you know you'll be hot and sweaty, such as while doing yard work or exercising, can stop a fungal infection before it starts.

While some experts recommend cornstarch as an alternative, others warn that this home remedy can backfire. Some strains of yeast that cause a rash similar to jock itch use cornstarch as food.

Already itchy? Use an antifungal product. Unless your rash is severe, start with an over-the-counter antifungal cream, gel, powder, or spray. There are plenty on the drugstore shelves. Over-the-counter products containing terbinafine or butenafine are as strong as prescription-strength antifungal creams. Once you've had jock itch, you may want to continue using an over-the-counter product intermittently as needed to prevent a recurrence.

Say "not tonight, honey." If your partner has jock itch, skin-to-skin contact could transmit the fungus to you during sex. Women are much less likely to develop jock itch than men, but it can happen. Ask him to use an antifungal cream until the infection is gone or use an antifungal cream yourself to prevent infection.

Prevention Boosters

Enlist your washer and dryer. Washing clothes and towels in hot water, then drying them on high heat in the dryer, kills fungus. A cold-water wash isn't enough.

Take your own towel to the gym. If you're still picking up jock itch despite taking all the other preventive measures here, try this strategy. It's possible that the gym isn't washing its towels in water that's hot enough to kill fungus.

Wrap yourself in a towel in the locker room. Don't sit naked on locker room benches. Instead, wrap your bottom in your towel after a shower and keep it on until you dress. It keeps a barrier between you and any lurking fungus.

WHAT CAUSES IT A family of fungi called dermatophytes. These tiny critters live on our skin normally, but when conditions are moist and warm, they can multiply quickly, causing an infection.

SYMPTOMS TO WATCH FOR Itchy skin in your groin area, buttocks, or inner thighs; a rash with slightly raised, brownish-red patches of dry, scaly, or bumpy skin. Jock itch usually doesn't occur on the penis or scrotum, but it can extend to the lower abdomen in severe cases.

NEWEST THINKING The fungus that causes jock itch could be living on the seats of stationary bikes, weight machines, and free-weight benches, warn experts from the Institute for Fungal Illness in Berlin, Germany. Before you sit down, clean equipment with the disinfectant spray at the gym, or use your own.

Kidney Disease

26%

The amount by which you could reduce your risk of kidney disease if you maintain normal blood pressure.

Considering how many people these days have high blood pressure, diabetes, or both, it's no wonder that chronic kidney disease is on the rise, since both conditions are leading causes. One out of six adults have it, yet many people with weak or failing kidneys have no idea that anything's wrong. Chronic kidney disease occurs when the kidneys gradually lose their ability to filter waste and toxins from the blood. It can eventually cause fatigue and shortness of breath, and it's the main reason people end up needing dialysis. Once you have chronic kidney disease, you can't get rid of it, but you can halt or slow its progression.

Key Prevention Strategies

Prevent diabetes and high blood pressure. Your risk of chronic kidney disease doubles if you have both of these conditions, which damage tiny blood vessels in the kidneys. Follow the prevention tips in the Diabetes and High Blood Pressure chapters, and you'll do your kidneys a big favor. If you already have high blood pressure, talk to your doctor about treating it with an ACE inhibitor. Studies find these drugs work best at preventing kidney disease or at the very least preventing it from advancing to the point where dialysis or a transplant is required. If you already have diabetes, keep your blood sugar levels as normal as possible. If you have both conditions, talk to your doctor about a medication called Coversyl Plus, which combines the ACE inhibitor perindopril and the diuretic indapamide. A study of 11,000 patients found it worked best to prevent kidney disease and its progression.

Get a simple kidney checkup. If you're at risk for kidney disease—you have diabetes or high blood pressure or a family history of kidney problems—your doctor should test your kidney function regularly. Many doctors use a blood test that measures a protein called creatinine. But because creatinine levels vary among individuals, the test can be somewhat unreliable. Instead, experts recommend screening kidney function with the glomerular filtration rate (GFR) test, a blood and urine test that measures how well the kidneys filter waste from the blood.

Buy a home blood pressure monitor. Pay special attention to your systolic blood pressure, the top number in your reading; it's a good indication of your vulnerability to kidney disease. A major study of 8,093 men who were followed for 14 years found that a systolic pressure between 130 and 139 mmHg increased the risk of kidney disease by 26 percent, and one of 140 mmHg or higher increased it by 69 percent.

Prevention Boosters

Prevent kidney stones. Blockages caused by kidney stones can increase the risk of chronic kidney disease. (See the Kidney Stones chapter for easy prevention tips.)

Spend the night in a sleep lab. If you snore loudly, your partner says you make loud choking or gasping noises while you sleep, and/or you're exhausted during the day, you could have a condition called obstructive sleep apnea, which may mean you're more likely to have chronic kidney disease. Experts aren't sure why. Being overweight and having high blood pressure increase the risk of both conditions, but researchers also note that people with sleep-related breathing disorders often have anemia, or low levels of oxygen-carrying blood cells, which increases the risk of chronic kidney disease. It can't hurt—and will certainly help your overall health—to take care of your apnea. The only way to diagnose obstructive sleep apnea for certain is with polysomnography, a test that evaluates your breathing as you sleep.

Skip dessert. Or find other ways to lose some weight. While being overweight makes existing kidney disease worse, it can also increase the risk of developing the condition. A study in 11,000 healthy men that found those whose body mass indexes, or BMIs, increased 10 percent or more over 14 years were 27 percent more likely to develop chronic kidney disease than those whose BMIs either dropped or increased just 5 percent. The risk remained even if the men had normal blood pressure and blood sugar and exercised regularly.

WHAT CAUSES IT Damage to blood vessels in the kidneys. The damage is most often caused by high blood pressure or diabetes but may also be the result of lupus; infections; inherited diseases; long-term use of acetaminophen, aspirin, or ibuprofen; kidney stones; an enlarged prostate that obstructs urine flow from the kidneys; or cancer.

SYMPTOMS TO WATCH FOR The early stages have no symptoms. In later stages, you may experience fatigue, frequent hiccups, feeling "flu-ish," itching, headache, foot and ankle swelling, nausea and vomiting, or weight loss. In the late stages, symptoms include blood in the vomit or stools, decreased alertness, reduced feeling in your hands or feet, easy bruising, an increase or decrease in urine, muscle twitching or cramps, seizures, or white crystals in and on your skin.

NEWEST THINKING A recent study found that people with gum disease were 60 percent more likely to have chronic kidney disease. Researchers suspect that the chronic inflammation caused by gum disease may play a role.

Kidney Stones

29-49%

The amount you can reduce your risk of kidney stones by drinking enough fluids to urinate about twice as much as most people do.

One out of every 10 adults will experience the excruciating pain of trying to pass a kidney stone at some point in their lives. Some say it's worse than the pain of childbirth. Kidney stones result from microscopic deposits in urine that eventually solidify, much like the salt left at the bottom of a glass of saltwater after the liquid evaporates. There are several types of kidney stones. If you've had a stone that passed, your doctor can test its composition and measure chemicals in your blood and urine to decide on the best way to prevent stones in the future.

Key Prevention Strategies

Drink up. Drinking more fluids is the best way to prevent all types of kidney stones. One study found that men who produced a prodigious 2.6 quarts or more of urine a day (the average is 1.5 quarts) were 29 percent less likely to develop symptomatic stones than those who excreted 1.3 quarts or less. In women, urinating 2.7 quarts or more reduced their risk by 49 percent compared with urinating less than 1.5 quarts a day. You'll need to drink 3.5 to 4 quarts of liquid a day (14 to 16 cups) to get there. This should make you urinate every two hours or so.

Spoon up some yogurt. Doctors used to warn all patients at risk for kidney stones to limit their calcium intake. After all, most kidney stones are composed primarily of calcium. Boy, were they wrong! It turns out that people who have the least calcium in their diets can have the highest risk of kidney stones. (A few patients, those with absorptive hypercalciuria, are still asked to reduce their calcium intake.) Note that we're talking about dietary calcium; there's no evidence that calcium supplements reduce your risk. In fact, in women, supplements could increase the risk of kidney stones by about 20 percent.

Researchers think that calcium protects against stones by binding to oxalic acid, a salt found in certain foods that contributes to kidney stones, thus preventing it from getting into urine. The best

drugs that PREVENT DISEASE

If you've had one or more calcium stones in the past, talk to your doctor about taking a thiazide diuretic (which reduces the amount of calcium in the urine) with potassium citrate (to replace the potassium the diuretic depletes) to slash your risk of future stones. Studies show these drugs are highly effective and can reduce new stone formation by 90 percent or more. Uric acid stones can be treated with other medications.

sources are low-fat milk, yogurt, and cheese. Edamame (green soybeans) are also calcium packed. An unexpectedly good source is whole grain cereal, which contains up to 1,000 milligrams in a single serving. Most people need 1,200 milligrams of calcium a day to protect their bones, although there is no specific level recommended to reduce the risk of kidney stones.

Limit high-oxalate foods. This is for those of you who have already had calcium stones. Researchers find that certain high-oxalate foods—spinach, rhubarb, beets, strawberries, nuts, chocolate, wheat bran, peanuts, and almonds—increase the risk of stones. If you can't bear to give up any of these foods, increase the amount of calcium you take in when you eat them. For instance, slice your strawberries into a bowl of cereal with milk, sprinkle your almonds over yogurt, and top your spinach salad with low-fat grated cheese.

Prevention Boosters

Drink a glass of orange juice every day. Experts have long prescribed tart (very lightly sweetened) lemonade as a way to keep stones at bay. But recent studies suggest that orange juice may be an even better choice. Both are great sources of potassium citrate, which is often prescribed to prevent kidney stones. Just stay away from grapefruit juice: It seems that quaffing as little as eight ounces a day can increase the risk of kidney stones, though researchers have no idea why. Apple juice may increase risk by 35 percent.

Lose weight if you need to. When researchers crunched the numbers, they found that men who weighed more than 220 pounds were 44 percent more likely to develop kidney stones than those who weighed less than 150 pounds. For women, the danger of being overweight was greater: Those who weighed more than 220 pounds were between 89 and 92 percent more likely to develop kidney stones than those under 150 pounds.

Avoid high-fructose corn syrup. It's not that easy to do since so many packaged foods and drinks these days contain it. But kicking the soda habit, avoiding sweetened fruit drinks, and eater fewer snacks out of boxes is a good start. Cutting back may significantly reduce your risk of stones. Researchers suspect the connection has to do with fructose's tendency to increase the amount of calcium in urine.

WHAT CAUSES IT Genetic disposition, urinary tract infections, kidney disease, chronic dehydration, and certain metabolic conditions that affect the makeup of urine. Certain medications, including diuretics and calcium-based antacids, can also contribute.

SYMPTOMS TO WATCH FOR Initially, none. In fact, the majority of stones pass without any symptoms. Larger stones, however, can cause sudden, intense pain in your back, side, and lower abdomen, as well as nausea and vomiting. You may also have some blood in your urine, feel that you have to urinate more often than usual, and/or feel burning when you urinate.

NEWEST THINKING People with metabolic syndrome— a constellation of symptoms that include high blood pressure and triglycerides, abdominal fat, insulin resistance, and low levels of "good" HDL cholesterol— have a much higher risk of developing kidney stones.

Knee Pain

The human knee is an amazing yet flawed piece of architecture. This complex joint is built to withstand forces four times greater than your body weight with each step—and to support you as you bend, twist, and jump. But the knee isn't perfect. Its rigging system of bones, ligaments, and tendons works best when the muscles around it are also strong and flexible. Let 'em go soft, and even a long day carting heavy packages at the mall can lead to pain. And time isn't always kind to knees either. Since aging, genetics, and injuries contribute to the wide variety of problems that can cause knee pain, it's no wonder that one in four people over age 55 complain of chronic knee pain. Here's how to avoid it.

Key Prevention Strategies

Drop extra pounds. Each pound of excess weight you lose reduces the pressure on your knees by 4 pounds. On a one-mile walk, that translates to 4,800 fewer pounds that your knees have to support. Exercising while you diet not only makes permanent weight loss much easier but also translates into bigger benefits for knees. In a study that followed 316 women and men with painful knees, those who took a knee-friendly low-impact aerobics and strength-training class for one hour three times a week and also lost weight reported a 30 percent drop in knee pain and a 24 percent improvement in their ability to easily do everyday things like climbing stairs and getting in and out of a car.

Don't smoke. Chemicals in tobacco smoke derail the process that heals torn ligaments, including those in the knees. University of Washington School of Medicine researchers found that smoking reduced the number of infection-fighting cells called macrophages that reported for duty at the site of ligament injuries. That's a problem because macrophages release chemical signals that summon other cells needed for making repairs. Why it matters: Tens of millions of people endure knee pain each year due to torn ligaments. A symptom of a torn ligament is pain, tenderness, or stiffness on the outside of the knee that you feel mostly when you're moving around.

Avoid high-impact exercise. If running, step aerobics, or even jumping jacks hurt, it's time to switch to a lower-impact fitness routine. Walking, swimming, biking, and water aerobics are great workouts that burn calories, boost cardiovascular fitness, and have even been shown to reduce knee pain in studies. Stop doing an activity if it hurts your knees.

Strengthen all the muscles that support your knees. Strong quadriceps (the big muscles the run down the fronts of your thighs) and hamstrings (at the backs of your thighs) act as shock absorbers that take some of the pressure put on your knees when you walk, jump, and bend. They also keep the bones in your knees better aligned, which reduces the risk of pain and excess wear and tear. In one study, women with stronger thigh muscles had 55 percent less chance of developing knee pain. (See the Arthritis chapter for exercises to strengthen both your quadriceps and hamstrings.)

But don't stop there. Strengthening your "core" abdominal and back muscles, as well as those in your hips and buttocks, is equally important for decreasing knee pain. (See the Back Pain and Hip Fracture chapters for some good exercises.)

Prevention Boosters

Wear joint-friendly footwear. The best shoes for your knees are flat and flexible, say researchers from Rush Medical College in Chicago. The scientists analyzed pressure on the knees of 16 volunteers as they walked in clogs, flip-flops, walking shoes, and "stability" shoes (stiff shoes often worn by older people with balance problems). The surprise winners: Flip-flops and walking shoes, which allowed the feet to bend and flex naturally with each step, taking pressure off the knees. We recommend the walking shoes. While flip-flops are comfortable on the beach, they don't protect your feet or stay in place very well as you walk.

If you have flat feet, slipping over-the-counter shoe inserts or custom-made orthotics into your shoes can help keep the bones in your knees better aligned, helping to prevent pain.

Measure your legs. Or better yet, ask your doctor to do it. Legs of unequal length can contribute to osteoarthritis as well as knee and hip pain, say researchers from the University of North Carolina at Chapel Hill School of Medicine. Having one leg just 1/3 inch shorter than the other can raise the risk of knee pain by 50 percent, they say. The fix: Ask your doctor about shoe inserts.

WHAT CAUSES IT
Osteoarthritis, rheumatoid arthritis, overweight, falls and accidents, overuse, weak muscles, or not warming up before starting a challenging exercise routine.

SYMPTOMS TO WATCH FOR Knee pain due to osteoarthritis is usually deep and achy, is felt around the knee joint, and is often worse at night. Sudden, severe pain can be the result of injured ligaments (which attach the bones in your upper and lower legs), irritation or inflammation of tendons (which attach muscle to bone), or a dislocated kneecap. Your knee may also lock in place, often due to a torn meniscus, the curved piece of cartilage inside your knee joint. If your knee swells (often called water on the knee), it may be a sign that fluid-filled sacs called bursae that act as joint cushions have become inflamed. You may also have pain just below the knee. Make a doctor's appointment if your knee is hot, swollen, or extremely painful, has locked in place, or if you can't stand or walk.

NEWEST THINKING Low vitamin D levels can make knee pain worse. If you have osteoarthritis of the knee, be sure you're getting 1,000 to 2,000 IU of vitamin D a day.

Lung Cancer

50%

The amount by which your risk of lung cancer drops 10 years after quitting smoking.

Unless you've been on a desert island for the past 40 years, you know that smoking is the leading cause of lung cancer (although 2 to 10 percent of lung cancers occur in people who never smoked, particularly women). To prevent it, don't smoke, and stay away from chronic smokers—one hour spent inhaling someone else's cigarette smoke damages your lungs as much as smoking four cigarettes yourself!

Key Prevention Strategies

Quit smoking. Your risk of developing lung cancer if you smoke a pack of cigarettes a day for 40 years is about 20 times that of someone who never smoked. We know it's not easy to quit; it typically takes several attempts before it sticks. Our advice: Make a doctor's appointment. Working with your doctor increases your odds of success by 75 percent versus going solo. The doctor will probably prescribe a nicotine replacement product. Whether you choose gum, a patch, lozenges, or a nasal spray, studies find that the products can double the odds of quitting successfully (defined as being smoke free for a year).

Your doctor may also prescribe bupropion (Zyban) or varenicline (Chantix), both of which help people quit. Only Zyban can be used in conjunction with nicotine replacement products.

Should you try to quit slowly or all at once? Research shows that quitting cold turkey works better.

Test your house for radon. Radon, a colorless, odorless gas that results from decaying radioactive elements in the earth, seeps into homes through basements and windows. It is the second leading cause of lung cancer. The only way to know if you have radon in your house is with testing. You can test with a home kit, available at hardware stores, or

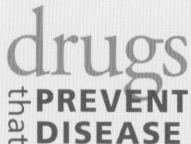

drugs that PREVENT DISEASE

Researchers evaluating the use of statins, drugs widely prescribed to reduce cholesterol, in nearly half a million patients found that taking the medication for at least six months reduced the risk of lung cancer by 55 percent. Researchers suspect that statins protect against the disease by taming inflammation in the body, which contributes to cancer development. The next step is clinical trials to confirm the findings.

Another drug that may help prevent lung cancer is the pain reliever celecoxib (Celebrex). In one study, researchers found that heavy smokers who took a high dose of the drug were less likely than those who didn't get the drug to develop the kind of precancerous cellular changes seen in smokers. Like statins, Celebrex reduces inflammation. Both drugs have potential side effects, so weigh the risks and benefits with your doctor.

call in a professional. If you find radon, it can be vented to the outside with a pipe and fan system.

Prevention Boosters

Load up on veggies. Start with broccoli, cabbage, and brussels sprouts. These cruciferous vegetables are high in compounds called isothiocyanates, which prevent lung cancer in animals. In humans, researchers find that eating these vegetables at least once a week could cut your risk of lung cancer by 33 percent.

Skip the burgers, steak, and ice cream. Sticking to poultry, fish, and low-fat or fat-free dairy foods and using olive oil instead of butter could pare your lung cancer risk threefold, and nearly fivefold if you're a smoker. Researchers don't know why saturated fat has such a strong impact on lung cancer risk; it could be related to high levels of inflammation seen in people who eat a lot of these fats.

Brush and floss regularly. Losing your teeth, which is usually due to bacterial infection in the mouth, increases your risk of lung cancer by 54 percent even if you don't smoke. The reason? It could be related to the inflammation that leads to gum disease and tooth loss or to the fact that people who lose their teeth don't have as healthy a diet as people with a full set.

WHAT CAUSES IT
Smoking causes 90 percent of lung cancers. Other causes are radon and exposure to asbestos, other chemicals, and secondhand smoke.

SYMPTOMS TO WATCH FOR Chronic cough, hoarseness, coughing up blood, weight loss, loss of appetite, shortness of breath, fever for no reason, wheezing, bouts of bronchitis or pneumonia, chest pain.

NEWEST THINKING
Vitamin E supplements don't protect against lung cancer and may even increase your risk. A large study involving more than 77,000 people found that taking a 400-milligram daily dose increased risk by 28 percent over 10 years. Don't worry about dietary vitamin E, however; there's no evidence that it—or levels of any other vitamin or mineral in food—increases the risk of lung cancer.

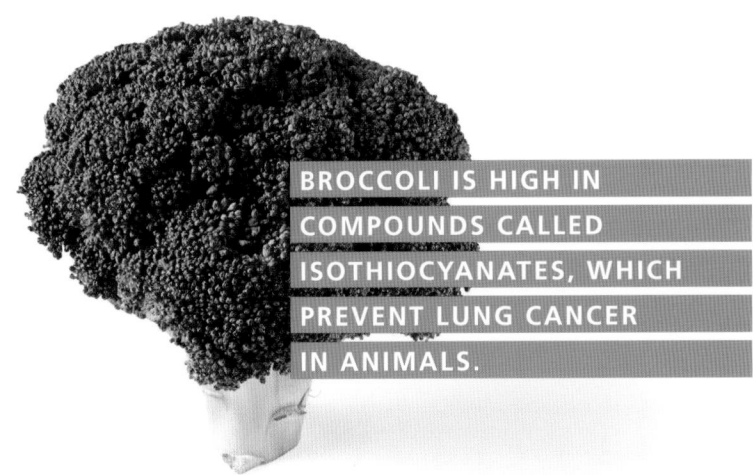

BROCCOLI IS HIGH IN COMPOUNDS CALLED ISOTHIOCYANATES, WHICH PREVENT LUNG CANCER IN ANIMALS.

Lyme Disease

40%

Who would have guessed that something about the size of a poppy seed could trigger such a big health problem? A single bite from a deer tick infected with the bacterium *Borrelia burgdorferi* is enough to cause Lyme disease and the various miseries that come with it. Most cases are easily cured with antibiotics, but if untreated, the disease can eventually lead to serious heart, joint, and nervous system complications. Since doctors first began reporting Lyme disease in 1991, its incidence has doubled in the United States and parts of Europe. Now, thanks to climate change, the geographic areas in which the ticks are found are expanding, putting millions more at risk. Follow these precautions to reduce your exposure.

Key Prevention Strategies

Cover up. You don't have to take a 10-mile hike in the woods to get Lyme disease. Most cases occur on a person's own property or near their house, particularly in grassy fields and heavily wooded areas. Regardless of the temperature, protect yourself with long pants tucked into socks, long-sleeved shirts, and light-colored clothing (the better to see any ticks). Dressing this way can reduce your risk of Lyme disease by 40 percent.

Spray yourself—and maybe your clothes. Using a tick repellent reduces your risk of infection by 20 percent. The most effective repellents contain 10 to 35 percent DEET. Products with 10 percent DEET work for about two hours; be sure to reapply after that. Don't use repellents with more than 30 percent DEET on children. If you expect to be heavily exposed to ticks, in addition to spraying yourself with DEET, consider spraying your clothing (especially socks and pants) with the pesticide permethrin, which lasts through several washings. This combination seems to be most effective against ticks. Never use permethrin on your skin.

Check yourself daily for ticks. Examine your whole body for any small, round, black or brown bumps. Don't forget to check between your toes, on the bottoms

what to do if you find a tick

The best way to remove a tick is with fine-point tweezers. Grab it with the tweezers as close to your skin as possible, near the tick's head or mouth, then pull the tick straight out—don't twist. Don't squeeze it, rub petroleum jelly on it, touch it with a hot match or cigarette, or pour kerosene or nail polish on it. Place the tick in a small jar or resealable plastic bag and take it with you to the doctor.

of your feet, and in your groin. Stand in front of a long mirror to look at your back, and have someone check your scalp. If you see a tick, don't panic. You have up to 24 hours to remove it before the infection is transmitted, and 96 percent of people who find and remove a tick in this timeframe don't get infected.

Know the signs of a tick bite. At first, a tick bite causes a hard bump. About 70 to 80 percent of people with Lyme disease develop a circular rash at the site of the bite within 3 to 30 days of being bitten. As the rash expands, the center may become lighter, creating a bull's-eye appearance. But you can have Lyme without developing the rash. Other early symptoms include fever, chills, body aches, and headache. If you've been bitten or suspect you have Lyme disease, go to your doctor for a dose of antibiotics. Studies find that a single, 200-milligram dose of doxycycline within 3 days of removing the tick can reduce the risk of serious disease by 87 percent. This treatment can help prevent the infection, but some experts recommend longer-term treatment even if a potential infection is caught early, just in case the infection has already taken hold.

Prevention Boosters

Stay in the middle of the trail. When you're hiking, avoid the trail edges. Ticks inhabit shrubby vegetation anywhere from ankle to waist high. If you avoid brushing against the greenery at the trail's edge, you're less likely to come home with a tick.

Do some landscaping. Get rid of any brush and leaf litter (where ticks love to hang out) and create a one-yard buffer zone of wood chips or gravel between any forest and your yard. Keep your lawn cut short. If you live in a very deer-prone area, consider installing deer fencing to keep the pesky animals away (deer carry ticks on their bodies).

WHAT CAUSES IT A bite from an ixodid ("deer") tick infected with *Borrelia burgdorferi* bacteria.

SYMPTOMS TO WATCH FOR Early symptoms include fever, headache, fatigue, and a characteristic skin rash. Left untreated, the infection can spread to the heart, joints, and nervous system. Complications include arthritis, heart rhythm abnormalities, encephalitis, and facial paralysis.

NEWEST THINKING The antibiotic doxycycline, used to treat the disease in its earliest stage, could one day be used to protect against it, perhaps as a slow-release patch that you put on before heading outside in tick-infested areas.

Macular Degeneration

35%

The drop in your risk of progressive vision loss if you keep your plate loaded with colorful fruits and vegetables.

There's no cure for this sight-robbing condition. Called age-related macular degeneration (AMD) by specialists because it usually strikes after age 60, it destroys the macula—the center of the retina, a whisper-thin layer of light-sensitive tissue in the eye. Vision erodes so gradually that you may not notice anything at first. Most people with AMD have this slow-moving "dry" form. But 1 in 10 develop "wet" AMD, in which blood vessels in the macula leak, and vision deteriorates rapidly. Your best move now: Regular eye exams plus the following measures to reduce your risk.

Key Prevention Strategies

Don't light up that cigarette. The more you smoke, the higher your risk. In fact, when University of Wisconsin scientists tracked the health of nearly 5,000 women and men for 15 years, they found that smoking raised risk by 47 percent. Smoking robs your eyes of antioxidants that protect against cell damage, reduces blood flow to the eyes, and may even affect the pigments in your retinas, which not only determine your eye color but also act as a natural sunscreen.

Eat the "vision veggies." Spinach, kale, and romaine lettuce are rich in the eye-protecting nutrients lutein and zeaxanthin. These compounds concentrate in the macula of the eyes, filtering out the sun's destructive blue light before it can harm delicate light-sensitive cells deeper in the retina. They also neutralize damaging free radicals produced when light hits the eye. Other top sources of these nutrients are turnip and collard greens, broccoli, zucchini, corn, peas, and brussels sprouts—as well as eggs. At this point, experts say there's no evidence that antioxidant supplements help prevent AMD, though they may slow its progression if you have it.

slowing vision loss with supplements

If you already have macular degeneration, taking an antioxidant supplement could cut your risk of deteriorating vision by 33 percent, says a recent British review of eight well-designed studies. (They didn't help prevent AMD in people whose eyes were healthy.) Consider taking a supplement if you have been diagnosed with intermediate or advanced AMD. The formula recommended by experts contains 500 milligrams of vitamin C, 400 IU of vitamin E, 15 milligrams of beta-carotene, 80 milligrams of zinc (as zinc oxide), and 2 milligrams of copper (as cupric oxide). The latter is added to prevent copper deficiency, which can occur if zinc intake is high.

Eat smarter carbs. Do you love to load up on white bread, white rice, potatoes, baked goods, or sweetened fruit drinks? You may be harming your eyes by sending your blood sugar on a rollercoaster ride. When Tufts University researchers checked the diets of 526 people with macular degeneration, they found that those who ate the most foods that make blood sugar spike were 2.7 times more likely to develop AMD than those who ate the fewest. The answer? Load up on fresh fruits, vegetables, and dried beans, choose whole grain bread and cereal, drink water or unsweetened tea, and skip the chips, crackers, and cookies. How it helps your eyes: Experts think lower blood sugar helps maintain a healthy flow of blood and oxygen to the eyes.

Dine on salmon, not cheeseburgers. In one Harvard Medical School study, eating two or more fish meals a week cut the risk of AMD by an impressive 60 percent. The researchers think that the omega-3 fatty acids in fatty fish promote good blood flow to the eyes and cool inflammation, an emerging risk factor for AMD. The catch: Fish helped only people who also limited the omega-6 fatty acids in their diet. These are found in corn, safflower, and sunflower oils as well as fried foods and margarines made with these oils.

More foods to avoid: Cheese, ice cream, hamburgers, and anything else rich in saturated fat. People who ate a ton of these foods had twice the risk that early macular degeneration would progress compared to people who ate a "skinnier" diet.

Prevention Boosters

Make nuts your snack of choice. The same Harvard study found that people with AMD who ate more than one serving of nuts each week cut their risk for the progression of AMD by 40 percent. (A serving is about 22 almonds, 16 cashews, or 12 walnut halves.) What do your peepers love about nuts? It could be resveratrol, an antioxidant found in nuts and other foods that can protect against cell damage, soothe inflammation, and promote healthy blood flow, the scientists speculate.

Watch your weight. Overweight people with AMD get worse up to twice as fast as people of normal weight. Research shows that exercising as part of your weight-control strategy pays dividends for your eyes. In a study, people with early AMD who got at least a half hour of vigorous exercise three times a week cut their risk of developing advanced AMD by 25 percent.

WHAT CAUSES IT Experts don't know what triggers the damage, but smoking and being over age 60, Caucasian, or female raises the risk.

SYMPTOMS TO WATCH FOR Distorted vision in one or both eyes; straight lines will look wavy. Over time, central vision grows worse, and it becomes difficult to see objects far away, to read or do close work, or even to distinguish faces and colors.

NEWEST THINKING Avoid secondhand smoke. Nonsmokers who lived with smokers raised their risk of AMD by 87 percent in one recent British study. Don't wait for your partner to quit in order to clear the air and guard your eyesight: Ask your spouse to smoke outside to protect your health.

Menstrual Cramps

600%

The amount by which you could reduce cramps by supplementing with vitamin E before and during your periods.

Compared to their ancestral grandmothers, who spent most of their reproductive years pregnant or breastfeeding, women today have about three times as many menstrual periods. The reality is that we don't *need* to menstruate. In fact, the manufacturers of birth control pills originally included one week of placebo pills mainly because they thought that women would find it "reassuring" to have their periods! Today women can choose continuous birth control that prevents periods—and cramps. Other approaches can also help.

Key Prevention Strategies

Start on birth control. If you're not trying to get pregnant, starting on oral contraceptives is the most effective way to prevent menstrual cramps. Standard birth control pills contain progestin, a synthetic hormone that thins the lining of the uterus over time. A thinner lining produces less arachidonic acid, which contributes to the production of prostaglandins, hormone-like chemicals that cause cramps.

If you want to avoid your period (and the resulting cramps) altogether, talk to your doctor about continuous oral contraception, in which you use the pill for up to a year without a break, or extended oral contraception, in which you use the pill for three months at a time, then have a period. Other contraceptive options that can reduce or prevent menstrual cramps include the vaginal ring (NuvaRing), injectable contraception (Depo-Provera), and the Mirena IUD.

Take painkillers early. Start taking an over-the-counter anti-inflammatory such as ibuprofen or naproxen, following the label directions, one to two days before your period is due. A review of 51 studies involving 1,649 women found that 72 percent experienced significant pain relief with this approach compared to women taking a placebo. Continue for the first two or three days of your period. These pain relievers prevent your body from making cramp-causing prostaglandins.

Prevention Boosters

Try a low-fat vegetarian diet. Researchers asked 33 women with bad cramps to follow such a diet (no animal products, fried foods, avocados, olives, or nuts, but plenty of grains, vegetables, legumes, and fruits) for two menstrual cycles, then eat their regular diet for two cycles and take a placebo pill. During the vegetarian diet phase, the duration and intensity of the women's menstrual pain dropped by about a third. And there was a bonus: They lost weight! The diet probably triggers beneficial changes in the metabolism of estrogen and/or cuts down on the production of prostaglandins.

Feast on fish or take fish oil. Fatty fish like mackerel and salmon are high in omega-3 fatty acids, which may help ease menstrual cramps and have the added benefit of improving your levels of blood fats, including cholesterol. A study of 181 Dutch women found that those with the lowest levels of omega-3 fatty acids in their diets had the greatest amount of menstrual pain.

Even if you don't like fish, you can still get your omega-3's by taking fish-oil capsules. A study of 70 women, half of whom received fish oil, found that pain levels in those taking the oil dropped by 33 percent compared to a 20 percent improvement in the women who took placebos. The women took two grams of fish oil every day for a month. The next month, they took two grams a day for eight days before their periods and two days after their periods. Check with your doctor before taking fish oil.

Supplement carefully with E. We don't recommend regular long-term use of vitamin E supplements, which may slightly increase the risk of early death. But some research suggests that taking it just before and just after your period begins can bring significant relief from cramps. One study involving 278 adolescent girls found that taking 400 IU of vitamin E a day beginning two days before their periods began and continuing for the first three days of their periods relieved cramps better than a placebo. After four months, girls who took the vitamin E had average pain scores nearly six times lower than those who took placebos, and their pain lasted an average of 1.6 hours compared to 17 hours in the placebo group. Vitamin E may help by affecting prostaglandins.

Run (or walk) it off. Ask a jogger in your office about her menstrual cramps. Chances are, she just doesn't have them. Studies find that women who exercise regularly—regardless of what kind of activity they do—are less likely to have pain during their periods.

WHAT CAUSES IT Hormonal changes during your menstrual cycle trigger the production of hormone-like chemicals called prostaglandins that make the uterus contract, causing cramps. You could also have bad cramps if you have endometriosis, a condition in which the tissue that lines the uterus grows outside the organ.

SYMPTOMS TO WATCH FOR Lower-abdominal pain during your periods.

NEWEST THINKING Menstrual blood may someday provide a rich source of stem cells, which can be used to create a variety of tissue ranging from nerves to kidneys to insulin-producing cells for people with type 1 diabetes.

Migraines

40%

The drop in the number of migraines among people who switched to a low-fat diet for eight weeks.

Migraines can be downright crippling. They're a problem for 1 in 6 women and 1 in 16 men. But half of all sufferers don't realize what's behind their debilitating head pain—and as a result, they're missing out on strategies that can stop the downward spiral before it starts. If your symptoms match some or all of those listed on the opposite page, you owe it to yourself to try these effective prevention measures.

Key Prevention Strategies

Avoid your personal migraine triggers. Certain foods, some medications, stress, changes in sleeping patterns, cigarette smoke, and a variety of other things can flip switches in your brain that turn on a migraine. Everyone's triggers are different; keeping a headache diary can help you determine yours. Record when you get a migraine and what you were taking, eating, drinking, feeling, and doing for the 24 hours before the pain began.

Common medication culprits include some antidepressants, bronchodilators, contraceptives, and diet pills. Food and drink triggers include caffeine (drinking too much—or abruptly giving it up), alcohol (vodka seems okay), aged cheese, processed meats, monosodium glutamate, nuts, dairy foods, many tropical fruits and most dried fruits (dried apples, cherries, peaches, and pears are usually okay), onions, fresh yeast breads, and aspartame.

Step off the painkiller merry-go-round. Taking painkillers of any kind more than twice a week can set you up for trouble. These drugs constrict swollen blood vessels, which makes your head feel better. But when they wear off, blood vessels swell again, and you could get a migraine as a result. End the cycle by stopping your pain medications. It will probably hurt at first, but experts say you'll start feeling better after a week to 10 days. Then you can focus on prevention strategies like the ones here.

drugs that PREVENT DISEASE

If you get two or more migraines each month, ask your doctor if you're a candidate for a migraine prevention medication such as propranolol (Inderal) or timolol (Blocadren). The right remedy could cut your risk of future migraines in half, but it can take four weeks to begin seeing improvements and up to six months to know whether a drug is really working for you.

You may even find relief by taking a low-dose aspirin every day or every other day, studies show.

Slash the fat in your diet. Drastically reducing the amount of fat you eat could cut the number of migraines you have by 40 percent. That was the finding from a Loma Linda University study that followed 54 migraine sufferers who stuck with extremely low fat diets (they got just 10 to 15 percent of their calories from fat each day) for eight weeks. When study volunteers did get headaches, they were 66 percent less intense and about 70 percent shorter than before. The participants also used 72 percent less headache medicine.

The researchers suspect that eating less fat improves the flexibility of blood vessels so they expand and contract more easily. They also discovered that study volunteers replaced fat with carbohydrate-rich foods like bread and pasta, which raise levels of the brain chemical serotonin, linked to lower migraine risk.

Not ready to go so low fat? Work on cutting back on saturated fat—the kind found in fatty meats, full-fat milk and cheese, and tropical oils (like palm and coconut oil)—and getting most of your fat from fatty fish, canola or olive oil, walnuts, and flaxseed. In some studies, these good fats reduced the frequency of migraines, perhaps by keeping blood vessels flexible.

Prevention Boosters

Give butterbur a try. When 245 people who got migraines took a butterbur product called Petadolex or a placebo for three months, 68 percent of those who took the herb saw the number of migraines they experienced drop by at least 50 percent. Butterbur extract may help by quieting spasms in blood vessel walls, soothing inflammation, or both. People who took 75 milligrams of butterbur extract a day got the most relief. Make sure you use a commercial product free of harmful compounds called pyrrolizidine alkaloids.

Ask your doctor about supplementing with riboflavin. In one Belgian study, 60 percent of people who took 400 milligrams of riboflavin (vitamin B$_2$) every day for three months had half as many migraines as before the study started.

Relax your mind and body. You can do this with yoga, meditation, deep breathing, or any other therapy that helps relieve tension. In one promising study from India, 72 migraine sufferers who practiced yoga for an hour five days a week reduced the frequency and intensity of their migraine attacks.

WHAT CAUSES IT No one's sure. Experts suspect that the trigeminal nerve system, which sends and receives pain signals involving the face and head, is involved, as is the brain chemical serotonin. Levels of serotonin fall during a migraine and may prompt the trigeminal nerve to send out chemicals that dilate blood vessels—causing pain.

SYMPTOMS TO WATCH FOR Moderate to severe pain on one or both sides of the head. It may throb or pulse, feel worse with physical activity, and come with nausea, vomiting, and sensitivity to light and sound. Some people experience auras just before the pain begins. These can include flashing lights, blind spots, tingling in arms or legs, or feeling extremely weak. (Migraines with auras also raise risk for cardiovascular problems, studies show, so follow our advice for preventing heart disease and stroke.)

NEWEST THINKING Think twice before using feverfew. It probably won't do any harm, but this popular anti-migraine herb did little to prevent migraines or lessen pain in a British review of five well-designed studies.

Neck Pain

54%

The amount by which doing stretching and relaxation exercises throughout the day could reduce your risk of neck pain.

The average human head weighs about as much as a bowling ball, yet it rests atop seven of the smallest, lightest vertebrae in your spinal column. Nature designed your neck to curve slightly backward to keep your head from flopping over. But years of bad posture, computer work, driving, and sleeping on sagging mattresses or big pillows can erase that curve, leading to pain. Injuries (think whiplash) and plain old stress also contribute. Here's how to prevent this literal "pain in the neck."

Key Prevention Strategies

Pull up on your string. Think of yourself as a puppet with a string coming out of the top of your head. Now imagine that someone's pulling on that string, causing you to sit (or stand) straight and hold your head high, with your chin tucked in slightly. That's the position you want to be in most of the time. Instead, many of us sit, drive, and even walk on the treadmill with our heads thrust forward, which puts strain on the neck. To help you sit up straight at the computer, use armrests and adjust your monitor so that your eyes are looking near the top of the screen. While driving, adjust your seat and headrest so you don't have to crane your neck forward to see the road.

Use music to keep your head held high. You don't need to listen to the music; all you need is the jewel case the CD came in. Place it on top of your head and see how long you can keep it there. Eventually, sitting straighter should become second nature.

Downsize your pillows. Sleeping on a big stack of pillows or just one high pillow inevitably means your neck will be out of line with the rest of your spine while you sleep. It's better to use a small pillow—and sleep on your back or side, not on your stomach. If you're prone to neck pain, a neck pillow is the best way to go (you'll need to sleep on your back to use it).

Move every 20 to 30 minutes. If you're e-mailing the kids, knitting a sweater, or working on that oil

help for a stiff neck

Wet a towel, wring it out, and warm it in the microwave for 30 seconds. Then wrap it around your neck and keep it on until it loses its heat. Do this before performing neck exercises to loosen up the muscles.

painting, it's easy to get lost in the flow and sit in an unnatural position for too long, straining your back, shoulder, and neck muscles. Set an alarm or kitchen timer to ring every 20 to 30 minutes. Each time it chimes, stand up, walk around for a few minutes, and practice the neck exercises on page 258. An Italian study found that when office workers were trained to practice relaxation and stretching exercises several times a day to stop "clenching" their neck and shoulder muscles, they had 54 percent less neck and shoulder pain compared with a control group, whose pain dropped by only 4 percent.

Prevention Boosters

Lighten the load. Carrying an overstuffed purse slung on one shoulder is a leading cause of neck pain for many women because it pulls the body out of balance. One doctor, tired of hearing his patients complain about neck pain, started weighing their purses and found that many tipped the scales at 7 to 10 pounds. If you must carry a lot of stuff, use a backpack to evenly distribute the weight.

Watch your phone posture. If you're talking on an old-fashioned home phone a lot, avoid scrunching the phone between your ear and shoulder. When using a cell phone, use an earpiece.

WHAT CAUSES IT Trauma, such as whiplash from a car accident; excessive strain on the neck or shoulder muscles; emotional stress that causes you to tighten your shoulder or neck muscles; and degenerative changes in the vertebrae and disks in your neck, which are common with age.

SYMPTOMS TO WATCH FOR Pain and difficulty turning your head to the right or left or moving it up or down; frequent headaches.

NEWEST THINKING Stainless steel disks can replace worn-out cervical disks in your neck, relieving pain while retaining mobility. The FDA approved the first one in late 2007. Surgery is, of course, a last resort when nothing else helps.

CARRYING AN OVERSTUFFED PURSE SLUNG ON ONE SHOULDER IS A LEADING CAUSE OF NECK PAIN.

Stretch and Strengthen Your Neck

That pain in your neck is often related to unconsciously tensing your neck, particularly when you're spending hours at the computer or in the car. Next time you're playing Spider Solitaire or knitting a sweater in time for Christmas, remind yourself to do these stretching exercises to relieve the tension and keep your neck limber. You can strengthen your neck simply by resisting all these motions with your hand.

Neck Rotation

1 Lie on the floor with a thick book under your head (a phone book is perfect).

2 Slowly turn your head to one side and hold for 10 to 20 seconds. Repeat on each side three to five times.

Head Tip

Sit straight and gently tilt your head forward as far as it will go. Hold for 10 seconds, then return to the starting position. Repeat five times.

Head Tilt

Stand or sit straight and hold the right side of the top of your head with your left hand. Let your right arm hang loosely at your side. Slowly pull your head to the left until you feel a gentle stretch in your neck. Hold for 10 seconds, then repeat on the other side.

Armpit Stretch

Stand or sit straight and hold the left side of the top of your head with your right hand. Let your left arm hang loosely at your side. Slowly pull your head to the right and down, stopping when you feel a gentle stretch in your neck. Hold for 10 seconds, then repeat on the other side.

Side Tip

Sit straight and turn your head to the right as far as it will go. Gently tilt your head forward until you feel the stretch. Hold for 10 seconds, then return to the starting position. Repeat five times on each side.

Shoulder Shrug

Stand or sit straight and raise your shoulders toward your ears until you feel slight tension in your neck and shoulders. Hold for 5 seconds, then relax. Repeat five times.

Obesity

22%

The amount by which you could reduce your risk of obesity over eight years simply by eating a bowl of cereal every morning.

Obesity is one of the most devastating conditions when it comes to your health. It's linked not only to an increased risk of the problems you'd expect—heart disease and diabetes, as well as joint pain—but also to numerous others you may not think of, such as cancer, hearing loss, Alzheimer's disease, and gastrointestinal problems. For some people, keeping extra weight off seems almost impossible—but it's not. Just don't make the mistake of relying on short-term "dieting," which is surprisingly ineffective. The trick is to combine smart portion control with exercise, something you simply can't leave out of the equation.

Key Prevention Strategies

Exercise 30 minutes a day. Exercise, even more than cutting calories, is key to losing weight and keeping it off. Any amount helps, but a good, easily reached goal is 30 minutes on most days. Surprisingly, a 30-minute workout is almost as effective as a 60-minute workout, according to a study published in the *Journal of the American Medical Association*. When 184 women walked either outside or on a treadmill at various intensities for 30 or 60 minutes a day, five days a week for a year, researchers found that it didn't matter how hard or how long the workout was—the women still lost nearly the same amount of weight. Those who exercised for an hour a day lost about 10 percent more than those who did it for a half hour a day. Given that the average weight loss was 19 pounds, that's a difference of only about 2 pounds. But why? The researchers speculate that the more you exercise, the more you think you can eat—and by eating more, you offset some of the weight loss you would have achieved. The moral of the story: Go ahead and get as much exercise as you can (some people will need more than 30 minutes a day to get rid of stubborn fat or keep weight off); just don't raid the cookie jar as a reward.

Eat breakfast. We've known for a long time that people who eat breakfast every day (we recommend a whole grain cereal with at least three grams of fiber per serving) are more likely to maintain a healthy weight or, if they're trying to lose weight, drop more pounds than those who don't have breakfast. The reason has to do with how your body reacts to any shortage of food, even a brief one. If you skip breakfast in the morning, not only do you feel like you're starving by lunchtime, your body actually thinks it's starving and reacts by slowing down metabolism to conserve calories. Most experts agree that eating breakfast every day is simply one of the best things you can do for your weight.

Some researchers now even think that your breakfast should be a big one—your biggest meal of the day, in fact. They point to research that suggests a big breakfast does a better job of controlling appetite and cravings for sweets and starches later in the day, helping you keep weight off.

Practice portion control. In the United States, we're eating as much as 25 percent more food per person than we did 40 years ago. One reason is "portion distortion"—we've become used to the vastly oversized servings at fast-food and sit-down restaurants, making it difficult for us to recognize a "normal" portion at home. Here's a new mindset to adopt: When you eat, think about quality over quantity, and consider yourself done eating when you're only 80 percent full. The point is to give your body the nutrition it needs, not to overstuff yourself as if food may never again be available (it will!). Try these tips.

- **Use smaller plates.** Studies find that if you use large plates, you not only put more food on the plate but eat more of what's in front of you.
- **Eat in the dining room.** Serve in the kitchen, then go to another room to eat. You'll be less likely to go for seconds if you have to get up and return to the kitchen to get them.
- **Slow down.** Most of us eat too fast. This doesn't give the brain time to receive the hormonal signals from the stomach that it's full. Along those lines, wait at least 20 minutes after eating before going for seconds or dessert. Chances are, you won't want either!

"fast food" from your freezer

Eating out—particularly fast food—is a major cause of weight gain. One study found that people who consumed fast food more than twice a week gained 10 pounds more over a 15-year period than those who ate fast food less than once a week. To reduce the incentive to eat out, keep the freezer stocked with these "convenience" foods.

- **Frozen shrimp**
- **Frozen fish (no sauce)**
- **Frozen vegetables (no sauce)**
- **Frozen edamame (green soybeans)**
- **Boneless skinless chicken breasts**
- **Homemade chili or soup**
- **Turkey burgers**
- **Frozen ravioli**
- **Pork loin (thinly sliced for quick cooking)**

Combine them with pantry items such as whole grain pasta, brown rice, vinegars, olive oil, bottled pesto, canned tomatoes, and beans, along with bagged salad greens from the fridge, and you have the makings of countless emergency meals.

Fill half of your plate with nonstarchy vegetables. Most vegetables, not including corn and potatoes, fill you up on very few calories—far fewer than whatever other food your plate contains. Fill another quarter of your plate with a carbohydrate such as pasta, brown rice, or corn and the rest with lean meat, chicken, fish, or another protein food. It's the easiest, simplest way we know to keep a lid on excess calories.

Join a weight-loss support group to keep weight off. If you've managed to lose weight and want to keep it off, it helps to have support, preferably in person (think Weight Watchers). When researchers compared people who attended support groups with those who received online help or just a newsletter about maintaining weight loss, they found that the live-meeting group regained an average of 5.5 pounds; the other two groups regained an average of 10 to 11 pounds. The online support did have some benefit, however; Just 54.6 percent of those participants regained weight compared with 72.4 percent in the newsletter group.

Prevention Boosters

Hang around healthy-weight people. You know the old saying that after a while, people start to look like their dogs? It turns out the same may be true when it comes to their friends. One major study that followed a group of people for more than 30 years found that a person's risk of obesity increased by 57 percent if they had a friend who became obese and by 37 percent if their spouse became obese. The moral of the story: Spend time with healthy-weight friends! If you or your spouse is gaining weight, hit the track/salad bar/Weight Watchers group together; studies find that buddying up like this can lead to both of you shedding more pounds than either of you would if you tried alone.

Weigh yourself often. It's much easier to lose 1 pound than 10, and unless you wear your clothes tight,

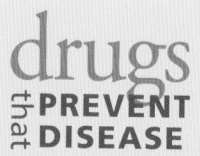

drugs that PREVENT DISEASE

Researchers are still searching for the proverbial "diet in a pill," but until they find it, some medications—coupled with lifestyle changes—can help you lose more weight than lifestyle tweaks alone. One of those drugs is sibutramine (Meridia). It works like many antidepressants by increasing the amount of serotonin and norepinephrine in your brain. These chemicals are involved in regulating not only mood but also appetite. Increasing them helps you feel full sooner, reducing the amount you eat.

If you take Meridia, it's important to also eat right and exercise. In one study, people who took the drug and changed their lifestyle lost an average of more than 26 pounds compared with the 11 pounds lost by those who only took the medication and 15 pounds lost by those who only made lifestyle changes. The researchers found similar results in people using the drug to maintain weight loss.

you may not notice that you've added a few. A study of more than 3,000 people found that the more often people weighed themselves, the more weight they lost or the less weight they gained.

Watch it when you're pregnant. One of the nice things about pregnancy is that you no longer have to hold in your stomach. Just watch out for exactly how much weight you gain. It turns out that pregnancy itself may leave a "legacy" of extra pounds. For instance, in one study, a year after women delivered, they still weighed between 4.5 and 6.6 pounds more than women of the same age who had not been pregnant. To maintain a healthy weight during pregnancy, continue to do some physical activity, weigh yourself regularly, and don't pretend that half gallon of Rocky Road is "for the baby."

Cut back on calories and up the exercise when you quit smoking. Nicotine suppresses weight gain, so if you're quitting smoking (which, as you know, you should), plan to get more exercise, and stock up low-calorie foods (carrot sticks, anyone?) you can use to help you through when you want to keep your mouth busy. Also, weigh yourself regularly to catch the pounds before they accumulate. The prescription drug bupropion (Zyban) may help you quit without gaining weight. (See page 39 for more information.)

Spring for professional advice. A registered dietitian will evaluate how you eat and live, help you set weight and health goals, and design a customized diet and exercise program to get you there. Such assistance works: A University of Minnesota study found that adults who met with a dietitian once a week for nearly three months lost 67 percent more weight than those who attended semi-weekly weigh-in meetings that didn't involve a dietitian. Your health insurance may cover the cost, but even if you have to pay out of pocket (figure about $60 for a one-hour appointment), it's cheaper than the medical costs associated with obesity.

WHAT CAUSES IT While genetics plays a role in weight, the greatest contributor is eating more calories than your body burns as energy. The excess is stored as fat.

SYMPTOMS TO WATCH FOR A body mass index (BMI) of 30 or more, which indicates obesity. You can figure your BMI at www.cdc.gov/nccdphp/dnpa/bmi/adult_BMI/english_bmi_calculator/bmi_calculator.htm.

NEWEST THINKING A virus known as human adenovirus-36 may be partly responsible for obesity in some people. A study involving 502 unrelated thin and obese people found that 30 percent of those who were obese had at one point been infected with adenovirus-36 compared with 11 percent of those who were not obese. The researchers also looked at 28 pairs of twins and found that people with antibodies to the virus (meaning that they had been infected at some point) tended to weigh more than their identical siblings who didn't have the antibodies.

Osteoporosis

40%

The amount by which you can reduce your risk of hip fracture by walking four hours a week.

After about age 30, the body breaks down old bone faster than it can build new bone. Since the hormone estrogen works to keep bones strong, women have even more rapid bone loss after about age 50 or when they reach menopause. Drugs are available to slow the process in people at high risk for fractures, but generally speaking, once bone is lost, it's gone for good. (And some bone-building drugs come with scary side effects, including an *increased* risk of certain fractures!) That's why prevention is so important. While about 60 percent of your bone density is determined by genetics, that still leaves 40 percent you can affect. Get crackin' before your bones do!

Key Prevention Strategies

Get enough calcium and vitamin D. If you're not getting enough calcium in your diet, your body steals what it needs from your bones, putting you at risk for osteoporosis. To protect your bones, add more low-fat dairy foods (such as fat-free milk and yogurt) to your diet. You'll need four dairy servings (generally a cup, or eight ounces) to achieve your target of 1,200 milligrams a day. (See "Eating Your Calcium" on page 266 for other sources.)

It's also critical to get enough vitamin D, which helps the body use calcium. Sunlight is the best source of the "sunshine vitamin," but because we're wearing more sunblock these days, many of us run low. Experts sometimes recommend getting 10 or 15 minutes of sunlight—without sunblock—a day. Unfortunately, as you age, your body's ability to synthesize the vitamin from sunlight fades, so it's not a bad idea to take a daily supplement of 400 IU of vitamin D, especially if you live in a northern climate or don't want to expose yourself to sunlight because of fears about skin cancer.

Although getting calcium from food is best, as insurance you might also consider calcium supplements.

drugs that PREVENT DISEASE

If you're a postmenopausal woman with a high risk of osteoporosis—because it runs in your family, you're underweight, you smoke or used to smoke, and/or you don't get much weight-bearing exercise (being Caucasian is also a risk factor, as is long-term use of corticosteroids for diseases like asthma or arthritis)—talk to your doctor about taking either raloxifene (Evista) or one of the bisphosphonate drugs, including ibandronate (Boniva), risedronate (Actonel), or alendronate (Fosamax). Evista works by mimicking estrogen in your body, which slows bone-destroying cells. Bisphosphonates work by suppressing the bone-destroying cells directly. These drugs have side effects, so be sure to ask for a frank assessment of their risks and benefits.

In the massive Women's Health Initiative study, women who took 1,000 milligrams of calcium and 400 IU of vitamin D every day for seven years had a hip bone density 1.06 percent higher than that of those who took a placebo, plus a 29 percent lower risk of hip fracture. You can take up to 1,200 milligrams of calcium a day in two doses (up to 600 milligrams each, which is all the body can absorb at one time). Calcium citrate, though it costs more than other forms of calcium, is absorbed better by your body, especially if you're taking a proton-pump inhibitor like omeprazole (Prilosec) or esomeprazole (Nexium) or an H2 blocker like famotidine (Pepcid) or ranitidine (Zantac), which reduce stomach acid that breaks down nutrients.

Stress your bones through exercise. When astronauts go into space, they lose up to 1.5 percent of their total bone mass for each month in orbit. Why? Because at zero gravity, there's no weight pressing on their bones, and bone-building cells do their work only when they feel some "strain." That, in a nutshell, sums up the reason that exercise is so important to bone strength. An analysis of 25 major studies on the effect of exercise on bone found it could prevent or reverse almost 1 percent of bone loss a year in the lower spine and hip for pre- and postmenopausal women. That may not sound like a lot, but it's enough to make a huge difference in your risk of fracture, given that with age, between 0.5 and 1 percent of bone density is lost per year.

The best kinds of exercise are those that tax your muscles (and therefore your bones), such as working hard in your garden, lifting weights, or jogging. You can even just hop up and down. When British researchers had premenopausal women hop on one leg for a few minutes (50 hops) for six months, they found increased hipbone density on the side of that leg compared to no change in the other hip. Plain old walking also helps. A study of more than 61,000 postmenopausal women found those who walked for four or more hours a week had a 40 percent lower risk of hip fracture than those who walked an hour or less a week.

Get treated for depression. If you have even mild depression—feeling less interested in things you usually enjoy, changes in your sleep and eating patterns, fatigue, and so on—your bones may suffer. It turns out that premenopausal women with even mild depression have less bone mass than women of the same age who aren't depressed. It doesn't seem to be related to antidepressants

"The best kinds of exercise are those that tax your muscles."

but to changes in the immune system that increase inflammation. In fact, some experts suggest that depression should be viewed as an early symptom of osteoporosis, a disease that typically has no symptoms. It seems to be just as serious a risk factor as low calcium intake, smoking, and lack of exercise. (Turn to the Depression chapter for prevention tips.)

Prevention Boosters

Stop smoking. By now you're probably sick of hearing this advice, but if you want to save your bones, it's time to stamp out the butts. Studies find that smoking increases the risk of a spinal fracture by

eating your calcium

Women who get most of their calcium from their diets do better bone-wise than those who rely on supplements. Four dairy servings will get you to 1,200 milligrams of calcium. Here are some other easy ways to get more calcium from food.

- **Start with cereal.** Just 3/4 cup of whole grain cereal (even without milk) provides 1,100 milligrams, thanks to the fact that cereals are enriched with added nutrients; add a half cup of fat-free milk, and you're up to 1,390 milligrams—all you need for the day!

- **Snack on yogurt.** An eight-ounce container of plain low-fat yogurt gives you 452 milligrams. To sweeten it, spoon in a tablespoon of blackstrap molasses, which adds about another 200 milligrams.

- **Get your greens at dinner.** One cup of kale contains 42 milligrams of calcium. Spinach is another top source of calcium, but your body has a tougher time absorbing all of it. With kale, your body takes in nearly the full amount. Soybeans are another good non-dairy source.

- **Open a tin.** Of sardines, that is. Three ounces of the oily fish (with bones) provides 325 milligrams. Consider substituting sardines for tuna in sandwiches.

- **Drink a glass of fortified OJ.** Eight ounces of orange juice fortified with calcium and vitamin D gives you 330 milligrams of calcium and about 45 IU of vitamin D.

- **Stick with soft cheeses.** How about low-fat ricotta cheese on whole grain crackers or toast for a healthy snack or breakfast? Two ounces provides about 167 milligrams.

- **Whip up a batch of cornbread.** One cup of cornmeal is packed with 483 milligrams.

- **Treat yourself to a smoothie.** Blend a banana, 1 cup milk, 1/2 cup strawberries, and a tablespoon of brown sugar on high for 30 seconds for a luscious drink that provides about 500 milligrams of calcium.

13 percent in women and 32 percent in men and ups the risk of a hip fracture by 31 percent in women and 40 percent in men. Once you quit, that risk begins to drop almost immediately.

Stock up on spinach. Spinach is packed with vitamin K, an often-forgotten vitamin important for preventing fractures. One study found that taking 45 milligrams of K a day reduced the rate of spinal fractures by 65 percent in women with osteoporosis compared to women who didn't supplement. Other studies find that as little as 1 to 10 milligrams a day can reduce the amount of bone that's lost. You can get about 1 milligram from a cup of most greens, including kale, collards, spinach, and turnip and beet greens.

TO PROTECT YOUR BONES, ADD MORE LOW-FAT DAIRY FOODS (SUCH AS FAT-FREE MILK AND YOGURT) TO YOUR DIET.

WHAT CAUSES IT Bone is constantly being built up by cells called osteoblasts and broken down by cells called osteoclasts. Until about your thirties, the osteoblasts are in the lead, but sometime during that decade you reach "peak bone mass," and for the next decade or so, the two run neck and neck. From about age 50 onward, as levels of estrogen (in women) and testosterone (in men) drop, the osteoclasts pull ahead.

SYMPTOMS TO WATCH FOR None. Osteoporosis is typically identified with a bone density scan or when you fracture a bone. If you have a fracture, particularly if it occurred as a result of something relatively innocuous like tripping over a step, ask your doctor for a scan to measure your bone density. Everyone should have a bone scan at least once at age 65, or earlier if your doctor recommends it.

NEWEST THINKING Men should also be screened for osteoporosis. The American College of Physicians now recommends that doctors evaluate risk factors for osteoporosis in men before age 65; if risks exist, men should have a scan to measure their bone density and start on medication if it's low. About 6 out of 100 men will have osteoporosis by age 65.

Ovarian Cancer

Don't shrug off persistent back or abdominal pain, especially if you've also been feeling bloated and tired. It could be a signal of ovarian cancer. While breast cancer is far more common in women, ovarian cancer is far more deadly. That's because most of the time, it isn't discovered until the late stages, when it's much more difficult to treat. The cancer isn't inevitable for women, however; researchers have found numerous steps you can take to reduce your risk.

Key Prevention Strategies

Take birth control pills. The link between oral contraceptives and a reduced risk of ovarian cancer is so strong that a recent editorial in a leading medical journal suggested that all women who can take the pills should. Just how strong is the link? An analysis of 45 studies from 21 countries found that women who had ever used oral contraceptives had a 27 percent lower risk of developing ovarian cancer than women who had never used them. Every five years of use reduced the risk by about 20 percent; after 15 years of use, the risk was halved. Even better? The protective effect of oral contraceptives lasts 30 years after a woman stops taking them. The downsides of oral contraceptives include a higher risk of blood clots.

Breastfeed your children. Because breastfeeding suppresses ovulation, it can also reduce your risk of ovarian cancer. One study of nearly 150,000 nurses found that women who had ever breastfed a child—no matter for how long—reduced their risk by 14 percent. Those who breastfed for 18 months or longer cut their risk by one-third. Overall, each month of breastfeeding reduced the risk of ovarian cancer by 2 percent.

Prevention Boosters

Get your tubes tied. Done having babies? Opt for a tubal ligation, an operation in which your fallopian tubes are cut and sealed shut. Many studies find that it reduces the risk of ovarian cancer by at least one-third overall and by up to 60 percent in women who carry the BRCA1 genetic mutation. One reason may be that when the tubes are closed off, cancer-causing chemicals and other toxins can't travel from the vagina and cervix through the tubes to the ovaries.

got the gene?

If your mother, sister, or mother's sister had ovarian cancer or breast cancer before menopause, talk to your doctor about the possibility that you might carry a mutation of the BRCA1 or BRCA2 gene. These mutations significantly increase your risk of developing ovarian cancer as well as breast cancer. If genetic screening shows you do carry the gene, you may want to consider having your ovaries removed, which studies find can reduce your risk of ovarian cancer by 96 percent and of breast cancer by 50 percent.

Avoid talcum powder. Made from magnesium silicate, talcum powder is linked with an increased risk of ovarian cancer in some studies and has even been found embedded in some ovarian cancers. One study found that women who used talcum powder in the genital area or on sanitary pads had a 50 to 70 percent increased risk of developing ovarian cancer. The link may be related to the inflammation that results if particles of talc travel through the reproductive tract to the ovaries or to the fact that decades ago, the powder was contaminated with asbestos, a known carcinogen. While today's manufacturers are careful to keep any asbestos fibers out of the powder, it's still worth finding another alternative for staying dry.

Shed some pounds. If you have a body mass index (BMI) of 30 or more, you also have about a 30 percent increased risk of developing ovarian cancer. And if you do get the cancer, your risk of dying from it is 50 percent higher than that of women with a healthier BMI. The reason is probably related to the fact that fat cells release chemicals that are eventually converted to estrogen, a hormone that fuels the growth of reproductive cancers like ovarian cancer.

BECAUSE BREASTFEEDING SUPPRESSES OVULATION, IT CAN ALSO REDUCE YOUR RISK OF OVARIAN CANCER.

WHAT CAUSES IT The precise cause is still under investigation, but there are two main theories. One is that ovulation leads to trauma and repair of ovarian cells; the more you ovulate, the more repair is required, providing more opportunities for genetic "mistakes" to occur when cells divide. The other theory suggests that long-term exposure to reproductive hormones like estrogen, which contribute to cell division, triggers those cellular mistakes.

SYMPTOMS TO WATCH FOR Bloating; pain in your pelvis, abdomen, or lower back; feeling full quickly; urinary symptoms, such as the urgent or frequent need to urinate; persistent fatigue. If these symptoms occur suddenly and are present nearly every day for several weeks, see your doctor.

NEWEST THINKING A simple blood test to detect early-stage ovarian cancer may soon be available. Researchers at the Yale School of Medicine have developed a test that is sensitive enough to detect the cancer in the early stage with 99 percent accuracy, though whether the test will have an acceptably low number of false-positive results when used in a large population of women remains to be shown. The test measures levels of proteins that are higher in the blood of women with ovarian cancer.

Peripheral Vascular Disease

33%

The reduction in your risk of peripheral vascular disease if you get 29 grams of fiber per day.

Think of peripheral vascular disease (PVD) as heart disease in your legs. The same factors that clog your coronary arteries with plaque, from eating double cheeseburgers to hugging the couch or chair all day, also pad the walls of your leg arteries with plaque. This can eventually shut off the blood supply to leg muscles and trigger intense pain when you walk. PVD is a big deal for two reasons: It causes circulation problems that keep you off your feet and raise your risk of getting tough-to-heal sores on your feet, and it's a warning sign that arteries throughout your body are being narrowed by plaque. People diagnosed with PVD have a one in five chance of having a heart attack or stroke within a year. These steps can keep the blood vessels in your legs clear.

Key Prevention Strategies

Stop smoking. Nothing's worse than tobacco smoke for the arteries in your legs. The thousands of toxic chemicals in cigarettes narrow your arteries so much that smokers have a tenfold higher risk for PVD than nonsmokers do. Nicotine and other chemicals in tobacco also stiffen the normally flexible inner lining of artery walls, raising blood pressure and helping to trigger changes in your cholesterol that prompt the buildup of plaque in artery walls. If you already have signs of PVD, such as leg pain, stopping smoking can double or triple the distance you can walk pain free.

Control your blood sugar. Having diabetes raises your risk of PVD 2.5 times higher than normal. Following all the advice in our Diabetes chapter will help. But if your blood sugar remains high (126 mg/dl or higher on a fasting blood sugar test), it's time for blood sugar–lowering medication. In a British study of people with diabetes, those who kept their blood sugar under tight control cut their risk of serious PVD problems—like leg pain or the need for blood vessel surgery or even amputation—by 22 percent.

Lower your bad cholesterol, raise your good. Unhealthy cholesterol levels clog the walls of arteries in your legs (or arms) just as they do in your heart. Having high total cholesterol (over 200 mg/dl) increases your odds for PVD by an incredible 90 percent. The best fix? The same strategies that protect the arteries in your heart and brain: reducing your "bad" LDL cholesterol and boosting your "good" HDL cholesterol. Follow all the smart advice in the High Cholesterol chapter—choose salmon instead of steak, switch from refined grains to whole grains, load your plate with fruits and veggies, and get some exercise most days of the week.

Follow all of your doctor's advice if you have heart disease or have had a stroke. A history of heart attack or stroke more than triples your risk of PVD. If you've survived one of these life-threatening events, it's time to pamper your entire cardiovascular system so that you can live well. That means getting regular physical activity, eating well, cutting stress, and taking any medications your doctor prescribes.

Deflate that spare tire. If you have a beer belly or any other form of extra fat around your middle, it's time to trim it. When Spanish researchers weighed and measured 708 men with and without PVD, they found that those carrying more fat around their middles had a 32 percent higher risk than those with trim, slim waists. Experts recommend waist measurements under 40 inches for men and under 35 inches for women.

Prevention Boosters

Go high fiber. Men who got 29 grams of fiber a day had a 33 percent lower risk of developing PVD compared to men who got just 13 grams a day (close to the amount the average person eats), report researchers from the Harvard School of Public Health who tracked the health of more than 44,000 men for 12 years. The guys who ate high-fiber foods got lots of whole grains, fruits, and vegetables; compared to men who ate low-fiber foods, they also tended to exercise more and eat less fat, all strategies that also keep blood vessels healthy.

WHAT CAUSES IT Deposits of plaque in the walls of the arteries that supply blood to your legs and/or arms. They narrow arteries and restrict the flow of blood to your muscles. They can also trigger the formation of artey-blocking clots.

SYMPTOMS TO WATCH FOR Numbness or weakness in your legs; cold feet or legs; sores that won't heal on your toes, feet, or legs; hair loss or changes in the color of the skin on your legs and feet; pain or cramping that starts when you're active and disappears after you stop. Half of the people with PVD have very mild symptoms or no symptoms.

NEWEST THINKING Exposure to lead and cadmium could raise PVD risk. In a Johns Hopkins University study, researchers found that those with the highest lead exposures—from sources such as lead paint, lead-glazed pottery, and contaminated drinking water—had a 65 percent higher risk than people with the lowest exposures. High exposure to cadmium, found in the emissions from coal-fired power plants and trash incinerators and in cigarette smoke, raised risk 86 percent compared to people with the lowest exposures. Steering clear of cigarette smoke and following safety advice for removing lead paint are some ways to limit exposure.

Poison Ivy

68%

The drop in your chances of getting a blistery rash if you slather on a poison ivy–blocking lotion before heading outdoors.

Itchy, itchy, itchy. There's no better description for the blisters that pop up—and keep popping up—after a run-in with poison ivy, poison oak, or poison sumac. The rash-provoking oil in these plants, called urushiol, rubs off not only on you but also on pets, garden tools, and clothes, putting you at risk even if you aren't outdoors. Knowing how to avoid the plants is key, of course. These strategies can protect your skin and, in case of unexpected exposure, help you get rid of the blister-raising oil fast.

Key Prevention Strategies

Know the enemy. Poison ivy, oak, and sumac crop up in surprising spots—in flowerpots, along sidewalks, or twined in trees and bushes. Know how to recognize them. Visit a local nature center and ask the naturalist to point out your local itch maker.

Cover up. Wearing high socks, long pants, and a long-sleeved shirt provides a barrier against itch-provoking plants. If you find yourself face to face with these botanicals often (perhaps you've got a dog who loves to chase squirrels through the underbrush), keep an extra pair of pants and a shirt in your car.

you touched it? do this to avoid blisters

If you can't wash with soap and water within 10 minutes after a brush with a "poisonous" plant, take these steps immediately.

Use a poison ivy wipe or wash. Formulated to remove urushiol, these products can whisk up to 95 percent of urushiol off the skin, studies show. Brands include Tecnu Outdoor Skin Cleanser and Cortaid Poison Ivy Care wipes.

No special products? Try cold water. Dash to a stream or pond and rinse well. Avoid getting rinse water on other parts of your body; some experts think using water without soap can spread urushiol around, while others maintain that a thorough rinsing is worthwhile because it can dislodge the oil.

Rewash with soap or an ivy wash when you get home. Washing with soap will remove any urushiol that hasn't attached itself to skin proteins yet. Even if you've taken emergency measures while outdoors, hopping into the shower or washing off your arms and legs in a sink within an hour after exposure can further cut your risk of itchy blisters.

If you have a poison ivy wash product at home, use it, following the label directions. (Some must be rubbed onto dry skin before you wash up.) The wash may help break urushiol's grip up to eight hours after you brushed against the wrong plant.

Slather on a urushiol-blocking lotion before you head outside.
In a study of 211 people, 68 percent of those who used a lotion
called IvyBlock had no rash after exposure to urushiol. Once the
oil gets onto your skin, it penetrates the top layer quickly and is
difficult to remove, especially if you're far from soap and water.
The most common active ingredient in this type of product,
bentoquatam, is a clay that stops absorption of urushiol.

Work carefully outdoors. Some people claim that urushiol can
penetrate latex and rubber (though we don't have confirmation),
so wear vinyl gloves when working outdoors. Consider wearing
a face mask when mowing or using a trimmer near these plants.
And treat dead or dormant plants as if they were alive—they still
contain the oils that cause rashes. Never burn poison ivy, oak, or
sumac; the urushiol can severely irritate your lungs.

Prevent out-of-control itching. Once the rash appears, it will
be there for a while. An over-the-counter antihistamine like
diphenhydramine (Benadryl) can help with the itching. Over-
the-counter hydrocortisone cream may help in milder cases, but
stronger prescription cortisone products provide greater relief.
Cortisone pills or injections can help control more severe outbreaks.

Prevention Boosters

Launder all outdoor clothing right away. If you suspect you've
brushed against itch-making plants, wash all clothing, including
outerwear, right away. The oil stays potent for months or even
years and can trigger a new outbreak if you come in contact with
the clothing later on.

Lather Fido and Fluffy. Dogs and cats don't develop poison ivy,
but they can transfer the oil to you. If you think your pet's been
exposed, put on vinyl gloves and give her a bath with pet shampoo.

Clean up garden tools, outdoor play equipment, and shoes, too.
Urushiol that's rubbed off on shovels, clippers, balls, boots, and
other objects can stay potent for at least a year in warm, humid
environments and for several years in drier climates. That raises
your risk of surprise outbreaks even if you haven't ventured
outdoors! Cleaning up with soap and water works, as does a
rubdown with rubbing alcohol or a solvent like xylene or acetone.

WHAT CAUSES IT An
allergic reaction to urushiol,
a sticky, irritating oil found
in poison ivy, poison oak,
and poison sumac plants.
An estimated 85 percent of
adults and children react;
the remaining 15 percent are
blissfully unaffected.

**SYMPTOMS TO WATCH
FOR** An itchy rash with red
patches and long streaks that
appears 8 to 48 hours after
exposure. Oddly, new blisters
can continue to appear for up
to three weeks after exposure,
as your skin continues to react
to the urushiol. The fluid in the
blisters does not spread the rash.

NEWEST THINKING Watch
out! Thanks to global warming,
poison ivy's more abundant
and may be itchier, too. Weed
experts from the USDA reported
recently that growth rates
for poison ivy have doubled
in the past 50 years, perhaps
thanks to slight increases in
carbon dioxide levels in the
atmosphere. The plants also
seem to be making a more
potent form of the rash-
triggering oil, urushiol.

Premenstrual Syndrome (PMS)

33%

The amount by which you may reduce your risk of PMS by getting at least 1,200 milligrams of calcium and about 400 IU of vitamin D from your daily diet.

About one in three women experience the bloating, breast tenderness, insomnia, headaches, and other symptoms of premenstrual syndrome (PMS) in the five to seven days before their periods. Another 3 to 8 percent experience a more severe version, premenstrual dysphoric disorder, or PMDD. Given that women will have, on average, 451 menstrual cycles in their lifetimes, feeling lousy for four or five days before each cycle adds up to more than six years of misery. Beat the averages with these tips.

got the gene?

In late 2007, researchers identified the first genetic link to PMS and its more severe cousin, premenstrual dysphoric disorder (PMDD). The gene in question affects how women respond to changes in estrogen levels; in women with PMS, mutations in the gene make them respond abnormally. The mutations also lead to reduced levels of dopamine, a brain chemical involved in mood. The findings may provide some peace of mind to women who now know that the mood swings and other symptoms of PMS are not in their heads but at least partly in their genes.

Key Prevention Strategies

Follow a bone-strengthening diet. That means one rich in calcium and vitamin D, which helps the body absorb calcium. No one is certain exactly why this combination works—it's possible that PMS actually stems from a lack of calcium—but it does help some women. A large study of about 3,000 women found that those who got about 1,200 milligrams of calcium and 400 IU of vitamin D from food were about a third less likely to have PMS than those who got considerably less. Fat-free milk is a great source of both nutrients, as is fortified orange juice. You can read more about good food sources of each in the Osteoporosis chapter.

While getting calcium from food provides the greatest benefit (both for preventing PMS and helping to keep bones healthy), there is also evidence that supplementing can help. One study of 248 women found that supplementing with 1,200 milligrams of calcium carbonate for three months slashed PMS severity nearly in half compared to taking a placebo.

Turn to chasteberry. Several studies find that an extract from the fruit of chasteberry trees works fairly well at preventing PMS symptoms. In one study of 170 German women, 86 received the dried herbal extract and 84 got a placebo. Researchers tracked six PMS symptoms—irritability, mood swings, anger, headache, breast fullness, and bloating—and found that symptoms improved by more than 50 percent in the majority of the women taking the herb compared to no improvement in those taking the placebo. Follow the dosage directions on the brand you purchase.

Prevention Boosters

Eat less fat and more vegetables. A study of 33 healthy women found that reducing the amount of fat in their diets from the typical 40 percent to 20 percent by following a vegetarian regimen reduced duration and intensity of pain, improved concentration, and reduced mood swings and bloating prior to menstruation. Overall, bloating incidence dropped from nearly 3 to 1.3 days, mood swings from 1.7 to 1.1 days, and concentration problems from nearly 2 days to less than 1 day.

Why does this type of diet help? It could be that it flattens the hormone rollercoaster by lowering levels of estrogen in the blood.

Consider these supplements. Various studies suggest that taking either 100 milligrams of vitamin B_6 a day or 200 to 360 milligrams a day of magnesium (in divided doses taken three times a day beginning 15 days after your period starts) can also relieve PMS symptoms. Check with your doctor before taking any of these supplements long term.

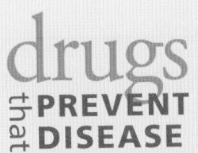

Two drugs are approved for preventing the more severe form of PMS known as premenstrual dysphoric disorder (PMDD). However, many doctors will prescribe them if you have PMS. The first is a low dose of the anti-depressant fluoxetine (best known as Prozac). In numerous studies, it relieved 60 to 75 percent of PMS/PMDD symptoms. The cyclical version of fluoxetine prescribed for PMDD is called Sarafem, and you take it only during the 14 days prior to your period. The second drug, YAZ, is an oral contraceptive that combines estrogen with a new form of progestin. It may help with premenstrual symptoms, and some studies find that it significantly decreases PMDD symptoms.

Even regular birth control pills, if taken for 24 days with 4 days off rather than the typical 21 days on and 7 days off, can reduce PMS symptoms. Discuss this option with your doctor.

WHAT CAUSES IT There is probably a link between hormonal changes during the menstrual cycle and mood-related chemicals in the brain called neurotransmitters, particularly serotonin and endorphins. There's some evidence that the autonomic nervous system, which manages involuntary processes like breathing and heart rate, also plays a role.

SYMPTOMS TO WATCH FOR Bloating, fatigue, breast tenderness, headaches, mood swings, irritability, depression, increased appetite, forgetfulness, trouble concentrating.

NEWEST THINKING Severe PMS may be a sign of a permanently depressed nervous system. Japanese researchers proposed this theory in late 2007 after measuring heart rates and hormone levels in 62 women and evaluating their physical, emotional, and behavioral symptoms before and during their periods. Women with PMS showed significant drops in heart rate variability, a sign of how well the autonomic nervous system functions.

Prostate Cancer

73%

The amount by which drinking three cups of green tea a day could reduce your risk of this cancer.

If you're a man and you live long enough, you'll develop prostate cancer. That's just one of the downsides of the hormone testosterone, which fuels the growth of prostate cells. The key is to keep this typically slow-growing cancer at bay long enough so that if you *do* get it, it remains so minuscule that it doesn't need treatment.

Key Prevention Strategies

Follow a prostate-protective diet. Here's what a typical day might look like.

Breakfast

- **Half a grapefruit.** It turns out that the pectin in citrus fruits—the stuff used to make jams and jellies gel—destroys prostate cancer cells. It's also an important form of soluble fiber, one that binds to hormones like testosterone to reduce the amount circulating in your body—and the amount your prostate cells are exposed to. Studies find lower levels of prostate-specific antigen (PSA), a protein released by prostate cells and often used to detect prostate cancer, in men whose diets are rich in soluble fiber (also found in peas, beans, and oats). Researchers suspect that high-fiber diets are one reason vegetarians are so much less likely to develop prostate cancer than meat eaters.

- **A cup of green tea.** Green tea contains hefty amounts of a powerful antioxidant called EGCG, which protects prostate cells from the type of biological damage that can lead to cancer. One study found that men who drank three cups a day of tea a day were 73 percent less likely to develop prostate cancer than those who didn't drink tea at all; men who drank this much tea for more than 40 years were 88 percent less likely to develop the cancer. Overall, the more tea the men drank and the longer they drank it, the lower their risk of prostate cancer. This area is so promising that the National Institutes of Health is studying a green tea extract as a way to prevent prostate cancer.

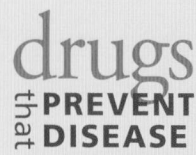

drugs that PREVENT DISEASE You may have heard of finasteride (Proscar), the drug used to treat prostate enlargement. It may help prevent prostate cancer, too. A major prostate cancer prevention trial involving nearly 20,000 men who didn't have prostate enlargement found that men who took the drug for seven years had about a 25 percent reduced risk of prostate cancer compared to men who took a placebo.

Lunch

Soup or salad with edamame. People in Asian countries tend to eat a lot of soy, and men there don't develop prostate cancer as often as Western men do. Soy products like edamame (immature soybeans still in their pods), tofu, and soy milk contain plant-based hormones called isoflavones that help reduce levels of sex hormones like testosterone. The less testosterone, of course, the less fuel is available to drive prostate cancer cell growth. Buy edamame frozen, thaw, and add to soups and salads, or steam lightly, sprinkle with a touch of salt, and enjoy as a snack.

Snack

- **A handful of almonds.** Next to wheat germ oil, almonds are the best food source of vitamin E in nature, providing 7.4 milligrams in a one-ounce serving—and vitamin E may reduce your risk of prostate cancer. A major study of 29,000 Finnish males found that men who took 50 IU of vitamin E (about 33 milligrams) in supplement form were 32 percent less likely than men not taking the supplement to develop prostate cancer and 41 percent less likely to die from it during a five- to eight-year period.

Dinner

- **Roasted salmon.** Salmon is an excellent source of omega-3 fatty acids, which you probably know because of their powerful heart benefits. They are also strongly linked with a lower risk of prostate cancer. A 30-year study of 6,000 Swedish men found that those who ate little or no fish had two to three times the risk of developing prostate cancer compared to those who ate moderate or high amounts of fatty fish. Mackerel is another fish rich in omega-3's.
- **Broccoli sautéed in olive oil.** Broccoli, along with cauliflower, cabbage, and brussels sprouts, contains the anticancer compound sulforaphane. One study found that men who ate three or more servings a week of these veggies were 41 percent less likely to develop prostate cancer than those who ate less than one serving a week. Why sauté (or oven-roast) it in olive oil? The oil is made primarily of good-for-you monounsaturated fat, versus the polyunsaturated fat in corn, safflower, and sunflower oil. Several studies found that men whose diets were high in polyunsaturated fats were more likely to develop prostate cancer.

> "The more tea the men drank and the longer they drank it, the lower their risk of prostate cancer."

Seek out selenium. The trace mineral selenium, found in grains (especially wheat flour and pearled barley), Brazil nuts, and many white fish, is linked to lower rates of prostate cancer. But since levels of selenium in the soil vary widely throughout the world, they vary widely in much of the food we eat. A study conducted with people living in the southeastern United States, where soil levels of selenium are very low, found nearly half the rate of prostate cancer in people who supplemented with 200 micrograms of selenium compared to those who didn't supplement. This and other studies find the benefits of selenium are even greater in ex-smokers.

Taking individual selenium supplements can be risky, though, since they can raise the risk of diabetes, according to new research (and side effects of excess selenium can include hair loss and brittle nails). We recommend sticking with the amount in your multivitamin, if you take one, and adding more fish to your diet if you haven't already. Your doctor can check your selenium levels through a blood test if you want to know if they are low.

Sit in the sun, sans sunscreen, for 10 minutes a day. You'll get valuable vitamin D, which the body manufactures when the sun's UVB rays strike the skin. Men in the United Kingdom—a country not known for its sunny days and where vitamin D deficiency is fairly common—who took regular holidays in sunny climates, sunbathed regularly, and had more overall exposure to ultraviolet rays had far less risk of prostate cancer than men who didn't do these things. Men with low levels of sun exposure also developed cancer younger (age 67.7) than those with more exposure (age 72.1). Of course, sun exposure raises your risk of skin cancer, so don't take this news as an excuse to sunbathe; 10 minutes is all you need. If you live in a low-sun climate, consider supplementing with 1,000 IU of vitamin D a day, especially during the winter months. (It's also good for your bones.)

Prevention Boosters

Ask your doctor about a PSA test. If your doctor suspects you have prostate cancer (or even if he doesn't), he may order a PSA test. This blood test measures levels of a protein called prostate-specific antigen, which is produced by prostate cells. The higher your levels, the more likely it is that you have prostate cancer. But the test isn't definitive; it sounds a lot of false alarms that can result in unnecessary needle biopsies. And since prostate cancer often grows so slowly that treating it isn't necessary, finding it early doesn't necessarily affect your risk of dying from it. That's why there's no consensus on whether doctors should use the test to screen men for the disease. Should you get screened? That's a decision you and your doctor should make based on your family history and your overall risk.

Another test that's used to detect prostate cancer is the digital rectal exam, often used in conjunction with the PSA test.

Order the chicken. If you are a black man, eating 23 or more ounces of red meat a week—no matter what type—means you are more than twice as likely to develop prostate cancer than if you eat less than 9 ounces. (The study showed a difference only in African-American men.) Bacon, sausage, and hot dogs pose the greatest risk. It's safe to load up on chicken and turkey.

SALMON IS AN EXCELLENT SOURCE OF OMEGA-3 FATTY ACIDS, WHICH ARE STRONGLY LINKED WITH A LOWER RISK OF PROSTATE CANCER.

WHAT CAUSES IT Aging. Over time, the cellular mechanisms that prevent abnormalities in dividing cells and destroy aberrant cells weaken. This increases the risk of cells whose "off buttons" don't work. When that happens, the cells divide relentlessly, fueled in part by male hormones such as testosterone. Two out of every three prostate cancers are found in men over 65.

SYMPTOMS TO WATCH FOR Frequent urination, particularly at night; problems urinating (starting or stopping the flow); painful urination; blood in the urine or semen.

NEWEST THINKING
Prostate cancer in many men does not require treatment. Older men with less aggressive forms of cancer can be simply followed through exams and blood tests. In a major study of 9,000 men, average age 77, with early-stage prostate cancer who did not undergo treatment, researchers found that 72 percent either died of other causes or didn't have enough cancer growth to warrant treatment. For the rest, about 10 years passed before the cancer grew enough to require treatment. Men with more aggressive forms of the cancer, however, do require treatment.

Psoriasis

57%

In psoriasis, skin cells mature almost 10 times faster than normal. They pile up, creating silvery scales and patches of thick, red, scaly skin on the elbows, knees, legs, scalp, and elsewhere. These steps can help you avoid the condition and, if you have it already, lower your odds of a flare-up.

Key Prevention Strategies

Quit smoking. Tobacco use triples your risk of plaque psoriasis, the most common form of this condition, Swedish researchers report. If you already have psoriasis, smoking scuttles your chances of having clear, calm skin. When researchers asked 104 people if their psoriasis had ever gone into remission, 77 percent of nonsmokers said yes, compared to just 9 percent of smokers.

Think before you drink. Alcohol boosts psoriasis risk. And Finnish scientists have found that for people who already had psoriasis, the amount of skin affected increased as their alcohol intake rose. If you're in the midst of a flare-up, abstaining makes sense. If your psoriasis is under control, and you find that an occasional drink doesn't aggravate your skin, enjoy in moderation.

Maintain a healthy weight. Gaining extra pounds raised risk by 40 percent in one Harvard Medical School study of more than 78,000 women. Doctors aren't certain how excess body fat contributes to psoriasis, but they do know that it can make existing skin problems worse and render psoriasis treatments less effective.

dead sea magic?

A month of sunbathing and swimming at one of the psoriasis spas along Israel's scenic Dead Sea is virtually guaranteed to improve or completely clear up your skin, studies show. A more affordable option: Fill your bathtub with warm water, sprinkle in Dead Sea salts (available at health food stores), and soak. In one German study, almost everyone who did this three or four times a week for a month saw their psoriasis improve significantly.

Try one of the newer treatments. If you have psoriasis, your goal is to prevent flare-ups. Older medications were often too messy or risky for many people. For people with just a few spots of psoriasis, newer sprays or foam products may be preferable. For more severe forms of psoriasis or for psoriatic arthritis, newer injectable medications are available. One of them, etanercept (Enbrel), improves psoriasis symptoms by 75 percent in 57 percent of the people who use it. Two others, adalimumab (Humira) and infliximab (Remicade), are even more effective.

Moisturize. Lubricating your skin every day can also help cut your odds for flare-ups prompted by dry skin. Go for a greasy cream or ointment. Even cooking oils and vegetable shortening are effective.

Stress less. Coping with psoriasis can be extremely stressful—and stress can trigger new flare-ups. Break the cycle by building relaxation into your day, even if it's just 10 minutes of quiet, calm breathing. Or try mindfulness-based stress reduction (MBSR). In one University of Massachusetts study, people with psoriasis who listened to an MBSR tape while undergoing light therapy saw their skin clear up twice as fast as those who didn't hear the tape, researchers report. Many hospitals offer MBSR classes.

Sunbathe, but safely. Exposing your skin to sunlight for a few minutes each day can reduce inflammation and scaling. Eighty percent of people with psoriasis who try daily sunbaths see an improvement. Don't overdo it, though; for about 1 in 10 people, sun exposure makes skin problems worse, and getting a sunburn raises the risk of skin cancer. Use a broad-spectrum sunscreen on skin that's not affected by psoriasis. Commercial tanning beds may help, but talk it over with your doctor first; some dermatologists still discourage their use.

Steer clear of these medications. Some prescription drugs can trigger a flare-up. If your doctor recommends anti-malaria pills, beta-blockers, indomethacin (Indocin), or lithium, ask whether a substitute is possible.

Prevention Boosters

Baby your skin. For about half of all people with psoriasis, it worsens 10 to 14 days after any sort of cut, bruise, bug bite, or scrape. Even shaving or removing an adhesive bandage could trigger a flare-up.

Check your reaction to gluten. In studies, people with celiac disease who avoided gluten, a protein found in wheat, barley, and rye, saw their psoriasis improve. Symptoms of gluten intolerance include diarrhea, abdominal pain, and gas.

WHAT CAUSES IT Genes raise your risk of psoriasis, but experts aren't certain what triggers the immune system malfunction that leads to the condition. It begins when infection-fighting T cells in the skin become too active, stimulating the overgrowth of skin cells.

SYMPTOMS TO WATCH FOR Patches of thick red skin with silvery scales on the elbows, knees, other parts of the legs, scalp, lower back, face, palms, and soles of the feet. Less often, they appear on the fingernails, toenails, and genitals and inside the mouth.

NEWEST THINKING In a recent survey, over half of people with moderate to severe psoriasis weren't getting the treatments that prevent future flare-ups. If your psoriasis isn't improving with lotions and topical medications, ask about light therapy and oral or injectable medications that help normalize the overactive immune responses that trigger psoriasis.

Rosacea

50%

The drop in the likelihood of a recurrence of symptoms if you use a prescription skin-calming cream for six months after antibiotic therapy.

Avoiding and treating flare-ups of this adults-only skin condition can help keep it from getting worse. Yet three out of four people don't recognize the early signs and symptoms. Flushing, blushing, and stubbornly red skin on your cheeks and nose are major clues, but other hints are burning, stinging, or itching facial skin as well as raised red patches and even swollen spots. In one survey, one in four people had signs of rosacea on the neck, chest, scalp, or ears, too. You may be more prone to rosacea if other family members have it or if you're of Irish or English descent.

Key Prevention Strategies

Avoid rosacea triggers. The most important step in avoiding outbreaks is learning what triggers them. Tops on most people's lists are sun exposure, emotional stress, and hot weather, but there are plenty more. In a survey of people with rosacea, about half said that wind, heavy exercise, drinking alcohol, taking a hot bath, cold weather, and spicy foods (including obvious hot stuff like chile peppers and Mexican food, as well as vinegar, white pepper, and garlic) set off a reaction.

To pinpoint your triggers, keep a rosacea diary (use a small notebook or even a desk calendar). Write down common triggers you're exposed to and record days when symptoms flare up. After two to four weeks, you should see a pattern; triggers usually jumpstart redness within a few minutes to a day.

Sidestep the sun. The sun's ultraviolet rays aggravate rosacea simply by reddening the skin. But that's not all. Dermatologists from Boston University have found that sunlight also seems to trigger the production of compounds that spur the growth of blood vessels close to the surface of the skin. Your best protection: Stay in the shade during the brightest hours of the day and wear a broad-brimmed hat and apply sunscreen to your face when you leave the house.

Don't let your sunscreen aggravate your skin, though. Choose a formula that contains dimethicone and cyclomethicone. In one study, these additives protected against the irritation caused by the sun-blocking ingredient Padimate O. Or try a sunscreen formulated for babies, which may be milder. Also look for the ingredients zinc oxide and micronized titanium oxide, which deflect some of the sun's heat and therefore help prevent rosacea flare-ups.

Maintain healthy skin with a prescription cream or gel.
Many doctors begin treatment by prescribing antibiotics such as tetracycline for 12 weeks or so to help reduce bumps and redness. But that's not a cure. In one study, two-thirds of the people who took a course of tetracycline for rosacea saw skin problems return within six months. That's why doctors also prescribe a skin-calming cream or gel containing metronidazole (Metrogel, Noritate) or azelaic acid for long-term use. In one study, people who used metronidazole for six months after antibiotic treatment were about half as likely to have redness or bumps return as those who didn't use it.

Consider the "rosacea antibiotic." For years, doctors have prescribed short courses of the antibiotic doxycycline for rosacea. Now there's a low-dose time-release version called Oracea, approved for long-term prevention of rosacea outbreaks. When 91 people with rosacea received Oracea or a 100-milligram dose of doxycycline daily for 16 weeks, the two were equally effective at reducing rosacea's bumps. The advantage: Just 5 percent of the Oracea group had gastrointestinal side effects like nausea, diarrhea, vomiting, or stomach discomfort compared to 26 percent of those who took doxycycline. Oracea seems to work by cooling inflammation rather than by killing microbes.

Prevention Boosters

Pamper your skin. Skin-care products such as cleansers, moisturizers, sunscreens, and makeup can easily irritate and redden your skin if you have rosacea. To avoid irritation, choose mild, hypoallergenic cleansers and moisturizers, wash with lukewarm (not hot) water, and avoid rough stuff like scratchy washcloths, loofahs, and abrasive skin-care products. If your skin tends to sting when you apply sunscreen, makeup, or medicated creams and gels, wait a half hour after washing so your skin is completely dry.

WHAT CAUSES IT Swelling of tiny blood vessels near the surface of the skin. Experts say that genetic factors and sun damage both play a role. There's also some evidence that microscopic mites that live in human hair follicles may clog oil glands and inflame skin.

SYMPTOMS TO WATCH FOR Reddened skin, especially on your cheeks and nose. As rosacea progresses, you may notice small, spidery blood vessels appearing in these areas as well as bumps on your nose, cheeks, forehead, and chin. You may also notice a gritty or burning feeling in your eyes. For a few people, rosacea triggers the buildup of tissue on and around the nose, too.

NEWEST THINKING Ask your dermatologist about a retinoid product. These vitamin A–based skin creams and washes speed cell turnover and are usually used to control acne and reduce wrinkles. Recent studies suggest they may reduce two visible signs of rosacea: redness and tiny blood vessels near the surface of the skin. Proceed with caution, though; retinoids can irritate the skin at first, so start with a low-dose product.

Sexually Transmitted Infections

90%
The amount by which you could reduce your risk of HIV by always using a condom.

The United States was shocked in early 2008 when researchers announced that an estimated one in four teenage girls had a sexually transmitted infection (STI). But don't think it's only kids who need to be careful. STIs—including genital warts, herpes (see the Herpes chapter), chlamydia, gonorrhea, and syphilis—are also increasingly common among people over 45. Since most STIs have no symptoms in the early or even late stages, simply asking or looking at your partner won't help you avoid them; the following steps will.

Key Prevention Strategies

Don't have sex. It's that simple. If you abstain from anal, oral, or vaginal sex until you are in a long-term monogamous relationship with someone who has tested negative for any sexually transmitted infections, it's highly unlikely you'll get an STI.

Use condoms. These simple sheaths have been around for more than 300 years, and they're still the best thing we have to protect against many STIs, including HIV, gonorrhea, chlamydia, and trichomoniasis (caused by a parasite). They're not perfect since they can break or slip off, and they don't protect completely. But in the case of AIDS, for instance, properly used latex condoms could prevent 80 to 90 percent of HIV infections. It's important, however, that a condom fit properly. If it doesn't, it's much more likely to slip or break. If the regular size isn't right for you, look for a bigger or smaller one.

Limit your partners. Do the math: The fewer people you have sex with, the fewer of their sexual partners you're exposed to. The less exposure,

the kindest cut?

A growing body of evidence suggests that circumcision may reduce the risk of STIs, particularly HIV, in men. For instance, a large Kenyan study showed that circumcision reduced men's risk of HIV infection from men or women by 53 percent, while a Ugandan study showed a reduced risk of 51 percent. Researchers think that circumcision protects against HIV because the foreskin of the penis contains a rich source of cells the virus likes to target; remove the foreskin, and you remove vulnerable cells. Other studies find that circumcised men have a lower risk of infection with syphilis and chancroid (a bacterial infection). There is still no good evidence that circumcised men are less likely to infect women with HIV than uncircumcised men are.

the less likely you are to catch an STI. Stick with one person at a time, preferably for a long time.

Get vaccinated for HPV. While progress on an HIV vaccine has been dismal, we do have a vaccine that prevents four of the most common types of human papillomavirus (HPV), including the ones that cause the majority of cervical cancers, not to mention genital warts. Called Gardasil, the three-dose vaccine is recommended for girls beginning at age 11, before they become sexually active, and is approved for women as old as 26. If you're past this age, think about the vaccine for your daughter or granddaughter.

Prevention Boosters

Get tested. If you're sexually active and not in a monogamous relationship, you should be screened at least once a year for STIs, particularly gonorrhea, chlamydia, and trichomoniasis. A large multinational study found that women infected with trich are 50 percent more likely to acquire HIV. Researchers don't know why, but they suspect that the infection may lead to minuscule areas in the vagina that provide more entry points for the HIV virus.

Nix the cigarettes. We already know that smoking increases the risk of cervical cancer, but there's also intriguing evidence that smokers have a greater risk of HIV infection than nonsmokers, with the increase ranging from 60 percent to more than threefold. Researchers suggest that the effects of tobacco smoke on the immune system may reduce the ability of immune cells to fight off the virus.

CONDOMS ARE STILL THE BEST THING WE HAVE TO PROTECT AGAINST MANY SEXUALLY TRANSMITTED INFECTIONS.

WHAT CAUSES IT Viruses, bacteria, or protozoa (in the case of trichomoniasis) that are spread through sexual intercourse, oral sex, or even skin-to-skin contact. Some, like HIV, are also spread through blood.

SYMPTOMS TO WATCH FOR Many STIs don't cause any symptoms in the early or even late stages; infections like chlamydia can spread and permanently damage parts of your reproductive system without you being aware of it. See your doctor if you have genital itching or discharge; painful sex or urination; pelvic pain; a sore throat (if you have oral sex) or a sore anus (if you have anal sex); sores, blisters, or scabs on your genital area, anus, tongue, and/or throat; a scaly rash on the palms of your hands and soles of your feet; dark urine, light-colored loose stools, and yellow eyes and skin; swollen glands, fever and body aches; or unusual infections, unexplained fatigue, night sweats, and weight loss.

NEWEST THINKING One reason that men are at greater risk for AIDS than women are may be an enzyme produced by the prostate and found in semen; it appears to increase the risk of HIV infection. The finding, from German researchers, could open up a new avenue for prevention.

Shingles

61%

The drop in your risk of getting this painful skin condition if you get the shingles vaccine.

Those blisters are long gone, but if you had chickenpox as a child (or an adult), the virus responsible for your illness never really left your body. Called the varicella-zoster virus, it can lie dormant for decades in a bundle of nerves at the base of your spine, only to raise a new red rash and blisters in middle age or later—and possibly cause excruciating skin pain. An estimated one in five older adults will develop this new infection, called shingles. You don't have to be one of them, thanks to a new vaccine and a host of smart, immunity-bolstering strategies.

Key Prevention Strategies

Get the shingles vaccine. A single dose of Zostavax cuts your risk of developing shingles by 61 percent. In studies of more than 38,500 women and men, the vaccine also reduced the severity of shingles outbreaks for people who developed it. And it cut the risk of the agonizing chronic nerve pain that sometimes occurs after an outbreak by two-thirds.

The vaccine is a high-potency form of the chickenpox vaccine given to children. It's currently approved in the United States for people age 60 and over, but researchers from the Mayo Clinic suggest that it may be a good idea for people as young as 50. When scientists reviewed more than 1,600 recent shingles cases, they estimated that 1 in 24 people between ages 50 and 59 will develop it.

The vaccine is designed for people who have already had chickenpox. If you somehow made it to adulthood without contracting this classic childhood illness, ask your doctor about a chickenpox vaccine, which contains the same virus but at a lower potency; experts say it protects against shingles and chickenpox. The shingles vaccine isn't recommended for people with weakened immune systems.

Act fast if you notice shingles symptoms. Shingles blisters heal in three to five weeks, but pain can linger for months or even years. Called post-herpetic neuralgia (PHN for short), this sharp, throbbing, or stabbing pain affects up to 40 percent of people who get shingles. PHN can make your skin so sensitive that wearing even the softest, lightest silk or cotton is agony. A kiss or a cool breeze can be excruciating. Living with this chronic pain can lead to depression, anxiety, sleeplessness, and even weight loss.

Your best option for avoiding PHN is getting the shingles vaccine. Your second-best strategy: Recognizing the early symptoms of a shingles outbreak and getting to your doctor for treatment within 72 hours. Studies show that the antiviral drugs acyclovir (Zovirax), famciclovir (Famvir), and valacyclovir (Valtrex) can lessen PHN pain and shorten its duration if taken early. These drugs seem to work by reducing the nerve damage caused by the virus. They also speed healing of the original shingles outbreak.

It sounds odd, but adding a tricyclic antidepressant, such as amitriptyline (Elavil), can help, too. In one study, people who took 25 milligrams of Elavil daily were 50 percent less likely to have lingering PHN pain after six months than those who got a placebo. Study volunteers began taking the antidepressant 2 days after the rash appeared and continued for 90 days.

Prevention Boosters

Feed your immune system more fruit and vegetables. In a British study of 726 people, those who ate more than three servings of fruit a day cut their risk of shingles in half compared to people who ate fruit less than once a day, report researchers from the London School of Hygiene and Tropical Medicine. Study volunteers who ate five daily servings of vegetables reduced their odds by 70 percent compared to people who had just one or two daily helpings.

Learn the ancient art of tai chi. In a UCLA study of 112 healthy adults ages 59 to 82, this gentle, flowing exercise form boosted immunity against shingles dramatically. Compared to participants who took health education classes, volunteers who practiced tai chi three times a week for four months developed antibodies to the shingles virus on a par with those found in 30- and 40-year-olds who had gotten the shingles vaccine.

No one's saying this type of exercise is a replacement for the vaccine, however; it works best in combination with immunization. When the researchers gave the shingles vaccine to everyone in the study and rechecked their immunity a few weeks later, they found that the tai chi group's immunity was 40 percent higher than that of the vaccine-only group.

WHAT CAUSES IT The varicella-zoster virus, the same virus responsible for chickenpox. Once you've had chickenpox, the virus lies dormant in a bundle of nerve cells called the sensory ganglia, located near the spinal cord. It can reemerge as shingles decades later, often triggered by lowered immunity, physical or emotional stress, an injury, or even dental work.

SYMPTOMS TO WATCH FOR Burning, tingling, or numb skin plus chills, fever, upset stomach, and/or headache; after a few days, a red rash develops on your body (especially the torso), neck, or face. The rash morphs into fluid-filled blisters, which dry up in a few days. Shingles clears up completely in three to five weeks, but for 25 to 50 percent of people who get it, severe nerve pain can linger for months or years afterward.

NEWEST THINKING Shingles in the family? Don't put off getting the vaccine. Having just one close family member with shingles increases your risk of developing it fourfold, say dermatologists at the University of Texas Medical School in Houston. They quizzed 500 people with shingles about their relatives and discovered that for 39 percent, it ran in the family. The more relatives who've had it, the higher your risk.

Sinusitis and Sinus Infections

72%
The potential reduction in your risk of chronic sinus infections if you rinse your nose with saline every day.

Hidden beneath the skin and bone of your face are eight hollow cavities: your sinuses. Their purpose remains a mystery, but their serious design flaw is well known: When tiny sinus drainage holes swell shut, trapped mucus causes pressure and pain—and provides a home where viruses and bacteria can breed. Stop your next sinus infection before it starts by avoiding colds and flu and treating or preventing respiratory allergy attacks. And follow these steps to ease congestion and promote drainage.

Key Prevention Strategies

Rinse with saline. For thousands of years, people have used saltwater or seawater rinses to prevent sinus problems. Now there's hard science to recommend this practice. When researchers from England's Royal National Throat, Nose, and Ear Hospital reviewed eight well-designed studies, they concluded that a daily saline rinse cuts the risk of chronic sinus infections by up to 72 percent. A rinse can also help prevent a cold from turning into a sinus infection. (Experts say you should use a decongestant first to reduce swelling so the fluid can drain out easily.)

You can buy a sinus-rinsing tool called a neti pot—it looks like a tiny watering can—at a health food store or use a bulb syringe to deliver the saline solution to your nose. Mix 1/4 teaspoon of table salt and 1/4 teaspoon of baking soda in eight ounces of lukewarm water. Lean over the sink. Tilt your head sideways and pour some of the solution into your upper nostril. Relax and keep breathing through your mouth as the liquid makes its way into the other nostril and back out. Spit out any that solution that drains into your mouth. Repeat until you've used all the solution.

Got a cold or the flu? Thin that mucus. Mucus trapped in your sinuses during a cold, bout of flu,

don't be a blowhard!

Blowing hard into a tissue is counterproductive because it triggers "reflex nasal congestion," experts say. This natural reaction, which happens when you sneeze, increases blood flow and makes nasal tissues swell. It serves a purpose by preventing noxious stuff from reentering your nose after an *A-choo!* or from traveling further up your nose. But it also happens if you blow too vigorously. The result: Your nose becomes even more stuffy. Blowing gently is a better way to keep nasal passages open.

or allergy attack is a breeding ground for viruses and bacteria. To keep it thin so it can drain, drink at least six to eight glasses a day of water, hot tea, or other clear liquids. Also consider an over-the-counter remedy that contains the mucus-thinner guaifenesin, such as Mucinex. If you prefer a natural approach, inhale some steam for 10 minutes. Simply lean over a bowl of hot water with a towel over your head to trap the steam, stand in a steamy shower, or sit in the steam room at the gym.

If your home or office is very dry, increasing the humidity can help. Use a humidifier or vaporizer; just be sure to clean it regularly according to the manufacturer's directions.

Warm your sinuses. Placing a hot washcloth on your cheeks and/or drinking a cup of hot tea feels good if sinus pressure is building. It may also nudge microscopic hairs in your sinuses into action. Called cilia, they normally sweep back and forth at a brisk 700 beats per minute to whisk mucus along. When you have a cold or the flu, the hairs move at a sluggish 300 beats per minute. Warmth seems to help them pick up the pace.

Use drugstore decongestants very sparingly. These pills and sprays make blood vessels in your nose constrict, opening swollen nasal passages. Early in a cold or flu, using a decongestant could help promote drainage. But it can backfire quickly, causing "rebound congestion" as each dose wears off. Few experts believe decongestants should be used to help prevent sinus infections at all. Our best advice: Never use an over-the-counter decongestant spray for more than three days, and use decongestants in pill form sparingly; they can thicken mucus.

For a severe acute infection or chronic infections, get medical treatment. If you develop severe pain in your face or jaw and/or a fever higher than 101°F when you have sinus congestion, talk with your doctor. You may need an antibiotic.

Ask about preventive drugs. If you have multiple episodes of sinus congestion or sinusitis in a year, or your colds or allergy attacks tend to turn into sinus infections, you may benefit from long-term courses of appropriate antibiotics or from prescription steroid nasal sprays. The sprays soothe inflammation, shrinking swollen nasal and sinus passages so they can drain, without the side effects of over-the-counter decongestant sprays.

WHAT CAUSES IT When swollen nasal and sinus passages cause congestion, trapped mucus can become a breeding ground for viruses and bacteria.

SYMPTOMS TO WATCH FOR Pressure and pain in your cheeks or behind your eyes (often on just one side) or in the upper teeth or jaw; green, yellow, or brownish nasal discharge; fever higher than 101°F; extreme fatigue; reduced sense of taste and/or smell, cough from postnasal drip, and new or unusual bad breath.

NEWEST THINKING Antibiotics inhaled as a mist via a device called a nebulizer could help if sinus surgery and other medical treatments don't cure chronic sinus trouble. In one Stanford University study of 42 people with repeated sinus infections, 76 percent saw significant improvement with 3 weeks of nebulized antibiotics, and they remained infection free for an average of 17 weeks. Before treatment, infections recurred about every 6 weeks.

Skin Cancer

40%
The amount by which you can reduce your risk of squamous cell skin cancer, the second most common form of skin cancer, by using sunscreen every day.

Sunlight improves our mood and provides us with all-important vitamin D. But everyone knows the downside of getting too much: skin cancer. Just consider the difference in skin cancer rates in different parts of the world. For instance, sunny Australia has a rate of about 1,035 cases per 100,000 men and 472 per 100,000 women, while gloomy Finland's rate is about 6 out of 100,000 in men and 4 out of 100,000 in women. Blame UVB rays, which cause the majority of skin cancers, as well as UVA rays, which make the damage worse (and may even cause cancer in their own right, new research suggests). Follow these strategies to keep your skin healthy.

Key Prevention Strategies

Slather on the sunscreen. If you're going to be in the sun for more than 10 or 15 minutes, make sure you're wearing sunscreen. Slather it on generously; most people don't use enough. It takes about a shot glass–full to cover you completely (for that day at the beach or pool) and about two tablespoons to cover your face and neck (don't forget the ears). We recommend keeping an actual shot glass (plastic if you can find one) in your beach bag or glove compartment so you always have a handy measuring tool. And pay special attention to the danger areas; 55 percent of skin cancers occur on the head or neck (balding men take note!), followed by the hands, forearms, and legs. Also use lip protection with an SPF rating of 15 or higher. Reapply every two hours.

Stay covered up. Wearing protective clothing and a hat when you're in the sun is also important. These days, you can even find clothing with built-in sun protection; it's not cheap, but

shopping for sunscreen

Stymied by the plethora of sunscreens on the drugstore shelf? Look for the following.

- **An SPF of at least 15.** These block 93 percent of all incoming UVB rays, assuming you reapply often. SPF 30 blocks an extra 4 percent, and SPF 50 an extra 6 percent. SPF doesn't measure protection from UVA rays, only UVB.
- **UVA-filtering ingredients.** Most sunscreens today offer "broad-spectrum" protection, meaning they protect against both UVA and UVB rays. But some may not provide adequate UVA protection. For extra insurance, look for avobenzone (Parsol 1789) or ecamsule (Mexoryl), both of which absorb UVA light. (Unfortunately, they also add—sometimes significantly—to a product's price tag.) Also look for titanium dioxide or zinc oxide, which both scatter rather than absorb UVA light. If you have sensitive skin, look for a PABA-free sunscreen.
- **An expiration date that will get you through the summer.**
- **The Skin Cancer Foundation's seal of recommendation.** It ensures that the product meets the highest standards of protection based on independent testing.

it's an excellent long-term investment in your health. An alternative is to add a product called SunGuard when doing laundry; the manufacturer claims it can boost the ultraviolet protection factor (UPF), a measure of how well a fabric keeps the sun's rays from reaching your skin. Using SunGuard supposedly increases the UPF of a white cotton T-shirt from a rating of 5 to a 30.

Use self-tanners, not tanning beds. Tanning beds, which use UVA rays to darken your skin, can increase your risk of melanoma by up to 75 percent, boost your risk of basal cell cancer by 50 percent, and more than double your risk of squamous cell cancer. Stick to self-tanning products, which safely provide a bronze glow.

Prevention Boosters

Stop the smokes. As with nearly every other cancer, your risk of skin cancer is higher if you smoke, with one study finding that the risk doubled in smokers.

Use more turmeric. This yellow spice, prominent in curry powder, contains the chemical curcumin, considered a strong cancer-fighting agent. Lab studies suggest it may help protect against melanoma in particular.

WEAR PROTECTIVE CLOTHING AND A HAT WHEN YOU'RE IN THE SUN.

WHAT CAUSES IT
Ultraviolet rays from the sun or radiation. Your risk of basal cell skin cancer, the most common type, and squamous cell skin cancer, the second most common type, depends on cumulative sun exposure throughout your life. Your risk of melanoma, the deadliest form of skin cancer, seems to depend more on the intensity of the sun exposure. Even a single bad sunburn could lead to melanoma.

SYMPTOMS TO WATCH FOR Pearly or waxy bumps; a flat, flesh-colored, or brown scar-like lesion on your chest or back; a red nodule on your face, lips, ears, neck, hands, or arms; a flat lesion with a scaly, crusted surface on your face, ears, neck, hands, or arms; a large brownish spot with darker speckles; a mole that changes color or size or bleeds; spots or lesions with irregular borders and red, white, blue, or blue-black spots; dark lesions on your palms, the soles of your feet, fingertips, and toes, or on mucous membranes lining your mouth, nose, vagina, or anus.

NEWEST THINKING A prescription skin cream in the works could protect against certain types of skin cancer by making the outer layers of skin less vulnerable to damage from UV rays. The active ingredient, myristyl nicotinate, is derived from the vitamin niacin.

Snoring

26%
The potential reduction in snoring due to obstructive sleep apnea if you're overweight and lose 10 percent of your body weight.

If you've ever been banished to another room for snoring too loudly, it's time to take action. Loud nighttime snorts and snurfles are a sign that tissue in the airway is vibrating with each breath at decibel levels that can keep a bed partner awake for hours. These steps can quiet the racket. An estimated 50 to 60 percent of loud snorers also have obstructive sleep apnea (OSA), in which flabby tissue blocks the airway over and over throughout the night, leading to dozens or even hundreds of unrecognized partial awakenings and an increased risk of high blood pressure, diabetes, heart disease, depression, weight problems, and dangerous daytime fatigue. OSA requires medical evaluation and therapy, though some of these measures also help.

Key Prevention Strategies

Prop yourself up. Instead of lying flat on your back, sleep with your head, shoulders, and upper back elevated on extra pillows or a foam wedge. Or elevate the entire head of your bed by about four inches by putting two wide, flat lengths of board (such as short pieces of a two-by-eight from the local home center) under the legs at the top end of your bed. Elevating your head may keep flabby tissue in your throat from collapsing into your breathing passages and vibrating all night, alleviating garden-variety snoring and even mild OSA.

Use the tennis ball cure. Snoring tends to be worse when you sleep on your back because your tongue and soft palate crowd the back of your throat, blocking your airway. Sleeping on your side can help. To keep you there, wear an old T-shirt to bed backward, with the pocket in the back, and put a tennis ball in the pocket, or put a ball in a fanny pack and wear it to bed.

Lose a little weight. When University of Wisconsin Medical

solving sleep apnea

In a recent Hungarian study of 12,643 people, those with obstructive sleep apnea had increased odds of high blood pressure (40 percent higher), of a heart attack (34 percent higher), and of a stroke (67 percent higher). The condition can also increase your odds for diabetes. A night of monitored sleep either with special devices brought to your home or in a sleep clinic, with monitoring of your breathing pattern, heart rate, and blood oxygen levels, can help doctors determine whether you have apnea. If you do, talk to your doctor about the snore-stopping strategies in this chapter that may improve mild cases. If you're overweight, losing weight will help, but it may take months or years, and treatment with medical solutions such as the ones here shouldn't wait.

School researchers tracked 690 Wisconsin residents for four years, they found that for people who started out without OSA, a gain of at least 10 percent in body weight increased the odds of developing it by sixfold. In people who already had it, whenever weight increased by 10 percent, OSA worsened by 32 percent. A 10 percent weight loss lessened apnea by 26 percent.

Almost any amount of weight loss helps OSA and garden-variety snoring. Extremely overweight people who underwent surgical weight-loss procedures to drop 25 to 50 percent of their body weight had a 70 to 98 percent drop in OSA in one study. And among people who lost just 7 to 9 percent of their body weight (14 to 18 pounds for someone weighing 200 pounds), OSA fell by about 50 percent.

Avoid alcohol, sleeping pills, and antihistamines at night. All act as sedatives, which trigger snoring and apnea by relaxing muscles in your mouth and throat. Sedatives like these also make OSA worse, possibly by altering your ability to rouse yourself when your airway is blocked and by making it more difficult to fall into deep, restorative stages of sleep.

Relieve congestion before you turn in. Inhale steam—in a hot shower, from a pot of hot water, or from the type of steam vaporizer that you can use as a facial sauna—to loosen mucus, then gently blow your nose. If you have seasonal allergies, keep the windows shut in your bedroom and use an air conditioner to filter the air. Keep pets out, too, and remove throw rugs—they can harbor allergens. Also, the next time you get new floor covering, choose something other than carpet.

Stop smoking. Tobacco smoke from cigarettes, cigars, and pipes irritates mucous membranes in your throat. The result: Tissue swells, narrowing your airway and making a nighttime vibrato more likely. Smoking also increases your risk of heart disease, breathing problems, and the irritation of seasonal allergies.

Sleep with an oral appliance. These devices, which look like a cross between a sports mouth guard and braces, reposition your jaw to prevent tissue in your mouth from flapping as you breathe. Custom-made versions, available from dentists, have a success rate of 70 to 80 percent for regular snoring (and may also be effective for mild to moderate OSA). Off-the-shelf versions, sold

"Elevating your head may keep flabby tissue in your throat from collapsing into your breathing passages and vibrating all night."

online and in stores, are much less effective, say experts from the Academy of Dental Sleep Medicine.

Ask about surgery. Have a deviated septum? Two surgical procedures, a submucous resection (SMR) and a septoplasty, can fix the ultra-loud snoring this nasal defect can trigger. Both involve removing cartilage from the bony divider between your left and right nasal cavity. In one small study from Thailand, septum surgery significantly quieted snoring for 28 out of 30 study participants.

Continuous positive airway pressure (CPAP). The "gold standard" treatment, CPAP uses a small, quiet air compressor to gently push air through a mask over the sleeper's nose and keep the airway open during sleep. Studies show that CPAP can ease daytime sleepiness by about 50 percent, boost blood oxygen levels, reduce high blood pressure, improve heart function, reduce memory problems related to apnea, lower blood sugar levels in people with diabetes and apnea, and cut the number of nighttime sleep disruptions.

Surgery. If CPAP and oral appliances don't work, surgical removal of excess tissue from your nose or throat might. The most widely used technique, uvulopalatopharyngoplasty (UPPP) trims tissue from the rear of your mouth and top of your throat; tonsils and adenoids are usually whisked out at the same time. The catch: It doesn't help everyone. UPPP improves apnea for just 40 to 60 percent of those who try it, say Israeli researchers who reviewed dozens of apnea studies—and it's impossible to predict who the lucky ones will be, they concluded.

Prevention Boosters

Try a nasal strip. These adhesive strips improve airflow through your nose by lifting the top of each nostril up. We'll be honest: Some research has found no benefit for snorers, but in one Swiss study, the strips quieted snoring after about two weeks of use. This inexpensive solution could work for you, especially if your snoring is caused by nasal congestion or mouth breathing.

Sing loud, long, and low. When 20 chronic snorers practiced singing techniques that shaped up their throat muscles, their snoring quieted, report researchers from England's University of Exeter. The snorers agreed to keep voice-activated tape recorders by their beds for a week before and after their three months of daily 30-minute singing sessions.

Belting out your favorites from *The Sound of Music* won't do the trick. Exercises that work—such as energetically singing "ung-gah" to familiar tunes—build strength in muscles that support your soft palate, the tissue at the back of your mouth that vibrates if you snore. You can order the program at www.singingforsnorers.com.

Play a wind instrument. When 25 snorers at a Swiss sleep clinic took up the didgeridoo, an ancient, breath-powered instrument from Australia that looks like a long, hollow tree branch, daytime sleepiness improved by 12 percent and snoring was lessened by about 22 percent. No access to a didgeridoo? Get that old clarinet, flute, or tuba out of the closet and honk away!

Rest your head on a snore-stopping pillow. These pillows have many different designs; some elevate the head, while others have a hump in the middle and slanting sides so that you simply cannot sleep on your back. Do they work? Experts say there's no guarantee, but some types may work for some people.

PLAYING A WIND INSTRUMENT CAN REDUCE SNORING BY ABOUT 22 PERCENT.

WHAT CAUSES IT The relaxation of your tongue as well as muscles in the roof of your mouth and throat during sleep, which causes throat tissues to vibrate as you inhale and exhale. They may even collapse against your airway, restricting or blocking the flow of air. Being overweight or having enlarged tonsils, thick tissue on the roof of your mouth, or an extra-long uvula increases the chances that you'll snore.

SYMPTOMS TO WATCH FOR Light snoring may not disrupt your sleep or your partner's. But if you snore loudly and feel tired or have a headache when you wake up in the morning, or you gasp and choke or stop breathing for short periods of time during sleep, you may have obstructive sleep apnea and should ask your doctor about testing and treatment.

NEWEST THINKING Obstructive sleep apnea's immediate health risk: Traffic accidents. People with OSA are twice as likely to be involved in crashes as those without the disorder, say Canadian researchers who tracked the car insurance records of 1,600 people. And they're not just fender-benders: OSA increased the odds of severe car crashes that caused physical injury and death three to five times higher than normal.

Stomach Bugs

96%

The percentage of stomach-bug virus particles removed from your hands if you wash vigorously with soap and water for 20 seconds.

What do mountain climbers in Alaska, guests at an Australian tea party, participants at a West Virginia family reunion, and British hospital patients have in common? All have been hit recently by nasty stomach bugs that cause cramping, fever, vomiting, and diarrhea, researchers report. The germ responsible for the misery: norovirus, the super-contagious virus that causes 90 percent of "stomach flu" outbreaks. Other viruses and bacteria can cause tummy distress, too, but these precautions can help you and your family sidestep the next outbreak.

Key Prevention Strategies

Wash your hands. You can easily get a stomach bug by touching a contaminated doorknob or shaking hands with someone who's sick. Your best defense: Soap, water, and 20 seconds of vigorous scrubbing and rinsing. In an Emory University study, hand washing removed 96 percent of viral particles compared to just 46 percent removed with an alcohol-based hand sanitizer. Not near a sink? An alcohol-based hand sanitizer is a good alternative.

Keep sick and recently sick people out of the kitchen. Many stomach-bug outbreaks have been traced to food prepared by people who had active or waning tummy infections. Shoo sick friends and relatives out of the kitchen. If you're not successful, wipe down counters and other kitchen surfaces with Lysol- or Clorox-type wipes or a solution of one teaspoon bleach in one quart warm water. If an ill friend or relative brings homemade food to a function, avoid it. Half of the attendees at one West Virginia family reunion came down with vomiting, cramps, and diarrhea after eating goodies prepared by two sick relatives, researchers report.

tummy-bug secrets revealed

Why the heck are stomach bugs so darn contagious? For starters, norovirus, a family of hardy germs responsible for most cases of stomach flu (which isn't really the flu because it's not caused by the influenza virus), is highly contagious before anyone has warning signs. Here are some good reasons to protect yourself all the time.

- **Number of viral particles it takes to become infected:** Less than 10
- **Percentage of infected people who are contagious but never have symptoms:** 30
- **Length of time someone is contagious after vomiting ends:** 2 to 3 weeks
- **Lifespan of the virus on floors, counters, and other hard surfaces:** 3 days
- **Lifespan on "soft" surfaces like rugs:** up to 12 days

Clean up fast after someone gets sick. After a bout of vomiting and/or diarrhea, fast cleanup can help prevent the spread of germs. Wipe down exposed surfaces with a mixture of bleach and water. Wear rubber gloves and use paper towels—and dispose of them outside the house. Wash the gloves before you take them off. Be sure the sick person also washes up and changes clothes right away, then wash the clothes separately from those of other household members on your washer's hottest setting. Use a little bleach if possible, following laundering directions.

Wash fruit and veggies and follow safe food-handling rules. Viruses and bacteria that trigger vomiting and diarrhea can live on virtually any food. Prevent trouble by washing, storing, and cooking foods safely, using the advice in the Food Poisoning chapter.

Stay safe at sea. Cruise ships aren't the only places you can contract tummy bugs like norovirus; they've just gotten a lot of publicity because these self-contained, highly social floating resorts provide the perfect environment for passing this bug around. Studies show that the risk of contracting the bug on board has increased somewhat over the past two decades. These steps can help you steer clear on your next shipboard vacation.

- **Wash your hands often.** In one recent Centers for Disease Control and Prevention study, people who contracted stomach bugs on cruise lines were less likely to wash up after using the restroom and less likely to use publicly available hand sanitizers even after an outbreak had started.
- **Use the cruise ship "handshake."** Whether you're greeting the captain or meeting the couple in the next cabin, employ the official shipboard alternative to clasped hands: knocking elbows together. Several cruise lines have encouraged this new nicety to help reduce the risk of virus transmission.

WHAT CAUSES IT Viruses and bacteria. Most "stomach flu" is the result of infection with norovirus.

SYMPTOMS TO WATCH FOR Nausea, vomiting, stomach cramps, and diarrhea that last for 12 hours to 3 days. Usually a bout of stomach flu is uncomfortable but not serious, but young children, older people, and anyone with a weakened immune system should be watched for signs of dehydration or lingering infection. Drink plenty of fluids and call the doctor if you see these signs: extreme thirst, dry mouth, dark or scanty urine, few tears, weakness, lethargy, dizziness.

NEWEST THINKING Cook those oysters! The largest stomach-bug outbreak in the history of New Zealand sickened 350 people who ate raw oysters during a party at a rugby match. While any food can carry viruses and bacteria that cause tummy troubles, bivalve shellfish can pose a special threat if they're uncooked. Substances in the oyster's gastrointestinal tract allow the norovirus to bind and accumulate, a recent USDA study showed, meaning you could get a big dose if you chomp on a contaminated one. If you love oysters, eat them steamed, boiled, baked, or fried; thorough cooking destroys the virus.

Stomach Cancer

Here's the good news about stomach cancer: Ever since we discovered that most ulcers and the most common form of stomach cancer (non-cardia) are caused by the bacterium *Helicobacter pylori* and began treating people who are infected with it with antibiotics, rates of stomach cancer have plummeted in most countries. Here's the not-so-good news: At the same time, rates of the other form of stomach cancer (cardia) are rising. Here's what you can do to keep both types out of your life.

Key Prevention Strategies

Avoid foods high in nitrites. Most studies evaluating what people eat and their risk of stomach cancer find that diets high in salted, pickled, or smoked foods (think pickled vegetables, herring, smoked salmon, etc.) and preserved or salt-cured meat (such as ham and bacon) significantly increase the risk of stomach cancer. These foods contain nitrites, which can form cancer-causing compounds called nitrosamides in the stomach.

Eat an orange a day. Eating plenty of fresh fruits and vegetables can reduce your risk of stomach cancer. You may get more bang for your produce buck from citrus fruits like oranges, grapefruits, lemons, and limes. One review of 14 studies found that three or more servings of citrus fruit a week reduced the risk of stomach cancer by 28 percent (though this may be a high estimate). Researchers suspect the antioxidants vitamin C and a carotenoid called beta-cryptoxanthin may protect stomach cells from cancer-causing damage.

Put the word whole in your diet. If your diet is loaded with refined grains in the form of white bread, pretzels, store-bought baked goods, and the like, and you avoid whole grains in the form of foods like barley and oats, you could be increasing your risk of stomach cancer by anywhere from 50 percent to more than sevenfold. Conversely, the more fiber you eat, the lower your risk, particularly for women.

Cut out the steaks, burgers, and cheese. A Mexican study of about 1,000 people found that those who ate an average of 25 grams of saturated fat (about the amount in a Double Whopper with cheese) a day were 3.3 times more likely to develop gastric cancer than those who kept their intake at 14 grams or less. Another study found that every 3.5 ounces of meat eaten per day—no matter what type—increased the risk of stomach cancer nearly 2.5 times overall and more than 5 times in people infected with *H. pylori*.

Prevention Boosters

Treat *H. pylori* infection early. Infection with this bug is the leading cause of ulcers; now we also know that it's the leading cause of stomach cancer. Researchers think that inflammation related to *H. pylori* infection leads to changes in the stomach lining that make the stomach less acidic, encouraging the formation of cancer-causing nitrosamides.

Getting rid of the infection can lower your risk. A Chinese study randomly assigned 1,630 people infected with the bacteria to take either a placebo or therapy designed to eradicate the bacteria. After 7 1/2 years, six people in the placebo group had developed stomach cancer compared to none in the treatment group. The traditional treatment for *H. pylori* infection is 7 to 14 days of treatment with a proton-pump inhibitor such as omeprazole (Prilosec) or esomeprazole (Nexium) and the antibiotics clarithromycin and either amoxicillin or metronidazole. Ask your doctor if you should be tested for the bug.

Kick the habit. The smoking habit, that is. As with so many other cancers, smoking increases your risk of stomach cancer; nearly one in five cases are related to smoking. Overall, European researchers found that people who had ever smoked had about a 40 percent increased risk of stomach cancer; those still smoking had a risk 73 percent (in men) to 87 percent (in women) higher than that of people who never smoked.

Wash your hands thoroughly and often. This is especially important before cooking and eating. Researchers suspect that one of the main ways *H. pylori* is transmitted is through person-to-person contact—such as inadvertently touching the vomit or stool of someone who's infected. The other main transmission route may be well water, so if you have a well, stick to bottled water for drinking.

WHAT CAUSES IT The bacterium *Helicobacter pylori* causes the most common form of stomach cancer, non-cardia gastric cancer, or cancer anywhere in the stomach except the top inch, where the stomach meets the esophagus. Cancer in that area is called cardia gastric cancer. Ironically, the presence of *H. pylori* seems to reduce the risk of cardia cancer. Other risk factors include chronic gastritis, or inflammation of the stomach; age; being male; a diet high in salted, smoked, or preserved foods and low in produce; smoking; certain types of anemia; and a family history of the disease.

SYMPTOMS TO WATCH FOR Internal bleeding; it may not be noticed unless you have a fecal occult blood test or the bleeding becomes extreme, causing anemia. Symptoms of more advanced cancer include an uncomfortable feeling in your abdomen that antacids don't improve and that worsens when you eat; black, tarry stools; vomiting blood; vomiting after meals; weakness, fatigue, and weight loss; feeling full after meals even if you eat less than normal.

NEWEST THINKING In the near future, we'll have a vaccine for *H. pylori*. It will have to be given early, however; studies have found children as young as age 7 who are infected with the bacteria.

Stroke

42%
The drop in stroke risk if you lower high blood pressure by just 5 points.

A tiny clot. A rip in a hair-thin blood vessel. The smallest things can trigger a stroke—a potentially life-altering brain attack that shuts off the flow of blood and oxygen, destroying precious brain cells. The harsh truth: Strokes kill at least five million people worldwide each year and disable millions more, yet most of us rank it dead last among our greatest health fears. The rest of the story: If you act now, there's plenty you can do to stop a brain attack before it starts.

Key Prevention Strategies

Lower your blood pressure. If your blood pressure is above 120/80, your risk of having a stroke is dramatically higher than that of someone with lower blood pressure. Why? Blood moves faster through your arteries and veins, and this breakneck pace poses a triple threat. It damages blood vessels in your brain and in the carotid arteries in your neck that supply brain cells with life-giving oxygen. It can also create fragile "bulges" in these arteries, which can rupture. And it can make arteries thicken to the point where they squeeze shut. Small wonder, then, that high blood pressure is the number one cause of stroke.

The good news: If your blood pressure is high, every 5-point drop can cut your stroke risk by 42 percent or more. The strategy works whether you're 45 or 95. In a notable British study of nearly 3,500 people over age 80 with high blood pressure, those who used medication to get their numbers down to 150/80 cut their risk of stroke by 53 percent compared to volunteers who received placebo pills. That's higher than the healthy target (120/80) we mentioned above, but it illustrates the benefits of lowering high BP. Ultimately, your own healthy BP goal should be set by your doctor.

You may not even need medication to reach an optimal level. If your blood pressure's top number (systolic) is between 120 and 139,

take TIAs seriously

Before a stroke, 30 to 40 percent of people get a strange warning sign: a brief mini-stroke known to doctors as a transient ischemic attack, or TIA. Symptoms can include loss of strength or sudden numbness in your face, arm, or leg; feeling confused or unable to speak; loss of vision; and/or an unusual headache. They stop as swiftly as they start, but that doesn't mean the danger has passed. Your risk of having a full-blown stroke in the next two days is 1 in 20, and over the next three months, it's 1 in 10, unless you take action.

What to do: Call your doctor immediately and explain what happened. He may put you on medications to prevent blood clots, lower cholesterol, and reduce blood pressure. In a British study, this combination cut the odds for a major stroke after a TIA by 80 percent.

or your bottom number (diastolic) is between 80 and 89, you have prehypertension—and stand a good chance of reducing your pressure with weight loss, exercise, and a healthy low-salt diet packed with fruits, veggies, and low-fat dairy foods. If your numbers stay above 140/90 despite lifestyle changes, your doctor should prescribe one or several medications to bring them down.

Reduce your "bad" cholesterol. Too much harmful LDL cholesterol whizzing around in your bloodstream starts the process that leads to the development of thick, fatty streaks of gunky plaque inside artery walls, including the important carotid arteries that feed your brain. These supply lines can eventually grow so narrow that the tiniest clot acts like a stopper in your kitchen sink.

Reducing LDL with a low-fat diet plus a statin drug shrinks this perilous plaque and protects the brain. In one study of 2,531 men with slightly elevated LDL levels, those who took cholesterol-lowering drugs cut their stroke risk by 31 percent.

Your best LDL-whittling strategy: Start with a diet low in saturated fat and rich in fruits, veggies, whole grains, and low-fat milk products. Go easy on fatty red meats, premium ice cream, and full-fat dairy products like cheese. Lose weight if you need to. And exercise! If your levels stay high (an ideal LDL reading is below 100 mg/dl; it's even lower, below 70 mg/dl, if you have diabetes or a history of heart disease), ask your doc about taking a statin. If you've already had a stroke, taking one can cut your risk of a second stroke by 16 percent.

Break a sweat regularly, and snack on walnuts. These strategies can raise levels of HDL cholesterol—the "cholesterol cop" that whisks LDL out of your bloodstream. The minimum healthy HDL level for women is 50 mg/dl and for men, 40 mg/dl. But higher is better for your brain. In one study, people with the highest HDL cut their risk for the type of strokes caused by fatty plaque buildup by a whopping 80 percent.

Skip the burgers and the beers. Until recently, experts didn't realize how dangerous triglycerides, another type of blood fat, were to brain health. But in one study, people with the highest levels tripled their stroke risk compared to those with the healthiest, lowest levels. A healthy triglyceride reading is below 150 mg/dl. You can tame high triglycerides by losing weight and skipping alcoholic beverages, having broiled or baked fish instead

> "If your blood pressure is high, every 5-point drop can cut your stroke risk by 42 percent or more."

of burgers, and using canola and olive oil in place of butter. Cutting back on refined carbohydrates (found in white bread, sweets, snack foods, and sugary drinks) is also important.

Stop smoking. Puffing as few as 10 cigarettes a day increases your stroke risk by 90 percent—even if your cholesterol and blood pressure levels are low. Nicotine, carbon monoxide, and a cocktail of other chemicals in burning tobacco stiffen arteries, pack more plaque into artery walls, and make blood stickier and more prone to clotting. Quit today, and your stroke risk begins to fall immediately; within as few as five years, your risk falls to that of someone who never smoked.

Fix a fluttering heart. Atrial fibrillation (called A-fib for short), when the upper chambers of the heart quiver instead of beating strong and steady, quadruples stroke risk. It affects 1 in 25 people over age 65 and 1 in 10 over age 80. A-fib allows blood to pool in the heart and form clots; a strong heartbeat can then hurl a clot into your brain, causing a stroke.

If you're over 65, ask your doctor to assess you for A-fib. Simply checking your pulse and listening to your heartbeat may be enough, or you may need a simple, low-cost test called an electrocardiogram (known as an EKG or ECG). If you have the condition, the usual fix is the blood thinner warfarin (Coumadin), which experts say could cut stroke risk by 69 percent. Yet many people who would benefit from this lifesaving medication never get it, in part because doctors are cautious about prescribing it to older people who may bruise or bleed more easily if they have a fall.

Take a daily low-dose aspirin. If you've already had a stroke or are a woman at high risk for a stroke, swallowing an 81-milligram aspirin tablet daily could protect your brain. In one study, aspirin cut women's stroke risk by 17 percent (but didn't lower most men's risk). If you're at above-normal risk for stroke—due to high blood pressure, out-of-balance blood fats, atrial fibrillation,

preventive surgery for strokes

If the arteries in your neck are full of plaque, your risk of a stroke skyrockets. A good surgical cleaning could cut your odds by 50 to 75 percent, studies show. You may be a candidate if you've already had a stroke or mini-stroke or if x-rays using special dyes or other tests reveal that an artery is 75 to 99 percent blocked. (Warning signs of a blockage include blurred vision, slurred speech, or weakness.) The tried-and-true surgical technique for clearing blocked arteries, called carotid endarterectomy, involves opening the artery and scraping away plaque. Newer, less invasive methods use tiny wire cages called stents to hold narrowed arteries open.

or even a family history of stroke—ask your doctor if low-dose aspirin therapy is appropriate for you.

Prevention Boosters

Walk five days a week. Taking a brisk hour-long walk five times a week cuts your odds of a stroke nearly in half, and a half-hour stroll reduces your odds by about 25 percent. Don't like walking? Any vigorous physical activity that will burn 1,000 to 3,000 calories per week will cut your risk. How about swimming, biking, or trying out that aerobics video that's been gathering dust?

Cultivate the fine art of resilience. Breathe deeply, sing your favorite song, take a break for yoga, or dance to your favorite song on the radio. Learning to let anxiety and stress roll off your back, in whatever way works best for you, could cut your stroke risk by an extra 24 percent, say researchers from England's University of Cambridge.

Put fish on your menu. Enjoying broiled or baked tuna or other fin foods one to four times a week could cut your stroke risk by 27 percent, possibly because healthy fats in fish can keep blood vessels flexible and discourage plaque. But skip the fish and chips and the crispy fast-food fish sandwiches: In a Harvard Medical School study, people who ate fried fish just once a week raised their stroke risk by 44 percent!

Enjoy a little alcohol, then stop. A few sips may lower your risk, but having too many drinks raises it. So say Chinese researchers who followed 64,000 men for nine years. Their conclusion: Having 1 to 6 drinks per week lowers stroke risk by 8 percent; having more than 21 per week raises it by 22 percent. And don't have all your drinks on Friday night; experts suggest no more than 1 drink a day for women and 2 for men.

Go for whole grains. Opt for oatmeal, whole wheat bread and cereal, and brown rice. Women who ate the most whole grains had a 40 percent lower risk of stroke than those who ate the fewest, according to a Harvard School of Public Health study.

WHAT CAUSES IT Nearly 90 percent of strokes are the result of a clot or bulging plaque that cuts off blood flow to part of the brain. The rest happen when a blood vessel in or near the brain ruptures, cutting off the supply of oxygen to surrounding brain cells.

SYMPTOMS TO WATCH FOR Classic signs are sudden numbness, weakness, or paralysis of the face, arm, or leg, usually on one side of the body; sudden difficulty talking or understanding speech; sudden blurred, double, or reduced vision; sudden dizziness, imbalance, or lack of coordination; sudden severe or unusual headache; confusion. Signs that may be unique to women: Loss of consciousness or fainting; shortness of breath; falls; sudden pain in the face, chest, arms, or legs; seizure; sudden hiccups, nausea, tiredness; sudden pounding or racing heartbeat.

NEWEST THINKING Your brain loves oranges, as well as strawberries, red bell peppers, and juicy grapefruit—all rich in vitamin C. When British scientists tracked 20,000 people for 10 years, they found that those with the highest blood levels of vitamin C had a 42 percent lower risk of stroke compared to those with the lowest levels.

Tinnitus

40%

The amount by which you could reduce the severity of the condition by using a device that desensitizes your brain to tinnitus.

Yes, you are hearing things! If it's a ringing, buzzing, or roaring sound, you have tinnitus, which strikes 1 in 20 people. One theory links it to hearing loss; because the brain doesn't get enough sound signals from the ear, it creates its own noise (nature hates a vacuum or, it appears, silence)—similar to the way people who've had a limb amputated still feel "phantom" pain. Most people go on just fine with occasional or even constant ringing, but for some, tinnitus can wreak havoc on their ability to lead normal lives. Whether you've never experienced it or it's just beginning to creep up on you, keep the worst at bay with these recommendations.

Key Prevention Strategies

Turn down the volume. One common culprit in tinnitus is noise-related hearing loss, even if the loss isn't severe enough for you to notice. Even being in a noisy place like a restaurant can stimulate your hearing system and temporarily make tinnitus louder. (Check out the Hearing Loss chapter for prevention tips.)

Walk away from the cotton swabs. Putting anything in your ear—including a finger or a Q-tip—can push wax against your eardrum, which can contribute to or worsen tinnitus. A better way to clear the wax is to put a drop or two of mineral oil in one ear and lie on the opposite side for an hour while the oil loosens the wax and brings it to the surface. When you turn over, have a napkin handy to catch the wax and oil.

Cut back on the aspirin. If you're popping the pills frequently for headaches or pain, talk to your doctor about other alternatives. Overuse can lead to tinnitus. If you're on daily low-dose aspirin therapy, though, don't worry; the amount isn't great enough to trigger tinnitus.

Relax your jaw. Tinnitus is a common symptom of temporomandibular joint disease (TMJ), in which the hinge that

already have tinnitus?

Neuromonics uses an MP3-like device to deliver a pleasant, customized sound to people with tinnitus as part of an overall treatment approach that includes counseling and support. One study, sponsored by the device's manufacturer, found that after six months, 86 percent of people using the device saw their tinnitus improve at least 40 percent, compared to just 47 percent of people who received counseling and listened to other types of noise, and 23 percent of those who received counseling only.

works the jaw and the muscles and ligaments that support it are stressed or misaligned. (See the TMJ chapter for prevention tips.)

Watch your meds. More than 200 medications are associated with tinnitus. If you're hearing ringing or buzzing, ask your doctor if one of your meds could be to blame and whether you can lower the dose or switch to another drug. Some of the worst culprits are those that injure the inner ear, like quinines (used for malaria and rheumatoid arthritis); diuretics (used for high blood pressure); certain antibiotics; and some chemotherapy drugs.

Control your blood pressure. High blood pressure can lead to tinnitus. You're more likely to hear blood whooshing through blood vessels when the pressure of the flow is strong. You should also try to keep your cholesterol in check, since narrowed arteries can cause turbulent—and loud—blood flow.

Prevention Boosters

Stay happy. Depression, anxiety, stress, and tinnitus seem to go hand in hand, although no one's sure which is the chicken and which is the egg. One study found that nearly half of people with disabling tinnitus also had major depression. People with tinnitus who take antidepressants or receive psychotherapy improve more than those who do neither.

Watch what you drink. There's some evidence that drinking too much alcohol or too many sodas or cups of coffee or tea (the caffeine is the likely culprit) can lead to tinnitus.

Hide the saltshaker. Consuming a lot of sodium can make tinnitus worse by increasing blood pressure. Using herbs and other nonsodium spices is one way to reduce sodium intake; the best way, however, is to stay away from processed foods.

Check your posture. Holding your neck in a hyperextended position, such as when you ride a bicycle, can lead to tinnitus. Look in the mirror and ask yourself: Do I look like a bird pecking for worms? If the answer is yes, your neck is hyperextended. (Read more about proper neck posture in the Neck Pain chapter.)

Get a blood test. Low blood levels of iron or thyroid hormones are associated with tinnitus.

WHAT CAUSES IT Loud noises, noise- and age-related hearing loss, excess earwax, infections, medications, tumors, allergies, heart and blood vessel problems, problems with the jaw and neck.

SYMPTOMS TO WATCH FOR A ringing, buzzing, roaring, hissing, or whistling noise in your ears. You may notice it only when you're in a quiet place.

NEWEST THINKING Electrodes implanted in the part of the brain responsible for hearing and then electrically stimulated can suppress the phantom noises of tinnitus. One study of 12 people who underwent the implants showed a 97 percent reduction in tinnitus.

TMJ

60%

The amount you can reduce jaw pain by doing isometric jaw exercises several times a day and taking an anti-inflammatory for four weeks.

Whenever you chew, yawn, or open your mouth really wide to have dental work or yell at your teenager, you dislocate your jaw. Don't worry; it pops back into place when you close your mouth. The joints responsible for this amazing feat are the temporomandibular joints, one on each side of your head, which keep your jaw attached to your skull. They're among the most complicated and commonly used joints in the body, able to move forward and backward and side to side. That means, of course, that they're more prone to problems. For instance, chewing too much, grinding your teeth, or having a misalignment in your teeth and/or jaw can all stress the joints or the muscles and ligaments that control them, leading to temporomandibular joint disorder, or TMJ. Prevent it with these suggestions.

Key Prevention Strategies

Rest your jaw. Chill out on the chewing (stop crunching ice, for instance) and halve the size of your sandwiches so you don't have to open your mouth as wide. If you open your mouth wider than the width of three fingers, that's too wide. It also helps to avoid chewing gum and especially chewy foods (think taffy).

See the dentist. Unlike elephants' teeth, ours were not meant to grind. If you grind your teeth (or your bed partner says you do), get to your dentist, who can fit you with a mouth guard or splint to wear at night to prevent this major cause of TMJ. You're also more likely to develop TMJ if your teeth don't come together neatly. If you have this problem (called malocclusion), talk to an orthodontist about braces to realign your teeth, improve your bite, and reduce your risk of TMJ.

Stop clenching. Some people hold tension in their jaws without realizing it, especially when they're under stress. That tension can contribute to or even cause TMJ so that it becomes painful even to eat. Here's how to learn to relax the muscles that control your jaw.

Put a cork in it. Hold a wine bottle cork between your front teeth and relax the muscles around it. Do this whenever you feel yourself clenching or until relaxing those muscles becomes automatic.

Try biofeedback. Electromyogram (EMG) biofeedback teaches you to relax your jaw and facial muscles. You start out with sensors attached to your forehead, jaw muscles, and shoulder muscles that signal you when they sense muscle tension. Then you're taught techniques to relax and reduce the tension. After practicing for a few weeks, you're able to reduce the tension without the sensors. Ask your doctor or dentist for a referral.

See a cognitive behavioral therapist. This type of therapy can help you realize and change factors, such as your response to stress and anxiety, that contribute to your TMJ. It provides you with skills to reduce your response to pain and works well for preventing the pain of TMJ. You don't need many sessions; one study found that pain improved by 50 percent in people who had just four sessions. Your doctor or health insurance company can help you find a specialist. Combining this type of therapy with biofeedback and a mouth splint works better than any of the three treatments alone.

Prevention Boosters

Exercise your jaw. Isometric jaw exercises can strengthen and stretch the muscles around the joints. Practice the exercises below several times a day. Hold each position for five seconds and repeat five times.
- **Opening.** Hold the back of your hand underneath your jaw to create resistance. Open your mouth about an inch, pushing against your hand.
- **Forward thrust.** Hold the back of your hand against the bottom of your jaw to create resistance. Push your jaw forward against your hand.
- **Sideways thrust.** Hold the palm of your hand against the side of your jaw that hurts. Push your jaw to that side.

WHAT CAUSES IT Stress, a misaligned jaw, clenching your jaw, grinding your teeth, degenerative joint disease.

SYMPTOMS TO WATCH FOR Jaw pain; neck, back, and facial pain; pain in and around the ear; headaches; ringing in the ear. You may hear a clicking sound when you chew.

NEWEST THINKING Injections of botulinum toxin (Botox), the same drug used to erase frown lines, into the muscles used to move the jaw significantly reduce pain in people with TMJ.

Ulcers

33%

The reduction in your ulcer risk if you eat seven servings of fruit and vegetables a day.

Once upon a time, people with stomach ulcers tried to soothe the gnawing pain by eating bland food and chugging thick, tummy-coating antacids. Today experts know that a tiny bacterium called *Helicobacter pylori* is responsible for two-thirds of all gastric ulcers (those in the stomach) and duodenal ulcers (those in the beginning of the small intestine). Using nonsteroidal anti-inflammatory drugs (NSAIDs) such as aspirin and ibuprofen causes almost all the rest. Here's how to lower your ulcer odds.

Key Prevention Strategies

Protect your stomach from common pain relievers. If you regularly take low-dose aspirin for your heart or use ibuprofen or naproxen for your arthritis, you're raising your risk of an ulcer. These drugs interfere with mechanisms that protect the lining of the stomach from corrosive stomach acids. They thin the stomach's protective mucus coating; reduce production of an acid-neutralizing chemical called bicarbonate (yes, it's similar to the stuff in baking soda); and reduce blood flow, which helps stomach cells repair themselves. NSAIDs can also interfere with blood clotting; if an ulcer bleeds, it may do so even more freely.

In a study of more than 3,000 people, British researchers found that those who had taken NSAIDs recently were 2 to 30 times more likely to have bleeding ulcers than those who avoided these pain relievers. What should you do? Experts suggest three strategies.

- **Switch to acetaminophen for chronic pain relief.** It's not an NSAID and won't harm the lining of your stomach. (To protect your liver, take no more than three grams per day, and avoid alcohol when you take it or risk liver failure).
- **Take the lowest possible dose of an NSAID as infrequently as possible.** Use this alternative if acetaminophen doesn't work for your pain.
- **Add a second, stomach-protecting drug.** Experts we consulted recommend the prescription drugs sucralfate (Carafate) and

treat an ulcer right

If you're relying on antacids and a bland diet to control ulcer pain, it's time to update your strategy. The only way to prevent dangerous complications such as bleeding and stomach perforation: Get tested to confirm a *Helicobacter pylori* infection, which causes most ulcers, then start treatment. A course of antibiotics, usually given along with an acid-reducing proton-pump inhibitor, is the only way to knock out the spiral-shaped germ, which burrows into the protective mucus layer lining the stomach wall, releasing toxins that burn holes in the stomach lining.

misoprostol (Cytotec) to shield the stomach lining from damage if you must take an NSAID on a daily basis. Important caution: If you are pregnant or planning to become pregnant, do not take Cytotec, which can cause miscarriage and birth defects.

Quit smoking. Nicotine in tobacco increases the amount of acid in your stomach and makes it more concentrated. Studies show that smoking raises the risk of ulcers seven times higher than normal. Some experts suspect that chemicals in tobacco smoke may somehow work with the *H. pylori* bacterium to create stomach ulcers.

Cut down on or cut out alcohol. Alcohol irritates and erodes your stomach lining and boosts acid production. While it may not cause ulcers all by itself, scientists believe that it boosts risk in people with an *H. pylori* infection and those who use NSAIDs regularly. Considering that half of all adults are infected with this bacterium by age 60, holding the line at happy hour sounds like a good idea.

Prevention Boosters

Wake up to a bowl of oatmeal with fresh fruit. In a Harvard study of more than 47,000 men, those who ate seven servings of fruit and vegetables a day had a 33 percent lower risk of developing ulcers than those who had less than three servings daily. Eating lots of soluble fiber—the type found in beans, barley, pears, and oatmeal—cut risk by a whopping 60 percent. Experts aren't sure why these foods are protective. One possibility is that soluble fiber becomes a thick, smooth gel in your digestive system and may help protect the walls of your upper small intestine from damage by digestive juices.

Eat your spinach and your beets. Veggies such as spinach, lettuce, radishes, and beets are rich in chemicals that raise levels of nitric oxide in the stomach. The ulcer connection: Swedish researchers say higher nitric oxide levels seem to strengthen the stomach's inner lining so it can better protect itself from digestive acids.

WHAT CAUSES IT The bacterium *Helicobacter pylori*; regular use of nonsteroidal anti-inflammatory drugs (NSAIDs) such as aspirin and ibuprofen.

SYMPTOMS TO WATCH FOR Burning pain in your abdomen that starts two to three hours after a meal, gets worse at night when your stomach is empty, and eases when you eat something. An ulcer may also take away your appetite, cause weight loss, or make you feel nauseated. Get immediate help if you notice blood in your stools or in vomit; a bleeding ulcer can be a medical emergency.

NEWEST THINKING Three antibiotics are better than two against the ulcer bug. In a review of 10 studies involving more than 2,800 people with ulcers, Italian researchers found that *H. pylori* was eliminated in 93 percent of the volunteers when they used a 10-day therapy that involved three different antibiotics. In contrast, 77 percent of those who got two antibiotics improved.

Urinary Tract Infections

20-40%
The amount by which your risk of recurrent urinary tract infections drops if you drink eight ounces of cranberry juice a day.

Blame female anatomy for the fact that women are twice as likely as men to experience urinary tract infections (UTIs). The route from the outside world (via the urethra) to the bladder is much shorter in women than in men, giving the bacteria responsible for these painful, often recurrent infections easier access. Plus, in women, that urethral opening is just a couple of inches from the rectum, making it far easier for bacteria from the bowel to slip in. About 6 out of 10 women will have at least one UTI, and about 2 out of 10 will experience them repeatedly. Prevent them with these measures.

Key Prevention Strategies

Practice good hygiene. Prevent bacteria from getting in by wiping from front to back after a bowel movement—never from back to front. Use a clean washcloth to wash the skin around your rectum (and especially between rectum and vagina) every day when taking a shower or bath.

sweet ways to get your cranberries

Cranberry juice for urinary tract infections is one of those folk cures that really work. An antioxidant compound in cranberries (and blueberries) prevents bacteria from adhering to bladder and urinary tract cells. Most studies on cranberries have been conducted with pure juice (buy unsweetened juice, not cranberry juice cocktail, which is loaded with sugar; if it's too tart, dilute it with water or seltzer) or dried cranberry extract pills. Here are five other ways to get this important fruit into your diet.

1. Sprinkle dried cranberries over salads or yogurt and mix them into pancake or muffin batter in place of raisins.

2. Use fresh cranberries with apples, blueberries, peaches, or cherries in pies.

3. Enjoy cranberry relish. Combine a bag of fresh cranberries, one cup sugar, the juice of one lemon, and a cinnamon stick in a medium saucepan and cook over medium-low heat until the cranberries pop. Cool and use to top pork loin or chicken breasts or thighs.

4. Whip up a cranberry smoothie. Blend a banana, one cup low-fat raspberry frozen yogurt, one cup cranberry juice, and one cup fresh or frozen blueberries.

5. Make ice pops. Mix equal amounts cranberry juice and seltzer water, pour into ice pop trays, and freeze.

Drink up. The more you drink, the more you urinate. The more you urinate, the more bacteria you flush out of your urinary tract. Any liquid will do, although unsweetened cranberry juice offers the best protection (see "Sweet Ways to Get Your Cranberries" on the previous page). Blueberry juice and other berry juices are also good choices.

Visit the bathroom before and after sex. When you're there, do two things: urinate to flush any bacteria from the urethra, and wash the area. Wet wipes designed for bathroom use are handy for this.

Wear cotton where it counts. Cotton breathes, keeping the area between the legs drier so it doesn't become a breeding ground for bacteria.

Skip douching. It's not necessary. All douches and vaginal sprays do is irritate the urethra and disrupt the natural balance of good and bad bacteria that keeps infections in check.

Prevention Boosters

Ask about antibiotics. If you're prone to UTIs, ask your healthcare provider about prophylactic antibiotics—antibiotics taken to prevent infection. Whether taken daily, only after sex, or every few weeks, they work to prevent UTIs, according to studies.

Choose your birth control carefully. Using a diaphragm and spermicide may increase the risk of UTIs in women with a history of repeated infections. Even condoms used with spermicide can up the risk. Skip the spermicide if you think it bothers you, or choose a birth control method that isn't inserted into the vagina, such as oral contraceptives or contraceptive injections.

Ration the intercourse. The more often you have sex, and the more people with whom you have sex in a year, the higher your risk of UTIs.

WHAT CAUSES IT Usually, infection with *E. coli* bacteria, which tend to originate around the rectum and spread to the bladder opening in the vagina, then make their way up to the bladder.

SYMPTOMS TO WATCH FOR Burning or pain during urination; feeling that you need to urinate more often than usual; feeling that you need to urinate but not being able to; leaking urine; cloudy, dark, smelly, or bloody urine.

NEWEST THINKING The bacteria that cause UTIs actually invade bladder cells, taking up residence there more or less permanently and leading to recurrent infections. This may be one reason that prophylactic (preventive) antibiotic therapy works so well. Previously, researchers didn't think the bacteria could get into bladder cells.

Varicose Veins

50%

The amount by which you could lower your risk of varicose veins by drinking a glass of wine most days.

Ingeniously designed one-way valves in the veins of your legs prevent blood from flowing backward. But if the veins stretch out or the valves weaken—due to genetics, inactivity, a job that keeps you on your feet, pregnancy, or other factors—blood can do just that, causing pooling that leads to twisted, bulging varicose veins and tired, achy, itchy, swollen legs. These steps can protect your legs and keep varicose veins from growing worse if you already have them.

Key Prevention Strategies

Don't stand when you can sit. Standing for long periods every day raises your risk of varicose veins by 60 percent, say researchers at Finland's Tampere University Hospital. Sitting down whenever possible helps by easing pressure on blood vessels. Plant your feet flat on the floor or cross your ankles when you sit; crossing your legs at the knees squeezes veins shut, further blocking blood flow.

Elevate your legs several times each day. Raising your legs prevents blood from pooling. If you already have varicose veins or simply want to give your legs veins extra help, lie down at home and raise your legs higher than the level of your heart by propping them on pillows or even against the wall. This allows gravity to work to move blood to your heart instead of having it pool in the veins of your legs and feet.

Lose those extra pounds. Being overweight puts extra pressure on the fragile veins just below the surface of the skin in your legs. Being overweight or obese raised the odds for varicose veins by as much as 58 percent in one large Scottish study. A great way to lose weight is by getting more exercise, which also reduces your risk of vein problems.

rein in vein pain

Horse chestnut seed extract (HCSE) is one alternative remedy for varicose vein discomfort that seems to really work. When Harvard Medical School doctors reviewed 16 well-designed studies of thousands of people with weak valves in their leg veins, they found that those who took the extract, sold in health food stores, had four times less pain than those who got a placebo. Half saw a decrease in swelling, and 70 percent had less itching. They also reported improvement in feelings of fatigue and heaviness in their legs. British researchers who reviewed seven HCSE studies say this safe botanical may be as effective as compression stockings. The active ingredient, called escin, has strengthened the walls of small blood vessels in lab studies.

The usual dose is 300 milligrams of HCSE (containing 50 to 75 milligrams of escin per dose) every 12 hours for up to 12 weeks.

Keep your legs on the move. Standing and even sitting still at a desk all day allows blood to pool. Push it back toward your heart as often as you can. How? If you're sitting, point and flex your feet to boost circulation. If you're on your feet, get the blood moving several times an hour by rising on your toes, shifting your weight from one foot to the other, bending your legs, and walking in place.

Don compression stockings. These long elastic socks squeeze your legs so blood can't pool as much. They can ease aching and swelling if you have varicose veins and may help prevent them, too. When Japanese researchers measured the legs of 20 people with varicose veins, they found that all grades of compression stockings reduced swelling, but medium- and strong-grade stockings worked best. These are labeled "22 mmHg" or "30–40 mmHg." British researchers found that this hosiery can reduce the amount of blood pooling in leg veins by about 20 percent.

Wear flats. Stilettos may not cause varicose veins, but wearing them makes your calf muscles less effective at pumping blood back toward your heart when you walk, say experts at Wake Forest University Baptist Medical Center in Winston-Salem, North Carolina.

Prevention Boosters

Stop straining. Working too hard to have a bowel movement increases pressure on veins in the lower legs. Researchers at Scotland's University of Edinburgh report that this behind-closed-doors pushing nearly doubled the risk of vein problems in men. To make bowel movements as easy and comfortable as possible, drink plenty of water during the day and increase your fiber intake.

Enjoy a glass of wine. Spanish researchers who analyzed the health records of 1,778 people found that those who enjoyed a glass of wine every day had a 50 percent lower risk of varicose veins than those who drank less—or more. Other research suggests that flavonoids and saponins in wine can help keep blood vessels flexible and healthy.

WHAT CAUSES IT
Weakened valves in leg veins, which allow blood to pool instead of traveling back to your heart. Age, genetics, lack of exercise, standing for long periods, and extra pressure due to overweight or pregnancy can all make the valves malfunction.

SYMPTOMS TO WATCH FOR Enlarged, bulging veins; swelling in your legs and ankles; a "heavy," painful, or crampy feeling in your legs; itching; discolored skin.

NEWEST THINKING
Exercise your legs even if you wear compression stockings. Scientists in Hong Kong recently discovered a design flaw in the stockings: As study volunteers moved around, their stockings sometimes squeezed tighter at the calves than at the ankles, which could actually promote blood pooling rather than prevent it. The researchers' conclusion: Compression stockings are still worth wearing if you're on your feet all day, but you should also plan to exercise your calf muscles to help keep blood moving.

Wrinkles

36%

The reduction in your odds of developing deep wrinkles if you eat several servings of vitamin C–rich fruits and vegetables every day.

There's plenty you can do, short of surgery, to reduce these signs of aging and prevent new ones from cropping up. The key? Pampering your skin's inner structure, the collagen and elastin fibers that keep your face looking firm.

Wear sunscreen every day. Sunlight causes 90 percent of age-related damage to your skin, making sun protection the most effective anti-wrinkle measure you can take. The culprits are UVA rays—the longer, more penetrating ultraviolet light that's constant throughout the year—and UVB, the rays that cause sunburn and are strongest in summer. Your best protection comes form clothing—including a broad-brimmed hat—and a broad-spectrum sunscreen with SPF 30 or higher. For the best protection from UVA rays, look for a product with mexoryl, avobenzone (Parsol 1789), ecamsule, zinc oxide, or titanium dioxide.

Kick the tobacco habit. When University of Utah researchers compared facial wrinkling in 109 smokers and 23 nonsmokers, they found that heavy smokers were five times more likely to have deep, craggy lines. Chemicals in cigarette smoke seem to dismantle the internal scaffolding—which includes connective tissue made of the proteins collagen and elastin—that keeps skin firm and smooth.

Put more fruits and vegetables on your plate. When British researchers checked the diets and wrinkles of 4,025 middle-aged women, they found that vitamin C–rich foods reduced the risk of significant wrinkles by 36 percent. This antioxidant vitamin may protect skin by mopping up free radicals, the unstable oxygen molecules that damage collagen. Increasing your intake of vitamin C is as easy as having berries or a glass of orange juice at breakfast, red peppers and grapefruit at lunch, and broccoli at

the anti-wrinkle diet

When dermatologists checked the skin and diets of 453 people from Australia, Greece, and Sweden, they found that while a healthy diet can't erase damage done by years of unprotected sunbathing or smoking, it can help. Here's what to eat and what to avoid.

Have More of These	And Less of These
Olive oil	Butter
Fish	Red meat
Low-fat milk	Full-fat milk
Water and tea	Soft drinks
Fruit and vegetables	Cakes and pastries
Eggs	Margarine
Nuts and nut butters	Potatoes
Beans	

dinner. Other studies show that the more produce of all kinds you eat, the lower your odds of wrinkling.

Order salmon when you're dining out. This bumps up your intake of the good omega-3 fatty acids that the researchers found reduced the risk of old-looking skin by 25 percent. Walnuts, canola oil, fish-oil capsules, and flaxseed are also great sources.

Cut back on white bread and sugar. Each 50-gram increase in your daily carbohydrate consumption (the amount in two eight-ounce soft drinks) increases your risk of wrinkles by 28 percent, according to the British study mentioned earlier. The link may be "advanced glycation end products," molecules made from sugars and proteins that attack collagen as well as elastin, the stretchy protein that keeps skin looking firm.

Prevention Boosters

Have a cup of sugar-free cocoa. In one study, antioxidants called epicatechin and catechin in cocoa protected skin from sun damage and boosted circulation to skin cells.

Use a facial cleanser instead of soap and water. Soap strips away barrier oils and moisture that protect skin from wrinkling.

Shop for a smart anti-wrinkle product. Confused by the countless anti-aging creams on the market? A recent test by *Consumer Reports* magazine reports that most do very little. But products containing these active ingredients may help.
- **Retinoids.** Available in prescription creams (such as Renova) and in weaker over-the-counter versions, this vitamin A derivative minimizes fine lines and helps build new collagen.
- **Alpha-hydroxy acids (AHAs).** These natural acids minimize the appearance of fine lines and wrinkles, especially around the eyes, by lifting off the top layer of dead skin on your face. At higher concentrations, they may even spur the production of new collagen.
- **Antioxidants.** Creams and lotions containing vitamin C, idebenone, and other antioxidants may help reduce fine lines and wrinkles by battling cell damage.

WHAT CAUSES IT Sun exposure, smoking, genetics, aging, skimping on produce and "good" fats, eating a diet high in saturated fat and refined carbohydrates, and other factors all conspire to erode collagen and elastin, the fibers that keep skin smooth, flexible, and firm.

SYMPTOMS TO WATCH FOR Fine lines around the eyes; furrows in the forehead and around the mouth; deepening wrinkles under the eyes.

NEWEST THINKING Driving your car could give you wrinkles. Dermatologists at the St. Louis University School of Medicine report an upswing in patients with mysterious, lopsided facial wrinkles. These signs of aging were usually worse on the left side than the right. The cause? Sun streaming through the driver's side window of the car—even for just a few minutes each day. The sun's UVA rays, which penetrate more deeply into the skin and cause more of the damage that leads to wrinkles, travel easily through window glass—a good reason to wear sunscreen every day.

Yeast Infections

33%

The amount by which you could reduce your risk of yeast infections by eating yogurt that contains live *Lactobacillus acidophilus* cultures every day.

Like a rainforest, the vagina is a complex and delicate ecosystem, home to a variety of microscopic organisms—in this case, mostly bacteria (both "good" and "bad") including the yeast-like fungus *Candida vulvovaginitis.* Candida resides in the vagina trouble free in up to half of all women. But disrupt the ecosystem, and it can overgrow, causing the itching, soreness, and burning of the all-too-common yeast infection. Keep yourself infection free with this advice.

Key Prevention Strategies

Favor cotton down below. Skip that ubiquitous nylon lingerie in favor of old-fashioned cotton, which lets air in and helps prevent yeast from breeding. And always wear undies under your pantyhose.

Keep the area dry. After a shower or bath, use a blow dryer on the coolest setting (be careful not to burn yourself) to dry your vaginal area before getting dressed. And change out of a wet swimsuit as soon as possible. Yeast loves damp environments.

Wipe the right way. After bowel movements, wipe from front to back, never back to front. One theory about yeast infections is that "bad" bacteria get into the vagina from the rectum, disrupting the environment that normally keeps yeast in check.

Spoon up some yogurt. Some studies suggest that eating eight ounces a day of yogurt that contains live, active bacteria cultures helps maintain a healthy vaginal environment and could reduce the risk of recurrent yeast infections.

Check your blood sugar. If you've ever made bread from scratch, you know that yeast needs sugar to grow. That's why women with diabetes are much more vulnerable to yeast infections. (See the Diabetes chapter for prevention tips.)

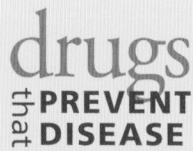
drugs that PREVENT DISEASE

Up to 30 percent of women taking antibiotics are prone to yeast infections. The drugs can kill off beneficial bacteria that keep vaginal flora in balance. If you're taking antibiotics and you're prone to yeast infections, consider taking an over-the-counter probiotic ("good" bacteria supplement) with bacteria such as lactobacillus to maintain the appropriate checks and balances, or eat a cup of yogurt with live, active cultures every day. Also keep some over the counter anti-yeast creams or suppositories (miconazole or clotrimazole) on hand and use at the first sign of vaginal itching.

Stick to regular sex. Nix the oral sex for a while if you're susceptible to yeast infections, or at least cut way back. Having your partner perform oral sex five or more times a month can increase your risk of yeast infections.

Prevention Boosters

Avoid dyes and perfumes. Skip colored or perfumed toilet tissue and scented sanitary pads and tampons, all of which can disrupt the normal vaginal environment.

Avoid most "feminine products." After you buy your tampons or pads, leave the feminine product aisle. There's simply no need to use douches, powders, or sprays, which can irritate the genital area.

Follow a low-GI diet. Just as women with diabetes are more prone to yeast infections, so too are women with insulin resistance. This condition occurs when cells become resistant to insulin, the hormone that allows glucose into cells, leading to higher than normal blood sugar levels. Foods made with sugar, high-fructose corn syrup, and white flour—which include most store-bought baked goods as well as crackers, cookies, chips, and sweetened drinks—all contribute to insulin resistance because they spike blood sugar. White bread and white rice do the same. Instead, eat foods with a low glycemic index (GI), which have less effect on blood sugar. These include most high-fiber foods like vegetables, legumes, and whole grains; "good" fats from olives, nuts, and avocados; and lean protein foods.

WHAT CAUSES IT Out-of-control growth of the yeast organisms that live on your skin, in your vagina, and in your mouth. The growth occurs when the normally acidic vaginal environment loses its acidity. Numerous things can disrupt vaginal harmony, including menstruation, pregnancy, diabetes, antibiotics, oral contraceptives, and steroids. Frequent sex, or anything that irritates the vagina, can trigger yeast growth.

SYMPTOMS TO WATCH FOR Itching and burning in the vagina and the surrounding area (the vulva), as well as vulval swelling; cottage cheese–like vaginal discharge; pain during intercourse.

NEWEST THINKING A tablet designed to help maintain the normal acidity of the vagina could one day be used to prevent recurrent yeast infections. It's currently under investigation.

disease preventing recipes

Long live the joy of food—and long live *you* when you dine on delicious food made at home with the help of these amazingly easy, amazingly healthful dishes. Don't forget dessert!

putting prevention on your plate

In the Disease Prevention Survey, when we asked doctors specially trained in preventive medicine the best way to avoid illness, we heard two pieces of advice loud and clear: Get more exercise and eat right. These experts weren't shy about telling us what "ingredients" go into a healthy diet either: plenty of fruits, vegetables, whole grains, and good fats, especially the omega-3 fatty acids found in many types of fish. Here we've transformed those ingredients into amazingly delicious recipes that put taste first (and health a close second). After all, eating great food is one of life's great pleasures, and we believe that nothing should take that joy away.

We designed this unique collection of easy, tasty dishes specifically to help you meet three goals central to disease prevention.

what's a serving?

It's easier than you think to get nine servings of produce a day. You can knock off one serving just by starting your morning with fruit juice, and three or four more by having a big salad at lunch. Here's what a "serving" actually looks like.

Fruit	Vegetables
1 medium piece of fruit	1 cup raw leafy vegetables
1/2 cup chopped, cooked, or canned fruit	1/2 cup other vegetables, cooked, chopped, or canned
1/4 cup dried fruit	3/4 cup vegetable juice
3/4 cup 100% fruit juice	1/2 cup dried beans

1. **Eat more fruits and vegetables.**
2. **Eat more whole grains.**
3. **Get more of your calories from good fats.**

These goals are right in line with advice that came up again and again from the doctors who participated in the survey. In their own words, they told us that people should "eat more plant-based foods," "avoid refined and processed foods," and "cut down on red meats and foods high in saturated fat." They also told us that it's more important to limit simple carbs than to focus on a low-fat diet!

Many noted one more goal: Eat less. Fortunately, thanks to smart ratios of protein, good fats, and whole grains, these recipes keep your belly full longer so you're not tempted to eat again as soon, a great strategy for staving off weight gain.

What you won't find is a lot of saturated fat, trans fat, or refined carbohydrates, all linked to an increased risk of disease. You won't find margarine either; many brands contain hydrogenated oils, which are terrible for your heart.

About Your Goals

Achieving all three goals will yield amazing health benefits. For starters, it will help you keep your blood sugar levels stable, improve your cholesterol ratio, lower your blood pressure, and even decrease your risk of cancer and possibly Alzheimer's disease. Here's a bit more guidance to help you meet these goals.

Your produce goal: Eat five servings of vegetables and four servings of fruit a day.
Most doctors and nutritionists agree that a plant-based diet—one full of produce, grains, and legumes—is the way to go to prevent most of today's major diseases. The fact is, if you're filling your plate with these foods, you aren't filling it with deadly saturated fat or an overabundance of calories. And you're getting hefty doses of vitamins, minerals, and other plant nutrients that fight against specific diseases. You're also hitting an important target: getting at least 25 grams of fiber per day.

Earlier in the book we recommended that you eat "at least" five servings of produce a day, based on the Disease Prevention Survey, but the truth is, nine servings a day is the ideal goal.

Your fat goal: Get about 25 percent of the calories you eat from good fats.
Leading nutrition experts now advocate getting 25 to 35 percent of your calories from fat. Here's the trick: Most of that should be healthy monounsaturated fats (the kind in nuts, avocados, and canola and olive oil) and omega-3 fatty acids, found in foods like salmon and flaxseed. Less than 7 percent of your calories should come from saturated fat (the kind in fatty meat, butter, and cheese), which promotes insulin resistance and heart disease. We also recommend limiting fat from corn, safflower, and sunflower oils, as these promote inflammation. See "Your Fat Targets" at right to find out how many grams of fat these recommendations amount to.

Your carbohydrate goal: Get three of your daily grain servings from whole grains.
Eating refined carbohydrates (think white rice, white bread, and other foods made with white flour) helps promote both weight gain and insulin resistance. Swapping these foods for slow-digesting whole grains (for instance, barley or bulgur instead of rice) is one key to preventing many of the chronic diseases that plague us today, from obesity to heart disease.

One of our very favorite pieces of advice from the survey is to "Stop and choose how you want to live life." That includes the way you eat. Start by choosing one of the dishes in this chapter. Each recipe includes a box that shows what the recipe contributes toward your three dietary goals. And if you don't have a problem with alcohol, enjoy this last tip: "Have a glass of wine or beer with dinner!"

Your Fat Targets

DAILY CALORIES	DAILY GOOD FAT GOAL	DAILY SATURATED FAT GOAL
1,600	44 grams	Less than 12 grams
1,800	50 grams	Less than 14 grams
2,000	55.5 grams	Less than 15.15 grams
2,200	61 grams	Less than 17 grams
2,400	66.6 grams	Less than 18.6 grams
2,600	72 grams	Less than 20 grams

Serves 11

PREP 5 minutes

COOK TIME (in slow cooker) 10 hours

3 cups unsweetened apple juice

1 cup steel-cut oats

1/2 cup hard wheat berries

1 cup dried fruit, such as raisins, dried cranberries, dried cherries, chopped dried apricots, chopped dried figs, or chopped pitted prunes

2 tablespoons packed brown sugar

1/2 teaspoon ground cinnamon

3/4 cup 1% milk or soy milk

Overnight Oat and Wheat Berry Hot Cereal

Cooking great-for-you grains takes something that's often in short supply: time. Now you can wake up to fragrant whole grain oatmeal that has cooked—almost magically—while you slept. Steel-cut oats, wheat berries, and fruit provide a healthy dose of fiber.

1 Coat a 4-quart or larger slow cooker with cooking spray. Combine the apple juice, 2 1/2 cups water, oats, and wheat berries in the cooker. Cover and cook on low until the wheat berries are tender and the cereal has thickened, about 10 hours.

2 Stir in the fruit, then cover and cook for 5 minutes. Sprinkle each serving with about 1/2 teaspoon brown sugar and a pinch of cinnamon. Top with about 1 tablespoon milk. One serving is 1/2 cup.

Tip: Be sure to use steel-cut oats (sometimes known as Irish oats), which are whole oat groats that have been cut into several pieces rather than rolled. Traditional rolled oats, even the old-fashioned variety, cook too quickly and may turn to mush with this slow-cooker method. Look for steel-cut oats in the natural foods section of your supermarket or in natural foods stores. You can find wheat berries in the bulk bins section of natural foods stores.

meeting your **goals**

Each portion provides 1.1 servings fruit, 1.1 servings whole grains, and 1 gram good fat.

NUTRITION • *Per serving*
178 calories, 4 g protein, 39 g carbohydrates, 3 g fiber, 1 g total fat, 0 g saturated fat, 1 mg cholesterol, 13 mg sodium

Spinach, Mango, and Black Bean Salad with Shrimp

This colorful protein-rich salad makes a satisfying lunch or light supper and gets you well on your way to meeting your fruit and vegetable targets for the day. For the best flavor, cook shrimp in their shells. However, to save time, you can purchase peeled cooked shrimp. *See photo, page 327.*

1 To make the dressing: In a jar with a tight-fitting lid or a small bowl, combine the orange juice, oil, vinegar, cumin, oregano, honey, garlic, salt, and pepper. Shake or whisk to blend.

2 To make the salad: Place a large bowl of ice water beside the stove. Bring 2 quarts lightly salted water to a simmer in a Dutch oven or deep sauté pan. Add the shrimp and simmer over medium-low heat until pink, 2 to 4 minutes. With a slotted spoon, transfer to the ice water to stop the cooking. Drain the shrimp, then peel.

3 In a medium bowl, combine the beans and 1/4 cup of the dressing and toss to coat. In a large bowl, combine the spinach, mangos, bell pepper, onion, and shrimp. Add the remaining dressing and toss to coat. Divide the salad among 4 plates and top each serving with about 1/3 cup beans. One serving is 3 cups.

meeting your **goals**

> Each portion provides 1.3 servings fruit, 2 servings vegetables, and 10 grams good fat.

salads

Serves 4

PREP 35 minutes
COOK TIME 2 to 4 minutes

DRESSING
1/4 cup orange juice

3 tablespoons extra-virgin olive oil

2 tablespoons apple cider vinegar

1 1/2 teaspoons ground cumin

1/2 teaspoon dried oregano

1 teaspoon honey

1 small clove garlic, minced

1/4 teaspoon salt, or to taste

Freshly ground black pepper to taste

SALAD
1 pound medium (51–60 count) shrimp, shells on

1 can (15 ounces) black beans, drained and rinsed

6 cups baby spinach, washed and dried

2 ripe mangos, diced

1 small red bell pepper, diced

1/2 cup finely diced red onion

NUTRITION • *Per serving*
325 calories, 20 g protein, 42 g carbohydrates, 9 g fiber, 13 g total fat, 2 g saturated fat, 108 mg cholesterol, 757 mg sodium

Serves 4

PREP 25 minutes

BAKE TIME 12 to 15 minutes

WALNUTS
1/4 cup walnuts, coarsely chopped

1 teaspoon olive oil

1 teaspoon honey

Pinch of salt

DRESSING
3 tablespoons walnut oil (see Tip) or extra-virgin olive oil

2 tablespoons finely chopped shallot (1 medium)

4 teaspoons white or red wine vinegar

1 teaspoon Dijon mustard

1/2 teaspoon salt, or to taste

Freshly ground black pepper to taste

SALAD
4 cups mixed baby salad greens (mesclun), washed and dried

1 Belgian endive, cored and cut crosswise into 1/2"-thick slices

1 ripe but firm red Anjou or Bartlett pear, peeled, cored, and thinly sliced

1 cup red seedless grapes, washed, patted dry, and halved

NUTRITION • *Per serving*
223 calories, 3 g protein, 20 g carbohydrates, 4 g fiber, 17 g total fat, 2 g saturated fat, 0 mg cholesterol, 365 mg sodium

Mixed Greens with Pears, Grapes, and Honey-Glazed Walnuts

Adding fresh fruit to a green salad is an easy way to give it pizzazz. A topping of nuts—rich in good fats—is the crowning touch and a much healthier option than store-bought croutons. Here, we toast the nuts with a honey glaze for a touch of sweetness.

1 To make the walnuts: Preheat the oven to 350°F. Coat a small baking dish with cooking spray. In a small bowl, combine the walnuts, oil, honey, and salt and stir to coat. Spread the mixture in the baking dish. Bake, stirring occasionally, until fragrant, 12 to 15 minutes. Let cool.

2 To make the dressing: In a jar with a tight-fitting lid or a small bowl, combine the walnut oil, shallot, vinegar, mustard, salt, and pepper. Shake or whisk to blend.

3 To make the salad: Just before serving, combine the greens, endive, pear, and grapes in a large bowl. Add the dressing and toss to coat well. Divide the salad among 4 plates and top each serving with about 2 tablespoons walnuts. One serving is 2 cups.

Tip: With a delicate nutty flavor, walnut oil is an excellent choice for dressing salads, especially when paired with nuts or flavorful cheese. It's also a good source of heart-healthy omega-3 fatty acids. You can find it in most large supermarkets and in specialty food stores. The oil is expensive, but a little goes a long way in distinguishing your salad. Refrigerate the bottle after opening.

meeting your **goals**

> Each portion provides 0.8 serving fruit, 1.2 servings vegetables, and 14 grams good fat.

Grilled Chicken and Peach Salad with Watercress

This main-dish salad is summer eating at its very best. The fruity dressing balances the peppery bite of watercress—a cancer-fighting cruciferous vegetable rich in beta-carotene and vitamin C—and infuses the chicken with flavor. The ginger helps fight inflammation. *See photo, page 335.*

1 To make the marinade and dressing: In a blender, combine the peach nectar, oil, vinegar, soy sauce, ginger, garlic, and pepper. Cover and blend until smooth.

2 To make the chicken and salad: Place the chicken in a zipper-seal bag. Add 1/4 cup of the juice mixture, seal the bag, and turn the chicken to coat. Refrigerate for at least 30 minutes or for up to 1 day. (Reserve the remaining marinade, covered, in the refrigerator, for dressing the salad.)

3 Set a fine-mesh vegetable grill topper on the grill. Preheat the grill to medium. Lightly oil the topper and grate by rubbing with a piece of oil-soaked paper towel. Brush the peaches and onion with the oil and place on the grill topper. Place the chicken on the grill grate. Cover the grill and cook, turning once halfway through cooking, until the chicken is browned and cooked through (an instant-read thermometer inserted in the center should register 170°F) and the onion and peaches are lightly browned, 10 to 12 minutes.

4 Cut the chicken into 1/4-inch-thick slices. Cut the peaches into wedges. Separate the onion rings. In a large bowl, combine the watercress, chicken, peaches, and onion. Add the reserved dressing and toss to coat well. One serving is 1 3/4 cups.

Tip: Look for unsweetened peach nectar in the natural foods section of your supermarket or in a natural foods store. Check to make sure that the juice has not been sweetened with high-fructose corn syrup.

meeting your **goals**

> Each portion provides 1 serving fruit, 1.7 servings vegetables, and 13 grams good fat.

Serves 4

PREP 25 minutes

MARINATE TIME 30 minutes to 1 day

COOK TIME 10 to 12 minutes

MARINADE AND DRESSING
1/3 cup unsweetened peach or apricot nectar (see Tip) or juice

3 tablespoons canola oil

4 teaspoons rice vinegar

2 teaspoons reduced-sodium soy sauce

2 slices (1/4" thick) fresh ginger, peeled and crushed

1 clove garlic, crushed and peeled

1/4 teaspoon crushed red pepper

CHICKEN AND SALAD
1 pound boneless skinless chicken breasts, trimmed

2 teaspoons canola oil

2 peaches, peeled, pitted, and halved

1 small red onion, cut into 1/2"-thick slices

6 cups trimmed watercress sprigs, washed and dried

NUTRITION • *Per serving*
294 calories, 25 g protein, 14 g carbohydrates, 2 g fiber, 16 g total fat, 2 g saturated fat, 63 mg cholesterol, 167 mg sodium

Asian Steak Salad

PREP 30 minutes

MARINATE TIME 6 hours
or overnight

COOK TIME 10 to
12 minutes

**MARINADE AND
DRESSING**

1/4 cup fresh lime juice

2 tablespoons rice vinegar

1 tablespoon fish sauce
(see Tip)

1 tablespoon sugar

2 teaspoons grated
fresh ginger

2 teaspoons minced
jalapeño or serrano
pepper

1 small clove garlic,
minced

STEAK AND SALAD

8 ounces flank steak,
trimmed

3 cups sliced romaine
lettuce (1 small head)

1 cup diced
red bell pepper

1 cup sliced cucumber

1/2 cup fresh mint leaves,
cut into thin slivers

1/4 cup chopped scallions

2 tablespoons unsalted
roasted peanuts, coarsely
chopped

Here, a green salad is utterly transformed into a mouthwatering
meal. A tangy Asian-flavored marinade turns lean, budget-friendly
flank steak tender and doubles as a dressing. If you're short on time,
use a strip loin steak and marinate it for just 20 minutes. *See photo,
next page.*

1 To make the marinade and dressing: In a medium bowl, whisk the
lime juice, vinegar, fish sauce, sugar, ginger, jalapeño, and garlic until
the sugar dissolves.

2 To marinate the steak: Place the steak in a zipper-seal bag. Add
1/4 cup of the lime juice mixture, seal the bag, and turn the steak to
coat. Refrigerate for at least 6 hours or overnight. (Reserve the remaining
marinade, covered, in the refrigerator, for dressing the salad.)

3 To cook the steak: Preheat the grill to medium-high or preheat the
broiler. Remove the steak from the marinade, discarding the excess.
If grilling, lightly oil the grill grate by rubbing it with a piece of oil-
soaked paper towel. If broiling, coat the broiler pan with cooking spray.
Grill or broil the steak until it reaches desired doneness, 5 to 6 minutes
per side for medium-rare (an instant-read thermometer should register
140°F). Transfer to a clean cutting board and let stand for 5 minutes.
Carve across the grain into thin slices.

4 To make the salad: In a large bowl, combine the lettuce, bell pepper,
cucumber, mint, and scallions. Add the steak and reserved dressing
and toss to coat. Sprinkle each serving with peanuts. One serving is
3 cups.

Tip: You can find fish sauce, made from salted fermented anchovies, in the
Asian foods section of most supermarkets. If it's not available, substitute reduced-
sodium soy sauce. For a more authentic taste, mix 1/8 teaspoon anchovy paste with
1 tablespoon soy sauce.

meeting your **goals**

**Each portion provides
0.2 serving fruit, 3.8 servings vegetables, and
17 grams good fat.**

NUTRITION • *Per serving*
311 calories, 30 g protein,
25 g carbohydrates, 7 g fiber,
12 g total fat, 3 g saturated
fat, 37 mg cholesterol,
781 mg sodium

Clockwise from top left: Quinoa Salad with Corn and Lime Dressing; Spinach, Mango, and Black Bean Salad with Shrimp; Asian Steak Salad; Spring Vegetable Soup

Serves 6

PREP 30 minutes

COOK TIME 18 to
20 minutes

3/4 cup quinoa, rinsed
thoroughly

3/4 teaspoon salt

2 ears corn, husked

1/4 cup plus 1 tablespoon
fresh lime juice

1 jalapeño pepper,
seeded and minced

1 small clove garlic,
minced

1 teaspoon ground cumin

Freshly ground
black pepper to taste

1/4 cup canola oil

2 cups cherry tomatoes or
grape tomatoes, halved

1/2 cup chopped scallions

1/2 cup chopped
fresh cilantro

2 Hass avocados, diced

Quinoa Salad with Corn and Lime Dressing

Grain salads are ideal for potlucks, picnics, and backyard barbecues. While quinoa (pronounced *keen-wa*) isn't technically a grain, it's used as one and contains plenty of fiber and considerable protein to boot. This lively Latin-inspired salad is terrific with grilled pork, chicken, or fish. *See photo, page 327.*

1 In a medium saucepan, combine the quinoa, 1 1/2 cups water, and 1/2 teaspoon salt. Bring to a simmer, then cover and cook over low heat until the quinoa is tender and most of the liquid has been absorbed, 12 to 15 minutes. Remove from the heat and let stand for 5 minutes. Fluff with a fork, transfer to a large bowl, and let cool.

2 Bring 1 inch of water to a boil in a large pot. Add the corn, cover, and cook until tender, about 5 minutes. Refresh under cold running water. Cut the kernels off the cobs (you should have about 1 cup).

3 Meanwhile, in a small bowl, whisk 1/4 cup lime juice, the jalapeño, garlic, cumin, pepper, and the remaining 1/4 teaspoon salt. Gradually whisk in the oil.

4 Add the tomatoes, scallions, cilantro, and corn to the quinoa. Add the dressing and toss to coat. The salad will keep, covered, in the refrigerator for up to 2 days. Just before serving, toss the avocados with the remaining 1 tablespoon lime juice in a small bowl. Garnish the salad with the avocados. One serving is a generous 3/4 cup.

meeting your **goals**

Each portion provides 1.2 servings fruit, 1.1 servings vegetables, 0.7 serving whole grains, and 16 grams good fat.

NUTRITION • *Per serving*
299 calories, 5 g protein, 29 g carbohydrates, 7 g fiber, 20 g total fat, 2 g saturated fat, 0 mg cholesterol, 309 mg sodium

Bulgur Salad with Dried Apricots and Mint

This fruity version of tabbouleh features dried fruit, colorful red bell pepper, and sweet mint in a lightly spiced citrus dressing. Bulgur is one of the most convenient whole grains. It doesn't even need to be cooked, just soaked. It raises blood sugar much less than rice does.

1 Bring about 2 1/2 cups water to a boil in a small saucepan. Place the bulgur and apricots in a large bowl and add enough boiling water to cover. Let stand for 20 minutes, then drain and press out excess water.

2 Meanwhile, toast the pine nuts in a small dry skillet over medium-low heat, stirring constantly, until golden and fragrant, 2 to 3 minutes. Transfer to a plate and let cool.

3 In a large bowl, whisk the orange juice, vinegar, garlic, cumin, coriander, salt, and pepper. Gradually whisk in the oil. Add the bulgur, bell pepper, scallions, and mint and toss to coat well. The salad will keep, covered, in the refrigerator for up to 2 days. Just before serving, sprinkle with the pine nuts. One serving is 2/3 cup.

meeting your **goals**

Each portion provides 1.3 servings fruit, 0.7 serving vegetables, 0.6 serving whole grains, and 10 grams good fat.

Serves 6

PREP 25 minutes

COOK TIME 20 minutes

3/4 cup medium bulgur, rinsed

1/2 cup dried apricots, diced

1/3 cup pine nuts

1/3 cup orange juice

3 tablespoons cider vinegar

1 small clove garlic, minced

1/2 teaspoon ground cumin

1/4 teaspoon ground coriander

1/4 teaspoon salt, or to taste

Freshly ground black pepper to taste

3 tablespoons extra-virgin olive oil

1 small red bell pepper, seeded and diced (1 1/2 cups)

1/2 cup chopped scallions

1/2 cup chopped fresh mint

NUTRITION • *Per serving*
239 calories, 5 g protein, 29 g carbohydrates, 6 g fiber, 13 g total fat, 1 g saturated fat, 0 mg cholesterol, 107 mg sodium

Spring Vegetable Soup

PREP 20 minutes

COOK TIME 25 minutes

1 tablespoon olive oil

1 medium sweet onion, such as Vidalia, sliced (2 cups)

1 all-purpose potato, peeled and sliced (1 cup)

1 clove garlic, minced

4 cups reduced-sodium chicken broth or vegetable broth

1 1/2 pounds asparagus, tough stems snapped off, cut into 1" lengths (3 cups)

4 cups (3 ounces) baby spinach, washed and dried

1 tablespoon fresh lemon juice

1/4 teaspoon salt, or to taste

Freshly ground black pepper to taste

1/3 cup low-fat plain yogurt

2 tablespoons 1% milk

1 tablespoon snipped fresh tarragon or chives

Welcome spring and take advantage of the first crop of vegetables by making this simple, fresh-tasting *potage* (a type of rustic French soup). It boasts a velvety consistency without using a drop of cream. *See photo, page 327.*

1 Heat the oil in a Dutch oven or soup pot over medium-high heat. Add the onion and cook, stirring often, until softened, 2 to 3 minutes. Add the potato and garlic. Cook, stirring, for 20 to 30 seconds. Add the broth and bring to a simmer. Reduce the heat to medium-low, cover, and simmer for 15 minutes.

2 Add the asparagus and increase the heat to medium. Cover and cook until tender, 4 to 5 minutes. Stir in the spinach and cook just until it starts to wilt, 30 to 60 seconds.

3 Working in batches, puree the soup in a blender or food processor. (Use caution when blending hot liquids. Do not fill the blender more than half full. Cover the lid with a kitchen towel and hold it securely in place.) Return the soup to the pot and heat through. Stir in the lemon juice, salt, and pepper. In a small bowl, whisk the yogurt and milk until smooth. Ladle the soup into bowls and drop small dollops of the yogurt mixture into each, then draw the tip of a knife or toothpick through the yogurt to make decorative swirls. Sprinkle with tarragon. One serving is 1 cup.

meeting your **goals**

Each portion provides 1.8 servings vegetables, 0.4 serving whole grains, and 10 grams good fat.

NUTRITION • *Per serving*
84 calories, 6 g protein, 11 g carbohydrates, 3 g fiber, 3 g total fat, 0 g saturated fat, 1 mg cholesterol, 496 mg sodium

3 Great Ways to Eat Barley

With a deliciously nutty flavor, barley's a great addition to soups, pilafs, and salads that won't raise your blood sugar the way rice can. It's also loaded with soluble fiber to lower your cholesterol.

Barley and Beet Salad

Serves 5

1/2 cup pearl barley
1/2 teaspoon salt
1/3 cup extra-virgin olive oil
3 tablespoons red wine vinegar
Black pepper to taste
1 1/2 cups (8 ounces) diced cooked beets
1/2 cup chopped scallions
1/2 cup crumbled feta cheese
3 tablespoons chopped fresh dill

In a small saucepan, combine 2 1/2 cups water, the barley, and 1/4 teaspoon salt. Cover and simmer over medium-low heat until tender, 40 to 45 minutes. Transfer to a large bowl and let cool. In a small bowl, whisk the oil, vinegar, the remaining 1/4 teaspoon salt, and pepper. Add to the barley along with the beets, scallions, feta, and dill. Toss to coat.

Bean and Barley Soup

Serves 10

2 cans cannellini beans, rinsed
1 tablespoon olive oil
1 medium-large onion, chopped
2 medium carrots, diced
1 ounce prosciutto, diced
4 cups shredded green cabbage
4 cloves garlic, minced
1/4 teaspoon crushed red pepper
4 cups reduced-sodium chicken broth
1/2 cup quick-cooking barley
Black pepper to taste
1 1/4 cups shredded reduced-fat Swiss or Jarlsberg cheese

Mash 1 1/2 cups of beans. Heat the oil in a large pot. Add the onion, carrots, and prosciutto. Cook until golden. Add the cabbage, garlic, and red pepper. Cook until the cabbage has wilted. Add the broth, 1 1/2 cups water, barley, and all the beans. Simmer 8 to 10 minutes. Season with pepper. Top each serving with cheese.

Chicken Soup with Barley and Root Vegetables

Serves 8

1 large onion, chopped
3 cloves garlic, minced
1 tablespoon canola oil
5 cups reduced-sodium chicken broth
1/2 cup pearl barley
12 ounces sliced boneless skinless chicken breast
2 cups diced root vegetables, such as carrots and parsnips
2 tablespoons fresh lemon juice
1/4 teaspoon salt
Black pepper to taste
Snipped fresh dill or parsley

In a Dutch oven, cook the onion and garlic in the oil until softened. Add the broth and barley, cover, and simmer for 25 minutes. Add the chicken and vegetables. Simmer, covered, about 20 minutes. Season with the lemon juice, salt, and pepper. Garnish with dill.

Serves 10

PREP 50 minutes
(including Basil Pesto)

COOK TIME 40 minutes

8 cups reduced-sodium chicken broth

8 cloves garlic, crushed and peeled

1/4 teaspoon crushed red pepper

2 tablespoons olive oil

2 medium leeks, white and pale green parts, washed, sliced (1 cup)

1 onion, chopped (1 cup)

4 medium carrots, peeled, halved lengthwise, and sliced (1 cup)

2 cups (6 ounces) cauliflower florets, cut into 3/4" pieces

2 medium tomatoes, seeded and diced (2 cups), or 1 can (15 ounces) diced tomatoes

1 cup (4 ounces) green beans, ends trimmed, cut into 1" pieces

1 cup (4 ounces) medium whole wheat pasta shells

1 small zucchini (8 ounces), quartered lengthwise and sliced (2 cups)

Freshly ground black pepper to taste

3/4 cup Basil Pesto or prepared basil pesto

NUTRITION • *Per serving*
218 calories, 9 g protein, 18 g carbohydrates, 4 g fiber, 14 g total fat, 2 g saturated fat, 4 mg cholesterol, 622 mg sodium

Late Summer Minestrone with Basil Pesto

There's nothing like a trip to a farmer's market when the stands overflow with truly fresh produce to motivate you to eat more vegetables. What to do with all those veggies when you get home? Simmer them into this delicious soup. You'll get more than 2 servings of vegetables in your bowl.

1 Bring the broth to a boil in a large saucepan. Add the garlic and red pepper. Partially cover the saucepan and simmer over medium-low heat for 15 minutes to intensify the flavors. Pour the broth through a strainer into a large bowl, pressing the cooked garlic through the strainer.

2 Heat the oil in a large Dutch oven over medium heat. Add the leeks and onion. Cook, stirring often, until softened but not browned, 2 to 4 minutes. Add the broth, carrots, cauliflower, tomatoes, and beans. Partially cover and simmer over medium heat for 10 minutes.

3 Meanwhile, make the Basil Pesto (recipe at right) if using homemade.

4 Add the pasta and zucchini to the soup. Partially cover and cook until the pasta and vegetables are tender, 10 to 15 minutes. Ladle into bowls and stir about 1 tablespoon pesto into each. The soup will keep, covered, in the refrigerator for up to 2 days. Add a little water when reheating if it seems too thick. One serving is 1 cup.

meeting your **goals**

**Each portion provides
2.2 servings vegetables and
2 grams good fat.**

Basil Pesto

Serves 10 (makes 3/4 cup)

PREP 10 minutes

COOK TIME 2 to 4 minutes

1/3 cup pine nuts

3 cups lightly packed fresh basil leaves, washed and dried

3 small or 2 large cloves garlic, crushed and peeled

1/4 teaspoon salt, or to taste

Freshly ground black pepper to taste

1/4 cup extra-virgin olive oil

1/2 cup freshly grated Parmesan cheese

There's hardly a more delicious way to enjoy good fats courtesy of pine nuts and olive oil. Use it on pasta, spoon a dollop into vegetable soup, drizzle over sliced tomatoes, try it as an omelet filling, or use it atop a vegetable pizza.

1 Toast the pine nuts in a small dry skillet over medium-low heat, stirring constantly, until golden and fragrant, 2 to 4 minutes. Transfer to a small bowl and let cool.

2 In a food processor, combine the basil, garlic, salt, pepper, and pine nuts and process until the pine nuts are ground. With the motor running, gradually add the oil through the feeder tube, processing until the mixture forms a paste. Add the cheese and pulse until blended. Transfer to a bowl. The pesto will keep, covered with a sheet of plastic wrap placed directly on the surface (to keep it from turning brown) in the refrigerator for up to 2 days or in the freezer for up to 6 months. One serving is 1 generous tablespoon.

Maple-Glazed Chicken with Root Vegetables

Serves 4

PREP 30 minutes

BAKE TIME 45 to 55 minutes

4 cups assorted diced (1/2" x 3/4" pieces) peeled root vegetables, such as carrots, parsnips, celery root (see Tip), rutabaga, and/or turnips (1 pound, 3 ounces)

1 tablespoon olive oil

1/2 teaspoon salt

1/2 teaspoon freshly ground black pepper

2 1/2 pounds bone-in chicken thighs and/or drumsticks, skin removed and fat trimmed

1 tablespoon Dijon mustard

1 tablespoon maple syrup

2 teaspoons chopped fresh thyme or 3/4 teaspoon dried thyme

1/2 cup apple cider

1/2 cup reduced-sodium chicken broth

Here is a perfect recipe for late fall and winter, when earthy-tasting root vegetables are at their best. A tasty maple glaze acts as a faux skin for the chicken, providing a delicious crust and keeping the chicken moist and juicy without saturated fat. *See photo, at right.*

1 Preheat the oven to 400°F. Coat a large roasting pan with cooking spray.

2 Place the vegetables in the pan and toss with the oil, 1/4 teaspoon salt, and 1/4 teaspoon pepper. Push the vegetables toward the outside of the pan. Sprinkle the chicken with the remaining 1/4 teaspoon salt and 1/4 teaspoon pepper and place skinned side down in the center of the pan. Bake, uncovered, for 15 minutes.

3 Meanwhile, in a small bowl, combine the mustard, syrup, and thyme.

4 Stir the vegetables and turn the chicken pieces. Brush the chicken with the mustard mixture. Bake, stirring the vegetables occasionally, until the vegetables are glazed and tender and the chicken is cooked through (an instant-read thermometer should register 180°F), 30 to 40 minutes. (If either the chicken or vegetables are done first, remove and keep warm.) Transfer to a platter or individual plates. Add the apple cider and broth to the roasting pan, place over 2 burners, and bring to a boil over medium-high heat. Boil for 2 to 3 minutes. Drizzle the sauce over the chicken and vegetables. One serving is 2 pieces of chicken and 1/2 cup of vegetables.

Tip Celery root, also known as celeriac, is gnarly looking, but it's easy to peel the rough skin with a sharp knife. The creamy flesh has a nutty flavor reminiscent of celery and parsley. It can be served raw (shredded and tossed with vinaigrette dressing) or cooked. It's delicious boiled and pureed (like mashed potatoes), sautéed, or roasted.

meeting your **goals**

Each portion provides 0.2 serving fruit, 2 servings vegetables, and 11 grams good fat.

NUTRITION • *Per serving*
370 calories, 33 g protein, 24 g carbohydrates, 4 g fiber, 16 g total fat, 4 g saturated fat, 108 mg cholesterol, 568 mg sodium

Clockwise from top left: Maple-Glazed Chicken with Root Vegetables; Grilled Chicken and Peach Salad with Water-cress; Brown Rice Paella; Lean Beef Burgers with Blue Cheese Nuggets

Turkey Meatloaf with Asian Flavors

Serves 8

PREP 30 minutes

BAKE TIME 1 hour 10 minutes to 1 hour 20 minutes

1 pound 99% lean ground turkey breast

2 cups shredded sweet potato (1 small)

1 cup chopped onion (1 medium)

3/4 cup whole wheat panko (Japanese-style bread crumbs) or fresh whole wheat bread crumbs (see Tip, page 339)

1 large egg, lightly beaten

2 large egg whites, lightly beaten

6 tablespoons prepared stir-fry sauce

1 tablespoon grated fresh ginger

1 clove garlic, minced

1/2 teaspoon freshly ground black pepper

The secret ingredient that makes this loaf moist and juicy is shredded sweet potato, one of the most nutritious vegetables in nature. Ginger, garlic, and prepared stir-fry sauce give it a lively and unexpected flavor. Serve with steamed broccoli or sautéed spinach.

1 Preheat the oven to 350°F. Line an 8 x 4-inch or 9 x 5-inch loaf pan with foil, leaving a 1-inch overhang along the two long sides. Coat with cooking spray.

2 In a large bowl, combine the turkey, sweet potato, onion, panko, egg, egg whites, 2 tablespoons stir-fry sauce, ginger, garlic, and pepper and mix well. Transfer to the pan and press into a loaf. Spread 1 tablespoon stir-fry sauce over the top.

3 Place the pan on a baking sheet and bake for 1 hour. Drain off the fat, then bake until firm and an instant-read thermometer inserted in the center registers 170°F, 10 to 20 minutes. Drain off the fat and let stand for 5 minutes.

4 In a small microwavable bowl, whisk the remaining 3 tablespoons stir-fry sauce and 3 tablespoons water. Cover with wax paper and microwave on high until heated through, about 1 minute.

5 Use the foil overhang to lift the loaf and transfer it to a cutting board, then slice. Drizzle a little sauce over each slice. Leftover meatloaf will keep, covered, in the refrigerator for up to 2 days. One serving is 4 ounces of meatloaf and about 2 teaspoons of sauce.

Tip: Ground turkey can be a leaner alternative to ground beef as long as you choose 99% lean ground turkey breast. Regular 93% lean ground turkey is made from a mixture of breast and leg meat or all leg meat and doesn't offer significant savings in calories or fat over extra-lean ground beef (ground round).

meeting your **goals**

Each portion provides 0.5 serving vegetables and 0.2 serving whole grains.

NUTRITION • *Per serving*
147 calories, 17 g protein, 14 g carbohydrates, 2 g fiber, 3 g total fat, 0 g saturated fat, 49 mg cholesterol, 165 mg sodium

Brown Rice Paella

Studded with colorful vegetables, seafood, and poultry, this dish is a complete, wholesome meal in one skillet. Be sure to use short- or medium-grain brown rice as it cooks up into the creamy but toothsome consistency characteristic of a great paella. *See photo, page 335.*

1 In a small saucepan, bring the broth and saffron to a simmer. Remove from the heat, cover, and set aside.

2 Heat 2 teaspoons oil in a large nonstick skillet or sauté pan over medium-high heat. Add the sausage and cook, turning once, until browned, 2 to 3 minutes. Transfer to a plate. Add the chicken and cook, turning occasionally, until browned, 3 to 5 minutes. Transfer to the plate with the sausage.

3 Add the remaining 2 teaspoons oil to the skillet along with the onion and bell pepper. Cook, stirring often, until softened and starting to brown, 3 to 4 minutes. Add the garlic and red pepper and cook, stirring, until fragrant, 20 to 30 seconds. Add the tomatoes and bring to a simmer. Cook, stirring and breaking up the tomatoes with a wooden spoon, until most of the liquid has evaporated, 3 to 5 minutes.

4 Add the rice and stir to coat well. Add the broth, sausage, and chicken and bring to a simmer. Reduce the heat to low, cover, and cook for 45 minutes. If the paella seems dry, add a little extra broth or water.

5 Stir in the shrimp, artichokes, and peas. Cover and cook until the rice is tender, the shrimp is pink, and much of the liquid has been absorbed, about 5 minutes. Remove from the heat. Let stand, covered, for 5 minutes. Serve with lemon wedges. One serving is 1 1/2 cups.

Tip: You can find short- or medium-grain rice, such as the brands Nishiki from Japan or Lundberg from California, in large supermarkets and natural foods stores.

meeting your **goals**

> Each portion provides 2.1 servings vegetables, 1.2 servings whole grains, and 6 grams good fat.

Serves 6

PREP 30 minutes

COOK TIME 1 hour to 1 hour 10 minutes

---

3 1/4 cups reduced-sodium chicken broth

1/4 teaspoon saffron threads, crumbled, or 1 teaspoon paprika

4 teaspoons olive oil

4 ounces (2 links) fully cooked andouille-style chicken sausage, cut into 3/8"-thick slices

10 ounces boneless skinless chicken thighs, trimmed and cut into 1 1/2" chunks

1 medium onion, chopped

1 small red or green bell pepper, seeded and diced

2 cloves garlic, minced

1/8 teaspoon crushed red pepper

1 can (14 ounces) diced tomatoes

1 cup short- or medium-grain brown rice (see Tip)

12 ounces medium-large shrimp, peeled

1 can (14 ounces) artichoke hearts, drained, halved or quartered

1 cup frozen green peas, rinsed under cold running water to thaw

Lemon wedges

NUTRITION • *Per serving*
350 calories, 26 g protein, 44 g carbohydrates, 7 g fiber, 9 g total fat, 2 g saturated fat, 83 mg cholesterol, 767 mg sodium

White Bean and Kale Casserole

Serves 6

PREP 35 minutes

COOK/BAKE TIME 35 to 48 minutes

2 slices whole wheat bread, crusts trimmed, torn into pieces

3 teaspoons olive oil

12 ounces kale, stems trimmed, leaves washed and coarsely chopped

8 ounces Italian turkey sausage

1 medium onion, chopped (1 cup)

4 cloves garlic, minced

1/8 teaspoon crushed red pepper

1/2 cup dry white wine

2 cans (15 ounces each) cannellini beans, drained and rinsed

1 can (14 ounces) no-salt-added diced tomatoes

1/2 cup reduced-sodium chicken broth

Freshly ground black pepper to taste

1/2 cup freshly grated Parmesan cheese

Kale, a form of cabbage, is a nutritional superstar, with cancer-fighting powers and an impressive roster of vitamins and minerals. This casserole will convince even reluctant greens eaters just how delicious earthy-tasting kale can be. It partners beautifully with creamy cannellini beans and gets a flavor boost from lean turkey sausage and Parmesan cheese.

1 Preheat the oven to 425°F. Coat a 9 x 13-inch (or similar 3-quart) baking dish with cooking spray.

2 Place the bread in a food processor and process until coarse crumbs form. Transfer to a medium bowl, add 2 teaspoons oil, and stir to coat.

3 Bring 1 inch of water to a boil in a large pot. Add the kale and stir to submerge. Cook, uncovered, until just tender, 4 to 5 minutes. Drain and refresh under cold running water, then press out excess water.

4 Cook the sausage in a large nonstick skillet over medium-high heat, crumbling with a wooden spoon, until browned, 3 to 4 minutes. Transfer to a paper towel–lined plate to drain.

5 Add the remaining 1 teaspoon oil to the skillet. Add the onion and cook over medium-high heat, stirring often, until softened, 2 to 3 minutes. Add the garlic and red pepper and cook, stirring, until fragrant, 20 to 30 seconds. Add the wine, bring to a simmer, and cook for 1 minute. Remove from the heat and add the beans, tomatoes, broth, pepper, kale, and sausage. Stir to mix well. Transfer to the baking dish and sprinkle with the Parmesan, then the bread crumb mixture. (If making ahead, cover and refrigerate for up to 2 days.)

6 Bake the casserole until bubbly and the top is browned, 25 to 35 minutes. One serving is 1 1/3 cups.

meeting your **goals**

Each portion provides 1.4 servings vegetables, 0.3 serving whole grains, and 5 grams good fat.

NUTRITION • *Per serving*
297 calories, 17 g protein, 34 g carbohydrates, 8 g fiber, 9 g total fat, 2 g saturated fat, 28 mg cholesterol, 753 mg sodium

Lean Beef Burgers with Blue Cheese Nuggets

Cheese-stuffed burgers on a healthy diet? You bet. The trick is to stretch the meat with grated vegetables and top your burger with plenty of tomato and greens (here we use spinach or peppery arugula). Hidden inside, a nugget of blue cheese. If you're not a fan, substitute shredded cheddar or mozzarella. *See photo, page 335.*

1 To make the patties: In a large bowl, mix the beef, egg white, zucchini, onion, panko, Worcestershire sauce, mustard, salt, and pepper. Form into 8 patties, 1/4 inch thick. Place about 1 tablespoon cheese on each of 4 patties and place a second patty on top to enclose the cheese. Press to seal in the cheese and form into 1/2-inch-thick patties.

2 To make the garnishes: Place the onion in a medium bowl, cover with ice water, and soak for 10 to 20 minutes. Drain.

3 Preheat the grill to medium-high. Lightly oil the grill grate by rubbing it with a piece of oil-soaked paper towel. Grill the patties until browned and cooked through (an instant-read thermometer inserted in the center should register 160°F), about 5 minutes per side. About 1 minute before the patties are done, place the muffins, cut side down, on the grill until lightly toasted, 30 to 60 seconds. Drain the onion.

5 To assemble the burgers: Divide the spinach and tomato slices among the muffin bottoms. Add the patties and top with the onion slices. Replace the muffin tops. One serving is 1 patty with 1 English muffin and garnishes.

Tip: To make fresh whole wheat bread crumbs, trim the crusts from 2 slices of whole wheat bread. Tear the bread into pieces and process in a food processor until coarse crumbs form. Makes about 2/3 cup.

meeting your **goals**

Each portion provides 2.3 servings vegetables, 2.8 servings whole grains, and 3 grams good fat.

---

meat

Serves 4

PREP 25 minutes

COOK TIME 10 minutes

PATTIES

8 ounces 95% lean ground beef

1 large egg white, lightly beaten

1 cup shredded zucchini (1/2 small)

1/3 cup finely chopped onion (1/2 small)

2/3 cup whole wheat panko (Japanese-style bread crumbs) or fresh whole wheat bread crumbs (see Tip)

1 tablespoon Worcestershire sauce

2 teaspoons Dijon mustard

1/4 teaspoon salt

1/4 teaspoon freshly ground black pepper

1/4 cup crumbled blue cheese

ROLLS AND GARNISHES

1 cup thinly sliced sweet onion or red onion

2 cups baby spinach or arugula, washed and dried

1 medium tomato, sliced

4 100% whole wheat English muffins, split

NUTRITION • *Per serving*
322 calories, 23 g protein, 43 g carbohydrates, 7 g fiber, 7 g total fat, 3 g saturated fat, 41 mg cholesterol, 909 mg sodium

meat

Serves 4

PREP 10 minutes

BAKE TIME 35 to 40 minutes

4 cups cubed (1" pieces) peeled butternut squash (1 pound, 2 ounces)

2 cups (8 ounces) whole shallots or cipollini onions, peeled

1 tablespoon plus 2 teaspoons olive oil

1/2 teaspoon salt

1/2 teaspoon freshly ground black pepper

1 teaspoon ground cumin

1 teaspoon brown sugar

1/2 teaspoon ground coriander

1/4 teaspoon ground red pepper (cayenne)

1 pound pork tenderloin, trimmed

3/4 cup unsweetened pomegranate juice

3/4 cup reduced-sodium chicken broth

1 teaspoon cornstarch

Roasted Pork with Pomegranate Sauce

Lean pork tenderloin is extra-delicious with pomegranate syrup, rich in antioxidants. Anytime you roast meat or poultry, take the opportunity to roast vegetables alongside. *See photo, at right.*

1 Preheat the oven to 425°F. Coat a large roasting pan or a baking sheet with sides with cooking spray.

2 In a medium bowl, combine the squash, shallots, 1 tablespoon oil, 1/4 teaspoon salt, and 1/4 teaspoon pepper and toss to coat. Spread the vegetables in the pan and bake for 15 minutes.

3 Meanwhile, in a small bowl, mix the cumin, brown sugar, coriander, red pepper, and the remaining 1/4 teaspoon salt and 1/4 teaspoon pepper. Pat the pork dry and rub with the spice mixture.

4 Heat the remaining 2 teaspoons oil in a large nonstick skillet over medium-high heat. Add the pork and cook, turning occasionally, until browned on all sides, about 4 minutes.

5 Stir the vegetables and push them to the outside of the pan. Place the pork in the center. Bake, stirring the vegetables occasionally, until the pork is just cooked through (an instant-read thermometer inserted in the center should register 155°F; the temperature will rise to 160°F during resting) and the vegetables are tender, 20 to 25 minutes.

6 Meanwhile, add the pomegranate juice to the skillet and bring to a boil. Boil until reduced to 2/3 cup, about 10 minutes. In a small bowl, mix 3 tablespoons water and the cornstarch, then add to the sauce and cook, stirring, until slightly thickened, about 1 minute.

7 Transfer the vegetables to a bowl and the pork to a cutting board. Let the pork rest for 5 minutes before carving. Cut into 1/2-inch-thick slices and serve with the vegetables and sauce.

meeting your **goals**

Each portion provides 0.3 serving fruit, 1.4 servings vegetables, and 8 grams good fat.

NUTRITION • *Per serving*
316 calories, 27 g protein, 31 g carbohydrates, 4 g fiber, 11 g total fat, 3 g saturated fat, 65 mg cholesterol, 452 mg sodium

Clockwise from top left: Roasted Pork with Pomegranate Sauce; Tuna-Bean Cakes with Arugula Salad; Braised Tofu in Peanut Sauce with Sweet Potatoes and Spinach; Hoisin-Glazed Salmon with Stir-Fried Bok Choy

Serves 2

PREP 15 minutes

COOK TIME 15 to
20 minutes

SALMON AND GLAZE
1 tablespoon hoisin sauce

1 1/2 teaspoons reduced-
sodium soy sauce

1 teaspoon rice vinegar

2 teaspoons grated
fresh ginger

1 small clove garlic,
minced

1/8 teaspoon crushed
red pepper

8 ounces salmon fillet,
cut into 2 portions

BOK CHOY
2 teaspoons sesame seeds

2 teaspoons canola oil or
peanut oil

1 teaspoon grated
fresh ginger

1 small clove garlic,
minced

8 ounces baby bok
choy, rinsed, stem ends
trimmed, halved or
quartered lengthwise,
depending on size

1 teaspoon reduced-
sodium soy sauce

1 teaspoon toasted
sesame oil

Lemon wedges

Hoisin-Glazed Salmon with Stir-Fried Bok Choy

This sophisticated yet easy dinner combines nature's best source of omega-3 fatty acids with bok choy, a fiber-rich, cancer-fighting member of the cabbage family. Hoisin sauce, a sweet and spicy Chinese condiment made from soybeans, makes a terrific base for the full-flavored glaze. *See photo, page 341.*

1 Preheat the oven to 450°F. Line a small baking pan with foil and coat with cooking spray.

2 To make the salmon and glaze: In a small bowl, whisk the hoisin sauce, soy sauce, vinegar, ginger, garlic, and red pepper. Place the salmon skin side down in the baking pan and spoon or brush the sauce over the salmon. Bake until the flesh is opaque and flakes when prodded with the tip of a knife or a fork, 15 to 20 minutes, depending on thickness.

3 To make the bok choy: Toast the sesame seeds in a small dry skillet over medium-low heat, stirring constantly, until golden and fragrant, 1 to 2 minutes. Transfer to a small bowl to cool.

4 Heat the oil in a large nonstick skillet or wok over medium-high heat. Add the ginger and garlic and stir-fry until fragrant, 10 to 20 seconds. Add the bok choy and stir-fry for 1 minute. Add 1/3 cup water, cover, and cook until crisp-tender, 4 to 5 minutes. Add the soy sauce and sesame oil and stir to coat. Divide the bok choy between 2 plates. Place a piece of salmon over each portion. (If the salmon skin sticks to the foil, just lift the fillets.) Sprinkle with sesame seeds and serve with lemon wedges. One serving is 1/2 cup of bok choy and 3 ounces of salmon.

Tip: You can substitute regular bok choy for the baby bok choy. To prepare it, separate the stalks from the leaves and rinse well. Cut the stalks into 3/4-inch pieces and coarsely chop the leaves. In step 4, stir-fry the stalks for 1 minute, then add the water, cover, and cook for 3 minutes. Add the leaves, cover, and cook until the stalks and leaves are crisp-tender, 2 to 3 minutes.

NUTRITION • *Per serving*
300 calories, 22 g protein, 9 g carbohydrates, 2 g fiber, 20 g total fat, 3 g saturated fat, 59 mg cholesterol, 452 mg sodium

meeting your **goals**

Each portion provides 1.6 servings vegetables and 15 grams good fat.

3 Ways to Use Canned Fish

We recommend eating fish at least twice a week. But when you can't get to the store for fresh fish, look to canned. Here are three simple ideas to help you make the most of this pantry staple.

Tuna Tapenade

Serves 4

1 can (6 ounces) tuna, drained

1/4 cup pitted black olives

3 tablespoons fresh lemon juice

2 tablespoons capers, drained and rinsed

1 teaspoon Dijon mustard

1/2 teaspoon anchovy paste

2 tablespoons extra-virgin olive oil

In a food processor, combine the tuna, olives, lemon juice, capers, mustard, and anchovy paste and process until puréed. With the motor running, gradually add the oil through the feeder tube. Transfer to a small bowl. Serve with crudités or use as a spread for whole grain crackers or toast or as sandwich filling. Makes 1 cup.

Greens with Salmon and Lemon Dressing

Serves 2

1/2 cup chopped red onion

2 tablespoons fresh lemon juice

1 small clove garlic, minced

1/8 teaspoon salt

Freshly ground black pepper to taste

1/4 cup extra-virgin olive oil

4 cups mixed salad greens, baby spinach, or arugula

1 cup sliced cucumber

1 can (6 ounces) salmon or tuna, drained and flaked

1/3 cup chopped fresh dill

In a small bowl, soak the onion in ice water for 10 to 15 minutes, then drain. In a large bowl, whisk the lemon juice, garlic, salt, and pepper. Gradually whisk in the oil. Add the greens, cucumber, salmon, dill, and onion and toss to coat.

Potato Salad with Salmon

Serves 4

1 pound baby red potatoes, scrubbed and quartered

1 teaspoon grated lemon zest

3 tablespoons fresh lemon juice

1 medium shallot, minced

1/2 teaspoon salt

Black pepper to taste

1/3 cup canola oil

2 cups sugar snap or snow peas, strings removed

1 can (6 or 7 ounces) salmon, drained and flaked

2 tablespoons chopped chives

Cook the potatoes until tender. In a bowl, whisk the lemon zest, lemon juice, shallot, salt, and pepper. Gradually whisk in the oil. Drain the potatoes and toss with the dressing. Cool. Steam the peas 2 to 4 minutes. Refresh under cold water. Add to the potatoes along with the salmon and chives and toss.

Serves 4

PREP **45 minutes**

COOK/BAKE TIME
25 minutes

TUNA CAKES
2 teaspoons olive oil

1 medium onion, chopped

2 stalks celery, chopped

1 can (15 ounces)
cannellini beans

1 can (6 ounces) water-
packed tuna, drained

2 large egg whites,
lightly beaten

1 1/2 cups whole wheat
panko (Japanese-style
bread crumbs)

2 tablespoons chopped
fresh dill or 1 1/2
teaspoons dried dill

1 tablespoon lemon juice

Salt and pepper to taste

SALAD AND DRESSING
3 tablespoons lemon juice

1 clove garlic, minced

Salt and pepper to taste

3 tablespoons olive oil

6 cups arugula, washed,
dried, and torn

1 cup cherry tomatoes or
grape tomatoes, halved

1 tablespoon reduced-fat
mayonnaise

2 teaspoons capers,
rinsed and chopped

NUTRITION • *Per serving*
381 calories, 22 g protein,
40 g carbohydrates, 8 g fiber,
16 g total fat, 2 g saturated
fat, 18 mg cholesterol,
464 mg sodium

Tuna-Bean Cakes with Arugula Salad

Canned tuna and cannellini beans team up to create delicious fish cakes. This recipe renders a crisp crust without using too much oil. Add a salad, and dinner's done. *See photo, page 341.*

1 To make the tuna cakes: Preheat the oven to 425°F. Coat a large baking sheet with cooking spray.

2 Heat 1 teaspoon oil in a large nonstick skillet over medium-high heat. Add the onion and celery and cook, stirring frequently, until softened, 3 to 5 minutes.

3 In a large bowl, mash the beans. Add the tuna, 1 egg white, 1/2 cup panko, the dill, lemon juice, salt, pepper, and the onion mixture. Mix.

4 Place the remaining 1 cup panko in a shallow dish and the remaining egg white in another shallow dish. Using a generous 1/4 cup per cake, form the bean mixture into 8 cakes, 3/4 inch thick. Coat each cake with egg white, then dredge in panko.

5 Heat 1 teaspoon oil in a large nonstick skillet over medium-high heat. Add the tuna cakes and cook until the undersides are browned, 2 to 3 minutes. Flip the cakes over onto the baking sheet and bake until browned and hot in the center, about 20 minutes.

6 To make the salad and dressing: In a small bowl, whisk the lemon juice, garlic, salt, and pepper. Gradually whisk in the oil. In a large bowl, toss the arugula and cherry tomatoes with 3 tablespoons of the dressing. Whisk the mayonnaise into the remaining dressing and stir in the capers.

7 Divide the salad among 4 plates. Top each serving with 2 cakes and spoon some dressing over each cake. One serving is 1 1/2 cups of salad and 2 tuna-bean cakes.

meeting your **goals**

Each portion provides 2.8 servings vegetables, 0.6 serving whole grains, and 12 grams good fat.

Quinoa-Stuffed Peppers

Colorful sweet bell peppers are perfect vessels for whole grain stuffing. This recipe features high-protein quinoa enlivened with the flavors of a Greek salad. Serve as a vegetarian entrée or a special side dish for chicken or pork. *See photo, page 347.*

1 Preheat the oven to 450°F. Coat a large baking sheet with cooking spray.

2 Place the pepper halves cut side down on the baking sheet and bake just until tender, 12 to 15 minutes. When cool enough to handle, discard the stems from 2 of the pepper halves and coarsely chop the peppers. Set aside. Reduce the oven temperature to 350°F.

3 Meanwhile, in a medium saucepan, combine the quinoa, 1 1/2 cups water, and salt. Bring to a simmer, cover, and cook over low heat until the quinoa is tender and most of the liquid has been absorbed, 12 to 15 minutes. Let stand for 5 minutes. Fluff with a fork.

4 Heat the oil in a large nonstick skillet over medium-high heat. Add the onion and cook, stirring frequently, until softened, 3 to 4 minutes. Add the garlic and oregano and cook, stirring, until fragrant, 20 to 30 seconds. Stir in the tomato and cook for 3 minutes. Remove from the heat. Stir in the quinoa, reserved chopped bell peppers, cheese, olives, parsley, and pepper and mix well.

5 Using about 2/3 cup per pepper shell, divide the quinoa mixture among the remaining 8 pepper halves. Place in a 9 x 13-inch baking dish. (If making ahead, cover and refrigerate for up to 2 days.)

6 Add 2 tablespoons water to the baking dish and cover with foil. Bake until the filling is heated through, 30 to 40 minutes. One main-dish serving is 2 filled pepper halves; one side dish serving is 1 filled pepper half.

meeting your **goals**

> Each main-dish portion provides 3.8 servings vegetables, 1.1 servings whole grains, and 8 grams good fat.

Serves 4 as a main dish or 8 as a side dish

PREP 40 minutes

COOK/BAKE TIME 1 hour

5 large red, yellow, and/ or orange bell peppers, halved lengthwise (leave stems intact) and seeded

3/4 cup quinoa, rinsed well

1/2 teaspoon salt, or to taste

2 teaspoons olive oil or canola oil

1 cup chopped red onion

3 cloves garlic, minced

1 teaspoon dried oregano

1 medium tomato, seeded and diced

1 cup crumbled feta cheese

1/3 cup pitted black olives, chopped

1/3 cup chopped fresh parsley

Freshly ground black pepper to taste

NUTRITION • *Per main-dish serving* 358 calories, 13 g protein, 44 g carbohydrates, 8 g fiber, 16 g total fat, 7 g saturated fat, 33 mg cholesterol, 929 mg sodium

NUTRITION • *Per side-dish serving* 179 calories, 6 g protein, 22 g carbohydrates, 4 g fiber, 8 g total fat, 3 g saturated fat, 17 mg cholesterol, 465 mg sodium

Serves 3

PREP 20 minutes

COOK TIME 10 to
14 minutes

1/3 cup walnuts, coarsely
chopped

1/4 cup lightly packed
fresh parsley leaves,
washed and dried

1 clove garlic, crushed
and peeled

1/2 teaspoon salt, or to
taste

Freshly ground
black pepper to taste

2 tablespoons extra-virgin
olive oil

3 tablespoons freshly
grated Parmesan cheese

1 1/2 cups (6 ounces)
whole wheat penne or
rigatoni pasta

2 cups (8 ounces)
green beans, stem
ends trimmed, halved
crosswise

Penne with Parsley-Walnut Pesto and Green Beans

Two time-honored pairings—green beans and walnuts and pasta and pesto—come together in this simple dish. Trading walnuts for the traditional pine nuts in a pesto sauce is an easy way to boost omega-3's. Green beans up the vegetable quotient. *See photo, at right.*

1 Bring a large pot of lightly salted water to a boil.

2 Toast the walnuts in a small dry skillet over medium-low heat, stirring constantly, until fragrant, 2 to 3 minutes. Transfer to a plate and let cool.

3 In a food processor, combine the parsley, garlic, salt, pepper, and 1/4 cup walnuts. Process until the walnuts are ground. With the motor running, gradually add the oil through the feeder tube. Add the cheese and pulse until mixed in.

4 Add the penne to the boiling water and cook for 3 minutes. Add the beans and cook until the penne is al dente (almost tender) and the beans are crisp-tender, 5 to 8 minutes. Reserve 1/2 cup of the cooking water, then drain the penne and beans and place in a large bowl. Add the pesto and reserved cooking water and toss to coat well. Sprinkle with the remaining toasted walnuts. One serving is 1 1/3 cups.

meeting your **goals**

Each portion provides 1 serving vegetables, 1.7 servings whole grains, and 9 grams good fat.

NUTRITION • *Per serving*
339 calories, 10 g protein,
48 g carbohydrates, 7 g fiber,
13 g total fat, 2 g saturated
fat, 4 mg cholesterol,
478 mg sodium

Clockwise from top left: Quinoa-Stuffed Peppers; Roasted Green Beans and Grape Tomatoes; Penne with Parsley-Walnut Pesto and Green Beans; No-Bake Whole Grain Breakfast/Snack Bars

Serves 9

PREP 1 hour 20 minutes
BAKE TIME 50 minutes

12 whole wheat lasagna
noodles (9 ounces)

1 pound Swiss chard

6 teaspoons olive oil

1 pound assorted
mushrooms, such as
cremini (baby bella),
shiitake (discard
stems) and/or oyster
mushrooms, wiped clean
and quartered (5 cups)

3 cloves garlic, minced

1/2 teaspoon dried
oregano

1/4 teaspoon crushed
red pepper

1/4 teaspoon salt

Freshly ground
black pepper to taste

1 large egg

15 ounces part-skim
ricotta cheese (2 cups)

2/3 cup freshly grated
Parmesan cheese

3 cups (24 ounces)
prepared marinara sauce

2 cups grated part-skim
mozzarella cheese

Whole Wheat Lasagna with Mushrooms and Swiss Chard

To give crowd-pleasing lasagna a healthy update, we've used whole wheat noodles and layers of vegetables rather than fatty meats. While preparing this dish requires a certain time commitment, you can't beat it for make-ahead convenience. To save time, you can substitute 16 ounces frozen spinach, cooked according to package directions, for the chard.

1 Bring a large pot of lightly salted water to a boil. Drop in the noodles and cook just until tender, 7 to 8 minutes. Using tongs or a slotted spoon, transfer to a large bowl of cold water to stop the cooking. Lay the noodles on a baking sheet, cover, and set aside.

2 Meanwhile, bring about 1 inch of lightly salted water to a boil in a large pot. Separate the stems from the Swiss chard leaves (see Tip). Wash the stems and leaves thoroughly. Cut the stems into 1/2-inch lengths and the leaves into 1-inch pieces. Add the stems to the boiling water, cover, and cook for 3 minutes. Add the leaves to the pot, cover, and cook until wilted and tender, 3 to 4 minutes. Drain, refresh under cold running water, and press out excess water.

3 Heat 2 teaspoons oil in a large nonstick skillet over medium-high heat. Add half of the mushrooms and cook, turning occasionally, until browned and tender, 4 to 6 minutes. Transfer to a large bowl. Add another 2 teaspoons oil to the skillet, sauté the remaining mushrooms, and transfer to the bowl.

meeting your **goals**

Each portion provides 3.3 servings vegetables, 1.1 servings whole grains, and 8 grams good fat.

NUTRITION • *Per serving*
374 calories, 23 g protein,
34 g carbohydrates, 7 g fiber,
17 g total fat, 7 g saturated
fat, 57 mg cholesterol,
774 mg sodium

4 Add the remaining 2 teaspoons oil to the skillet. Add the garlic, oregano, and red pepper and stir until fragrant, 5 to 10 seconds. Add the chard and turn to coat. Transfer to the bowl with the mushrooms. Season with 1/8 teaspoon salt and pepper and toss to mix.

5 In a medium bowl, whisk the egg, ricotta, 1/3 cup Parmesan, the remaining 1/8 teaspoon salt, and pepper.

6 To assemble the lasagna: Preheat the oven to 400°F. Coat a 9 x 13-inch baking dish with cooking spray. Spread about 1/2 cup marinara sauce in the baking dish and arrange 3 noodles over the sauce. Spread about 2/3 cup ricotta mixture over the noodles and scatter about 1 1/3 cups vegetables on the ricotta. Spoon another 1/2 cup sauce over the vegetables and sprinkle with 1/2 cup mozzarella. Add another layer of noodles and repeat the layering with the ricotta, vegetables, sauce, mozzarella, and noodles 2 more times. Spread the remaining sauce evenly over the final layer of noodles. (Reserve the remaining Parmesan and mozzarella.) Cover with a sheet of parchment paper and then foil. (If making ahead, cover and refrigerate for up to 2 days.)

7 Bake, covered, for 35 minutes. Sprinkle with the remaining 1/3 cup Parmesan and 1/2 cup mozzarella. Bake, uncovered, until the noodles are tender and the lasagna is bubbly, about 15 minutes. Let stand for at least 5 minutes before serving. One serving is 1 rectangle, 4 1/2 x 3 inches.

Tip: To prepare Swiss chard, fold each leaf in half lengthwise. Place a chef's knife at a slight angle to the stem and cut off the stem, including the thicker portion in the leaf area. Wash the stems and greens in several changes of water. Trim the ragged ends of the stems, then cut the stems as desired. Stack several leaves, then roll. Using a chef's knife, cut the leaves into ribbons, then turn the ribbons and cut again.

Serves 10

PREP 20 minutes

COOK TIME 40 to
50 minutes

4 tablespoons extra-virgin
olive oil

2 medium onions,
chopped (2 cups)

1 cup diced carrots
(3–4 medium)

6 cloves garlic, minced

1 1/4 cups brown lentils,
rinsed and picked over

1 teaspoon dried thyme

6 cups reduced-sodium
chicken broth or
vegetable broth

1 bay leaf

1 1/4 cups whole wheat
orzo

1 can (14 ounces) diced
tomatoes

8 cups (6 ounces) baby
spinach, washed and
dried

2 tablespoons fresh
lemon juice

1/2 teaspoon salt,
or to taste

Freshly ground
black pepper to taste

Lentil and Whole Wheat Orzo Ragout with Spinach

This warm, hearty ragout features cholesterol-lowering lentils and nearly two servings of vegetables per portion. A drizzle of olive oil gives the simple, comforting dish a delicious finish; this is a time to splurge on good-quality olive oil.

1 Heat 1 tablespoon oil in a large Dutch oven over medium heat. Add the onions and carrots and cook, stirring frequently, until softened, 4 to 6 minutes. Add the garlic and cook, stirring, for 30 seconds. Add the lentils and thyme and stir to coat. Add the broth and bay leaf and bring to a simmer. Reduce the heat to low, cover, and simmer for 20 minutes.

2 Add the orzo and simmer, covered, stirring occasionally, until the orzo and lentils are almost tender, 10 to 15 minutes.

3 Add the tomatoes and simmer, covered, until the lentils and orzo are tender and the mixture has thickened, 5 to 10 minutes. Discard the bay leaf. Add the spinach and cook, stirring, just until wilted, about 1 minute. Stir in the lemon juice and season with the salt and pepper. The ragout will keep, covered, in the refrigerator for up to 2 days. Top each serving with a drizzle of the remaining oil. One serving is 1 cup.

meeting your **goals**

Each portion provides
1.8 servings vegetables,
0.3 serving whole grains,
and 5 grams good fat.

NUTRITION • *Per serving*
241 calories, 12 g protein,
36 g carbohydrates, 10 g fiber,
6 g total fat, 1 g saturated
fat, 0 mg cholesterol,
540 mg sodium

Quick-and-Easy Mac 'n Cheese with Veggies

This homey pasta dish is almost as easy as packaged macaroni and cheese, but it's far better for you! A generous quantity of vegetables cooks seamlessly alongside the whole wheat pasta. The calcium-rich sauce is made right in the pasta pot, making this a one-pot meal. Just add a salad.

1 Bring a large pot of lightly salted water to a boil.

2 In a small skillet, combine the panko and oil. Cook over medium-low heat, stirring constantly, until golden and crisp, 2 to 3 minutes. Transfer to a small bowl and let cool.

3 In a small bowl, combine the cornstarch, mustard, and cayenne.

4 Add the cauliflower and macaroni to the boiling water and cook just until tender, about 7 minutes (the macaroni will continue to cook while you make the sauce). Add the spinach and stir to submerge, then drain immediately.

5 Return the macaroni and vegetables to the pot. Add the cornstarch mixture and stir to coat. Stir in the milk. Cook over medium-high heat, stirring, until the milk starts to bubble and thicken, 2 to 3 minutes. Remove from the heat, add the cheese, and stir until melted and smooth. Season with the salt and pepper. Sprinkle each serving with 1 tablespoon toasted bread crumbs. One serving is 1 cup.

Serves 5

PREP **15 minutes**

COOK TIME **10 minutes**

1/4 cup whole wheat panko (Japanese-style bread crumbs) or fresh whole wheat bread crumbs (see Tip, page 339)

1 teaspoon olive oil

2 tablespoons cornstarch

1 1/4 teaspoons mustard powder

1/8 teaspoon ground red pepper (cayenne)

3 cups (9 ounces) cauliflower florets (1" pieces)

2 cups (8 ounces) whole wheat macaroni

6 cups baby spinach (5 ounces), washed and dried

1 1/2 cups 1% milk

1 1/2 cups (4 ounces) shredded sharp cheddar cheese

1/4 teaspoon salt, or to taste

Freshly ground black pepper to taste

meeting your **goals**

Each portion provides 2.1 servings vegetables, 1.7 servings whole grains, and 2 grams good fat.

NUTRITION • *Per serving*
367 calories, 18 g protein, 46 g carbohydrates, 6 g fiber, 14 g total fat, 8 g saturated fat, 34 mg cholesterol, 429 mg sodium

Serves 10

PREP 30 minutes

COOK TIME 45 to
50 minutes

---

1 1/2 cups brown rice

Pinch of salt

1 tablespoon canola oil

1 medium onion, chopped

3 cloves garlic, minced

2 jalapeño or serrano
peppers, seeded and
minced (2–3 tablespoons)

1 tablespoon curry powder

2 packages (14 ounces
each) firm tofu, drained,
patted dry, and cut into
1" cubes

2 1/2 cups vegetable
broth or reduced-sodium
chicken broth

1 can (14 ounces) diced
tomatoes

1 medium sweet potato,
peeled and cut into
1/2" pieces

1/2 cup natural
peanut butter

12 cups baby spinach,
washed and dried

2 tablespoons lime juice

2/3 cup unsalted roasted
peanuts, coarsely
chopped

Hot pepper sauce

Lime wedges

NUTRITION • *Per serving*
356 calories, 16 g protein,
38 g carbohydrates, 6 g fiber,
17 g total fat, 3 g saturated
fat, 0 mg cholesterol,
310 mg sodium

Braised Tofu in Peanut Sauce with Sweet Potatoes and Spinach

If you're looking for ways to turn yourself and your family on to tofu, this recipe is just the ticket. Peanut butter lends delicious richness to the sauce, while vivid orange sweet potato and green spinach add color and powerful nutrients. *See photo, page 341.*

1 In a Dutch oven, combine the rice, 3 3/4 cups water, and salt. Bring to a simmer, then reduce the heat to low, cover, and simmer until the rice is tender and most of the liquid has been absorbed, 45 to 50 minutes.

2 Meanwhile, heat the oil in a large Dutch oven over medium-high heat. Add the onion and cook, stirring often, until softened, 2 to 3 minutes. Add garlic, jalapeños, and curry powder and cook, stirring, until fragrant, about 20 seconds. Add the tofu and stir to coat. Add the broth, tomatoes, and sweet potato. Bring to a simmer, then reduce the heat to low, cover, and simmer until the sweet potato is tender, 20 to 25 minutes.

3 Add the peanut butter and stir until blended. Gradually add the spinach, stirring until it has wilted. Stir in the lime juice. Spoon the stew over the rice and sprinkle each serving with about 1 tablespoon peanuts. Serve with lime wedges and hot pepper sauce. The stew will keep, covered, in the refrigerator for up to 2 days. One serving is 1/2 cup of rice and 1 cup of stew.

meeting your **goals**

**Each portion provides
2 servings vegetables,
1.1 servings whole grains,
and 13 grams good fat.**

Napa Cabbage Slaw with Peanut Dressing

With its delicate flavor and crisp texture, napa cabbage (also known as Chinese cabbage) makes an appealing alternative to traditional green cabbage in a slaw. Instead of a saturated fat–laden mayonnaise dressing, this slaw is dressed with a spicy peanut dressing rich in good fat.

1 Place the peanut butter in a large bowl and gradually whisk in the hot tea. Add the soy sauce, vinegar, brown sugar, hot sauce, and garlic and whisk until smooth.

2 Add the cabbage, carrots, and scallions and toss to coat well. Sprinkle with the peanuts. One serving is 2/3 cup.

Tip: This slaw gets watery as it sits, so it's best to toss it with the dressing shortly before serving. However, you can prepare the vegetables and dressing up to 1 day ahead and store them in separate covered containers in the refrigerator.

sides

Serves 6

PREP 20 minutes

1/3 cup natural peanut butter

1/4 cup hot brewed black or green tea

4 teaspoons reduced-sodium soy sauce

4 teaspoons rice vinegar

1 1/2 teaspoons brown sugar

1 teaspoon hot sauce, such as Sriracha, chile-garlic sauce, or Tabasco

1 clove garlic, minced

4 cups thinly sliced napa cabbage

1 cup shredded carrots

1/2 cup chopped scallions

1/3 cup unsalted roasted peanuts

meeting your **goals**

Each portion provides
1.8 servings vegetables and
9 grams good fat.

NUTRITION • *Per serving*
158 calories, 7 g protein,
11 g carbohydrates, 3 g fiber,
11 g total fat, 2 g saturated
fat, 0 mg cholesterol, 226
mg sodium

Serves 4

PREP 20 minutes

BAKE TIME 20 to
25 minutes

**4 cups (12 ounces)
green beans, stem ends
trimmed**

2 teaspoons fennel seed

1 clove garlic, minced

4 teaspoons olive oil

1/2 teaspoon salt

**Freshly ground
black pepper to taste**

**1 pint grape tomatoes or
cherry tomatoes**

Roasted Green Beans and Grape Tomatoes

Roasting vegetables in a hot oven is an excellent way to bring out their inherent sweetness. Green beans are delicious when roasted, but to become tender, they must be blanched before roasting. The tomatoes roasted alongside form a light but flavorful sauce for the garlicky beans. *See photo, page 347.*

1 Bring a large saucepan of lightly salted water to a boil. Preheat the oven to 450°F. Coat a large rimmed baking sheet with cooking spray.

2 Cook the beans in the boiling water until crisp-tender, 3 to 4 minutes. Drain and refresh under cold running water.

3 Place the fennel seeds on a cutting board and crush with the bottom of a saucepan to bring out their fragrance. Transfer to a medium bowl. Add the garlic, 2 teaspoons oil, 1/4 teaspoon salt, and beans and toss to coat. Spread the beans on one end of the baking sheet. In the same bowl, combine the tomatoes, the remaining 2 teaspoons oil and 1/4 teaspoon salt, and pepper. Toss to coat. Spread on the other end of the baking sheet.

4 Bake the vegetables until the beans are tender and browned in spots and the tomatoes start to collapse, 20 to 25 minutes. Toss the beans and tomatoes together. One serving is 3/4 cup.

meeting your **goals**

Each portion provides
1.9 servings vegetables and
5 grams good fat.

NUTRITION • *Per serving*
81 calories, 2 g protein,
9 g carbohydrates, 4 g fiber,
5 g total fat, 1 g saturated
fat, 0 mg cholesterol,
300 mg sodium

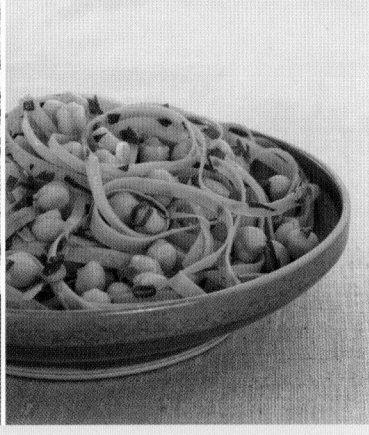

3 Great Ways to Eat Carrots

Sturdy carrots are great keepers, so stock up. They're a superb source of beta-carotene, a proven cancer fighter that also guards against diseases like macular degeneration, cataracts, and even arthritis. These simple recipes demonstrate how delicious and versatile the common carrot can be.

Carrot-Ginger Soup

Serves 5

4 cups reduced-sodium chicken broth

3 cups peeled baby carrots

1 cup chopped onion

2 tablespoons grated fresh ginger

1 clove garlic, minced

1/4 teaspoon curry powder

1/3 cup orange juice

In a large saucepan over medium-low heat, simmer the broth, carrots, onion, ginger, garlic, and curry powder until very tender, 25 to 35 minutes. Working in 2 batches, puree the soup in a blender. Return to the pan and stir in the orange juice.

Lemony Roasted Carrots

Serves 2

3 cups carrot sticks

2 teaspoons olive oil

1/4 teaspoon salt

Freshly ground black pepper to taste

1 tablespoon chopped fresh parsley

1 teaspoon grated lemon zest

1 tablespoon fresh lemon juice

Preheat the oven to 450°F. Lightly oil a rimmed baking sheet. In a medium bowl, toss the carrots with the oil, salt, and pepper. Spread on the baking sheet and bake, stirring once or twice, until tender and lightly browned, about 20 minutes. Toss with the parsley, lemon zest, and lemon juice.

Carrot and Chickpea Salad

Serves 4

3 tablespoons olive oil

2 tablespoons fresh lemon juice

1 small clove garlic, minced

1 teaspoon ground cumin

1/4 teaspoon salt

Freshly ground black pepper to taste

2 cups shredded carrots

1 can (7 ounces) chickpeas, drained and rinsed

2 tablespoons chopped fresh parsley

2 tablespoons chopped scallions

In a medium bowl, whisk the oil, lemon juice, garlic, cumin, salt, and pepper. Add the carrots, chickpeas, parsley, and scallions and toss to coat.

Serves 24

PREP 25 minutes

COOK TIME 5 to
10 minutes

1 cup old-fashioned
rolled oats

1/4 cup whole flaxseed

1 cup whole grain puffed
rice, puffed wheat, or
toasted oat cereal

1 cup dried blueberries or
cranberries

1/2 cup unsalted roasted
peanuts

1/2 cup almonds, coarsely
chopped

1/2 cup nonfat dry milk

1/4 teaspoon salt

3/4 cup natural peanut
butter, almond butter, or
cashew butter

2/3 cup honey

1 teaspoon vanilla extract

No-Bake Whole Grain Breakfast/Snack Bars

Keep these bars on hand for days when you don't have time for a sit-down breakfast. They're also perfect as energy-boosting snacks, and they're infinitely more healthful than bars you'll find in the supermarket. With this easy homemade version, you're guaranteed to get whole grains, fruit, and good fats—and no hydrogenated oils. *See photo, page 347.*

1 Line a 7 x 11-inch or 9 x 9-inch baking dish with foil, leaving a 1-inch overhang on each long side. Coat with cooking spray.

2 Toast the oats in a medium skillet over medium-low heat, stirring constantly, until aromatic and golden, 3 to 4 minutes. Transfer to a large bowl. Toast the flaxseed in the skillet over medium-low heat until aromatic and starting to pop, 2 to 3 minutes. Transfer to a small bowl and let cool. Grind the flaxseed into a coarse meal in a spice grinder (such as a clean coffee grinder) or blender. Add to the oats. Add the cereal, blueberries, peanuts, almonds, dry milk, and salt and stir to mix.

3 In a small saucepan, combine the peanut butter and honey. Cook, stirring, over low heat until blended and smooth. Stir in the vanilla. Add to the oat mixture, mix well, and transfer to the baking dish. Use a piece of plastic wrap to press the mixture firmly into an even layer. Cover with plastic wrap and refrigerate until firm, about 30 minutes. Using the foil overhang, lift the bars and transfer to a cutting board. Cut into 24 bars. Store the bars, covered or individually wrapped, in the refrigerator for up to 2 weeks. One serving is 1 rectangle, 1 3/4 x 2 inches.

Tip: Toasting rolled oats brings out their nutty flavor. Make extra and have some on hand to sprinkle over fruit and yogurt. Store in a zipper-seal bag for up to 2 weeks. If you prefer, toast the oats in a small baking dish in a 350°F oven for 10 to 15 minutes.

meeting your **goals**

Each portion provides 0.3 serving fruit, 0.2 serving whole grains, and 6 grams good fat.

NUTRITION • *Per serving*
171 calories, 5 g protein,
20 g carbohydrates, 3 g fiber,
8 g total fat, 1 g saturated
fat, 1 mg cholesterol,
78 mg sodium

Oatmeal–Whole Wheat Scones with Apples and Dried Cranberries

The monster scones you find in coffee shops are often loaded with butter or shortening and refined carbohydrates. These are appropriately sized and are made with 100 percent whole grains, fruit, and good fats like canola oil and nuts. Serve with a dollop of honey or no-sugar-added fruit spread.

1 Preheat the oven to 400°F. Line a large baking sheet with parchment paper or a nonstick baking mat, or coat with cooking spray.

2 In a large bowl, whisk the flour, 1/4 cup sugar, cinnamon, baking soda, baking powder, and salt. In a measuring cup, mix the yogurt, apple juice, and egg with a fork until blended.

3 Add the cream cheese to the flour mixture and blend with a pastry blender or your fingers until it forms small balls the size of peas. Add the oil and toss with a fork to coat. Stir in the apple, cranberries, and oats. Add the yogurt mixture to the flour mixture and stir with a fork until a soft dough forms. Using a 4-ounce scoop or 1/2-cup measure, drop the dough onto the baking sheet, leaving 2 inches between scoops. Sprinkle with nuts, pressing lightly so they adhere, then sprinkle with the remaining 1 teaspoon sugar.

4 Bake until lightly browned and firm to the touch, 20 to 25 minutes. Transfer to a rack to cool slightly before serving. One serving is 1 scone.

Tip: White whole wheat flour is a special variety of hard wheat. Although it has a lighter color and sweeter flavor than regular whole wheat flour, it has all the benefits of whole grain flour because it is milled from the entire wheat berry.

meeting your **goals**

Each portion provides 1.2 servings fruit, 1.2 servings whole grains, and 5 grams good fat.

---

baked goods

Serves 10

PREP **20 minutes**

BAKE TIME **20 to 25 minutes**

1 1/2 cups white whole wheat flour (see Tip) or whole wheat pastry flour

1/4 cup plus 1 teaspoon sugar

1 teaspoon ground cinnamon

1/2 teaspoon baking soda

1/4 teaspoon baking powder

1/4 teaspoon salt

1/3 cup low-fat plain yogurt

1/3 cup unsweetened apple juice or apple cider

1 large egg, lightly beaten

2 ounces (1/4 cup) reduced-fat cream cheese (Neufchâtel), cut into pieces

2 tablespoons canola oil

1 cup diced peeled firm cooking apple, such as Cortland, Granny Smith, Northern Spy, or Jonagold

3/4 cup dried cranberries

1/2 cup old-fashioned rolled oats

1/3 cup chopped walnuts or pecans

NUTRITION • *Per serving*
225 calories, 6 g protein, 35 g carbohydrates, 4 g fiber, 8 g total fat, 1 g saturated fat, 25 mg cholesterol, 165 mg sodium

Serves 12

PREP 25 minutes

BAKE TIME 20 to
25 minutes

1/2 cup walnuts or
pecans, chopped

1/3 cup unsweetened
"natural" cocoa powder
(not Dutch-process)

1 1/2 cups white whole
wheat flour or whole
wheat pastry flour

1 teaspoon baking soda

1/4 teaspoon salt

1 large egg

1/2 cup granulated sugar

3/4 cup low-fat
buttermilk

3/4 cup mashed banana
(2–3 very ripe bananas)

1/3 cup canola oil

2 teaspoons vanilla
extract

1/2 cup bittersweet
(60% cacao) chocolate
chips

Nutty Whole Wheat Banana-Chocolate Muffins

Treat yourself and your family to this winning combination of banana and chocolate! The cocoa and bittersweet chocolate chips contribute a delicious flavor as well as antioxidant health benefits. These whole grain muffins are exceptionally tender and moist, thanks to the canola oil and mashed banana. *See photo, at right.*

1 Preheat the oven to 400°F. Coat 12 standard-size (2 1/2 x 1 1/4-inch) muffin cups with cooking spray.

2 Spread 1/4 cup walnuts in a small baking pan. Toast in the oven until fragrant, 6 to 8 minutes. Let cool.

3 Sift the cocoa into a large bowl and add the flour, baking soda, and salt. Whisk to blend. In a medium bowl, whisk the egg, sugar, buttermilk, banana, oil, and vanilla. Add to the flour mixture and mix with a rubber spatula just until the dry ingredients are moistened. Stir in the chocolate chips and toasted walnuts. Scoop the batter into the muffin cups and sprinkle with the remaining 1/4 cup walnuts.

4 Bake until the muffins are lightly browned and the tops spring back when touched lightly, 20 to 25 minutes. Let cool in the pan on a rack for 5 minutes. Loosen the edges of the muffins and turn out onto a wire rack to cool. One serving is 1 muffin.

Tip: Use "natural" cocoa such as Ghirardelli or Hershey's in this recipe. Dutch-process cocoa is treated with alkali. When mixed with another alkaline element like baking soda, the Dutch-process cocoa may develop a soapy taste.

meeting your **goals**

Each portion provides 0.1 serving fruit, 0.8 serving whole grains, and 9 grams good fat.

NUTRITION • *Per serving*
249 calories, 5 g protein, 31 g carbohydrates, 3 g fiber, 12 g total fat, 2 g saturated fat, 18 mg cholesterol, 177 mg sodium

Clockwise from top left: Oatmeal-Apricot Chocolate Chip Cookies; Dark Chocolate Celebration Cake with Raspberries; Old-Fashioned Fruit Cobbler; Nutty Whole Wheat Banana-Chocolate Muffins

Serves 6

PREP 10 minutes

COOK TIME 25 minutes
(including soaking time)

1/3 cup fine or medium
bulgur, rinsed

1/4 teaspoon ground
cardamom

1 1/4 cups 1% milk

2/3 cup seedless golden
raisins or seedless dark
raisins

1/4 cup granulated sugar

1 large egg

2 teaspoons freshly
grated lemon zest

1/2 teaspoon vanilla
extract

1/3 cup chopped peeled
pistachios or slivered
almonds

Bulgur Pudding with Golden Raisins and Pistachios

Creamy and comforting, this Middle Eastern–inspired pudding
is simply a whole grain version of rice pudding. It has a delicate
perfume of cardamom, an accent of fresh lemon zest, and a
crowning touch of pistachios. It's an easy, delicious—and healthy—
dessert.

1 In a medium saucepan, combine the bulgur, cardamom, and 2 cups
water. Bring to a simmer over medium-high heat. Immediately
remove from the heat, cover, and let stand until the bulgur is tender,
about 20 minutes. Drain and press out excess water. Return the bulgur
to the pan.

2 Add the milk, raisins, and sugar and bring to a simmer, stirring
often, over medium-high heat. Reduce the heat to medium-low and
cook, stirring, for 2 minutes.

3 Whisk the egg in a medium bowl. Gradually stir in the bulgur
mixture. Return to the pan and cook, stirring, over medium-low
heat, until slightly thickened, 1 to 2 minutes. (Do not boil. You can use
an instant-read thermometer to gauge readiness; the pudding should
reach a temperature of 160°F.) Transfer to a clean bowl and stir in
the lemon zest and vanilla. Let cool slightly, then cover and refrigerate
until chilled. Sprinkle each serving with a scant 1 tablespoon pistachios.
The pudding will keep, covered, in the refrigerator for up to 2 days.
One serving is 1/3 cup.

meeting your **goals**

**Each portion provides
0.9 serving fruit, 0.3 serving
whole grains, and 3 grams
good fat.**

NUTRITION • *Per serving*
195 calories, 6 g protein,
33 g carbohydrates, 3 g fiber,
5 g total fat, 1 g saturated
fat, 37 mg cholesterol,
76 mg sodium

Old-Fashioned Fruit Cobbler

A cobbler with a tender biscuit topping is a nice way to showcase the fruits of the season. We've replaced the butter in the topping with a mixture of low-fat cream cheese and canola oil. Flaxseed adds a nutty flavor and boosts fiber and good fat. *See photo, page 359.*

1 Preheat the oven to 400°F. Coat an 8 x 8-inch baking dish with cooking spray.

2 To make the filling: In a large bowl, combine the rhubarb, strawberries, sugar, cornstarch, and orange zest and toss to mix. Spread in the baking dish.

3 To make the topping: Grind the flaxseed into a coarse meal in a spice grinder or blender. Transfer to a large bowl. Add the flour, 1/4 cup sugar, baking soda, baking powder, and salt and whisk to blend. Add the cream cheese and blend with a pastry blender or your fingers, until the mixture resembles coarse crumbs. Add the oil and toss with a fork. Gradually add the buttermilk, stirring with a fork until the dough clumps. Transfer to a lightly floured surface and knead several times. Pat into a 1/2-inch-thick square and cut into 9 pieces. Arrange the pieces over the fruit, leaving a little space between them. Sprinkle with the almonds and remaining 1 teaspoon sugar.

4 Bake until the fruit is bubbly and the biscuit is golden and firm, 35 to 40 minutes. Let cool slightly. Serve warm.

Tip: If you don't have buttermilk, substitute 1/4 cup 1% milk plus 1 teaspoon lemon juice.

meeting your **goals**

> Each portion provides 1.2 to 1.6 servings fruit, 0.25 serving whole grains, and 7 grams good fat.

Serves 8

PREP 30 minutes

BAKE TIME 35 to 40 minutes

FILLING
3 cups chopped (1/2" pieces) rhubarb

2 cups halved strawberries

1/4 cup granulated sugar

3 tablespoons cornstarch

1 1/2 teaspoons grated orange zest

TOPPING
1/4 cup whole flaxseed

1/3 cup whole wheat flour

1/3 cup all-purpose flour

1/4 cup plus 1 teaspoon sugar

1 teaspoon baking soda

1/2 teaspoon baking powder

Pinch of salt

2 ounces (1/4 cup) reduced-fat cream cheese

2 tablespoons canola oil

1/4 cup low-fat buttermilk

3 tablespoons sliced almonds

NUTRITION • *Per serving*
213 calories, 4 g protein, 31 g carbohydrates, 4 g fiber, 9 g total fat, 1 g saturated fat, 4 mg cholesterol, 258 mg sodium

Oatmeal-Apricot Chocolate Chip Cookies

Makes 4 1/2 dozen

PREP 25 minutes

BAKE TIME 14 to 16 minutes (4 to 5 batches)

1 cup dried apricots, coarsely chopped

3 tablespoons orange juice

1/2 cup almonds, coarsely chopped

1 cup white whole wheat flour or whole wheat pastry flour

1/2 teaspoon baking soda

1/4 teaspoon salt

1 cup drained canned cannellini beans, rinsed

1 large egg

2 large egg whites

2/3 cup packed light brown sugar

2/3 cup granulated sugar

1/2 cup canola oil or light olive oil

2 teaspoons vanilla extract

2 cups old-fashioned rolled oats

1 cup bittersweet (60% cacao) chocolate chips

1/4 cup crystallized ginger, finely chopped

Everyone loves a good oatmeal cookie. There's a secret ingredient in these: canned beans! They do a superb job of standing in for butter, and no one will notice the difference. Dried apricots contrast beautifully with dark chocolate, while toasted nuts add good fat. Store these treats in the freezer so you don't eat them all at once! *See photo, page 359.*

1 Preheat the oven to 350°F. Line several baking sheets with parchment, nonstick baking mats, or coat with cooking spray.

2 In a small bowl, combine the apricots and orange juice. Cover with vented plastic wrap and microwave on high for 1 minute. Set aside to plump and cool.

3 Spread the almonds in a small baking dish and bake until golden and fragrant, 10 to 12 minutes. Transfer to a plate and let cool.

4 In a large bowl, whisk the flour, baking soda, and salt.

5 Puree the beans in a food processor. Add the egg, egg whites, brown sugar, granulated sugar, oil, and vanilla. Process until smooth, stopping once or twice to scrape down the sides of the bowl. Scrape into the flour mixture and mix with a rubber spatula. Stir in the oats, chocolate chips, ginger, apricots, and almonds.

6 Drop the batter by tablespoons 2 inches apart on the baking sheets. Bake 1 batch at a time until the edges of the cookies are golden, 14 to 16 minutes. Let cool on the baking sheet for 2 minutes. With a wide metal spatula, transfer to a wire rack to cool completely. One serving is 1 cookie.

meeting your **goals**

Each portion provides 0.2 serving fruit, 0.3 serving whole grains, and 2 grams good fat.

NUTRITION • *Per serving*
95 calories, 2 g protein, 14 g carbohydrates, 1 g fiber, 4 g total fat, 1 g saturated fat, 4 mg cholesterol, 30 mg sodium

Slow-Cooker Apple and Pear Compote

A slow cooker works magic on hearty fall and winter fruits. In this compote, the fruit takes on a tender, almost custard-like consistency, and the natural sweetness of the fruit intensifies during the long slow cooking. Enjoy it for breakfast or dessert.

1 Coat a 4-quart or larger slow cooker with cooking spray. Add the apples, pears, sugar, lemon juice, lemon zest, and ginger and toss to mix well. Cover and cook until the fruit is very tender and almost translucent but not pureed, 2 1/2 to 3 1/2 hours on high or 6 to 7 hours on low. Discard the lemon zest. Gently stir in the vanilla, Transfer to a medium bowl and let cool slightly. Cover and refrigerate until chilled. The compote will keep, covered, in the refrigerator for up to 4 days or in the freezer for up to 4 months.

2 Meanwhile, toast the almonds in a small dry skillet over medium-low heat, stirring constantly, until golden and fragrant, 3 to 4 minutes.

3 Top each serving with a dollop of yogurt and sprinkle with almonds. One serving is 1/2 cup of compote, 1 tablespoon of yogurt, and 1/2 tablespoon of almonds.

desserts

Serves 8

PREP 25 minutes

COOK TIME (in slow cooker) 2 1/2 to 3 1/2 hours on high or 6 to 7 hours on low

2 pounds firm cooking apples, such as Granny Smith, Empire, Northern Spy, or Rome, peeled, cored, and sliced (7 cups)

1 pound ripe but firm pears, such as Bosc or Anjou, peeled, cored, and sliced (2 1/2 cups)

1/4 cup granulated sugar

1 tablespoon fresh lemon juice

2 strips (about 3/4" x 2 1/2") lemon zest

1 teaspoon grated fresh ginger

1 teaspoon vanilla extract

1/4 cup sliced almonds

1/2 cup low-fat plain or vanilla yogurt

meeting your **goals**

Each portion provides 1 serving fruit and 1 gram good fat.

NUTRITION • *Per serving*
131 calories, 2 g protein, 29 g carbohydrates, 3 g fiber, 2 g total fat, 0 g saturated fat, 1 mg cholesterol, 11 mg sodium

Serves 16

PREP 20 minutes

BAKE TIME 35 to
45 minutes

8 ounces bittersweet
(60–70% cacao) chocolate,
chopped, or 1 1/2 cups
bittersweet (60% cacao)
chocolate chips

2 cups drained canned
black beans, rinsed

4 large eggs,
lightly beaten

1 cup granulated sugar

1/2 teaspoon
baking powder

2 teaspoons
vanilla extract

Confectioner's sugar

8 cups fresh raspberries,
rinsed, or sliced
strawberries or orange
sections

Dark Chocolate Celebration Cake with Raspberries

This cake has the intense chocolate flavor and fudgy texture that's so appealing in a rich flourless chocolate cake, but it contains a fraction of the saturated fat. Put your skepticism about the unconventional ingredient—canned black beans—aside. You can't taste them, and the fiber and protein from the beans help balance the carbohydrates. *See photo, page 359.*

1 Preheat the oven to 350°F. Coat a 9-inch round layer cake pan with cooking spray. Line the bottom with a circle of parchment paper or wax paper.

2 Melt the chocolate in a double boiler, stirring often, over hot (not simmering) water.

3 Puree the beans in a food processor. Add the eggs, sugar, baking powder, and vanilla. Process until smooth and creamy, stopping several times to scrape down the sides of the bowl. Add the chocolate and pulse several times until thoroughly blended. Scrape the batter into the pan.

4 Bake until the top springs back when touched lightly, 35 to 45 minutes. (The cake will look cracked.) Let cool in the pan on a wire rack for 5 minutes. Loosen the edges, invert the cake onto the rack, and peel off the paper. Let cool. Dust with confectioner's sugar. Serve slightly warm or at room temperature for the fudgiest texture, accompanied by the raspberries. One serving is 1/16th of the cake and 1/2 cup of raspberries.

Tip: For a special presentation, place a paper doily over the cake before dusting with confectioners' sugar. You can also create your own stencil with strips of wax paper.

meeting your **goals**

**Each portion provides
1 serving fruit and 3 grams
good fat.**

NUTRITION • *Per serving*
193 calories, 4 g protein,
36 g carbohydrates, 6 g fiber,
6 g total fat, 3 g saturated
fat, 53 mg cholesterol,
195 mg sodium

Chocolate "Truffles" with Almonds and Figs

Chocolate truffles in a book on disease prevention? Yes! But instead of a cream filling high in saturated fat, these confections get their rich flavor from almonds and dark chocolate, both of which offer health benefits. Dried figs provide the sweetness, along with valuable fiber.

1 Preheat the oven to 350°F. Spread the almonds in a small baking pan and toast in the oven until fragrant, 10 to 15 minutes. Transfer to a plate and let cool.

2 Melt the chocolate in the top half of a double boiler over hot (not simmering) water, stirring often.

3 Place the almonds and cinnamon in a food processor and pulse until coarsely chopped. Add the figs and pulse until the figs and almonds are finely chopped. Add to the chocolate and mix with a wooden spoon, adding a few drops of water if necessary to make the mixture adhere.

4 Place the sugar in a shallow dish. Form the chocolate mixture into 1-inch balls and roll in the sugar. The truffles will keep, in a covered container in the refrigerator, for up to 2 weeks. One serving is 1 truffle.

desserts

Serves 20

PREP 15 minutes

BAKE TIME 10 to 15 minutes

3/4 cup whole almonds, unpeeled

3 ounces bittersweet dark (70% cacao) chocolate, coarsely chopped

1/4 teaspoon ground cinnamon

3/4 cup dried Calimyrna figs

2 tablespoons granulated sugar

meeting your **goals**

Each portion provides 0.3 serving fruit and 3 grams good fat.

NUTRITION • *Per serving*
77 calories, 2 g protein, 9 g carbohydrates, 2 g fiber, 5 g total fat, 1 g saturated fat, 0 mg cholesterol, 1 mg sodium

Symptoms You Should Never Ignore

Getting frequent headaches? Bowel movements looking a little funny? Have a cough that won't go away? When your body speaks, you should listen. Most people aren't very good at it, though, and it's tempting to ignore a problem that could signal something bad. After all, if you don't get that lump looked at, you won't have to hear a cancer diagnosis (you'll just die early instead). Even if you do pay attention to your symptoms, it's not easy to know what they mean. That's why diagnosis is a job for a doctor. But you can use the information here to help you decide how urgently you need to see one.

Abdominal pain

DESCRIPTION	POSSIBLE CAUSES	RESPONSE
A burning sensation just below the breastbone, particularly after a large meal	Heartburn (reflux)	Take over-the-counter antacids and avoid large, greasy meals. If pain persists for several weeks, see your doctor.
Pain around and below your navel accompanied by gas	Constipation or flatulence	Take an over-the-counter laxative or anti-gas medication. If pain persists for more than two weeks, see your doctor.
Sudden pain around your navel; may be accompanied by nausea, fever, vomiting, loss of appetite, pressure to have a bowel movement, or stiffening of the abdominal muscles	Appendicitis	Go to the hospital. Appendicitis must be treated quickly or the appendix will rupture and leak infected fluid into other parts of the abdomen. Stiffening of abdominal muscles is a sign that infection is starting to spread.
Sudden pain in your right abdomen that may radiate to other parts of your abdomen or your back	Gallstones or gallbladder inflammation	If pain persists or worsens after eating greasy foods, see your doctor.
Sudden pain below your navel that radiates to either side of the navel	A colon disorder, a urinary tract infection, or pelvic inflammatory disease	If pain continues to worsen, call your doctor, who may order diagnostic tests or advise you to go to the emergency room.

DESCRIPTION	POSSIBLE CAUSES	RESPONSE
Sudden sharp pain near your lower ribs that radiates down your groin	Kidney stones or, if accompanied by fever, a kidney or urinary tract infection	Increase your water intake and call your doctor. Most kidney stones eventually pass on their own, although in rare cases, surgery is necessary. If you also have a fever, call your doctor.
Sudden pain and tenderness in your lower left abdomen may be accompanied by fever, nausea, or vomiting	Crohn's disease, ulcerative colitis, or diverticulitis	See your doctor, who may recommend a CT scan. Long-term treatment may include surgery and a change in diet.
Sudden pain accompanied by bloody diarrhea, blood in the stool, or vomiting blood	A blockage in the bowel, a perforated appendix, or bleeding from the bowel	These are symptoms of internal bleeding; go right to the hospital.
Mild pain or discomfort that comes on slowly and continues or recurs for weeks or months, sometimes accompanied by diarrhea, constipation, bloating, or flatulence	A chronic ailment such as lactose intolerance, irritable bowel syndrome, ulcers, food allergies, Crohn's disease, ulcerative colitis, or celiac disease	See your doctor, who may refer you to a gastroenterologist for follow-up.

Black or bloody stools

DESCRIPTION	POSSIBLE CAUSES	RESPONSE
Black or tarry stools; may be accompanied by a burning in the stomach and esophagus	An ulcer in the upper gastrointestinal tract	See your doctor, who will probably order an endoscopy for visual inspection and to take tissue samples for biopsy.
Maroon or black stools with no other worrisome symptoms	Consuming black licorice, blueberries, lead, iron pills, Pepto-Bismol, tomatoes, or beets	Stop eating the suspicious food to see if stool color returns to normal. If not, call your doctor. If you've ingested lead or iron, notify your doctor.
Maroon or bright red stools accompanied by pain and pressure while moving your bowels	Anal fissures (small tears around the anus) or hemorrhoids (swollen blood vessels near the rectum that can rupture)	Over-the-counter hemorrhoid creams, ointments, or pads can bring relief; surgery may be necessary for persistent hemorrhoids. If bleeding continues, see your doctor.
Maroon or bright red stools accompanied by discomfort in the lower abdomen and other GI symptoms, such as gas, constipation, diarrhea, or pain	A serious condition such as ulcerative colitis, Crohn's disease, diverticular disease, a tumor, or benign or cancerous polyps	See your doctor, who will order diagnostic tests such as colonoscopy, biopsy, ultrasound, or x-ray and may refer you to a gastroenterologist for follow-up and treatment.

Bloody urine

DESCRIPTION	POSSIBLE CAUSES	RESPONSE
Blood in the urine after starting a new medication	A side effect of drugs such as aspirin, some antibiotics, blood thinners, and cancer drugs	Talk with your doctor about whether a different drug should be substituted. Side effects sometimes disappear after a few days or weeks of taking a new medication.
Pink, red, or brownish urine accompanied by pain, burning during urination, a frequent strong urge to urinate, or foul-smelling urine	A urinary tract infection	See your doctor, who will order diagnostic urinalysis. Treatment is usually an oral antibiotic.
Blood in the urine, usually accompanied by fever and back pain	A kidney infection	See your doctor. An antibiotic is prescribed when a bacterial infection in the urinary tract moves to the kidneys.
Blood in the urine accompanied by severe pain	Kidney stones	See your doctor, who will order a CT scan or abdominal x-ray. Many kidney stones pass on their own when the patient drinks up to 3 quarts of water per day. If they don't pass, they may need to be surgically removed or shattered with shock waves.
In men, blood in the urine accompanied by difficulty urinating or a strong need to urinate often	Prostate enlargement	See your doctor, who will order diagnostic ultrasound or other imaging tests. Treatment includes medication or laser therapy to destroy excess prostate tissue.
Unexplained blood in the urine with no other symptoms	Bladder cancer, kidney cancer, or a genetic kidney disorder	See your doctor, who will order diagnostic ultrasound, CT scans, and other imaging tests.

Changes in appetite

DESCRIPTION	POSSIBLE CAUSES	RESPONSE
Decreased appetite accompanied by fatigue, hair loss, or decreased cold tolerance	Hypothyroidism (underactive thyroid)	See your doctor, who will order a diagnostic blood test. If your thyroid is underactive, treatment is thyroid hormone replacement pills.
Decreased appetite accompanied by other symptoms, including changes in bowel habits; fatigue; nausea; or bloody stools, urine, or vomit	Cancer	See your doctor, who may order diagnostic tests.
Decreased appetite after starting a new medication	A side effect of medications such as cancer drugs, some antibiotics, narcotic pain relievers, and some cough and cold preparations	Talk with your doctor about whether a different drug should be substituted. Side effects sometimes disappear after a few days or weeks of taking a medication.
Increased appetite accompanied by insomnia, excessive thirst, increased sweating, more frequent bowel movements, or hair loss	Hyperthyroidism (Graves' disease) or other hormone imbalance	See your doctor, who will order diagnostic blood tests. If your thyroid is overactive, prescription medication can slow it down.
Increased appetite accompanied by excessive thirst, fatigue, increased urination, or poor wound healing	Diabetes	See your doctor, who will order a test to measure your blood sugar.
Increased appetite after starting a new medication	A side effect of medications such as corticosteroids, some antidepressants, and some allergy medications	Talk with your doctor about whether a different drug should be substituted. Side effects sometimes disappear after a few days or weeks of taking a medication.

Chest pain

DESCRIPTION	POSSIBLE CAUSES	RESPONSE
Squeezing, tightening pain that usually occurs around the breastbone and may radiate to the jaws, back, or teeth and worsens with exertion; may come on suddenly (unstable) or regularly during exertion (stable)	Angina, which occurs when the heart is not getting enough blood or oxygen	Go to the emergency room; unstable angina can be very dangerous. Stable angina usually goes away within a couple of minutes if you stop the exertion that brought it on, but it is still a serious condition that requires a doctor's care.
Pain accompanied by shortness of breath, coughing, or wheezing	Asthma	If you have an inhaler, use it. If you don't, make an appointment with your doctor. If you can't breathe, go to the emergency room.
Sharp pain that worsens when you cough or take a deep breath; may be accompanied by flu-like symptoms; sometimes hurts when you press your hand against your chest	A lung condition such as pneumonia, a blood clot in the lung, a collapsed lung, inflammation of the lung's lining, or inflammation of ribcage cartilage	Call your doctor or, if you can't breathe, go to the emergency room, where doctors will order chest x-rays and other diagnostic tests.
Burning pain accompanied by GI symptoms such as indigestion or reflux	An ulcer, pancreatic disease, or an inflamed gallbladder	See your doctor, who may recommend diagnostic tests or refer you to a gastroenterologist.
Crushing, squeezing, tightening pressure on your chest that comes on suddenly; may be accompanied by pain that radiates from your chest to your jaw, back, neck, shoulders, or arm, particularly your left arm; may also be accompanied by nausea, racing pulse, or shortness of breath	Heart attack	Call 911 or have someone drive you to the hospital immediately. If your doctor has prescribed nitroglycerin pills to have on hand, take the suggested dose. After you call 911, chew one regular aspirin (325 milligrams) or four low-dose aspirin (81 milligrams each) right away.
Pain accompanied by anxiety, racing pulse, or shortness of breath	Panic attack	Breathe deeply and try to relax. If symptoms persist, call your doctor. Panic attack symptoms can mimic those of more serious conditions such as heart attack. If you have reason to believe it's more than a panic attack, call your doctor or go to the emergency room.

Chronic cough

DESCRIPTION	POSSIBLE CAUSES	RESPONSE
A cough accompanied by postnasal drip, repeated throat clearing, nasal discharge, or excessive phlegm	Allergies or a sinus infection	See your doctor, who may prescribe allergy medication or refer you to an allergist for diagnosis and treatment. If you have a sinus infection, your doctor may prescribe an antibiotic.
A nighttime cough that brings up no mucus and may end with wheezing or a rattling sound	Asthma	See your doctor, who may prescribe a bronchodilator, inhaled corticosteroid, or other medication to control asthma.
A cough after starting to take an ACE inhibitor	A drug side effect; ACE inhibitors cause dry cough in 5 to 10% of patients	Talk with your doctor about whether another drug should be substituted.
A dry cough accompanied by shortness of breath	Chronic obstructive pulmonary disease, a condition that includes chronic bronchitis and emphysema and is almost always caused by smoking	See your doctor, who may do a test to measure lung capacity and order a chest x-ray. There is no cure, but symptoms can be treated.
A cough accompanied by bouts of heartburn that occur more than twice a week	Gastroesophageal reflux disease (GERD), a condition involving chronic heartburn	See your doctor, who will prescribe antacids and drugs that inhibit stomach acid production and may recommend gastroscopy to assess damage to the esophagus.
A cough that worsens over time and may be accompanied by fatigue, chest pain, coughing up blood, hoarseness, or shortness of breath	Lung cancer	See your doctor, who will order diagnostic tests such as a chest x-ray, CT scan, MRI, and blood tests.

Confusion and memory loss

DESCRIPTION	POSSIBLE CAUSES	RESPONSE
Sudden confusion; may be accompanied by blurred vision, slurred speech, sudden numbness on one side of the body, or sudden severe headache	Stroke or transient ischemic attack (TIA)	Go to the hospital immediately. Prompt treatment can save your life, lessen damage to your brain, and reduce your risk of permanent disability.
Sudden confusion or memory loss after an accident	Head injury or concussion	Go to the hospital immediately.
In the elderly, **memory loss or confusion** that begins gradually but doesn't worsen quickly or interfere with everyday life	Normal age-related memory loss	Keep your mind active with crossword puzzles and other mental challenges. Use a detailed date book, always put keys and other items in the same place, and repeat a person's name to yourself several times when you meet.
In the elderly, **memory loss or confusion that begins gradually, starts to worsen quickly, and interferes with the functions of everyday life**	Alzheimer's disease, a neurodegenerative disorder, or a brain tumor	Talk with your doctor, who will determine whether testing is needed.
Confusion that comes on gradually after a period of vomiting, diarrhea, or significant exposure to heat or sunlight	Dehydration	Rehydrate by drinking at least 8 ounces of water every half hour for 4 hours. If dehydration is caused by vomiting or diarrhea, choose nondairy beverages or an over-the-counter electrolyte solution. Call your doctor if you can't keep liquids down or confusion persists.
Memory loss or confusion after starting a new medication	A side effect of medications such as barbiturates and benzodiazepines	Talk with your doctor about whether a different drug should be substituted. Side effects sometimes disappear after a few days or weeks of taking a medication.
Confusion that comes on rather suddenly; may be accompanied by hunger or lightheadedness	Low blood sugar	Have a sweet snack or drink.

Constipation

DESCRIPTION	POSSIBLE CAUSES	RESPONSE
Occasional constipation may be accompanied by bloating, a feeling of fullness, and the need to strain to have a bowel movement	Poor diet (low in fiber and fluids and high in fat), not enough exercise, or too much alcohol or caffeine	Symptoms usually clear up once you resume a healthy diet with plenty of fiber and fluids. Natural fiber supplements can also ease symptoms; be sure to drink plenty of water if you take them.
Constipation after starting a new medication	A side effect of medications such as painkillers, antacids that contain aluminum and calcium, calcium channel blockers, drugs for Parkinson's disease, antispasmodics, antidepressants, iron supplements, diuretics, and anticonvulsants	Talk with your doctor about whether a different drug should be substituted. Side effects sometimes disappear after a few days or weeks of taking a medication.
Constipation that occurs regularly and is accompanied by abdominal pain and bloating; may occur during periods of stress	Irritable bowel syndrome	See your doctor, who may prescribe medication, fiber supplements, physical activity, or stress reduction techniques like meditation to help reduce symptoms.
Constipation during or after pregnancy, travel, or other lifestyle changes	A temporary reaction to change	Symptoms should clear up on their own.
Constipation accompanied by bloating, gas, or pain	A disease or condition of the colon or rectum, such as diverticular disease, tumors, or scar tissue in the intestines	See your doctor, who will order diagnostic tests.
Constipation accompanied by excessive thirst, increased urination, fatigue, depression, weight gain, or headache	A metabolic or endocrine disorder such as diabetes, hypothyroidism (underactive thyroid), or hypercalcemia (too much calcium in the blood)	See your doctor, who will order diagnostic tests.

Diarrhea

DESCRIPTION	POSSIBLE CAUSES	RESPONSE
Diarrhea that comes on suddenly for no apparent reason; may be accompanied by fever, vomiting, cramping, or headache	A viral infection (stomach flu)	Symptoms usually clear up on their own within a few days. During that time, stay well hydrated. Drink nondairy, noncaffeinated beverages or an over-the-counter electrolyte solution throughout the day.
Diarrhea after eating certain foods, such as milk or eggs	Food allergy	Eliminate the trigger food from your diet and talk with your doctor about whether to have allergy tests.
Diarrhea starting 2–6 hours after a meal	A bacterial infection caused by spoiled, undercooked, or contaminated food; most cases of food poisoning are due to common bacteria such as staphylococcus or *E. coli*	Symptoms usually clear up on their own within 12–48 hours. Avoid solid food until your stools return to normal. Call your doctor if symptoms last more than two or three days or if you're unable to stay hydrated; you may need intravenous fluids. If you ate contaminated mushrooms or shellfish, go to the emergency room; your stomach may need to be emptied.
Diarrhea while traveling in a foreign country	An infection caused by contaminated water; most often due to common bacteria and sometimes parasites	Symptoms usually clear up on their own in one to two days. If they persist or are accompanied by other symptoms such as persistent vomiting and headache, see your doctor, who may prescribe an antibiotic or anti-parasitic medication.
Diarrhea while taking medications	A side effect of medications such as antibiotics, diuretics, laxatives that contain magnesium, or cancer drugs	Talk with your doctor about whether a different drug should be substituted. If you're taking an antibiotic, eat yogurt with active cultures to replenish the "good" bacteria in your gut.
Diarrhea that lasts more than four weeks	A chronic condition such as lactose intolerance, Crohn's disease, ulcerative colitis, irritable bowel syndrome, or celiac disease (intolerance to gluten, a protein found in wheat, rye, and barley)	See your doctor, who may refer you to a gastroenterologist and/or dietitian.

Dizziness

DESCRIPTION	POSSIBLE CAUSES	RESPONSE
Dizziness accompanied by dry mouth, thirst, dark urine, and decreased urination	Dehydration	Rehydrate with noncaffeinated beverages or an over-the-counter electrolyte solution. Call your doctor if you can't keep liquids down and dizziness persists.
Dizziness accompanied by ear pain, reduced ability to hear, and fever	An ear infection	See your doctor, but know that most ear infections clear up on their own within a few days. Use an over-the-counter pain reliever or a heating pad to reduce pain.
Dizziness accompanied by blurred vision, slurred speech, sudden numbness on one side of the body, or sudden severe headache	Stroke or transient ischemic attack (TIA)	Go to the hospital immediately. Prompt treatment can save your life and reduce your risk of permanent disability.
Sudden severe dizziness accompanied by chest pain, racing pulse, shortness of breath, sweating, or pain	Heart attack	Call 911. If your doctor has prescribed nitroglycerin pills to have on hand, take the suggested dose. After you call 911, chew one regular aspirin (325 milligrams) or four low-dose aspirin (81 milligrams each) right away.
Sudden severe dizziness accompanied by chest pain, shortness of breath, racing pulse, or fainting	Heart arrhythmia (irregular heartbeat)	An unusually fast or slow heartbeat is usually harmless, but the symptoms of arrhythmia are so similar to those of heart attack that only a trained medical professional can tell them apart. If you've never had them before, call 911.
Dizziness triggered by standing up	Positional vertigo (an inner ear disorder)	Sit or lie still until the dizziness passes. Avoid standing up quickly.
Dizziness after starting a new medication	A side effect of various medications, especially those for diabetes, high blood pressure, depression, and anxiety	Talk with your doctor about whether a different drug should be substituted. Side effects sometimes disappear after a few days or weeks of taking a medication.
Dizziness accompanied by anxiety, racing pulse, or shortness of breath	Panic attack	Breathe deeply and try to relax. If symptoms persist, call your doctor. Frequent panic attacks can be treated with therapy, medication, and relaxation techniques such as meditation.

Excessive thirst

DESCRIPTION	POSSIBLE CAUSES	RESPONSE
Thirst accompanied by chest pain, increased or decreased urination, appetite loss, nausea, vomiting, swelling or numbness in the hands or feet, muscle cramps, trouble concentrating, shortness of breath, or dizziness	Heart, liver, or kidney failure	Call your doctor immediately. A variety of diagnostic tests can determine the existence and extent of these conditions.
Thirst possibly accompanied by insomnia, unexplained weight loss, increased sweating, more frequent bowel movements, or hair loss	Hyperthyroidism (Graves' disease) or other hormone imbalance	See your doctor, who will order a diagnostic blood test. If your thyroid is overactive, prescription medication can slow it down.
Thirst after starting a new medication	A side effect of drugs such as diuretics, antihistamines, some antidepressants, cancer drugs, steroids, and heart disease medications	Talk with your doctor about whether to continue the medication, but don't stop it without a medical okay. Check the package inserts or call your pharmacist for advice on whether/how much to increase your fluid intake.
Thirst possibly accompanied by increased urination, unexplained weight loss, increased hunger, or blurred vision	Hyperglycemia (high blood sugar) or diabetes	See your doctor, who will order a test to measure your blood sugar levels.
A strong desire to drink with no other physical symptoms	Psychogenic polydipsia, a mental disorder	See your doctor, who may refer you to a mental health professional.
Thirst accompanied by excessive urination	Central diabetes insipidus, a rare disorder caused by a deficiency of certain kidney proteins necessary to manage fluid balance	See your doctor, who will order diagnostic blood tests.

Fatigue

DESCRIPTION	POSSIBLE CAUSES	RESPONSE
Sudden fatigue accompanied by viral symptoms	An illness such as a cold or the flu	Rest while your body fights off the virus.
Fatigue accompanied by loss of interest in favorite activities, unintentional weight gain or loss, irritability, feelings of hopelessness, or trouble concentrating	Depression or anxiety	Seek support from friends and family and see your doctor, who may refer you to a mental health professional. Long-term depression or anxiety, common in older people, can be treated with therapy, medication, or both.
Fatigue while taking medication	A side effect of drugs such as beta-blockers, antihistamines, anti-anxiety medications, cough and cold remedies, and some antidepressants	Ask your doctor or pharmacist if fatigue is a common side effect of any of the medications you take. If the answer is yes, talk with your doctor about whether a different medication should be substituted.
Fatigue that lasts more than two weeks	A problem such as infection, allergies, a sleep disorder such as apnea, anemia, heart disease, diabetes, kidney disease, or liver disease	See your doctor, who will order diagnostic tests and may refer you to a specialist.
Fatigue accompanied by unexplained weight gain, dry skin, hair loss, change in sleep patterns, constipation, or depression	Hypothyroidism (underactive thyroid)	See your doctor, who will order a diagnostic blood test. If your thyroid is underactive, treatment is thyroid hormone replacement pills.
Severe, persistent, unexplained fatigue accompanied by muscle aches or difficulty concentrating	Chronic fatigue syndrome (CFS)	See your doctor, who will rule out other possible causes. There is no cure, but symptoms can be controlled with various medications. Be sure your doctor has experience treating CFS.

Fever

DESCRIPTION	POSSIBLE CAUSES	RESPONSE
A small increase in body temperature (1–2°F) with no other symptoms	Exercise, menstruation, heat, heavy clothing, intense emotion	Normal body temperature is about 98.6°F. In adults and children over age 6, a variation of 1 to 2 degrees is normal. To reduce your temperature, turn on air conditioning, loosen clothing, drink fluids, or bathe in lukewarm water.
A rapid, dramatic increase in body temperature after exposure to heat, sun, or intense exercise; may be accompanied by rapid pulse, nausea, and disorientation	Heatstroke or heat exhaustion	Move to a cool place and spray yourself with and drink cool water. If symptoms are extreme (temperature of 106°F or higher), call an ambulance. Heat exhaustion is less serious; heatstroke is a medical emergency.
A moderate fever (100.5–104.5°F); may be accompanied by nasal discharge, sore throat, cough, earache, vomiting, or diarrhea	A viral or bacterial infection such as a cold, the flu, strep throat, an ear infection, bronchitis, or a urinary tract infection	Acetaminophen or ibuprofen can reduce the fever. If your fever is above 103°F or lasts more than three days, call your doctor. If you have a bacterial infection, your doctor may prescribe an antibiotic. Stay hydrated with water or an electrolyte solution.
A high fever (105°F or higher); may be accompanied by confusion, stiff neck, difficulty breathing, hallucinations, or convulsions	A viral or bacterial infection or pneumonia, a kidney infection, mononucleosis, or other serious condition	Go to the emergency room, especially if the patient seems lethargic or unresponsive. Acetaminophen or ibuprofen can reduce the fever, as can bathing in lukewarm water. Stay hydrated by drinking water or an over-the-counter electrolyte solution.
Fever after starting a new medication	A side effect of medications such as some antibiotics, antihistamines, barbiturates, anti-seizure medications, and hypertension drugs	Talk with your doctor about whether a different drug should be substituted. Side effects sometimes disappear after a few days or weeks of taking a medication.
A mild fever that occurs after a vaccination	A side effect of some routine immunizations, such those for diphtheria, tetanus, and pneumonia	Fever usually subsides in a day or two; take ibuprofen or acetaminophen to reduce discomfort.
A fever that occurs with other unexplained symptoms, such as weight loss, muscle or joint aches, or stomach pain, and may come and go	A wide variety of conditions and diseases, such as cancer, ulcerative colitis, Crohn's disease, lupus, HIV/AIDS, rheumatoid arthritis, and autoimmune disorders	See your doctor, who may order diagnostic tests.

Headache

DESCRIPTION	POSSIBLE CAUSES	RESPONSE
Dull pain in your head, neck, or shoulders that comes on gradually; may feel like a vise around your forehead, temples, or back of your head and neck	Tension headache; can be triggered by stress, fatigue, anger, or depression or can have no known trigger	Take aspirin, ibuprofen, or acetaminophen.
Pain after physical exertion such as running, sexual intercourse, coughing, or bowel movements	Exertion headache; related to cluster headaches, migraines, or, rarely, to aneurysms, tumors, or malformed blood vessels	Pain usually goes away in less than an hour. It can be treated with aspirin or medications for migraines or cluster headaches. If headaches persist, see your doctor.
Throbbing pain that comes on several days after consuming a large amount of caffeine	Caffeine withdrawal	Reduce or eliminate caffeine intake.
Throbbing pain, usually on one side of the head, often accompanied by nausea and sensitivity to light and sound; occasionally accompanied by flashing lights, blind spots, or tingling in the arm or face prior to head pain	Migraine; occurs more commonly in women and can be triggered by menstruation, ovulation, or menopause	Migraines typically last from 4 hours to three days. Take an over-the-counter painkiller or a prescription migraine medication if you have one, and lie down in a dark room. If you have more than two migraines a month, see your doctor, who may recommend preventive medication.
Sudden sharp, severe pain on one side of the head, sometimes around the eye; may be accompanied by excessive sweating, tearing, and nasal congestion	Cluster headache; 90 percent of sufferers are men	Headaches may last anywhere from a few minutes to several hours but are likely to recur later that day. See your doctor, who may prescribe medication to treat them. There are also preventive medicines that help ward off attacks. Avoid alcohol.
Unexplained pain that becomes progressively worse; may be accompanied by blurred vision, confusion, or loss of consciousness	Cancer; infection; high blood pressure; a disease or disorder of the brain; disorders of the eyes, ears, or nose; blood clots; or aneurysms	See your doctor, who may order diagnostic tests or refer you to a specialist.
Sudden severe pain; may be accompanied by numbness on one side of the body, dizziness, blurred vision, headache, or confusion	Stroke or transient ischemic attack (TIA)	Go to the hospital immediately. Prompt treatment can save your life, lessen damage to your brain, and reduce your risk of permanent disability.

Nausea and vomiting

DESCRIPTION	POSSIBLE CAUSES	RESPONSE
Nausea and vomiting in women in early pregnancy	Morning sickness	See your doctor, who may recommend ginger or vitamin B_6.
Nausea and vomiting after starting a new medication	A side effect of a medication	Talk with your doctor about whether a different drug should be substituted. Side effects sometimes disappear after a few days or weeks of taking a medication.
Nausea or vomiting accompanied by sudden pain in your upper right abdomen that may radiate to other parts of your abdomen or your back	Gallstones or gallbladder inflammation	If pain persists or worsens after eating greasy foods, see your doctor.
Nausea or vomiting starting 2–6 hours after a meal	A bacterial infection caused by spoiled, undercooked, or contaminated food; most cases of food poisoning are due to common bacteria such as staphylococcus or *E. coli*	Symptoms usually clear up on their own within 12–48 hours. Call your doctor if symptoms last more than two or three days or if you're unable to stay hydrated; you may need intravenous fluids. If you ate contaminated mushrooms or shellfish, go to the emergency room; your stomach may need to be emptied.
Nausea or vomiting accompanied by crushing, squeezing, tightening pressure on your chest that comes on suddenly; pain that radiates from your chest to your jaw, back, neck, shoulders, or arm, particularly your left arm; racing pulse; or shortness of breath	Heart attack	Call 911 or have someone drive you to the hospital immediately. If your doctor has prescribed nitroglycerin pills to have on hand, take the suggested dose. After you call 911, chew one regular aspirin (325 milligrams) or four low-dose aspirin (81 milligrams each) right away.
Nausea or vomiting after an accident, sports injury, or fall	A concussion or brain injury	If symptoms continue to worsen, call your doctor or go to the emergency room.
Nausea or vomiting accompanied by black or tarry stools, a burning sensation in the stomach and esophagus, indigestion, or reflux	An ulcer in the upper GI tract or gastroesophageal reflux disease (GERD)	See your doctor, who will probably order an endoscopy, in which a scope is inserted through your mouth and into your upper GI tract for visual inspection and to take tissue samples for biopsy.
Nausea or vomiting accompanied by other unexplained symptoms, such as fatigue, pain, or weight changes	Cancer	See your doctor, who will order diagnostic tests.

DESCRIPTION	POSSIBLE CAUSES	RESPONSE
Nausea or vomiting after eating certain foods, such as milk or eggs	Food allergy	Eliminate the trigger food from your diet and talk with your doctor about whether to have allergy tests.
Nausea or vomiting that comes on suddenly; may be accompanied by pain around your navel, fever, loss of appetite, or pressure to have a bowel movement	Appendicitis	Go to the hospital. Appendicitis must be treated quickly or the appendix will rupture and leak infected fluid into other parts of the abdomen.
Nausea or vomiting accompanied by excessive thirst, fatigue, increased urination, or poor wound healing	Poorly controlled diabetes	See your doctor, who can help you get your diabetes under control.
Nausea or vomiting that comes on gradually and continues or recurs for weeks or months; may be accompanied by pain or discomfort in the abdomen, diarrhea, constipation, bloating, flatulence, and other GI symptoms	A chronic condition such as lactose intolerance, irritable bowel syndrome, ulcers, food allergies, Crohn's disease, ulcerative colitis, or celiac disease	See your doctor, who may refer you to a gastroenterologist.
Nausea and vomiting accompanied by chest pain, excessive thirst, increased or decreased urination, appetite loss, swelling or numbness in the hands or feet, muscle cramps, trouble concentrating, shortness of breath, or dizziness	Heart, liver, or kidney failure	Call your doctor immediately. A variety of diagnostic tests can determine the existence and extent of these serious conditions.
Nausea or vomiting accompanied by throbbing headache on one or both sides of the head and sensitivity to light and sound; may be accompanied by flashing lights, blind spots, or tingling in the arm or face prior to head pain	A migraine	Migraines typically last from 4 hours to three days. Take an over-the-counter painkiller or a prescription migraine medication if you have one, and lie down in a dark room. If you have more than two migraines a month, see your doctor, who may recommend preventive medication.

Numbness and tingling

DESCRIPTION	POSSIBLE CAUSES	RESPONSE
Numbness and tingling along your arm or down the back of your leg, sometimes after an accident or fall	An injury to a nerve in the neck or back	See your doctor.
Pain in the lower back radiating to the buttock or down the back of the leg that may include numbness in the leg or foot	Sciatica caused by pressure on the spinal nerve from a herniated disk in the back	Avoid activity that hurts, but do exercise, or the muscles around the disk will weaken. Over-the-counter painkillers and physical therapy can also help.
Numbness or tingling in the hand, wrist, and fingers that develops over time, usually due to overuse of the hands for repetitive motion; may be accompanied by loss of feeling in the fingers	Carpal tunnel syndrome	See your doctor. Treatment options include wrist splinting, stretching exercises, nonsteroidal anti-inflammatory drugs, corticosteroids, and, in some cases, surgery.
In people with diabetes, numbness and tingling, usually in the feet; may be accompanied by a reduced ability to feel pain, heat, or cold; loss of balance; or sharp pains that worsen at night	Diabetic neuropathy	See your doctor. There is no cure, but symptoms can be managed with medication. To prevent progression, keep your blood sugar and blood pressure under control and take your diabetes medication as prescribed.
Numbness or tingling that comes on suddenly and affects one side of the body; may be accompanied by dizziness, blurred vision, headache, or confusion	Stroke or transient ischemic attack (TIA)	Go to the hospital immediately. Prompt treatment can save your life and reduce your risk of permanent disability.
Numbness or tingling that comes on gradually in your fingers, hands, and lower extremities; may be accompanied by fatigue or muscle weakness anywhere in the body	Abnormal levels of calcium, potassium, sodium, or vitamin B_{12}	See your doctor, who may suggest a supplement; be sure to discuss any other supplements you take.
Numbness or tingling in the limbs or face possibly accompanied by flu-like symptoms, joint pain and swelling, or rash; occurs weeks, months, or even years after a bite from an infected deer tick	Lyme disease	See your doctor, who will order a diagnostic test. Depending on the severity and duration of the symptoms, treatment can include either oral or intravenous antibiotics.

Painful urination

DESCRIPTION	POSSIBLE CAUSES	RESPONSE
A burning sensation during urination; may be accompanied by a frequent need to urinate	A urinary tract infection	See your doctor, who will order diagnostic urinalysis. Treatment is usually an antibiotic.
A burning sensation during urination accompanied by fever over 101°F and back pain	A kidney infection	See your doctor. An antibiotic is prescribed when a bacterial infection in the urinary tract moves to the kidneys.
Itching and burning during urination; may occur after antibiotic treatment	A yeast infection	See your primary care physician or gynecologist, who may collect a mucus specimen from your vagina to check for the presence of yeast.
Painful urination after starting a new medication	A side effect of medications such as ibuprofen and some antidepressants, osteoporosis drugs, and cancer drugs	Talk with your doctor about whether a different drug should be substituted. Side effects sometimes disappear after a few days or weeks of taking a medication.
Pain or pressure in the bladder area with difficulty emptying the bladder completely	An ovarian cyst pressing against the bladder	See your doctor, who will order tests such as an ultrasound and may biopsy the cyst if cancer is suspected.
Severe pain in the back and side; may be accompanied by a frequent need to urinate, inability to urinate, bloody urine, fever, chills, or foul-smelling urine	Kidney stones	See your doctor, who will order a CT scan or abdominal x-ray. Many kidney stones pass on their own when the patient drinks up to 3 quarts of water per day. If they don't pass, they may need to be surgically removed or shattered with shock waves.
Painful urination possibly accompanied by sores, blisters, scabs, or pustules in the genital area; painful intercourse; and unusual discharge from the vagina or penis	A sexually transmitted infection such as genital herpes, genital warts, syphilis, gonorrhea, or HIV/AIDS	See your doctor; prompt treatment can often prevent more serious symptoms. Avoid intercourse until you've seen your doctor.

Shortness of breath

DESCRIPTION	POSSIBLE CAUSES	RESPONSE
Sudden shortness of breath accompanied by chest pain or pressure, pain that radiates outward from the chest, or sweating	A heart attack, arrhythmia, or a blood clot that travels from the legs to the heart	Call your doctor or go to the emergency room.
Sudden shortness of breath after inhaling a piece of food, a liquid, or other foreign object; may be accompanied by frequent cough, fever, the feeling that something is stuck in your throat, or pain when trying to take a deep breath	Airway obstruction or infection (acute pneumonia) caused by aspiration of a foreign object	If the person is choking, perform the Heimlich maneuver. Otherwise, go to the emergency room, where a bronchoscope or laryngoscope can be used to remove a foreign object. If infection is present, antibiotics may be prescribed.
Sudden shortness of breath after exposure to an allergen such as nuts, shellfish, or eggs; may be accompanied by itching, hives, swelling of the tongue, or reddened skin	Anaphylactic shock	Go to the hospital immediately. Use an Epi-pen if your doctor has prescribed one.
Sudden shortness of breath after exposure to a known trigger such as dust, pollen, or pet dander	Asthma or an environmental allergy	Use an inhaler if you have one; take an antihistamine.
Shortness of breath before, during, or after a very stressful or anxiety-provoking experience; may come on suddenly; may be accompanied by sweating, hyperventilation, nausea, chest pain, or tightness in your throat	A panic attack	If you are hyperventilating, breathe through pursed lips (as if you were going to blow out a candle) or cover your mouth and one nostril and breathe through the other nostril. If it's your first panic attack, go to the emergency room to make sure you're not having a heart attack. If attacks continue, see your doctor, who may recommend medication or behavioral therapy.
Shortness of breath that comes on gradually, lasts for a week or more, and is accompanied by fever or cold or flu symptoms	Bronchitis or pneumonia	See your doctor, who will check the oxygen level in your blood. Treatment options include antibiotics, antifungal medication, and oxygen therapy.
Shortness of breath that comes on gradually and becomes chronic	Asthma, chronic obstructive pulmonary disease, cardiovascular disease, emphysema, tumors, pulmonary hypertension, muscular dystrophy, or amyotrophic lateral sclerosis (ALS)	See your doctor, who will order diagnostic tests.

Unintentional weight gain

DESCRIPTION	POSSIBLE CAUSES	RESPONSE
Gradual weight gain with no other symptoms	Decrease in exercise, increased calorie intake, or aging	Eat less and get more exercise. As you age, your calorie needs decrease.
Weight gain accompanied by swelling, chest pain, or shortness of breath	Heart or lung disease	See your doctor, who will order diagnostic tests.
Weight gain accompanied by fatigue, hair loss, decreased cold tolerance, constipation, or depression	Hypothyroidism (underactive thyroid)	See your doctor, who will order a diagnostic blood test. If your thyroid is underactive, treatment is thyroid hormone replacement pills.
Weight gain after starting a new medication	A side effect of medications such as corticosteroids, lithium, tranquilizers, and some antidepressants	Talk with your doctor about whether a different drug should be substituted. Side effects sometimes disappear after a few days or weeks of taking a medication.
In women, gradual weight gain possibly accompanied by irregular or nonexistent periods, excess hair growth, acne, or infertility	Polycystic ovary syndrome	See your doctor, who can prescribe medications to control symptoms; in some cases, surgery is necessary.
Weight gain during a period of high stress or anxiety	Anxiety or intense stress	Look for ways to change whatever is causing the stress or anxiety. Relaxation techniques such as meditation, yoga, and visualization can help you cope. Longer-lasting anxiety can be treated with therapy, medication, or both.
Weight gain accompanied by sadness, fatigue, loss of interest in enjoyable activities, or thoughts of suicide	Depression	See your doctor, who may refer you to a mental health professional for medication, therapy, or both.
Weight gain after quitting smoking	Emotional eating and the slowing of metabolism that comes with smoking cessation	Suck on sugarless candies, snack on raw vegetables, drink plenty of water, and start an exercise regimen. The drug bupropion (Zyban) seems to help decrease weight gain after quitting.
Weight gain accompanied by excessive thirst, fatigue, increased urination, or poor wound healing	Diabetes	See your doctor, who will order a test to measure your blood sugar levels.

Unintentional weight loss

DESCRIPTION	POSSIBLE CAUSES	RESPONSE
Weight loss accompanied by insomnia, unusual thirst, increased sweating, increased bowel movements, hair loss	Hyperthyroidism (Graves' disease) or other hormone imbalance	See your doctor, who will order a diagnostic blood test. If your thyroid is overactive, prescription medication can slow it down.
Weight loss after starting a new medication	A side effect of medications such as sedatives, SSRI antidepressants, and narcotic pain relievers	Talk with your doctor about whether a different drug should be substituted. Side effects sometimes disappear after a few days or weeks of taking a medication.
Weight loss during a period of high stress or anxiety	Anxiety or intense stress	Look for ways to change whatever is causing the stress or anxiety. Relaxation techniques such as meditation, yoga, and visualization can help you cope. Longer-lasting anxiety can be treated with therapy, medication, or both.
Weight loss accompanied by feelings of sadness, fatigue, loss of interest in enjoyable activities, or thoughts of suicide	Depression	See your doctor, who may refer you to a mental health professional for medication, therapy, or both.
Weight loss accompanied by GI complaints such as bloating, gas, constipation, or diarrhea	Celiac disease, an autoimmune disorder in which the gluten in wheat, rye, and barley damages the intestines and decreases the body's ability to absorb nutrients	See your doctor, who will order a diagnostic blood test or gastroscopy. Switching to a gluten-free diet is the only treatment.
Weight loss accompanied by intestinal pain and diarrhea or loose stools	Ulcerative colitis or Crohn's disease, which prevent digestion and absorption of some of the food you eat	See your doctor, who may recommend dietary changes, surgery, or medication that reduces inflammation.
Weight loss accompanied by excessive thirst, fatigue, increased urination, or poor wound healing	Diabetes	See your doctor, who will order a test to measure your blood sugar levels.
Weight loss with no other symptoms or accompanied by unexplained GI symptoms such as bloating, abdominal pain, bloody urine, bloody stools, or nausea	Gastrointestinal cancer	See your doctor, who will order diagnostic tests.

Vaginal bleeding or discharge

DESCRIPTION	POSSIBLE CAUSES	RESPONSE
Fishy-smelling discharge from the vagina; may be accompanied by swelling, redness, itching, or burning	Bacterial vaginosis, an inflammation of the vagina caused by bacteria	See your doctor or gynecologist, who will prescribe an oral antibiotic or an antibiotic cream or suppositories; these can clear up the symptoms within a few days.
Yellow or greenish bubbly discharge with a foul odor; may be accompanied by pain during intercourse; symptoms worsen after a menstrual period	Chlamydia, gonorrhea, trichomoniasis, or other sexually transmitted infection	See your doctor, who will prescribe antibiotic shots or pills. Ask whether your partner should also receive treatment, and avoid intercourse until the infection clears up.
White, cheese-like discharge; may be accompanied by swelling, pain during intercourse, and itching; may occur shortly after beginning a course of oral antibiotics	A yeast infection	See your doctor, who will order a diagnostic test and prescribe an antifungal drug to be administered orally or vaginally.
Bleeding between menstrual periods	Uterine fibroids or cancer of the uterus, vagina, endometrium, or ovaries	See your doctor, who will order diagnostic tests.
Bleeding between menstrual periods, possibly accompanied by excess hair growth, acne, or infertility	Polycystic ovary syndrome	See your doctor, who may prescribe medications to control symptoms; in some cases, surgery is necessary.
Bleeding while using an IUD	IUD use can cause occasional spotting	See your doctor if bleeding continues or becomes heavy.
In postmenopausal women, bleeding after intercourse	Irritation of vaginal walls that are dry because of decreased estrogen	Use an over-the-counter vaginal lubricant or see your doctor for prescription estrogen cream to decrease irritation.
Bleeding during pregnancy	A miscarriage, ectopic pregnancy, or other serious complication	Call your doctor immediately.
Bleeding or discharge; may be accompanied by fever or pain in the pelvic or lower abdominal area	Pelvic inflammatory disease, an inflammation or infection of the ovaries, fallopian tubes, or uterus; can be caused by sexually transmitted bacteria	See your doctor. Prompt treatment with antibiotics can prevent damage to your reproductive system that could contribute to infertility, ectopic pregnancy, and other reproductive disorders.

Vision loss

DESCRIPTION	POSSIBLE CAUSES	RESPONSE
Sudden loss of vision that occurs after an accident, sports injury, chemical burn, or contact with irritating foreign material	An injury to the retina, cornea, or nerves, including corneal abrasion and torn retina	Sudden vision loss is always an emergency. Go to the hospital immediately.
A sudden change in vision accompanied by confusion, slurred speech, sudden numbness on one side of the body, or sudden severe headache	Stroke or transient ischemic attack (TIA)	Go to the hospital immediately. Prompt treatment can save your life and reduce your risk of permanent disability.
A gradual decrease in your ability to focus on nearby objects	Presbyopia, an age-related change that typically begins around age 40	Buy drugstore reading glasses or see an eye doctor for bifocals.
Blurred vision, burning, dryness, irritation, or a gritty feeling in the eyes; often occurs in women during menopause	Dry eyes	Use over-the-counter or prescription eyedrops. In severe cases, a doctor can insert plugs into the tear ducts to maintain moisture in the eye.
Blurred vision and dry eyes after starting a new medication	A side effect of medications such as diuretics, beta-blockers, antihistamines, sleeping pills, and some pain relievers	Talk with your doctor about whether a different drug should be substituted. Side effects sometimes disappear after a few days or weeks of taking a new medication.
In people with diabetes, blurred or spotty vision	Diabetic retinopathy, in which blood vessels in the retina are damaged	See your doctor. Surgery (laser or conventional) can reduce loss of vision.
In older people, blurred, cloudy vision; may be accompanied by faded appearance of colors, glare or halos around lights, poor night vision, or double vision	Cataracts, a condition in which the eye's lens is clouded by clumps of protein	See your doctor. Clouded lenses can be surgically removed and replaced with artificial ones, improving vision in 90 percent of cases.
Blank spots in your field of vision possibly accompanied by blurred vision, loss of peripheral vision, eye pain, headache, and rainbow-colored halos around lights	Glaucoma, a disease caused by pressure within the eye that damages the optic nerve	See your doctor. Surgery and medication (eyedrops or pills) can slow glaucoma's progression but can't bring back lost vision.
Blurriness or loss of central vision; may be accompanied by straight lines appearing wavy, difficulty recognizing faces, and the need for extra light while reading	Age-related macular degeneration, a disease that occurs when the macula, the central part of the eye, breaks down or is damaged	See your doctor. Treatments include laser surgery, photodynamic therapy (medication combined with light therapy), and medications that are injected into the eye as often as every month. Treatment can't restore lost vision but can usually delay further loss.

Wounds that won't heal

DESCRIPTION	POSSIBLE CAUSES	RESPONSE
Cuts or bruises that heal unusually slowly but do not appear infected	Weakened immunity, which can be caused by poor nutrition, vitamin K deficiency, steroid medications, or cancer treatment	Talk with your doctor about vitamin supplementation or changes in steroid use; follow-up with a registered dietitian may be useful.
A wound that is swollen, red, or hot or has pus or red lines radiating from it; may be accompanied by fever	Cellulitis (a bacterial infection of the skin) or a foreign object stuck in the wound	See your doctor, who may prescribe an antibiotic. If symptoms are worsening quickly, go to the emergency room. Cellulitis can cause serious infection that can spread.
Poor wound healing accompanied by chest pains, shortness of breath, and changes in urinary habits	A disease of the heart, lungs, kidneys, or other major organs	See your doctor, who will probably order diagnostic tests.
Poor wound healing accompanied by excessive thirst, increased urination, unexplained weight loss, increased hunger, or blurred vision	Undiagnosed or poorly controlled diabetes	See your doctor, who will order a test to measure your blood sugar levels. If you have diabetes that is poorly controlled, you may need to switch from a family doctor to an endocrinologist.
In people with diabetes, poor wound healing in the feet; may be accompanied by a reduced ability to feel pain, heat, or cold; loss of balance, or sharp pains that worsen at night	Diabetic neuropathy	See your doctor. There is no cure, but symptoms can be managed with medication. To prevent progression, keep your blood sugar and blood pressure under control and take your diabetes medication as prescribed.
Sores on the legs or feet that won't heal, accompanied by cold feet, leg or foot pain or numbness, or changes in the toenails or amount of hair on the legs or feet	Peripheral arterial disease, a restriction of blood flow in the arteries of the leg caused by accumulation of arterial plaque	See your doctor. Circulation can be improved with exercise, smoking cessation, and a heart-healthy diet; in some cases, medication or surgery is needed.
A sore in the mouth or on the lip or skin that doesn't heal; may be accompanied by other symptoms, such as unexplained weight loss	Oral cancer or skin cancer	See your doctor, who may order diagnostic tests.

Index

A

abdominal pain, 113, 120, 139, 143, 157, 175, 181, 183, 203, 227, 243, 299, 309, 315, 373, 380, 381
  in diverticular disease, 158, 161, 367
  in irritable bowel syndrome, 232, 233, 234, 235, 367
  menstruation and, 252–53
  in ovarian cancer, 268, 269
  possible causes of, 366–67

absorptive hypercalciuria, 242

accidents, 15, 65–66, 245, 257, 295
  nausea or vomiting after, 380
  numbness or tingling after, 382
  sudden confusion or memory loss after, 372
  vision loss after, 388

ACE inhibitors, 141, 240, 371

acetaminophen, 69, 225, 241, 308, 378, 379

acetylcysteine (Mucomyst), 116

Achilles tendinitis, 119

acid-blocking medications, 94

acid reflux, 109, 117, 194–97

Aciphex (rabeprazole), 196

acne, 72–73, 283, 385, 387

ACTH hormones, 28

activated carbon filters, 59

Actonel (risedronate), 264

acupuncture, 197

acute angle-closure glaucoma, 185

acyclovir (Zovirax), 204, 286, 287

adalimumab (Humira), 281

adapalene (Differin), 73

Advil, 198

aerobic exercise, 17, 118, 150, 186, 212, 244, 303

African Americans, 25, 45, 184, 278, 279

age-related macular degeneration (AMD), 148, 250–51, 388

aging, 25, 30, 53, 163, 213, 257
  Alzheimer's and memory loss as caused by, 78, 81, 372
  cancer-risk as increased with, 139, 299
  hearing and vision loss as caused by, 192, 388
  joint issues as caused by, 84, 119
  varicose veins as caused by, 313
  wrinkles as caused by, 192, 388

AIDS, 284, 285, 378, 383

air conditioners, 58, 76, 163, 167, 169, 293, 378

air filters, 58, 75, 169, 293

air quality maintenance, 57–58, 251
  alleries and, 57–58, 74–75, 76, 92–93, 166, 293
  asthma and, 57, 92–93, 94, 95
  carbon monoxide detection in, 57–58
  carpets as infringing on, 57, 58, 74, 166, 293
  chronic obstructive pulmonary disease and, 133
  eczema and, 166
  lung cancer and, 58, 246–47
  peripheral vascular disease and, 271
  radon testing in, 57, 246–47
  snoring and, 293

air travel, health tips for, 62–63, 69, 135, 163, 177

alcohol, 11, 33, 64, 156, 170, 175, 215, 232, 254, 282, 293, 301–2, 308, 321, 373, 379
  Alzheimer's prevention with, 80
  aspirin and, 47
  BPH risk as increased with, 111
  cancer risks as increased with, 115, 137–38
  dehydration and, 63, 66

  gallstone prevention with, 183
  gout risk and, 187
  gum disease risk as increased with, 189
  heartburn and GERD as linked to, 195, 196, 197
  heart-related risks as lowered with, 146–47, 213, 303
  infertility risk as increased with, 223
  insomnia and, 230
  psoriasis risk as increased with, 280
  tinnitus and, 305
  ulcerative colitis relapses due to, 225
  ulcer risk increased with, 309
  varicose vein prevention with, 312, 313

alcohol, ethanol, 135

alcohol, ethyl, 177

alcohol, rubbing, 273

alendronate (Fosamax), 264

Aleve (naproxen), 198, 225, 252, 308

allergic rhinitis, 77

allergies, 34, 74–77, 121, 166, 273, 289
  air quality maintenance and, 57–58, 74–75, 76, 92–93, 166, 293
  anaphylactic shock due to, 384
  diet and prevention of, 76–77, 94
  eczema and, 165–66, 167
  insomnia as caused by, 230
  and reducing risks in children, 77
  shots and medications for, 74, 75, 94, 166, 369, 371, 384
  symptoms of, 75, 367, 371, 374, 377, 381, 384
  to food, 74, 75, 166, 281, 381, 384
  to mold, 58, 74, 75
  to pets, 74, 75, 76, 165, 166, 293, 384

allergists, 95, 166

almonds, 76, 172, 182, 212, 243, 277, 365

healthy recipes with, 356, 360–63, 365

alosetron (Lotronex), 233

alpha-1-antitrypsin deficiency, 133

alpha-hydroxy acids (AHAs), 72, 73, 315

alpha linolenic acid (ALA), 145

alprazolam (Xanax), 195

Altace (ramipril), 141

Altate (tolnaftate), 97

altitude sickness, 64

aluminum, 143, 160, 373

Alzheimer's disease, 15, 78–81
    brain exercises in prevention of, 78–79
    causes and contributing factors of, 27, 31, 35, 79, 80–81, 151, 260
    diet in prevention of, 17, 78, 79–81, 320
    genetics and, 79, 81
    symptoms of, 81, 372

Ambien (zolpidem), 230, 237

amitriptyline (Elavil), 233, 287

amoxicillin, 299

amputation, 270

amyloid precursor protein (APP), 80

amytrophic lateral sclerosis (ALS), 384

anaphylactic shock, 384

anemia, 191, 241, 299, 377
    iron-deficiency, 121, 172, 199

aneurysms, 379

angina, 147, 370

animals, 193, 247
    allergies to, 74, 75, 76, 92, 165, 166, 293
    avian flu and, 65

ankle swelling, 140, 141, 241, 313

antacids, 143, 160, 175, 197, 243, 299, 308, 371, 373

anti-arrhythmia drugs, 214

antibacterial products, 63, 65, 120, 188, 387
    soaps as ineffectual, 134, 156, 164, 177

antibiotics, 66, 378, 383, 384, 387, 389

heartburn and GERD as possibly caused by, 197
irritable bowel syndrome treatment and, 232–33, 249, 382
possible side effects of, 72, 157, 175, 197, 214–15, 305, 316, 317, 368, 369, 374, 378, 383
presurgery, 67–68
see also medications; specific ailments

anticonvulsants, 373

antidepressants, 15–16, 52, 83, 148, 254, 262, 265, 305, 385, 386
    hot flashes prevention with, 218–19
    irritable bowel syndrome as controlled with, 233
    for PMS and PMDD, 275
    quitting smoking as aided with, 39, 263, 385
    shingles symptoms as helped with, 287
    side effects of, 143, 160, 163, 189, 197, 214, 215, 230, 254, 369, 373, 375, 376, 377, 385, 386

antifungal sprays or powders, 97, 239

antihistamines, 75, 143, 230, 273
    side effects of, 143, 160, 163, 191, 293, 376, 377, 378, 388

anti-malaria pills, 281

antioxidants, 42, 43, 144, 187, 193, 340
    allergy prevention with, 76
    Alzheimer's disease prevention with, 80
    anxiety prevention with, 83
    bladder health increased with, 112, 310
    cancer prevention with, 112, 137, 276, 298
    joint health increased with, 86, 187
    lung health increased with, 133, 169
    male fertility and, 223
    prostate health increased with, 110, 276
    vision loss prevention with, 129, 250, 251
    wrinkle prevention with, 314–15

antispasmodic drugs, 233, 373

anti-wrinkle products, 315

anxiety, 82–83, 191
    causes and contributing factors to, 46, 83, 287, 370, 375

depression as linked to, 149–50
health conditions caused by, 82, 124, 142, 167, 305, 307
insomnia and, 229–30, 231
medications for, 82, 375, 377, 384, 386
panic attacks and, 83, 370, 375
symptoms of, 83, 385, 386
treatments and therapy for, 82, 83, 150, 235, 303, 375, 384, 385, 386

aphthous ulcers, 120–21

appendix, 366, 367

appetite, 27, 28, 369
    controlling of, 261, 262
    increase in, 155, 275, 369, 376, 389
    loss of, 69, 141, 169, 191, 203, 227, 247, 309, 366, 369, 376, 381
    sleep deprivation and, 46, 128

apple(s), 76, 77, 159, 161, 175, 187, 211, 212, 254, 310, 357, 363

apple cider, 334, 357

apple juice, 243, 322, 357

apricot(s), 159, 161, 322
    dried, bulgur salad with mint and, 329
    -oatmeal chocolate chip cookies, 359, 362

arms, 115, 167, 271
    dry or scaly skin on, 167, 291
    numbness in, 300, 303, 382
    pain in, 370, 380
    skin cancer spots on, 291
    squeezing pressure in, 147
    tingling in, 255, 379

arrhythmia, heart, 375, 384

arsenic, 59, 112

arthritis, 84–91, 150, 191, 203, 225, 264, 308, 355
    causes of, 85, 249
    exercises for prevention of, 88–91
    psoriatic, 280–81
    rheumatoid (RA), 34, 85–86, 122, 123, 129, 163, 245, 305
    symptoms of, 85, 122, 245, 378

artificial sweeteners, 208, 232

arugula, 339, 343
    salad, tuna-bean cakes with, 341, 344

treatment of, 113, 114, 173, 215, 223, 279, 305, 389

water treatment in home and, 59

Candida vulvovaginitis, 316

candy, 157,172, 175

canker sores, 120–21

canned foods, 145, 146, 207

beans, 51, 174, 212, 344, 362, 364

fish, three ideas for, 343

storing of, 62

tomatoes, 62, 261, 332, 337, 338, 350

cannellini beans, 331, 338, 344

canola oil, 33, 51, 145, 154, 163, 183, 210, 213, 225, 255, 302, 315, 321, 361, 362

in healthy recipes, 325, 328, 342, 343, 345, 352, 357–58,

car accidents, *see* traffic accidents

Carafate (sucralfate), 308–9

carbohydrates, 12, 51, 155, 175, 222, 255, 262, 315, 321, 364

simple or refined, 30, 73, 111, 133, 146, 302, 315, 320, 321, 357

"smart" sources of, 51, 146, 251

carbon dioxide, 175, 273

carbon monoxide, 38, 145, 302

prevention and detectors for, 57–58

cardiac rehabilitation programs, 140

cardia gastric cancer, 298, 299

cardiovascular disease, *see* heart disease

Cardura (doxazosin), 110

carotid endarterectomy, 302

carpal tunnel syndrome, 122–27, 382

carpets:

air quality compromised by, 57, 58, 74, 76, 166, 293

dry steam cleaning of, 74

removal of, 58

carrot(s), 43, 110, 159

healthy recipes with, 331, 332, 334, 350, 353, 355

casserole, white bean and kale, 338

Cataflam (diclofenac), 198

cataracts, 128–29, 214, 355, 388

cats, 74, 75, 77, 165

fungal infections as carried by, 96

poison ivy carried by, 272, 273

cauliflower, 112, 232, 277

healthy recipes with, 332, 351

Celebrex (celecoxib), 225, 246

celecoxib (Celebrex), 225, 246

celery root (celeriac), 334

Celexa (citalopram), 233

celiac disease, 120, 367, 374, 381, 386

cell phones, 67, 257

cellulitis, 389

central diabetes insipidus, 376

central-line catheters, 68

cereals, 51, 77, 111, 121, 142, 146, 151, 155, 159, 172, 183, 193, 227, 243, 251, 260, 266, 356

overnight oat and wheat berry hot, 322

cervical cancer, 18, 130–31, 285

cetylpyridinium chloride, 188

chamomile tea, 229

Chantix (varenicline), 246

chasteberry, 199, 274–75

cheddar cheese, 50, 351

cheese, 50, 113, 120, 154, 155, 172, 183, 207, 210, 227, 243, 251, 254, 255, 266, 301, 321

healthy recipes with, 331, 333, 338, 339, 345, 348–49, 351

quick-and-easy mac 'n, with veggies, 351

chemoprevention, 114

chemotherapy, 68, 113, 149, 173, 305

cherries, 186–87, 310

dried, 254, 322

cherry tomatoes, 328, 344, 354

chest, scaly skin or rash on, 167, 287

chest pain, 109, 144, 195, 197, 247, 371, 375, 376, 381, 384, 385, 389

types and possible causes of, 147, 370, 380, 384

chicken, 50, 65, 79, 124, 157, 159, 180, 186, 210, 261, 262, 279, 334-35, 345

chickenpox, 286, 287

chickpea(s), 138, 151

and carrot salad, 355

children, 248, 299

allergy prevention in, 77, 94

asthma and, 92, 94, 95, 176

breastfeeding of, 77, 94, 268, 269

canker sores in, 121

chronic bronchitis in, 117

developmental disorders in, 58, 59

diet of, 77, 94, 166, 224

eczema and, 166, 167

food poisoning in, 181

hepatitis vaccinations for, 202, 203

sneezing and, 177

stomach bugs in, 297

tonsil removal in, 121

chile peppers, *see* peppers, hot

chills, 69, 117, 135, 249, 287, 383

chlamydia, 223, 284, 285, 387

chlorhexidine, 67, 120

chlorine, 59, 164

chloroform, 59

chocolate, 120, 157, 175, 194, 195, 225, 232, 243

-banana muffins, nutty whole wheat, 358, 359

dark, *see* dark chocolate

"truffles" with almonds and figs, 365

chocolate chip(s), 358

cookies, oatmeal-apricot, 359, 362

in dark chocolate celebration cake with raspberries, 359, 364

choking, 384

cholesterol, HDL, 27, 31, 32, 33, 55, 123, 144, 147, 183, 210–13, 243, 253, 271

cholesterol, LDL, 24, 27, 31, 32, 33, 50, 111, 144, 147, 183, 210–13, 271, 301

cholesterol ratio, bad, 12, 16, 32–33, 42, 210–13, 301, 302

Alzheimer's link to, 80–81

BPH as possibly linked with, 111

causes and contributing factors of, 24, 27, 31, 32, 36, 44, 45, 210–11, 212, 213, 270

exercise in lowering or preventing of, 16, 32, 33, 212–13, 301

gallstones as caused by, 182, 183

eggs, 128, 213, 250, 314, 336, 348, 357, 358, 360, 362, 364
allergy to, 374, 381, 384

egg whites, 336, 339, 344, 362

Elavil (amitriptyline), 233, 287

electrocardiogram (EKG or ECG), 302

electrolytes, 156, 372, 374, 375, 378

electromyogram (EMG), 307

Elidel (pimecrolimus) cream, 166–67

emphysema, 11, 15, 132, 168–69
symptoms of, 169, 371, 384

Enbrel (etanercept), 280–81

encephalitis, 63, 249

endocrine disorders, 373

endocrinologists, 389

endometrial cancer, 199, 387

endometriosis, 223, 253

endoscopies, 367, 380

EPA, 145–46, 163

epicatechin, 315

Epi-pens, 384

erectile dysfunction, 15, 170–71

eructio nervosa, 109

erythromycin, 72

Escherichia coli, 62, 181, 311, 374, 380

escitalopram (Lexapro), 233

esomeprazole (Nexium), 94, 196, 265, 299

esophagus, 367
cancer in, 38
heartburn and GERD in, 194–97, 371, 380

estrogen, 110, 111, 114, 115, 131, 199, 218, 219, 253, 264, 267, 269, 274, 275, 387

etanercept (Enbrel), 280–81

ethanol (ethyl alcohol), 65, 135, 177

Evista (raloxifene), 114, 264

exercise, 11, 13, 14, 16, 36, 37, 40–41, 63, 155, 251, 282, 320, 378, 382
blood pressure lowered with, 12, 25, 48, 144, 208, 301

bone strength increased with, 214, 264, 265, 266
for brain, 78–79, 372
breathing, 54, 82–83, 121, 169, 191, 196, 231, 281, 303, 375
bursitis and tendinitis risk in, 118–19
calorie-burning rates in, 111
heart-related health as helped with, 389
introducing daily regimen of, 40–41
isometric jaw, 306, 307
Kegel, 220
lack of, 12, 14, 25, 26, 30, 32, 34, 98, 101, 154, 155, 170, 213, 312, 313, 373
showers after, 67, 96, 97
stretching, 84, 102–7, 118, 119, 123, 125–27, 231, 256, 257, 258–59, 382
weight loss and, 40, 98, 219, 244, 245, 260, 262, 263, 385
weight training as, 40, 85, 118, 119, 150, 265
see also specific ailments; specific forms of exercise

exertion headaches, 379

eyedrops, 129, 162, 163, 184-85, 388

eye exams, 45, 129, 184, 185, 214

eyelids, inflammation of, 163

eye masks, 229, 236

eyes, 69, 128, 129, 162-63, 191, 379
blurred vision in, 129, 163, 185, 191, 285, 303, 315, 372, 375, 376, 379, 382, 388, 389
burning in, 283, 388
cataracts in, 128–29, 214, 355, 388
glaucoma in, 184–85, 388
high blood pressure and damage to, 25, 48
injuries to, 184, 388
itchy, 75, 162–63
macular degeneration in, 148, 250–51, 355, 388
vision problems in, 25, 48, 148, 302, 303, 372, 388

ezetimibe (Zetia), 16

ezopiclone (Lunesta), 230

F

face:
dry or scaly skin on, 167, 281, 291
numbness or tingling in, 302, 379, 382
pain in, 303
paralysis in, 249, 301
reddened skin on, 283, 287, 291

face masks, 69, 168, 169, 273

facial cleansers, 315

fainting, 303, 375

fallopian tubes, 268, 387

famciclovir (Famvir), 204, 287

family history, *see* genetics

famotidine (Pepcid), 94, 196, 265

Famvir (famciclovir), 204, 287

fast food, 34, 50, 154, 207, 211, 261, 298–99, 303

fat(s), 111, 115, 144, 159, 162, 213, 263, 373
calories from, 50, 111, 155, 210, 255, 320, 321
diets low in, 210, 252–53, 254, 255
hydrogenated oils or, 32, 33, 34, 35, 50, 77, 155, 210–11, 320, 356
intra-abdominal, *see* intra-abdominal fat
polyunsaturated, 277
saturated, *see* saturated fat
trans, 51, 94, 154, 210–11, 320

fatigue, 58, 85, 109, 141, 203, 227, 237, 249, 285, 289, 292, 303, 312, 379, 382
prevention and reduction strategies for, 172–73
types and possible causes of, 377
see also specific aliments

fats, good, 32, 33, 51, 94, 139, 145, 151, 154, 160, 163, 211, 212, 213, 277, 315, 317, 320
daily serving goals for, 320, 321
monounsaturated as, 32, 170, 211, 212, 277, 321
omega-3 fatty acids as, *see* omega-3 fatty acids
recipes with good sources of, 322–65

fecal occult blood test, 299

gastrointestinal infections, 235, 260, 381

gastroscopy, 371, 386

gels, 72, 165, 283
  sanitizing, 65, 116, 117, 135, 177

generalized anxiety disorder, 83

genetics, 11–12, 19, 44, 45, 84, 85, 243, 312, 313, 315, 368
  see also specific ailments

genital herpes, 204, 205, 383

genital warts, 284, 285, 383

germs, *see* bacteria

ghrelin, 46, 155

ginger, 175, 380
  healthy recipes with, 325, 336, 342, 355, 363

ginkgo biloba, 47

glaucoma, 184–85, 388

glomerular filtration rate (GFR), 240–41

glucocorticoid drugs, 226

glucose (blood sugar), 30, 31, 42, 68, 154, 155, 190, 317, 331, 372, 389
  impaired fasting, 128

gluten intolerance, 120, 174, 175, 281, 374, 386

glycemic index (GI), 317

gonorrhea, 284, 285, 383, 387

gout, 186–87

grapefruit, 62, 276, 298, 303

grapefruit juice, 243

grapes, 42, 62, 76, 77, 175, 187
  mixed greens with pears, and honey-glazed walnuts, 324

grape tomatoes:
  healthy recipes with, 328, 354
  roasted green beans and, 347, 354

Grave's disease, 369, 376, 386

green beans, 77
  healthy recipes with, 332, 346, 347, 354

greens with salmon and lemon dressing, 343

green tea, 76, 153, 276, 353

grilled chicken and peach salad with watercress, 325, 335

grinding teeth, 306, 307

guaifenesin, 116, 289

gum, 157, 175, 195, 306
  nicotine, 38–39, 112, 246

gum disease, 30, 34, 35, 147, 241, 247
  prevention strategies for, 188–89
  symptoms of, 189

gyms, 40, 85, 115, 183, 219, 228
  guarding against infection at, 67, 96–97, 238–39

H

H$_2$ blockers, 94, 175, 196, 265

hair growth, excess, 385, 387

hair loss, 271, 278, 369, 376, 377, 385, 386

Halcion (triazolam), 195

hallucinations, 378

ham, 133, 159, 180, 298

hands, 167
  exercises for, 125–27
  numbness in, 123, 241, 381, 382
  pain in, 85, 123
  scaly skin on, 167, 281, 285, 291
  skin cancer spots on, 291
  swelling in, 85, 376, 381
  washing of, 65, 66–67, 68–69, 116–17, 134, 156, 177, 179, 181, 203, 296, 297, 299

hay fever, 74, 76

HDL cholesterol, 27, 31, 32, 33, 55, 123, 144, 147, 183, 210–13, 243, 253, 271

headaches, 15, 143, 151, 177, 225, 237, 241, 249, 257, 274, 275, 287, 302, 303, 307, 372, 373, 374, 375, 382, 388
  cluster, 190, 191, 379
  possible causes and treatments for, 191, 379, 381
  prevention strategies for, 190–91
  tension, 53, 190, 191, 379
  see also migraines

head injuries, 80, 372, 380

health:
  clean hands and, 65, 66–67, 68–69, 116–17, 134, 135, 156–57, 177, 179, 181, 203, 296, 297, 299
  diet and, *see* diet
  disease prevention strategies for, *see* prevention strategies
  emotional well-being as linked to, 11, 13–14, 16, 17
  exercise and, *see* exercise
  finding inner strength and motivation for, 14, 16–17
  germ-fighting and removal for, 60–61, 65, 66–68, 116–17, 134, 135, 156–57, 177, 180–81, 296–97, 299
  higher sense of purpose and religion in, 13, 14, 36, 37, 55, 83
  relationships and social interaction as contributing to, 13–14, 36, 37, 49, 53–54, 55, 83, 149, 150, 173
  screenings for, 11, 36, 37, 44–45
  sleep requirements and, 13, 35, 37, 46
  stress as detrimental to, 12, 14, 16, 17, 25, 26, 28, 29, 34, 36, 53
  symptoms that should never be ignored in, 366–89
  traveling tips for, 62–66, 69, 135, 156, 163, 177, 297, 374
  see also mental health; *specific diseases or ailments*

hearing loss, 192–93, 375
  tinnitus and, 304, 305

hearing tests, 45

heart arrhythmia, 375, 384

heart attacks, 12, 16, 38, 44, 48, 50, 82, 144, 147, 187, 270, 271, 292
  aspirin and, 47, 370, 375, 380
  congestive heart failure risk after, 140, 141
  symptoms of, 370, 375, 380, 384
  top six causes of, 24, 25, 27, 29, 33, 35, 206, 210
  see also heart disease

heartbeat, racing, 82, 83, 141, 303, 370, 375, 378

heartburn, 109, 175, 370, 371, 380
  prevention strategies for, 194–97
  symptoms of, 197, 366

wound healing and, 389

see also inflammation; *specific health conditions or diseases*

immunomodulator creams, 166–67

immunotherapy, 74, 94, 166

Imodium (loperamide), 233, 235

impaired fasting glucose, 128

implants, for tinnitus, 305

impotence, 15, 170–71

incontinence, 220–21

indapamide, 240

Inderal (propranolol), 82, 254

indigestion, 109, 183, 237, 370, 380

see also heartburn

Indocin (indomethacin), 281

indomethacin (Indocin), 281

infants, vaccinations for, 202, 203

infections, 30, 141, 158, 189, 377, 379

in ear, 375, 378

fungal, 96–97, 238–39

germ-fighting tips for prevention of, 60–61, 65, 66–69, 96–97, 116–17, 134

from hospitals, 16, 66, 67–68

inflammation due to, 34

sexually transmitted, 223

sinus, 117, 133, 191

staph, 16, 61, 66–68

stomach ulcers, 34, 47, 109

of wounds, 389

see also specific types of infection

infertility, 57, 222–23, 385, 387

inflammation, 15, 34–35, 246

asthma and, 95

in brain, 78, 79

causes and contributing factors of, 26, 28, 30, 34, 46, 77, 116, 141, 147, 154, 188, 266, 269, 321

health risks and conditions caused by, 30, 31, 35, 46, 47, 138, 147, 170, 187, 246, 247, 251, 269, 299

intestinal, 158, 160, 161, 224–27, 386

in joints and ligaments, 34, 84–91, 186, 187, 245

of liver due to hepatitis, 202–3

prevention strategies for, 35, 47, 144, 152, 247, 251, 255

see also specific ailments

inflammatory bowel disease, 139, 224–27

food irritants for, 227

genetics and, 225, 227

medications for, 129

infliximab (Remicade), 281

influenza, *see* flu

inhalers, 132

for asthma, 94, 95, 370, 371, 385

nicotine, 38, 39

injuries, 65–66, 121, 244, 245, 287, 295, 382

arthritis due to, 84, 85

bone fractures, 29, 40, 214–17, 226, 264, 265, 266–67

bursitis and tendinitis, 118–19

to eye, 184, 388

head, 80, 372, 380

in heart, *see* heart disease; *specific heart-related conditions*

inflammation due to, 34, 118–19

to joints, 84, 118–19

insect repellent, 63, 248

insects, 92

allergies to, 74, 75, 92–93

insoles, 85, 119, 245

insomnia, 46, 53, 83, 172, 228–31, 369, 376, 386

anxiety and depression in, 151, 228, 229–30, 231

sleeping pills and, 163, 195, 230, 388

insulin, 28, 30, 30, 31, 81, 139, 146, 152, 154, 155, 183

insulin resistance, 12–13, 30–31

causes and contributing factors of, 12, 27, 30, 31, 35, 153, 154, 155, 183, 321

health risks and conditions caused by, 12, 27, 31, 123, 152, 153, 155, 183, 243, 317

prevention strategies for, 12–13, 31

see also diabetes

intensive care unit (ICU), 68

internal bleeding, 367

intestinal gas, *see* flatulence; gas, intestinal

intestinal viruses, 65

intestines:

diverticular disease and, 158, 159, 161, 373

gas in, *see* flatulence; gas, intestinal

gluten intolerance and, 120, 174, 175, 281, 374, 386

inflammatory bowel disease and, 175, 224–27, 367, 374, 378, 381, 386

irritable bowel syndrome and, 156, 174, 175, 232–35, 367, 373, 374, 381

ulcers in, 15, 308, 309

see also digestion; *specific gastrointestinal conditions*

intra-abdominal fat, 12–13, 26–27

causes of, 14, 26, 28, 53

health risks caused by, 12, 27, 30, 31, 34, 79, 123, 147, 152, 154, 155, 182, 206, 243, 271

prevention strategies for, 12–13, 27

in vitro fertilization (IVF), 223

iron, low levels of, 172, 173, 305

iron-deficiency anemia, 121, 172, 199

iron supplements, 143, 160, 197, 199, 367, 373

irregular heartbeat, 375

irritability, 83, 151, 191, 274, 275, 377

irritable bowel syndrome (IBS), 156, 232–35

foods as triggers of, 232–33

medications for, 232–33, 235, 373

symptoms of, 174, 175, 235, 367, 373, 374, 381

ischemic strokes, 25

itching, 77, 164–67, 241, 384

athlete's foot and, 64, 96–97, 238

in eyes, 75, 162–63

jock itch and, 96, 238–39

poison ivy and, 272–73

vaginal, 316–17, 383, 387

varicose veins and, 312, 313

IUDs, 198–99, 252, 387

IvyBlock, 273

J

jalapeño peppers, 326, 328, 352

jaundice, 203

jaw pain, 147, 289, 304-7, 380

jet lag, 236–37

jock itch, 96, 238

jogging, 17, 111, 150, 160, 183, 193, 228, 253, 265

joints, 87, 99
   arthritis in, *see* arthritis
   bursitis and tendinitis in, 118–19
   gout and, 186, 187
   injuries to, 84, 118–19
   knee pain and, 244–45
   pain in, 43, 187, 203, 378, 382
   TMJ and, 304–5, 306–7

juice:
   pasteurized, 181
   urinary tract infection prevention with, 310, 311
   see also specific types of juice

junk food, 14, 43, 151, 183, 194-95, 207, 224, 225, 251, 261, 315
   cancer risk as increased with, 247, 298–99
   cholesterol as raised by, 210–11, 212
   diverticular disease risk as increased with, 159
   healthy substitutes for, 51, 153–54, 159, 210, 212, 224–25, 247, 251, 261, 301–2
   hydrogenated fats or oils in, 34, 35, 51, 210–11
   inflammation as caused by, 34, 35, 154, 247
   insulin resistance and high blood sugar as caused by, 31, 111, 153, 154–55, 251
   soda as, 51, 53, 209, 225, 315
   stroke risk increased with, 301–2, 303
   see also saturated fat

K

kale, 112, 128, 250, 266, 267
   casserole, white bean and, 338

Kegel exercises, 220

kidney beans, *see* cannellini beans

kidney cancer, 38, 368

kidney disease, 15, 240–41, 243
   symptoms of, 241, 377, 389

kidney failure, 140, 187, 203
   high blood pressure as cause of, 25, 48
   symptoms of, 376, 381

kidney infections, 367, 368, 378, 383

kidneys, 206, 368

kidney stones, 241, 242–43
   symptoms of, 243, 367, 368, 383

knee, 85, 118, 213, 281

knee pain, 244–45

L

Lachesis, 219

lactalbumin, 187

lactase tablets, 227

lactobacillus bacteria, 134, 157, 161, 226, 235, 316

lactose intolerance, 174, 175, 367, 374, 381

Lamisil AT (terbinafine), 97, 239

Lamisil Ultra (butenafine), 97

lansoprazole (Prevacid), 196

laryngitis, 197

laryngoscopes, 384

lasagna, whole wheat, with mushrooms and Swiss chard, 348–49

laser therapy, 368

LASIK surgery, 163

late summer minestrone with basil pesto, 332–33

laundry detergent, 167

laxatives, 175, 233, 374

LDL cholesterol, 24, 27, 31, 32, 33, 50, 111, 144, 147, 183, 210–13, 271, 301

lean beef burgers with blue cheese nuggets, 335, 339

left ventricular hypertrophy, 141

legs, 303

numbness or weakness in, 271, 302, 382, 389
pain in, 270, 271, 303, 313, 389
peripheral vascular disease in, 270–71
scaly skin on, 281
sores on, 271, 371, 389
swelling in, 140, 141, 312, 313
tingling in, 255
unequal length in, 245
varicose veins in, 312–13

legumes, 139, 159, 170, 252, 317, 321

lemon(s), 298, 337, 342, 343

lemon juice, 330, 331, 343, 355, 363

lentil(s), 79, 138, 151, 193
   and whole wheat orzo ragout with spinach, 350

levamisole, 121

Levitra (vardenafil), 171

levonorgestrel, 198–99

Levsin (hyoscyamine), 233

Lexapro (escitalopram), 233

lifestyle factors, 10–22, 161, 163, 196, 373
   diseases as linked to, 11–14; *see also specific diseases and ailments*
   memory and mental clarity as affected by, 17
   mental health and, 11, 13–14, 16, 17, 36
   motivation and inner strength in changing of, 14, 16–17, 41
   obesity as caused by, 261, 262
   quiz on rating health and, 19–22
   relationships and social interaction in, 13–14, 29, 36, 37
   sedentary habits in, 12, 14, 25, 26, 30, 32, 34, 98, 101, 154, 155, 170, 213, 312, 313, 373
   sleep as, 13, 35, 37, 46
   smoking and, *see* smoking
   working with doctors on advice for, 17–18
   see also diet; exercise; health; prevention strategies

light box, 236

light bulbs, 215

light therapy, 73, 281

nitric oxide, 25, 309

nitrites, 59, 60, 133, 169, 298

nitroglycerin pills, 370, 375, 380

nitrosamides, 298, 299

nizatidine (Axid), 196

n-nitroso compounds (NOCs), 137

non-cardia gastric cancer, 298, 299

non-Hodgkin's lymphoma, 122, 123

nonsteroidal anti-inflammatory drugs (NSAIDs), 78, 198, 225, 308–9, 382

norepinephrine, 28, 262

Noritate (metronidazole), 283, 299

Norpramin (desipramine), 233

nose, 379
    blowing of, 288
    nasal sprays or rinses for, 75–76, 134, 135, 246, 288–89
    runny, 58, 75, 109, 135, 370, 378
    sense of smell and, 38, 289
    stuffy, *see* congestion

notriptyline (Pamelor), 233

NSAIDs (nonsteroidal anti-inflammatory drugs), 78, 198, 225, 308–9, 382

numbness, 123, 241, 271, 287, 303, 372, 375, 388, 389
    types and possible causes of, 382

nursing homes, 214, 215, 220

nutritional deficiencies, 121, 389

Nutrition Facts labels, 51

nuts, 32, 33, 51, 79, 94, 111, 113, 117, 128, 145, 154, 161, 170, 172, 182, 207, 212, 213, 224, 243, 251, 252, 254, 314, 317, 321, 384
    see also specific types of nuts

NuvaRing (vaginal ring), 252

O

oak, poison, 272–73

oat bran, 193, 208

oatmeal, 32, 51, 142, 146, 172, 200, 210, 211, 309

oats, 33, 276, 298, 356, 362

obesity, 11, 43, 79, 140, 201, 203, 260–63, 321
    asthma symptoms worsened with, 93, 95
    BPH risk as increased with, 111
    breast cancer risk as increased with, 114–15
    bursitis and tendinitis risk as increased with, 119
    colorectal cancer risk increased with, 139
    congestive heart failure risk as increased with, 140
    diverticular disease risk as increased with, 161
    gallstone risk as increased with, 182
    gum disease as possibly linked to, 189
    infertility risk as increased with, 222
    losing weight and prevention of, 260–63
    sleep deprivation as contributing to, 46, 155, 228
    see also weight, excessive; weight loss

obstructive sleep apnea (OSA), 27, 172, 231, 292–95
    diagnosing of, 241
    health risks due to, 208–9, 241, 292, 294
    prevention and treatment of, 292–94
    symptoms of, 295, 377
    see also snoring

ocular rosacea, 163

oils, 145, 238, 281
    fish, 77, 82, 94, 137, 145, 146, 160, 163, 225, 315
    flaxseed, 163
    hydrogenated, 33, 35, 50, 51, 77, 155, 210–11, 320
    in poison ivy, 272–73
    in skin, 72, 315
    unhealthy versions of, 51, 151, 251, 255, 277, 321

olive oil, 32, 33, 50, 51, 77, 132, 133, 139, 154, 170, 183, 210, 213, 224, 247, 255, 261, 277, 302, 314, 321
    in healthy recipes, 323, 324, 329, 331, 333, 337–38, 340, 343, 345–46, 348–51, 354–55, 362

olives, 43, 252, 317

omega-3 fatty acids, 55, 251, 320, 321
    in Alzheimer's disease prevention, 78
    in depression prevention, 151
    dry eyes prevention with, 162, 163
    for healthy or wrinkle-free skin, 166, 315
    heart benefits of, 145, 277
    inflammation prevention with, 160, 166, 224–25, 251
    in intestinal infection prevention, 160, 224–25
    in menstrual cramp relief, 253
    in prostate cancer prevention, 277, 279
    recipes as good sources of, 324, 342, 346

omega-6 fatty acids, 151, 251

omeprazole (Prilosec), 94, 196, 265, 299

onions, 76, 110, 137, 180, 195, 254
    healthy recipes with, 323, 325, 330–32, 336–40, 343–45, 350, 352, 355

ophthalmologist, 129, 162, 184, 185

Oracea, 283

oral appliances, 293–94

oral cancer, 389

oral contraceptives, *see* birth control pills

oral sex, 285, 317

orange juice, 42, 207, 213, 243, 266, 274, 314
    in healthy recipes, 323, 329, 355, 362

orange peppers, 86, 345

oranges, 62, 77, 86, 146, 159, 161, 189, 298, 364
    mandarin, 128

orthotics, 119

orzo ragout, lentil and whole wheat, with spinach, 350

oseltamivir (Tamiflu), 69, 177

osteoarthritis, 84, 85, 87, 245

osteoporosis, 56, 133, 264–67
    causes and contributing factors of, 29, 35, 133, 264, 265–66
    depression as raising risk of, 29, 265–66

hip fractures and, 214, 215, 264, 265, 267
inflammatory bowel disease as raising risk of, 226
medications for, 197, 226, 264, 383
screening tests for, 44, 45, 267
ovarian cancer, 268–69, 387
ovarian cysts, 223, 383
ovaries, inflammation or infection in, 387
oxycodone, 143
oxygen therapy, 384

P

PABA-free sunscreen, 290
packing suitcases, 63–64
Padimate O, 282
paella, brown rice, 335, 337
painkillers, 143, 160, 197, 225, 252, 369, 373, 382
for migraines, 254, 379, 381
see also specific pain killers
pain relievers, 191, 198, 225, 386, 388
see also aspirin; ibuprofen; specific pain relievers
palm oil, 51, 255
pancakes, 152, 200, 310
syrup for, 157, 175
pancreas, 26, 28, 30, 31
pancreatic disease, 370
pandemic, flu, 68
panic attacks, 83, 370, 375, 384
panic disorder, 82
panko, healthy recipes with, 336, 339, 344, 351
pantoprazole (Protonix), 196
Pap tests, 45, 130
paralysis, facial, 249
Parkinson's disease, 171, 230, 373
Parmesan cheese, 333, 338, 346, 348
paroxetine (Paxil), 16, 219, 233
parsley, 331, 345, 355
Parsol 1789 (avobenzone), 290, 314

pasta, 73, 175, 255, 261, 262
patches, nicotine, 38, 39, 246
Paxil (paroxetine), 16, 219, 233
peach(es), 86, 159, 161, 175, 254, 310
peak flow meters, 94–95
peanut(s), 75, 79, 154, 243
dressing, napa cabbage slaw with, 353
in healthy recipes, 326, 341, 352, 356
peanut butter, 83, 172
in healthy recipes, 352, 353, 356
peanut oil, 342
pear(s), 32, 146, 175, 187, 212, 233, 309
and apple compote, slow-cooker, 363
dried, 254
peas, 86, 138, 146, 159, 250, 276
in brown rice paella, 337
canned, 62
snow, 343
pelvic exams, 45
pelvic inflammatory disease, 223, 366, 387
pelvic pain, 131, 285
penis, 239, 285, 383
penne with parsley-walnut pesto and green beans, 346, 347
Pepcid (famotidine), 94, 196, 265
peppermint, 173
peppermint-oil capsules, 234
peppers, bell, 110, 137
peppers, bell, green, 336
healthy recipes with, 326, 329, 337, 345
peppers, bell, red, 43, 86, 189, 303, 323
healthy recipes with, 325, 326, 329, 332, 337, 342, 345, 348
peppers, hot, 43, 282
healthy recipes with, 326, 328, 351, 352
see also specific types of hot peppers
peptic ulcers, 109, 236
Pepto-Bismol, 64, 156, 367
perfumes, 164, 167, 317
perindopril, 240

periodic fever, aphthousstomatitis, pharyngitis, and adenitis (PFAPA) syndrome, 121
periods, heavy, 198–99
peripheral vascular disease (PVD), 25, 270–71, 389
permethrin, 63, 248
pesticides, 57, 59, 63, 74, 94, 248
Petadolex, 255
pets, 49, 77, 150, 157
allergies to, 74, 75, 76, 165, 166, 293, 384
poison ivy carried by, 272, 273
phlegm, *see* mucus
photodynamic therapy, 388
physical therapy, 119, 382
phytoestrogens, 110–11, 218
Pilates, 100
pillows, 256, 295
pimecrolimus (Elidel) cream, 166–67
pineapple, 62, 137
pine nuts, 329, 333, 346
pinto beans, 182, 208, 212
pipe smoking, 132, 168
pistachios, bulgur pudding with golden raisins and, 360
plane travel, health tips for, 62–63, 69, 135, 163, 177
plantain, 208
plaque:
brain, 78, 80, 81
in heart and arteries, 16, 24, 27, 29, 33, 35, 48, 133, 144, 145, 147, 170, 171, 210, 212, 270, 271, 301, 303, 389
tooth and gum, 188, 189
pneumonia, 15, 16, 18, 188, 247
acute, 384
symptoms of, 370, 378, 384
vaccination for, 44, 64, 68, 117, 132, 168, 378
poisoning, food, 61
poison ivy, 272–73
pollen, 75, 76, 165, 167, 230, 384
pollution, 42, 57, 74, 116, 117, 133
polychlorinated biphenyls (PCBs), 58

polycystic ovary syndrome (PCOS), 223, 385, 387

polyethylene glycol (Miralax), 233

polyps, colon, 136, 367

polysomnography, 241

polyunsaturated fats, 277

pomegranate juice, 80, 340

Ponstel (mefenamic acid), 198

pores, skin, opening of, 72–73

pork, 50, 159, 232, 261
    healthy recipes with, 340, 345
    safe temperature reading for, 62, 180

portion control, 43, 220, 260, 261–62, 320

post-herpetic neuralgia (PHN), 286–87

posture, 98–99, 122, 257, 305

potassium, 156, 197, 207, 242, 382

potassium citrate, 242, 243

potato(es), 12, 51, 120, 159, 175, 190, 207, 227, 251, 314

potatoes, sweet, 42, 76
    healthy recipes with, 336, 352

poultry, 50, 62, 79, 121, 159, 247, 340
    cooking and storing of, 62, 157, 178, 179–80, 181
    recipes for, 334–38
    safe temperature reading for, 62, 157, 179, 180, 325, 334, 336
    see also specific types of poultry

powders, antifungal, 97, 239

prediabetes, 152, 155
    see also blood sugar, high; insulin resistance

prednisone, 226

pregnancy, 122, 123, 142, 145, 176, 252, 309, 317, 373
    allergy prevention and, 77
    asthma prevention and, 94
    eczema prevention and, 166
    hemorrhoids due to, 200, 201
    incontinence and, 220, 221
    miscarriages in, 59, 223, 309, 387
    morning sickness in, 380
    varicose veins in, 312, 313

water treatment and, 59
    weight gain and, 263

prehypertension, 24, 44, 48, 209, 301

premenstrual dysphoric disorder (PDD), 274, 275

premenstrual syndrome (PMS), 274–75

presbyopia, 388

prescription medications, 15–16, 39, 63, 69, 73, 82, 96, 97, 116, 120, 142, 143, 160, 162, 163, 173, 177, 191, 196–97, 198, 201, 204–5, 214–15, 225, 239, 263, 273, 281, 289, 291, 308–9, 315, 369, 379

Prevacid (lansoprazole), 196

prevention strategies, 11–18, 36–55
    for accidents and injuries, 65–66
    air quality maintenance and, *see* air quality maintenance
    air travel and, 62–63, 69, 135, 163, 177
    aspirin regimen as, 11, 37, 47, 78, 254
    for bad cholesterol ratio, 16, 33, 36, 41, 50–51, 55, 210–13, 271
    clean hands and, 65, 66–67, 68–69, 134, 135, 156–57, 177, 179, 181, 203, 296, 297, 299
    flu bacteria and, 68–69
    food safety tips, 61–62, 156, 157, 178–81, 297, 299
    germ-fighting and removal, 60–61, 65, 66–69, 116–17, 134, 135, 180–81, 238, 296–97, 299
    for heart disease, 11, 12–13, 16, 25, 33, 36, 37, 41, 43, 47, 140, 144–47
    for high blood pressure, 12–13, 25, 37, 41, 48, 55, 145, 146, 206–9, 240
    higher sense of purpose and religion as, 13, 14, 36, 37, 55, 83
    prescription drug regimens and, 15–16
    quitting smoking in, *see* smoking
    relationships and social interaction as, 13–14, 36, 37, 49, 53–54, 83, 149, 150, 173
    simple lifestyle adjustments as, 11–14, 36–43, 46, 50–51, 53–56

stress management in, 12, 13–14, 16, 17, 27, 29, 36, 37, for traveling, 62–66, 69, 135, 156, 177, 297
    vaccinations as, 11, 13, 18, 44, 64, 68
    water testing and treatment in home as, 59–60, 112, 113
    see also specific diseases and ailments

Prilosec (omeprazole), 94, 196, 265, 299

probiotics, 134, 157, 160–61, 166, 226, 235, 316

progestins, 131, 198–99, 218, 252, 275

progressive muscle relaxation, 228, 229, 234

propanolol (Inderal), 82

prophylactic antibiotics, 311

propranolol (Inderal), 82, 254

Proscar (finasteride), 110, 276

prostaglandins, 198, 252, 253

prostate:
    benign prostatic hyperplasia (BPH) of, 110–11
    enlargment of, 241, 276, 368

prostate cancer, 44, 111, 112, 221, 276–79

prostate-specific antigen (PSA) tests, 45, 276, 278–79

Protonix (pantoprazole), 196

proton-pump inhibitors (PPIs), 94, 196, 197, 265, 299, 308

Protopic (tacrolimus) cream, 166–67

Prozac (fluoxetine), 15–16, 219, 233, 275

pseudoephedrine, 143, 160

psoriasis, 54, 280–81

psychogenic polydipsia, 376

psyllium (Metamucil), 227

pulmonary disease, *see* chronic obstructive pulmonary disease (COPD)

pulmonary hypertension, 384

pulsed-dye lasers, 73

pumpkin seeds, 163, 182, 193, 208

punctal plugs, 162, 163

Homemade

how to make hundreds of everyday products fast, fresh, and more naturally

Reader's
Digest

The Reader's Digest Association, Inc.
New York, NY • Montreal

The Magic of Homemade

Many of us have a similar shopping ritual. Once a week we go to the grocery store, grab a cart, and load up with a box of this, a bottle of that, and a carton of those and these. Add to that a visit to Wal-Mart, Kmart, or Target for extra supplies, or to the warehouse club for bulk items. It's a whole lot of shopping—and spending—week after week after week.

What do we get with all these packaged products? Sure, good things like reliability and convenience. But there's more. Many everyday items are filled with incomprehensible chemicals and preservatives. You get an overflow of wasteful packaging, too (funny how our garbage cans are so much fuller these days). You also get to see your name-brand products on TV—your dollars pay for all those commercials. And, you get lots of choices—supermarket aisles are packed with mind-boggling variations of the same product.

All of this is modern life, you say. Maybe. But when it gets to the point that a window cleaner has to offer citrus orange or mountain berry flavors to get our attention, consumerism seems a bit out of control.

Our proposed solution: Make things yourself. The little-known truth is that you can replace almost everything you buy at the grocery store with a homemade version that will be cheaper, healthier, yet equally effective. That is exactly what *Homemade* is all about. On these pages, you'll find more than 700 replacement recipes for the most common items bought in stores. Not just food, mind you. Cosmetics, pet supplies, toiletries, cleaners, even everyday medicines can be made at home, easily, quickly, and effectively.

I say this with wholehearted conviction. In our home, my young sons make the barbecue and spaghetti sauces we eat all the time. My wife whips up all-natural mayonnaise, salad dressings, jams, and salsas that make us hum with delight. I whip up cleaners, bread mixes, ice cream, soup stocks, and other pantry items, sometimes just to relax. We save a lot of money. We also have great fun and get a real sense of pride.

You should do the same. These recipes are easy, clever, and unlike those you'll see in other books. You'll love the quality, you'll love the savings, and most of all, you'll love the feeling of accomplishment.

Neil Wertheimer
EDITOR IN CHIEF,
READER'S DIGEST BOOKS

contents

Part Two

*health and
beauty care
for you and
yours*

*

contents

introduction

The Joy of
Homemade Living

Homemade shampoo? Homemade ketchup? Yes, we know it sounds strange, even weird, to make your own shampoo or your own ketchup. After all, most of us are not such dedicated environmentalists or back-to-basics fundamentalists that we feel we must make every product we use from scratch like our homesteading pioneer forebears did a century and a half ago. And picking up a bottle of shampoo or ketchup at the supermarket or drugstore is not that much trouble—and in the grand scheme of things neither seems particularly expensive. And if you are buying a name brand, or even a discount house brand, you can feel relatively confident that you are getting products of reliably consistent quality that will do the job that you want them to do—a shampoo that cleans your hair with lots of bubbly lather or a condiment that will add a tangy sweetness and a bit of extra juiciness to the often dry, bland taste of your burger and fries. The giant multinational food and home products corporations are very adept at putting out innocuous uniform products with a long shelf life and eye-pleasing packaging.

So why bother to make them yourself? There are a great number of reasons that we'll explore on the following pages. For the record, these are not "replication" recipes. We don't claim to have the formula for Formula 409 or the secret of making Coca-Cola. Our versions of everyday products won't smell or look like many of the name-brand products they are replacing. But rest assured that they work—and work terrifically well.

The Rewards of Making It Yourself

As we said earlier, there are a lot of good reasons to make many common household products yourself. The first and most important reason is the real, tangible difference between your homemade product and the manufactured product it replaces. In most cases, you'll find that the quality of the homemade item is outstandingly superior to the store-bought item. Once you have made shampoo or ketchup for yourself, you will immediately know that your homemade version offers rewards that can't be duplicated by the average factory-made product—whether it be the relaxed, more natural feel of your hair after using your homemade shampoo or the richer, more exotic taste of your homemade ketchup.

The same is true of hundreds of other everyday food, beauty, health, cleaning, household, gardening, and even pet products that you routinely pick up at the supermarket, drugstore, or big-box outlet. These include salad dressings, pancake mixes, fresh pasta, pickles, cookies, breads, skin toners, lip balm, aftershave, gargles, toothpaste, pet bird treats, furniture polish, fabric softener, and pest repellents for both the house and garden. All told, you'll find recipes for more than 700 such products in this book.

Another significant reason for making these products yourself is that you'll save money—a lot of money, actually. It may not seem like much for each individual item as you buy it. Just a few dollars here and a few dollars there. But those dollars add up quickly as you buy more and more items. And with savings that range up to more than 90 percent for the homemade replacement versus a name-brand item, cumulative savings can mount rapidly.

But getting better quality and saving money are not the only rewards to be gained by creating your own homemade products. When you make something yourself, you know exactly what goes into it. So you have the enormous satisfaction of knowing that the product you made consists of ingredients that are all natural and healthful—or at least not harmful. And you know for sure that it contains no questionable extenders, stabilizers, or other artificial ingredients. Another reward of making things yourself is that you can adjust the recipe to meet your own needs or taste—making your shampoo less likely to dry out your hair or your ketchup sharper tasting.

When you make something yourself, you also create a lot less waste. And ultimately, when you create an item yourself rather than buying it, you gain a reward that can't be duplicated by anything you buy—a great feeling of self-satisfaction, the self-reliant joy brought on by the realization that you actually made the product yourself.

Here is a more detailed look at these rewards of homemade living.

Saving Money

Although it may seem like a trifling sum at times, you should not overlook the savings when you make something for yourself, because the amount you

424

save really grows the more items you make. And there are very good reasons for this. Every time you buy a bottle of ketchup for the table, shampoo for your hair, salve for an itch, or even liver snaps for your dog, only a very small percentage of the money that you pay goes to cover the costs of making the product. Indeed, if you leave out the actual cost of manufacturing, the ingredients in most products account for only pennies of the purchaser's dollar. What happens to the rest of the money that you plop down at the cashier? It goes to cover the costs of advertising, packaging, shipping, the retailer's rent and light bills, and of course the cashier's salary and her boss's bottom line. Paying a healthy chunk of your shopping dollar for advertising is especially irksome, considering advertising's well-known penchant for grossly inflating the image of a product to entice buyers. If it weren't for the happy faces, cheery jingles, and promises of better living in ads, why else would so many of us, who are otherwise rational, thrifty people, pay good money for cola drinks? After all, they are little more than fizzy water doctored up with sugar, caffeine, artificial flavoring, and brown dye. Actual lab analysis shows that colas are 99.5 percent sugar water; only 0.5 percent is flavoring and color. You can make any number of healthier, more satisfying, better-tasting thirst quenchers in your own kitchen for just a few cents each.

Similarly, a lot of the money you pay for a product goes for packaging—in many cases, the cost of the packaging surpasses the cost of the product itself. So saving your hard-earned cash for better uses is certainly a major reason for making products yourself whenever you can. The chart on page 12 gives some typical examples of how much you can save on a wide variety of products by making them yourself. Try it and watch the savings pile up.

Healthier and More Natural

Saving money, however, is not the only reason for producing your own homemade products. Even more disturbing are the compromises that have to be made to a commercial item's integrity to ensure that it will survive the weeks or months from the time it is manufactured, then shipped and stored, left on the retailer's shelf, and finally picked up and used by you. Depending on the type of product, it is pumped full of stabilizers, plasticizers, extenders, fillers, and other man-made chemicals.

Not all of those additives are there to extend shelf life. Some are added to facilitate the manufacturing process, making the product move faster, release from a mold easier, or create less interference to the smooth flow of production. Other artificial ingredients are added to help the item withstand heat and cold and to be less likely to clump, precipitate, or adhere to packaging.

Still other questionable chemicals are used to cut the cost of using natural ingredients. The best-known villain here is artificial flavoring. Why use expensive, perishable, and difficult-to-handle real strawberries when you can just add a few pinches of a chemical compound that simulates the smell and

real-life examples of savings

Before we started working on this book, we undertook a survey to see what kind of savings you could expect if you created your own homemade replacements for a wide range of brand-name items. Here are the results, and they speak for themselves. The savings are based on typical prices in early 2006 for brand-name items at mainstream suburban outlets near a major Northeastern city versus the comparable cost of ingredients to produce similar quantities of the homemade replacements.

Food	Store Price	Homemade Replacement	Savings
Chi Chi's salsa (16 ounces)	$2.79	$1.38	50%
Smucker's peanut butter (26 ounces)	$4.29	$1.24	71%
Starbucks Frappuccino (38 ounces)	$5.99	$.82	86%
Hershey's cocoa mix (7 ounces)	$3.49	$2.68	23%
Manischewitz chicken noodle soup (15 ounces)	$2.49	$1.15	53%
Aunt Jemima frozen waffles (16 waffles)	$2.99	$1.41	52%
Stubb's barbecue sauce (18 ounces)	$3.89	$1.92	50%
Pepperidge Farm croutons (16 ounces)	$1.79	$.53	70%
Hellmann's mayonnaise (32 ounces)	$3.39	$1.57	53%
Ore-Ida steak fries (28 ounces)	$3.39	$2.20	35%
Häagen-Dazs raspberry sorbet (1 pint)	$3.69	$1.18	68%
Edy's Whole Fruit Bar pops (16 ounces)	$2.75	$1.69	38%

Health, Beauty, and Pet Supplies			
Oil of Olay all-day moisturizer (6 ounces)	$9.29	$1.68	82%
Curél moisture therapy lotion (13 ounces)	$7.99	$4.62	42%
Aqua Velva aftershave (3.5 ounces)	$3.69	$.35	90%
Secret Platinum deodorant (2.7 ounces)	$3.69	$.50	86%
Robitussin cough syrup (4 ounces)	$4.69	$2.30	51%
Hall's Plus cherry lozenges (25 lozenges)	$1.99	$.33	83%
Sudafed decongestant (36 pills)	$8.99	$.65	92%
Milk-Bone dog biscuits (19 ounces)	$2.89	$1.91	33%
Whisker Lickins tuna cat treats (4.6 ounces)	$2.08	$.55	73%
Hartz parakeet food (28 ounces)	$3.99	$.87	78%

Household Compounds			
Lysol bathroom cleaner (29.3 ounces)	$3.19	$.15	95%
Cascade dishwasher soap (75.2 ounces)	$4.89	$2.96	39%
Pledge lemon furniture spray (12.5 ounces)	$3.79	$2.08	45%
Windex window cleaner (26 ounces)	$3.39	$.15	95%
Elmer's school glue (7.6 ounces)	$1.69	$.19	88%

taste of the berries? Chemical laboratories that support the food, cosmetic, and other industries actually have "sniffing" rooms lined with bottles, each containing a carefully concocted compound and labeled with the name of the fruit, flower, or other natural odors that it emulates. You didn't really believe that "lemon fresh" cleaner contains lemons, did you? No, no more than that "strawberry flavored" ice cream or candy contains real strawberries. They think that you can't taste the difference. But try the real thing side by side with the imitation and there's no question about which is the winner.

In short, anything that you make yourself is likely to be much more natural and more healthful for you than the great majority of manufactured products you buy—whether it's a food, a cosmetic, or a cleaning compound. And in the case of food, it's going to taste a lot fresher.

Suit Your Own Needs

Another great advantage of making products yourself is that you can customize them so that they are just the way you want them. If you like your moisturizer to be fresh smelling and restorative without being greasy and overwhelmingly perfumy, no problem. If you like your chocolate chip cookies to be moist and really chocolaty, no problem. If you want your spaghetti sauce tangier, your gumbo thicker, your ketchup smoother flowing, your mustard spicier, your frozen yogurt tarter, or if the doctor told you to cut back on the salt or sugar, no problem. Even if you are worried that Fido is not getting the right nutrients, no problem. Nearly all of the recipes in this book are flexible and can be readily adjusted to fit your wants or needs. Indeed, we invite you to experiment until you get a product just the way you like it. (Bread and cakes being notable exceptions; always follow the recipe for such baked goods exactly.)

Make Less Waste

In the process of making your own staples, you are going to greatly reduce the amount of useless, environment-damaging waste and garbage you produce. A lot of this is the result of all the packaging you won't be throwing away and all the spray bottles, jars, and such that you will be recycling. But you will also be cutting waste by making your products in batches small enough so that you can easily use them up without having to toss out the last part when it goes bad. For cleaning, laundering, and polishing, you will also be using compounds that are much gentler and less damaging to surfaces and fabrics—and to drains and sewage and septic systems. So when you make it yourself, you do your bit to save the world!

Get Personal Satisfaction

Last but not least among the rewards of making a product yourself is the great sense of personal satisfaction and accomplishment it brings. It's very gratifying to know not only that you can make a staple yourself, but also that you are not dependent on giant corporations and their vulnerable supply chains to satisfy your everyday needs. Being able to fashion our own food, cleaning, and other staples links us with traditions that helped shape us as a people and a nation—traditions of resourcefulness, ingenuity, independence, and self-reliance that stood our ancestors well as they struggled to fashion homes in a strange new land, tame frontiers, and endure the constraints of wartimes and depressions.

Expect to be pleasantly surprised by how really simple and easy it is to make many of the products that you are accustomed to buying ready-made—whether they be peanut butter or pancake mix at your local supermarket, chicken nuggets at a fast-food outlet, lip balm at the cosmetics counter, foot powder at the drugstore, liver snaps at the pet store, furniture polish and bug spray at the home and garden center, or gumdrops at the newsstand. Recipes for these products and more than 700 others are in the chapters that follow. None of the recipes are difficult to make and none call for a lot of ingredients. But first here are some tips that will make your homemade efforts easier and more successful.

Creating Your Own Food Products

The recipes in Part 1 of this book cover some 400 commonly purchased food products that you can make in your own kitchen. There are recipes for making items to stock your pantry, refrigerator, and freezer—or for creating fast on-the-spot replacements for such items. And there are recipes that let you make many foods that you would normally buy already prepared—and spend a great deal of money in the process. All told, they cover condiments, seasonings, sauces, pickled and preserved foods, baked goods, snack food, drinks, convenience dishes, candy, ice cream, and other sweets.

You don't need a large kitchen or a whole battery of equipment to be a good cook, but there are certain well-designed tools that will make your work in the kitchen go faster and more smoothly. Shop for new equipment at a reputable kitchen supply store. Good, sturdy kitchen tools will serve you well for a long, long time and are well worth the initial investment. A Well-Equipped Kitchen (page 16) shows a listing of the pots, pans, and other gear for food preparation and cooking that make life in the kitchen easier.

Before You Start ...

Take stock of your pots and pans. You want your pots and pans to conduct heat evenly (hot spots cause burning and uneven cooking), and you want at least one skillet and one pan with a nonstick interior coating for low-fat cooking. Here are your choices:
- Cast-iron cookware heats slowly and evenly, but needs special care to prevent rust. It is porous and absorbs flavors and reacts badly to some foods, especially acidic ones.

- Enameled cast iron has all the advantages of cast iron, plus it is nonreactive, but it is heavy to lift and you must take care not to chip the enamel.
- Aluminum conducts heat well, but reacts badly with acidic food, and lightweight aluminum pans tend to dent and warp easily.
- Anodized aluminum is a better choice because it is heavier and less prone to warping. Its surface finish makes it less reactive than plain aluminum.
- Clad metal pots are made of several metals fused together to take advantage of each one's properties—copper for even heat and stainless steel for easy cleaning, for example.
- Tin-lined copper pots are beautiful to look at and cook as well as or better than other pans; they are also very expensive and their maintenance is labor-intensive. Not only must they be polished frequently on the outside, but they also must be regularly re-tinned on the inside.

Check out your large appliances. Use an oven thermometer to check that your oven actually registers the heat it is set for. If it is only 5 to 10 degrees off, you can compensate by setting it higher or lower than the recipe requires. If the settings are more than 10 degrees off, call in a repairperson to recalibrate the stove.

Also check the temperatures of your freezer and refrigerator with a refrigerator/freezer thermometer. The freezer should read 0°F and the refrigerator 40°F. If either of them is above those standards, use a colder setting. Also check the door gasket for wear and consider putting in a new gasket to make the door seal tighter. You don't want to risk freezing lots of foods in a freezer that isn't as cold as it should be or risk the deterioration of refrigerated foods that are stored above 40°F.

Evaluate your freezer space. Making your own food is most efficient when you do it in batches large enough to last for a while. When you make a large pot of stock, for example, it will be most useful if you freeze some of it in ice cube trays and the rest in 1-cup or 2-cup containers. If you put the frozen stock cubes in a freezer bag, you will find it easy to add a little stock to a sauce or gravy to make it more flavorful. Save the larger 1- or 2-cup containers for making soups and stews that call for homemade stock.

You also need space for containers of Savory Meat Mix (page 166), which gives you a head start on many fast dinners. Use plastic containers (square ones use freezer space more efficiently than round ones) or heavy-duty plastic zipper bags, which take up even less space. Extra pancakes or waffles or muffins can also be frozen in freezer bags to make speedy but delicious breakfasts. Freezing the best summer and fall offerings of your local farmers' market will require more room too. Once you start stocking up on a regular basis, you may want to consider an auxiliary freezer. But be sure not to locate it in a place where it will be exposed to below-freezing temperatures—like a porch, carport, or unheated garage; freezers, surprisingly, don't work properly when ambient temperatures drop below freezing.

a well-equipped kitchen

When making the food recipes in this book, you don't need any specialized equipment beyond what you would ordinarily use for preparing meals. Here is a list of items that any well-outfitted kitchen should have.

Pots and Pans

10-inch skillet with a tight-fitting lid

7-inch skillet

3-quart saucepan with a tight-fitting lid

1-quart saucepan with a tight-fitting lid

4- to 5-quart Dutch oven or heavy kettle

4-gallon stock pot/pasta pot

Roasting pan, 13 x 9 x 2 inches with rack

Broiler pan with rack

Baking Equipment

2 baking sheets

1 jelly-roll pan

Loaf pan, 9 x 5 x 3 inches

1-quart microwave-safe casserole

2-quart microwave-safe casserole

3 nesting mixing bowls

2 six-cup muffin pans

8-inch or 9-inch cake pans

8-inch or 9-inch pie pans

2 wire cooling racks

Knives

8- to 10-inch chef's knife

2- to 4-inch paring knife

9- to 10-inch serrated bread knife

6-inch utility knife

Small Appliances

Blender or food processor

Coffee maker

Ice-cream maker

Microwave oven

Slow cooker

Waffle iron

Accessories

Candy thermometer

Can opener

Citrus juicer

Colander

Corkscrew

Cutting board

Expandable steamer

Flour sifter

Funnels

Grater

Knife sharpener

Ladle

Long-handled spoon

Measuring cups (dry and liquid)

Measuring spoons

Pancake turner

Pastry blender

Pepper mill

Rolling pin

Rubber spatulas

Salad spinner

Sieves

Slotted spoon

Tongs

Vegetable parer

Whisks

Whistling teakettle

Wooden spoons

As a Precaution ...

- When you preserve any foods by canning them, be especially careful to use only jars intended for canning. Be sure to sterilize the jars and treat the preserves in a hot-water bath (page 72) and to use only fresh seals on the jars. Canning is very safe as long as you observe these simple precautions. This applies to condiments and pickles as well as jams and jellies.
- Keep your knives sharpened. Most kitchen cutting accidents are the result of dull knives. Store knives in a wooden block or on a magnetic rack. Knives in drawers get nicked and lose their sharp cutting edges.
- Take special precautions with raw eggs; salmonella is still a problem; you need to cook the eggs at 160°F for a minute or two to be safe.
- Identify and date everything that you freeze or can. Try to put new packages below the older packages in the freezer and behind the newer jams or pickles on the cupboard shelf.
- If anything you have frozen or canned has an "off" color or odor when you open the package, discard it immediately.

Store leftover foods in covered containers or plastic bags and put them in the refrigerator right away. Never leave cooked meat, poultry, or fish at room temperature for more than two hours, including mealtime. This rule applies to the Thanksgiving turkey too. Foods in a slow cooker are kept at 165°F, just hot enough to kill harmful bacteria.

Creating Health and Beauty Products

Part 2 of this book covers more than 225 homemade beauty and health products and similar products you can make for your pets. You may at first be skeptical about making your own cosmetics or home remedies. It's only natural. Commercial over-the-counter medications and beauty products are both so expensive (and well advertised) and promise so much that you may feel reluctant to compete—or to compromise your skin, hair or health, or that of your pet.

But you should have no such trepidations. Both home remedies and home-made beauty products have a long and honored tradition. And truth be told, many commercial products are little more than dressed-up versions of classic home preparations—whether it be a cough syrup or a spa skin treatment. In the case of homemade cosmetics, it's best to start slowly—with a single mois-turizer, for example, and see how it feels and smells on your skin. Try treating your hair after a shampoo with a vinegar hair rinse. Then try one of the facial masks and a toner. Little by little, you will be won over to these fresh, natural products and want to make more and more of them on a regular basis.

Being able to instantly create your own home remedies is reassuring. You don't have to run to the drugstore or call the doctor every time you or another family member feels a little off. In this book, you'll find more than 100 remedies for the most common ailments that can slow you and your family down—remedies that make life a little more pleasant by making everyday ailments less irritating and long-lived. Hopefully, they'll keep you out of the doctor's office or the emergency room. But remember, home remedies do not take the place of conventional medicine; they complement it. If you don't respond to a home remedy, see a doctor. Let the doctor know how you have treated yourself. Talk to your doctor about the home remedies that have helped you and your family. Doctors will often offer you a few of their own to add to your repertory.

Making your own pet supplies gives you control over the quality of the food and care that your animals receive. Making nontoxic flea dips and ear oils, for example, will keep your dogs and cats healthier and make them less dangerous to the people who pet them. Commercial flea collars and at-the-shoulder dabs are poisonous to people too.

Follow the recipe closely. Read the recipes carefully and don't be tempted to use more of any ingredient than what is called for. Make sure you know the difference between regular oils and essential oils. Regular, or "fixed," oils, such as olive oil or canola oil, are the same nonvolatile mostly seed-derived oils that we use for cooking, while essential oils, such as geranium, lavender, or lemon oils, are highly concentrated volatile distillations of leaves and flowers much like perfume (see page 240). They are called essential because they capture the essence of the plant. Most essential oils must be diluted in a regular fixed oil before they are applied to the skin. In this case the regular oil is known as a carrier oil. Essential oils are expensive—it takes many, many pounds of leaves or petals to make even a few ounces of these concentrated oils. You need very little essential oil in each recipe; to conserve your supply, keep it in a cool, dark place. Many people keep them in the refrigerator, but this is not recommended if there is any chance that someone may mistake these oils, which are toxic, for a food and ingest them.

Find your ingredients. You can buy the ingredients for most home remedies and beauty products in health food stores, the supermarket, drugstores—or these days on the Internet. Even specialized ingredients are no longer as difficult to find as they once were. But because herbs and essential oils are not regulated by the government, make your purchases at a reputable store to ensure quality. You can buy many dried herbs at the supermarket, but ideally you will eventually grow and dry your own. You can buy seeds or seedlings for many fresh herbs at garden centers and nurseries; plant them in a sunny patch of soil or in pots on a sunny windowsill. If local gardening outlets don't have an herb you want, you can find many mail-order sources on the Internet.

The ingredients for pet foods and care products are found in groceries, pet shops, natural food stores, garden centers, and for a couple of recipes, liquor stores. None of the ingredients are particularly exotic or difficult to locate.

Take care with equipment. Although you use ordinary cookware to make home remedies or beauty products, it is best to keep this equipment separate from your regular kitchenware—to avoid contaminating foodstuffs. A list of the items you may need is given in Home Remedies and Cosmetics Gear (opposite). You can probably pick up whatever you need at garage sales or stores that sell odd lots of equipment for reduced prices. Making pet products doesn't involve any special equipment other than what you probably already have in your kitchen.

Select safe storage jars and dispensers. While shopping, look for small opaque jars with wide mouths and tight-fitting lids for storing your beauty creams or skin ointments. Because they have no preservatives, they need to be kept away from light and air. Any tinted or colored glass—amber, white, or blue—protects creams from light. Keeping a cream in a small container that it fills almost completely protects it from air. In fact, when you use up half a jar of cream, decant the remaining cream into a smaller jar to protect it further. Tight-fitting lids are important to keep out air and prevent evaporation. Cork lids are too porous to be safe.

Also be on the lookout for spray bottles and pint-size bottles with tight lids for mouthwashes and such. Many of the jars that you need you can probably recycle from your regular kitchen and bathroom supplies. It is smart to sterilize any storage jars before you use them (page 72). Wash plastic spray bottles thoroughly in soap and hot water, rinse thoroughly, and let them air-dry.

As a Precaution …

- If you are taking a prescription drug, talk to your doctor about possible interactions between it and any herbs or essential oils suggested here.
- If you have allergic reactions to any foods or medications, consult your doctor before taking any home remedy that might contain the allergen.
- If you are pregnant, don't take any herbal medications without consulting your doctor.
- Although side effects from using natural cosmetics are uncommon, allergic reactions can occur in susceptible people. If you have a reaction, immediately stop using the product.
- If you are planning to use an herb that is new to you, patch-test it first. Rub the herb against the tender skin on the underside of your arm right above the elbow or in the crease of the elbow. Wait overnight. If redness or another irritation occurs, don't use it.
- Essential oils should not be used on young children or pregnant women. Check with a doctor before using products with essential oils if you have a chronic or acute disorder such as heart disease, epilepsy, asthma, diabetes, or kidney disease.
- Do not swallow or even taste essential oils. Keep bottles and jars sealed and out of the reach of children. Don't keep them in the refrigerator if you have children.
- If an essential oil is accidentally swallowed, do not induce vomiting. Call a poison hotline or get the person to an emergency room immediately.

home remedies and cosmetics gear

You will need nonreactive equipment to protect your health or beauty products from chemical changes in color and odor. That means avoiding uncoated aluminum, iron, or copper cookware.

To make either beauty or health products, you need:

- Glass, stainless steel, or enameled double boiler
- Set of nonreactive mixing bowls
- Stainless steel or ceramic funnel
- Stainless steel measuring and stirring spoons
- Wooden stirring and mashing spoons
- Stainless steel or ceramic lemon squeezer
- Teakettle
- Ceramic tea bowls and cups
- Tea strainer
- Candy thermometer (for cough drops)

Be sure to label each new jar or bottle of a beauty product as you fill it. The label should give the product's name and the date on which it was prepared. If you are planning to give a homemade beauty product as a gift, list its ingredients as well (you don't want to inadvertently cause an allergic reaction). Labeling is important because many of these preparations look alike in the bottle and many have a limited shelf life.

Store natural products in a cool, dark place (page 255), preferably a dry one, and check them often. Heat, moisture, light, and contact with air can all cause deterioration. Particularly in the summer, the refrigerator is probably the safest place to store homemade cosmetics (again, though, not if you have young children). Even in the refrigerator, you should inspect them regularly to be sure they have not lost their potency. If a product is discolored or has a funny smell, chances are it is past its prime. Discard it and make a new batch.

Most of the home remedy recipes are for products that are intended to be used immediately or within a few days, so if you store a remedy at all, the safest place is in the refrigerator. You can keep some ointments and other remedies for longer; each recipe will advise you. If you do keep remedies longer, label and date them.

Making Products for the House and Garden

Part 3 of this book covers more than 115 useful household and gardening products that you can make—including cleaning and polishing compounds, glue and craft supplies, indoor and outdoor pest repellents, weed killers, fertilizers and soil conditioners, even houseplant food and whitewash. Having simple, nontoxic aids and remedies for house and garden undertakings and problems makes maintenance chores much more pleasant—and much, much cheaper. And none of these recipes are difficult to produce.

Cleaning and polishing your home or getting rid of weeds and pests in the garden may produce very gratifying results, but the processes involved can hardly be described as fun. So, it is no wonder that most of us are tempted by heavily promoted new products that promise to make cleaning and polishing, doing the laundry, or weeding and pest control easier and longer lasting. To avoid the drudgery and tedium of cleaning or weeding, such promises seem worth every penny, no matter what the price. But whether you are dealing with a cleanser, a polish, a bleach, a weed spray, or an insecticide, the problem with many of those commercial products is that they contain harsh and toxic chemicals that may be hard on grime, tarnish, stains, bugs, and other undesirable things, but they are also hard on furniture, floors, clothes, and shrubs—and hard on your skin, eyes, and lungs as well.

The good news is that there are many inexpensive, time-proven products that will make help your garden flourish and your house sparkle, smell good, and gleam invitingly without such toxic effects. You probably already have most of the ingredients for these homemade products on hand. Try making up one of the cleaning recipes and using it. It won't take long, cost much money, or require excessive elbow grease. Expect to be happily surprised.

Once you accept that there are easy, inexpensive ways to foil the pests that have plagued your woolens in the past, you won't find putting away winter clothes so onerous. Keeping ants and roaches out of the cupboards is no problem either when you get out the borax. And as you discover inexpensive, nontoxic ways to keep pests out of a summer garden, you may finally be able to raise the herbs and vegetables you have dreamed about with enrichment from your own compost heap. Or you may finally put together the container garden that you have pictured in your sunroom.

Before You Start …

Find your ingredients. None of the ingredients required for the cleaning, polishing, crafts, gardening, and other household recipes are particularly exotic. If you don't already have them, you can buy most of them at your local supermarket or hardware store. Just keep these tips in mind:

- Get the largest, cheapest sizes of baking soda, cider vinegar, and white vinegar. House brands are fine. You don't need giant sizes of chlorine bleach or ammonia, however, because the recipes that do use them call for very little of either.
- You'll find borax and washing soda among the detergents in a supermarket.
- Look for castile soap, glycerin, and essential oils at health food stores and on many Internet sites.
- Rubbing alcohol is also called isopropyl alcohol, and you can find an inexpensive house brand at any drugstore.
- Boiled linseed oil and materials needed for paints and finishes are available at paint, art supply, or hardware stores. You can find equipment and tallow for candle making at craft stores.
- One traditional cleaning-compound ingredient that you won't be able to find easily or inexpensively is, surprisingly, soap flakes. The last major national brand of soap flakes (Ivory Snow) was converted to a mild detergent more than 30 years ago. But it is very simple to make your own soap flakes by simply lightly grating a bar of pure soap (such as Ivory) on a coarse grater.

Make garden puttering easier. You will need some large containers for mixing soil and making compost tea. You can use plastic garbage cans or find large buckets at janitorial supply stores—or even better, yard sales. If you have unusually clayey, sandy, or other problematic soil, it's best to have the soil tested before adjusting it with homemade nutrients. To get your soil tested, contact your local Cooperative Extension Service—usually affiliated with a state university's agriculture school or listed on the government pages under the U. S. Department of Agriculture.

For potting and taking care of container plants, it's a good idea to devise a potting table, where you can work on your plants and keep extra pots, homemade fertilizers and pesticides, potting soil, and other planting supplies. Like a kitchen counter, the table should be waist high and have shelves above for storage of fertilizers and pesticides out of the reach of children and shelves below for large containers of compost, vermiculite, or sand. You can make such a gardening workstation in the garage or on a covered porch.

As a Precaution ...

- Never combine chlorine bleach and ammonia. While either of these powerful cleaning ingredients is perfectly safe to use alone, they can form a deadly noxious gas if they are mixed together.
- Label any cleaning compounds, pesticides, compost teas, and other fertilizers that you make and keep the containers out of the reach of children.
- Wear vinyl gloves to protect your hands when you are mixing and using household and gardening products.
- It is unlikely that anyone might ingest the essential oils used in homemade air fresheners in Chapter 10, but if an essential oil is accidentally swallowed, observe the same precautions noted earlier: Don't induce vomiting; call a poison center or rush the patient to an emergency room.

When You Are Done ...

Most of the cleaning and polishing compounds, craft supplies, pest repellents, and other household and gardening compounds in this book are best prepared just before you use them so that you get the maximum potency and best results out of them. Most are so simple to make, anyway, that you can whip them up in only a couple of minutes. But as the recipes advise, you can store some products, such as scouring powders and some cleaning and bug-control compounds, for periods ranging from a few days up to a couple of weeks. When you do, be sure to put them in tightly closed labeled and dated jars or spray bottles.

recycle rags and spray bottles

There are many ways to keep down the cost of household supplies besides using the recipes in the following chapters. One is to recycle worn or outgrown family clothing as rags for cleaning, polishing, and crafts. Cloth diapers make famously good rags. Old cotton T-shirts and underpants are also very good candidates. Well-worn terrycloth towels absorb water better than anything. And best of all, these rags can be tossed in the washer and used over and over again. Also, finish cleaning windows with newspaper. So, you may never buy paper towels again (at least for cleaning) or expensive disposable rags.

Wash out old empty spray bottles and reuse them for your homemade household or gardening products. (If you do need to buy some, try a garden center or a janitorial supply store; they are listed in the yellow pages.)

Part One

in the kitchen

*

Replacements for Pantry Staples

Nowhere do the benefits of making your own pay off more generously than in the kitchen, especially in making replacements for the cereals, condiments,

salad dressings, seasonings, sauces, and mixes that line your pantry shelves. To give them an almost indefinite shelf life, these manufactured staples are more likely than any other food products to be packed with fillers, preservatives, stabilizers, and other unnatural taste-degrading ingredients. In this chapter, you will not only learn how easy it is to make your own all-natural versions of these staples but also discover how much better a homemade creation tastes. Homemade stock has real flavor. And there is nothing like freshly ground peanut butter that melts in your mouth or fresh pasta so delectably light that it makes any sauce seem tastier.

None of the staple substitutes here have the extraordinary shelf life of manufactured products. But you will find healthy nutty breakfast cereals that will keep their fresh taste for weeks, as well as everyday condiments, ranging from ketchup and mustard that will last for months to fresh salsas that are best eaten in a day or two. Most salad dressings and both savory and sweet sauces are also best if used right away—they only take a minute to whip up anyway—but several will keep in the fridge for a couple of days, and there are salad dressing mixes you can prepare ahead. Most herbs and seasonings and dry mixes will keep for weeks or months, as will fresh pasta and stocks if frozen.

breakfast cereals

Toasted Muesli
This is a favorite Swiss-German morning cereal based on oats and fruit. Packaged versions are quite pricey and not nearly as good.

2 cups old-fashioned oats

1/4 cup sunflower kernels

1/4 cup sliced almonds

1/3 cup finely chopped dates

2 tablespoons oat bran

1 cup bran flakes

1/4 cup toasted wheat germ

1/4 cup raisins

1 tablespoon sugar

1. Preheat the oven to 350°F. In a 15 x 10-inch baking pan, combine the oats, sunflower kernels, and almonds. Bake for 10 to 15 minutes or until the almonds are almost golden.

2. In a large bowl, combine the dates and oat bran, and stir to coat the fruit with the bran. Add the toasted oat mixture, bran flakes, wheat germ, raisins, and sugar. Stir to gently combine all the ingredients.

3. Place the muesli in an airtight container or a self-sealing plastic bag. Label and date, and store in a cool, dry place.

Makes 3 1/2 cups (about 7 servings)

Helpful Hint

Why Make Your Own Breakfast Cereals?
Cereals are a frequent drain on the family budget. The homemade alternatives that are shown here have less sugar and salt and more fiber, making them a much healthier choice for you and your family. They are also generally cheaper, if you look for good prices on grains, nuts, seeds, and dried fruits in the bulk aisles of discount health food supermarkets.

Fruit and Nut Cereal
Packed with protein and high in complex carbohydrates, this tasty mix will keep you going well into lunchtime.

2 cups 1-minute oatmeal

1 cup crumbled shredded wheat

1 cup bran or bran cereal

1 cup wheat germ

1 cup unsalted walnuts, almonds, pecans, or cashews

1/2 cup chopped pitted dates

1 cup chopped dried prunes, apricots, pears, apples, or bananas

1 cup light or dark raisins

1 cup instant nonfat dry milk

1. In a large bowl, combine the oatmeal, wheat flakes, bran, wheat germ, and nuts. Add the dates and dried fruit, and toss to combine the ingredients and coat the fruit with the oatmeal mixture. Add the raisins and dry milk, and stir gently to combine the ingredients thoroughly.

2. Place the cereal in an airtight container or self-sealing plastic bag. Label and date, and store for up to 2 months in the refrigerator.

Makes about 9 1/2 cups

Granola

Packed with nutrition and good taste, granola is the ultimate win-win combination. Eat it with milk for breakfast; sprinkle it on fruit, yogurt, or ice cream; incorporate it into crumble toppings for cobblers; crush it to make crusts for pies or cheesecakes—or just grab a handful for a healthy, energy-boosting snack. To cut the cost of homemade granola, check out the bulk sales aisles of health food supermarkets, such as Whole Foods, Sunflower, or Wild Oats.

4 cups old-fashioned rolled oats

1 cup natural wheat and barley cereal

1 cup sliced unblanched almonds

1/2 cup firmly packed light brown sugar

1 teaspoon salt

1 teaspoon ground cinnamon

1/4 cup frozen apple juice concentrate, thawed

1/4 cup water

2 tablespoons butter, melted

2 tablespoons vegetable oil

2 tablespoons honey

1 teaspoon vanilla

Grated zest of 1 orange

1 cup dried pitted cherries

1 cup light seedless raisins

1. Preheat the oven to 300°F. Lightly coat a 15 x 10-inch jelly-roll pan with nonstick cooking spray and set aside.

2. In a large bowl, combine the rolled oats, cereal, almonds, brown sugar, salt, and cinnamon; set aside. In a small bowl, whisk together the apple juice concentrate, water, butter, oil, honey, vanilla, and orange zest. Pour the juice mixture over the oat mixture and toss until all the ingredients are well combined. Spread the mixture evenly in the prepared pan.

3. Bake, stirring every 15 minutes, until golden and slightly crunchy, about 1 hour.

4. Remove the pan to a rack to cool completely, about 1 hour. When cooled, stir in the cherries and raisins. Store in an airtight container.

Makes 7 cups

Oatmeal Mix

Ready-to-eat oatmeal mixes are a godsend on busy mornings when you need a healthy breakfast in a hurry. The prepackaged mixes are pricey. So whip up your own—and vary it depending on your family's tastes.

6 cups quick-cooking oats

1 1/3 cups dry milk

1 cup dried diced or small apples, apricots, banana slices, prunes, raisins, or mixed dried berries

1/4 cup sugar

1/4 cup brown sugar

1 tablespoon ground cinnamon

1 teaspoon salt

1/4 teaspoon ground cloves

1. In a large bowl, combine all the ingredients and toss to mix well.

2. Store the oatmeal mix in an airtight container or self-sealing plastic bag. Label, date, and store in a cool, dry place for up to 6 months.

To use: Shake the mix well before using. In a saucepan, bring 1/2 cup water to a boil. Slowly stir in 1/2 cup of oatmeal mix. Reduce the heat and cook, stirring, for 1 minute. Remove the pan from the heat, cover, and let stand for 1 minute more or until the oatmeal is the desired consistency.

Makes 8 cups

condiments and spreads

Ketchup
Forget about buying this American staple—homemade is so much better and an inspired way to use up those extra tomatoes at the end of summer.

4 quarts (about 24) ripe tomatoes, peeled, cored, and chopped

1 large yellow onion, chopped

1 large red bell pepper, cored, seeded, and chopped

1 1/2 teaspoons celery seed

1 teaspoon mustard seed

1 teaspoon whole allspice

1 stick cinnamon

1 cup firmly packed brown sugar

1 tablespoon salt

1 1/2 cups cider vinegar

1 tablespoon paprika

1. In a large, nonreactive saucepan or Dutch oven over moderate heat, combine the tomatoes, onion, and red bell pepper, and cook until the vegetables are soft. Using a food mill or a sieve, press the vegetables through to make a puree. Return the vegetable puree to the saucepan.

2. Over high heat, cook the vegetable puree rapidly until it is thick and the volume is reduced by about half, about 1 hour.

3. Cut a 4-inch square of cheesecloth. Place the celery seed, mustard seed, allspice, and cinnamon stick in the center, gather up the corners to form a bag, and secure with kitchen string. Add the spice bag, brown sugar, and salt to the tomato mixture. Over low heat, cook the mixture gently for 25 minutes, stirring frequently.

4. Stir in the cider vinegar and paprika. Continue to cook, stirring frequently, until the mixture is thick.

5. Spoon the ketchup into 3 hot, sterilized pint jars, leaving a 1/8-inch space between the top of the ketchup and the rim of the jar. Wipe the rims, cover, and process for 10 minutes in boiling water (see Safe Canning with a Hot-Water Bath, page 72). Cool and test for airtight seals. Label, date, and store in a cool, dark place for up to one year; the ketchup will be ready to eat in 1 week. Once a jar has been opened, store the ketchup in the refrigerator.

Makes 3 pints

Cocktail Sauce
The zesty side to shrimp and other seafood. To dial up the heat, add more horseradish or hot red pepper sauce. This is not only cheaper than bottled cocktail sauce, but you can mix ingredients to suit your taste.

1 cup Ketchup (above) or bottled chili sauce

1 tablespoon prepared horseradish

1 tablespoon lemon juice

1/2 teaspoon Worcestershire sauce

1/8 teaspoon hot red pepper sauce

1. In a small, nonreactive bowl, combine all the ingredients and stir until well blended. Cover the bowl and refrigerate for at least 1 hour before serving.

2. Store in an airtight container in the refrigerator for up to 1 month.

Makes about 1 cup

Mustard

Named for the plant that produces the seeds from which the powder is made, this versatile condiment is easily made and adjusted to suit a particular taste or use. The basic mix includes 2 to 3 tablespoons of a liquid (vinegar, wine, water, flat beer) to about 1/4 cup dry mustard. Other additions can include turmeric (which gives a bright yellow tint), garlic, tarragon, sugar or honey, salt, and more. Use it to spice up hot dogs, hamburgers, or sandwiches, or brush over meats before grilling or roasting.

1/3 cup mustard seed

3 tablespoons dry mustard

1/2 cup cider vinegar

1/2 cup dark beer

2 garlic cloves, minced

1/4 cup firmly packed light brown sugar

3/4 teaspoon salt

1/2 teaspoon ground ginger

1/4 teaspoon ground allspice

1. In a small bowl, combine the mustard seed, dry mustard, and cider vinegar. Cover the bowl with plastic wrap and let the mustard mixture stand at room temperature for 3 hours.

2. In a small saucepan, combine the dark beer, garlic, brown sugar, salt, ginger, and allspice. Stir in the mustard mixture. Over moderate heat, bring the mixture to a boil; reduce the heat to low and simmer for 5 minutes, stirring occasionally.

3. Spoon the mustard into a hot, clean canning jar and seal tightly. Let the mustard cool to room temperature. Store in a cool, dark place and in the refrigerator after opening.

Makes about 2 cups

Mayonnaise

Homemade mayonnaise tastes so good that it improves all the salads and sandwiches it gets used in. Our version is boiled, eliminating any fear of salmonella contamination from raw eggs. You can experiment with lemon juice for the vinegar and different oil. You also might try cayenne for the white pepper.

4 egg yolks

2 tablespoons water

1 tablespoon white wine vinegar

1 1/2 cups vegetable oil (or a combination of vegetable and olive oils)

Pinch ground white pepper

1. In the bowl of a food processor or blender, combine the egg yolks, water, and vinegar, and whirl just until the ingredients are combined. With the motor running, drizzle in the oil *very slowly*; if the oil is added too quickly, it will become a liquid dressing.

2. Transfer the egg mixture to the top of a double boiler and cook until a thermometer placed in the sauce registers 160°F. Stir in the white pepper. Store in the refrigerator for up to 5 days.

Makes 2 1/3 cups

Aioli (Garlic Mayonnaise)

Traditionally served with poached fish, aioli (pronounced eye-oh-lee) can also be used as a dip for fresh vegetables or seafood, or as a salad dressing. Homemade is delicious and much less pricey.

4 egg yolks

2 tablespoons water

1 tablespoon white wine vinegar

1 garlic clove, minced

1/2 cup fresh white bread crumbs

1 1/2 cups extra-virgin olive oil

Pinch ground cayenne pepper

1. In the bowl of a food processor or blender, combine the egg yolks, water, vinegar, garlic, and bread crumbs, and whirl just until the ingredients are combined. With the motor running, drizzle in the oil *very slowly*; if the oil is added too quickly, it will become a liquid dressing.

2. Transfer the egg mixture to the top of a double boiler and cook until a thermometer placed in the sauce registers 160°F. Stir in the cayenne pepper. Store in the refrigerator for up to 5 days.

Makes 3 cups

Tartar Sauce

When you have tasted a homemade version of this classic fish accompaniment, you won't waste your money on prepared tartar sauces.

1/2 cup Mayonnaise (page 29)

1/2 cup reduced-fat sour cream

6 scallions, minced

1/4 cup chopped Bread-and-Butter Pickles (page 67)

2 tablespoons lemon juice

1 tablespoon capers, drained

1 tablespoon minced parsley

1 tablespoon Dijon mustard

1. In a medium bowl, combine all the ingredients and stir until well blended.

2. Cover the bowl and refrigerate for 2 hours or overnight before using. Store in the refrigerator for up to 5 days.

Makes 1 1/4 cups

Spicy Tomato Salsa

Once relegated to Mexican and Southwestern cuisine, salsa has moved permanently into the mainstream. The spiciness can vary from very mild to tongue-burning hot, depending on the variety of chiles used and how many are included. Experiment until you get it just right for your taste. The zesty mix of tomatoes, scallions, and jalapeño peppers in this basic recipe is not just for tortilla dipping; dollop it on grilled chicken breasts, firm fish, in skirt or flank steak fajitas, or omelets.

3 medium ripe tomatoes, cored, seeded, and chopped

3 small scallions, trimmed and coarsely chopped

1 medium jalapeño pepper, cored, seeded, and finely chopped (wear gloves when handling; they burn)

1 garlic clove, minced

3/4 teaspoon salt

1/3 cup coarsely chopped fresh cilantro

1. In a large, nonreactive bowl, combine the tomatoes, scallions, jalapeño pepper, garlic, and salt. Toss to combine all the ingredients well. Let the salsa stand for 1 hour to let the flavors mellow.

2. Just before serving, toss in the chopped cilantro. Serve immediately or store in the refrigerator for up to 2 days.

Makes 3 1/2 cups

Tomato Basil Salsa

An Italian variation on the old favorite, this salsa may tickle your tastes too.

1 pound ripe tomatoes, peeled and chopped

1 small red onion, peeled and chopped

1 garlic clove, crushed

1 tablespoon extra-virgin olive oil

1/4 cup chopped fresh basil

Salt and freshly ground pepper, to taste

1. In a large, nonreactive bowl, combine the tomatoes, onion, garlic, olive oil, and basil; toss to combine all the ingredients. Add salt and pepper.

2. Cover the bowl and refrigerate for 2 to 4 hours to allow the flavors to develop. The salsa is best eaten on the day it is made but will keep, covered, in the refrigerator for 2 to 3 days.

Makes 2 to 3 cups

Salsa Verde

This green homemade salsa is a mixture of fresh herbs, garlic, capers, and salty anchovies that is sensational with seafood.

2/3 cup flat-leaf parsley

2/3 cup fresh basil leaves

1 garlic clove, halved

1/4 cup capers, drained

2 tablespoons chopped anchovies

3 tablespoons red wine vinegar

1/3 cup extra-virgin olive oil

1/2 teaspoon Dijon mustard

Freshly ground black pepper, to taste

1. Combine the parsley, basil, garlic, capers, and anchovies in the container of a food processor or blender. Whirl until the mixture is very smooth.

2. Stir in the vinegar, olive oil, and mustard. Add pepper. Serve immediately or store in the refrigerator for up to 2 days.

Makes about 1 cup

the story behind peanut butter

This will come as no surprise to nutritionists, but peanut butter was originally sold as a health food—which indeed it is, being an excellent source of protein, fiber, and B vitamins. Unlike today, when peanut butter is a staple of most average households, in its early years, it was mostly eaten by wealthy folks who frequented health spas.

Using ground peanuts as a food spread can be traced back to early Native American and African peoples, but for the modern face of marketed peanut butter, you find a name usually associated with another product: cereal. John Harvey Kellogg of Battle Creek, Michigan, was granted the first U.S. patent in 1895 to process peanuts.

Peanut Butter
This American staple can really eat up your budget. Surprisingly, peanut butter is not only cheaper to make at home, but healthier too.

4 cups shelled, salted dry-roasted peanuts

1 tablespoon plus 1 teaspoon safflower or other mild-flavored vegetable oil

For creamy style: Using a food processor or blender, and working in batches, process the peanuts and the oil until the desired consistency is reached. Stop and scrape down the processor container sides as needed.

For chunky style: Using a food processor or blender, coarse chop about 1/3 of the peanuts; set aside. Working in batches, process the remaining peanuts with the oil until the desired consistency is reached. Scrape down the processor container sides as needed. Stir in the chopped peanuts.

To store: Scrape the peanut butter into a clean container with an airtight lid. Store in the refrigerator for up to 1 month.

Makes 1 cup

Apple Butter
Try spreading this on raisin bread or bran muffins—yum! Some apples to use for this butter: Cortland, McIntosh, or Northern Spy. You can buy it, but homemade is much, much better.

3/4 cup unsweetened apple cider or juice

1/3 cup firmly packed light brown sugar

1 teaspoon ground cinnamon

1/2 teaspoon ground cloves

1/2 teaspoon ground allspice

3 pounds (6 medium) apples, peeled, quartered, and cored

1. In the bowl of a food processor or blender, combine the apple cider, brown sugar, cinnamon, cloves, and allspice. Whirl until all the ingredients are well blended. Add the apple quarters, 2 or 3 at a time, and whirl until the apples are pureed.

2. Pour the apple mixture into a large, nonreactive saucepan. Over moderately high heat, bring the mixture to a boil; reduce the heat to low, cover the saucepan, and cook for 1 hour, stirring occasionally. Uncover the saucepan and cook until the apple mixture is thickened, about 1 to 1 1/2 hours longer.

3. Spoon the apple butter into 2 widemouthed, warm, sterilized half-pint jars, leaving a 1/2-inch space between the top of the jam and the rim of the jar (see Safe Canning with a Hot-Water Bath, page 72). Wipe the rims, cover, label, and date. Store the jam in the refrigerator for up to 3 weeks or in the freezer for up to 1 year.

Makes 2 half-pint jars

salad dressings

Classic Vinaigrette

The classic salad dressing that can be (and should be) whipped up just before serving, then used sparingly over the freshest mixed greens. Since all the ingredients used in vinaigrette are pantry staples, this is a gourmet touch that is quick and easy to make and not costly at all.

1/4 cup extra-virgin or virgin olive oil

4 teaspoons vinegar (white wine, red wine, tarragon, etc.) or fresh lemon juice

1/2 teaspoon salt

Freshly ground pepper, to taste

In a small, nonreactive bowl, whisk together all the ingredients until well blended. Use immediately.

Makes 1/4 cup

Herb Vinaigrette

Fresh herbs give a heightened taste to this vinaigrette that you will never get from a bottled version.

1/4 cup extra-virgin or virgin olive oil

4 teaspoons vinegar (white wine, red wine, tarragon, etc.) or fresh lemon juice

1 tablespoon minced fresh herb, such as tarragon, basil, chives, or parsley

1/2 teaspoon salt

Freshly ground pepper, to taste

In a small, nonreactive bowl, whisk together all the ingredients until well blended. Use immediately.

Makes 1/4 cup

Mustard Vinaigrette

This is a classic dressing often served in good French restaurants.

1/4 cup extra-virgin or virgin olive oil

4 teaspoons vinegar (white wine, red wine, tarragon, etc.) or fresh lemon juice

1 teaspoon Dijon mustard

1/2 teaspoon salt

Freshly ground pepper, to taste

In a small, nonreactive bowl, whisk together all the ingredients until well blended. Use immediately.

Makes 1/4 cup

Garlic Vinaigrette
Experiment with different vinegars and/or lemon juice when you make this dressing.

1/4 cup extra-virgin or virgin olive oil

4 teaspoons vinegar (white wine, red wine, tarragon, etc.) or fresh lemon juice

1 clove blanched and chopped garlic or 1 clove pressed garlic

1/2 teaspoon salt

Freshly ground pepper, to taste

In a small, nonreactive bowl, whisk together all the ingredients until well blended. Use immediately.

Makes 1/4 cup

---

flavored oil

Surprisingly easy to make and packing a powerful flavor punch in salads, flavored oils make fabulous gifts too. Make these oils in small quantities, because they are perishable. Lower-moisture herbs such as rosemary, thyme, or summer savory, or spices such as coriander seed or chiles are the best choices.

To make a flavored oil, all you need are several sprigs of fresh herbs or whole spices and olive oil (enough to fill bottles).

1. Spread the herbs or spices on a clean work surface. Using a rolling pin, gently press down on the herbs or spices just to lightly bruise them.

2. In a small saucepan over low heat, warm the olive oil. Add the herbs or spices, and let steep for several minutes. Using a slotted spoon, transfer the herbs or spices to sterilized bottles, distributing them equally. Pour the warm oil on top of the herbs or spices, leaving a 1/4-inch space between the top of the oil and the rim of the bottle. Wipe the rims, cover tightly, and refrigerate for at least 2 days to allow the herbs or spices to infuse the oil.

3. Strain the oil into a new set of sterilized bottles, adding a fresh herb sprig or whole spice to each bottle. Wipe the rims, cover, label, and date. Store in the refrigerator for up to 1 month. Keep refrigerated after the oil is opened.

Balsamic Vinaigrette
Use the best balsamic vinegar and olive oil that you can afford for this dressing.

1/4 cup extra-virgin or virgin olive oil

4 teaspoons balsamic vinegar

1 tablespoon minced fresh basil

1/2 teaspoon salt

Freshly ground pepper, to taste

In a small, nonreactive bowl, whisk together all the ingredients until well blended. Use immediately.

Makes 1/4 cup

Replacements for Pantry Staples **449**

Orange and Almond Oil Dressing

A delicate variation on a classic vinaigrette base, this dressing uses orange juice in place of vinegar.

3 tablespoons orange juice

4 tablespoons almond oil

2 tablespoons canola, sunflower, or extra-virgin olive oil

Salt and freshly ground pepper, to taste

1. In a small, nonreactive bowl, combine the orange juice, almond oil, and vegetable or olive oil. Whisk together until the ingredients are well blended. Add salt and pepper. Whisk vigorously again just before using.

2. Store in an airtight container for up to 1 week in the refrigerator; bring to room temperature and whisk well before using.

Makes about 1/2 cup

Raspberry Vinaigrette

Sweet, tart, tangy—this will quickly become a family favorite. Homemade is better and half the price of the bottled version.

2 jars (12 ounces each) seedless raspberry preserves

1 1/4 cups sugar

1/4 cup water

1/3 cup chopped sweet onion

1/4 cup balsamic vinegar

1 tablespoon dried tarragon

1 tablespoon curry powder

1 teaspoon ground white pepper

1 teaspoon ground black pepper

1 cup extra-virgin or virgin olive oil

1. In a large, nonreactive saucepan over high heat, combine the raspberry preserves and 3/4 cup of the sugar to a boil. Remove the saucepan from the heat and let cool slightly. Pour the raspberry mixture into the bowl of a food processor or blender. Add the water, onion, vinegar, tarragon, curry powder, white pepper, black pepper, and the remaining sugar.

2. Cover and whirl, adding the olive oil in a slow, steady stream, until the ingredients are well blended and the dressing has a smooth consistency. Use immediately or store in an airtight container in the refrigerator for up to 1 week. Bring to room temperature and whisk vigorously before using.

Makes about 4 cups

Buttermilk Dressing Mix

This mix is easy to make and keep on hand for whenever you need a creamy dressing for salad or dip for crudités. It is cheap and convenient and wonderful.

4 1/2 cups buttermilk powder

1 1/2 cups freeze-dried chives

1/2 cup dried dill, crumbled

1/2 cup sugar

1/4 cup dry mustard

1. Whisk together all the ingredients until well blended.

2. Store the mix in an airtight, 2-quart jar in the refrigerator for up to 1 month.

Makes about 7 cups

Buttermilk Dressing

This is a delicious dressing for any tossed green or Caesar-style salad as well as for bean or pasta salads.

10 tablespoons Buttermilk Dressing Mix (opposite)

1 cup warm water

1/4 cup cider vinegar

2 tablespoons sour cream or plain yogurt

1. Whisk together all the ingredients until well blended.

2. Let the mixture stand at room temperature for 1 hour, then stir until all the ingredients are well blended and the dressing is a smooth, creamy consistency.

Makes about 2 cups

flavored vinegar

It's easy to make your own herb-flavored vinegars, which add a great subtle taste to salads, especially ones dressed with just oil and vinegar. But remember, the finished results depend on using a high-quality vinegar as the base.

To make flavored vinegar, you only need:

Several sprigs fresh herbs as desired

High-quality vinegar (enough to fill the desired number of bottles)

Here's how to proceed:

1. Spread the herbs on a clean work surface. Using a rolling pin, gently press down on the herbs just to lightly bruise them enough to release their flavor. Place 1 sprig in each sterilized bottle.

2. In a large, nonreactive saucepan over high heat, bring the vinegar to a boil. Pour the hot vinegar over the herb sprigs in each bottle. Cover the bottles and place them in a sunny windowsill for at least 2 weeks to allow the herbs to infuse the vinegar. Turn each bottle daily.

3. Place a fresh herb sprig into each of a new set of sterilized bottles. Strain the vinegar, discarding the old herbs. Pour the flavored vinegar into the new set of bottles, over the fresh herb sprigs. Cover, label, and date. Store the flavored vinegar in a cool, dark place for up to a year; the vinegar will be ready for use in 2 weeks. Store the flavored vinegar in the refrigerator after opening.

Herb Dressing Mix

All the taste—none of the preservatives! That's what makes this mixture such a delicious bargain.

1/2 cup dried parsley, crumbled

1/4 cup dried oregano, crumbled

1/4 cup dried basil, crumbled

1/4 cup dried marjoram, crumbled

1/4 cup sugar

2 tablespoons fennel seed, crushed

2 tablespoons dry mustard

1 tablespoon ground black pepper

1. In a large, 1-quart jar, combine all the ingredients. Cover the jar and shake until all the herbs are well mixed.

2. Store the Herb Dressing Mix in a cool, dry, dark place for up to 6 weeks.

Makes 2 cups

Herb Dressing
You can adjust the strength of this eye-opening dressing by increasing or decreasing the amount of Herb Dressing Mix you add.

2 tablespoons Herb
  Dressing Mix (page 37)

1 1/2 cups warm water

2 tablespoons olive oil

5 tablespoons white or
  tarragon vinegar

2 garlic cloves, crushed

1. In a small, nonreactive bowl, whisk together all the ingredients until well blended. Let the dressing stand at room temperature for 30 minutes; whisk vigorously again and use.

2. Store the dressing in an airtight jar or bottle in the refrigerator for up to 1 week.

Makes 2 cups

Ranch Dressing Mix
Classic, creamy, dreamy—this mix makes it easy to whip up some ranch dressing on demand, for tossing with salads, dipping with crudités, or soothing the fires of Buffalo wings.

2 tablespoons plus 2 teaspoons
  dried minced onion

1 tablespoon dried parsley,
  crumbled

2 1/2 teaspoons paprika

2 teaspoons sugar

2 teaspoons salt

2 teaspoons pepper

1 1/2 teaspoons
  garlic powder

1. In a small, airtight container, combine all the ingredients. Cover and shake vigorously to blend.

2. Store in a cool, dry, dark place for up to 1 year.

Makes about 6 tablespoons

Helpful Hint | Make Your Own Cost-Effective Croutons

A wonderful way to use up stale bread, croutons are so easy to prepare it makes no sense to spend extra money to buy them. Cut bread slices into 1/2-inch cubes. In a large skillet over moderate heat, heat extra-virgin olive oil. Add the bread cubes and sauté, stirring constantly, until the cubes are well coated, golden in color, and crisp. Transfer the cubes to paper towels and let drain. Add to salads or float on soups. Store in airtight containers.

To add more flavor to your croutons, sauté garlic slices or sprigs of herbs or even chile peppers in the olive oil. Remove and discard the flavorings before adding the bread cubes to the flavored oil.

Ranch Dressing

To make a lower-fat version of this dressing, substitute fat-free mayonnaise for the regular mayonnaise. Buttermilk is made from skim milk, so it is already low in fat and calories. If you don't use buttermilk often, buy a box of dry buttermilk powder and simply make as much as you need when you need it. If you'd like a thicker consistency for dipping, stir the Ranch Dressing Mix into 1 cup sour cream or plain yogurt.

1 container Ranch Dressing Mix (opposite)
1 cup mayonnaise
1 cup buttermilk

In a small, nonreactive bowl, whisk together all the ingredients until the dressing has a smooth, creamy consistency.

Makes about 2 cups

Blue Cheese Dressing

You can make this tangy treat or any of the other prepared salad dressings that follow from scratch and keep them on hand in the refrigerator. They are all easy to make and cost very little compared to commercial brands.

1 1/2 cups mayonnaise
1/2 cup sour cream
1/4 cup cider vinegar
4 teaspoons sugar
1/2 teaspoon dry mustard
1 teaspoon minced fresh garlic
2 teaspoons minced onion
1 cup (4 ounces) crumbled blue cheese

In a small, nonreactive bowl, combine all the ingredients except the blue cheese. Whisk to blend until the dressing has a smooth, creamy consistency. Gently stir in the blue cheese. Cover the bowl and refrigerate for at least 2 hours before serving. Store, covered, in the refrigerator.

Makes 2 cups

Light Blue Cheese Dressing

Rich and creamy and loaded with flavor—you won't guess this is a lower-fat cousin. And it is much better than lower-calorie commercial dressings.

1/2 cup fat-free mayonnaise
2 tablespoons 1% milk
1 tablespoon lemon juice
1/2 teaspoon sugar
1 teaspoon minced fresh garlic
1/4 teaspoon dry mustard
1/2 cup (2 ounces) crumbled blue cheese

In a small, nonreactive bowl, combine all the ingredients except the blue cheese. Whisk to blend until the dressing has a smooth, creamy consistency. Gently stir in the blue cheese. Cover the bowl and refrigerate for at least 2 hours before serving. Store, covered, in the refrigerator.

Makes about 1 cup

French Dressing

You probably have all the ingredients for this creamy favorite in your pantry. It takes just a few minutes to prepare and is much more delicious than the pricey bottled variety.

1 cup ketchup
1/2 cup reduced-fat mayonnaise
3 tablespoons cider vinegar
3 tablespoons honey
2 tablespoons water
1 tablespoon olive oil
1 teaspoon lemon juice
1/2 teaspoon dry mustard
1/4 teaspoon salt

In the bowl of a food processor or blender, combine all the ingredients. Whirl until all the ingredients are well blended and the dressing has a smooth, creamy consistency. Store in an airtight container in the refrigerator.

Makes 2 1/2 cups

Italian Dressing

Nothing tastes better—or is more pleasing to the pocketbook—than homemade Italian dressing.

1/4 cup extra-virgin or virgin olive oil
1/4 cup red wine vinegar
1 garlic clove, minced
1 teaspoon finely chopped onion
1/2 teaspoon dry mustard
1/2 teaspoon celery seed
1/2 teaspoon paprika
1/4 teaspoon Italian Herb Blend (page 42)
2-4 tablespoons sugar or sugar substitute equivalent

In a small, airtight container, combine all the ingredients. Cover and shake vigorously to blend all the ingredients well. Use immediately or store in the refrigerator overnight.

Makes 2/3 cup

Thousand Island Dressing

For a lighter version of this dressing, substitute low- or nonfat mayonnaise or nonfat yogurt for the regular mayonnaise. If you use homemade mayonnaise, it will please both your palate and your budget. In many parts of the country, this is called Russian dressing.

2 cups mayonnaise
1/4 cup chili sauce
1/4 cup pickle relish

1. In a small, nonreactive bowl, stir together all the ingredients until well blended and the dressing has a smooth, creamy consistency.

2. Store in an airtight container in the refrigerator.

Makes 2 1/2 cups

seasonings

Bouquet Garni

This famous combination uses either fresh herb sprigs or dried leaves. It can be added to soups, stews, and any moist-heat cooked meat and poultry dishes.

1/2 bay leaf
2 sprigs parsley
1 sprig thyme

1. Cut a piece of cheesecloth about 4-inches square. Lay the herbs in the center of the cheesecloth, then bring the corners of the cloth together to form a bundle around the herbs. Tie the top of the bundle with kitchen string.

2. Add herb bundle to soup or stew. Once the cooking is finished, the bundle can easily be removed and discarded.

Fines Herbes

This classic blend of four herbs enhances the flavor of fish, poultry, egg dishes, or cooked vegetables.

4 tablespoons dried parsley, crumbled
4 teaspoons dried tarragon, crumbled
4 teaspoons dried chervil, crumbled
4 teaspoons dried chives, finely chopped

1. In a self-sealing plastic bag or container with a tight-fitting lid, combine all the herbs.

2. Label and date, and store at room temperature. Use within 3 months.

how to dry herbs

With a little attention, herbs will grow for almost anyone and in almost any climate. And drying fresh herbs that you have grown yourself will really save you money at the grocery store. For best flavor, try to use dried herbs within 4 to 6 months after preserving them.

Air-drying: Pick fresh herbs. Gather the herbs in bunches and tie each bunch of stems with string, leaving a long end. Using the long end, hang the herb bunches upside down in a cool, dry place until they are completely dried.

Drying in an electric oven: Preheat oven to 100°F. Spread the herbs in a single layer over a baking sheet with a rim. Set the baking sheet in the oven until the herbs are completely dried, about 50 minutes.

Drying in a gas oven: Preheat oven to 200°F, then turn off the oven. Place the baking sheet with the herbs in the warm oven, close the door, and let the herbs sit until completely dried, about 50 minutes.

Herbes de Provence

This popular French mixture can be sprinkled over meats, fish, or poultry before grilling; stirred into rice, couscous, or other grain mixtures; added to omelets or scrambled eggs; or whisked with oil and vinegar for a lovely salad dressing.

6 teaspoons dried oregano, crumbled

3 teaspoons dried basil, crumbled

3 teaspoons dried sweet marjoram, crumbled

3 teaspoons dried thyme, crumbled

1 1/2 teaspoons dried mint, crumbled

1 1/2 teaspoons dried rosemary, crumbled

1 1/2 teaspoons dried sage leaves, crumbled

1 teaspoon fennel seed, crumbled

1. In a mortar, blender, or food processor, combine all the herbs. Crush or pulse-chop them to the consistency desired.
2. Place the herb mixture in a self-sealing plastic bag or airtight container, label, and date. Keep in a dry place at room temperature. Use within 3 months.

Italian Herb Blend

This well-loved herb mix is almost essential in pasta dishes and sprinkled on pizza. It is also delicious with chicken or firm fish.

6 tablespoons dried basil, crumbled

3 tablespoons dried oregano, crumbled

2 tablespoons dried parsley, crumbled

2 tablespoons dried thyme, crumbled

1 teaspoon dried garlic

1. In a self-sealing plastic bag or airtight container, combine all the ingredients.
2. Label and date, and store in a dry place at room temperature. Use within 3 months.

freezing herbs

Freezing herbs protects their flavor even more than drying them, in the opinion of many knowledgeable cooks. How you freeze an herb depends on whether you want to freeze it as a whole sprig or as chopped leaves frozen in an ice cube.

Whole sprigs: Wash and spin-dry sprigs of bushy herbs using a salad spinner. Pack in self-sealing freezer bags, label, date, and freeze. Remove leaves as needed, returning the sprigs to the bags, resealing, and refreezing.

Chopped leaves in ice cubes: Chop leaves of herbs such as chive or parsley. Place 1 tablespoon of the chopped herb into each container in an ice-cube tray. Pour just enough water into each container to cover the herbs and freeze. Pop out the frozen herb cube, place in self-sealing freezer bags, label, date, and freeze. When using in a recipe, just add the cube and let it melt.

Chili Powder

You don't have to pay fancy prices for fancy spice mixes. Make your own and then slowly start adding a little more of one ingredient or a little less of another until you have your own favorite variation. You can adapt this recipe to your own taste, making it spicier by adding more cayenne pepper or milder by adding less, and adding more or less of each spice.

- 3 tablespoons ground chile peppers or paprika
- 1 tablespoon ground cumin
- 1 teaspoon ground turmeric
- 1 teaspoon dried oregano, finely crumbled
- 1 teaspoon garlic powder
- 1/8-1 teaspoon ground cayenne pepper
- 1/4 teaspoon salt
- 1/4 teaspoon ground black pepper

1. Combine all the ingredients in an airtight container. Shake until all the spices are well blended.

2. Store in a cool, dark place for up to 6 months.

Makes about 1/4 cup

Creole Seasoning Mix

This is a spice sensation to sprinkle over popcorn or freshly baked pretzels, French fries, chicken pieces, or to use in Creole or Cajun dishes.

- 2/3 cup ground cayenne pepper
- 1/2 cup plus 2 teaspoons salt
- 1/4 cup garlic powder
- 1/4 cup onion powder
- 1/4 cup chili powder
- 2 tablespoons plus 2 teaspoons ground black pepper

1. Combine all the ingredients in an airtight container. Shake until all the spices are well blended.

2. Store in a cool, dark place for up to 6 months.

Makes 2 cups

Replacements for Pantry Staples **457**

Southwest Seasoning Mix

Sprinkle this taste of the Southwest over meats or seafood before grilling, over veggies, or over freshly popped popcorn. Stirring 1 tablespoon of this seasoning mix into 1 cup sour cream, then chilling, makes a fabulous dip.

1/4 cup chili powder

1/4 cup onion powder

2 tablespoons ground cumin

2 tablespoons ground coriander

2 tablespoons dried oregano, crumbled

2 tablespoons dried basil, crumbled

1 tablespoon dried thyme, crumbled

1 tablespoon garlic powder

1. Combine all the ingredients in a container with a tight-fitting lid. Shake until all the spices are well blended.
2. Store in a cool, dark place for up to 6 months.

Makes 1 cup

Make It a Gift

Give a Useful Jar of Herbs

Jars of herb mixtures are always welcome in a cook's home, especially if you have grown the herbs yourself. You can even make herb or spice bags with cheesecloth and kitchen twine, then place the bags in a mason jar—all the cook needs to do is pull out a bag and pop it into whatever's cooking to add fabulous flavor.

Seasoned Coating Mix

This is a fabulous addition to fried or baked chicken and pork recipes.

2 cups sifted all-purpose flour

1 tablespoon paprika

2 teaspoons dried marjoram, crumbled

2 teaspoons dried thyme, crumbled

2 teaspoons onion powder

2 teaspoons garlic powder

1 teaspoon dried rosemary, crumbled

1/2 teaspoon salt

1/4 teaspoon ground black pepper

1. In a self-sealing plastic bag, combine all the ingredients. Seal the bag and shake it to mix the ingredients thoroughly.
2. Label and date the bag, and store in a cool, dry place for up to six months.

Makes enough to coat 20 pork chops or four chickens

Caribbean Spicy Meat Rub

A pungent sweet and spicy blend to rub onto just about any kind of meat before grilling, this meat rub can also be added to sauces and stews. Or stir 4 tablespoons of the rub into 2 tablespoons vegetable oil and heat just until the aromas are released, then add to any marinade for tougher cuts of meat.

3 tablespoons brown sugar

2 tablespoons paprika

2 teaspoons dry mustard

2 teaspoons garlic salt

1 1/2 teaspoons dried basil, crumbled

1 teaspoon ground coriander

1 teaspoon dried savory, crumbled

1 teaspoon dried thyme, crumbled

1 teaspoon black pepper

1 teaspoon ground cumin

1 crushed bay leaf

1. Combine all the ingredients in an airtight container. Shake until all the spices are well blended.

2. Store in a cool, dark place for up to 6 months.

Makes about 1/2 cup

Green Curry Paste

This recipe and the one that follows are two staples of Thai cooking. You'll be surprised how often you'll find yourself reaching for these pastes to add a little exotic, exuberant flavor to your meals. You can find many of the ingredients in Asian cooking specialty stores. Stir this paste into poultry or vegetable dishes, or add to more delicately flavored meat dishes. To really release the flavors, sauté the paste in a little vegetable oil before using it.

4 shallots, chopped

1 teaspoon shrimp or anchovy paste

3 garlic cloves, quartered

2 dried kaffir lime leaves, crushed, or 1 teaspoon lime zest

1 piece (4 inches long) fresh lemongrass, inner stalk chopped

1 tablespoon coriander seeds

1 tablespoon sliced fresh ginger

1 teaspoon freshly grated nutmeg

1 teaspoon cumin seeds

1 teaspoon white peppercorns

6 green chiles, seeded and quartered

3-4 tablespoons coconut cream

1. In the container of a food processor or blender, combine all the ingredients. Whirl until all the ingredients are well blended and the mixture is smooth.

2. Use the paste at once or place in an airtight container, cover with vegetable oil, and store in the refrigerator for up to 4 days. Or pack the paste into an ice-cube tray, freeze, pop out the paste cubes, and store in a self-sealing, freezer-safe plastic bag in the freezer, and use the cubes as needed in recipes.

Makes about 3/4 cup

Red Curry Paste

Keep the milk handy when you dine on this spicy Thai delight—though you can adjust the heat by adding or subtracting the fresh red chiles. (Milk puts out chile fires better than water.) As with the Green Curry Paste (page 45), sautéing the paste in a little oil before using it allows the flavors to be fully released.

3-6 fresh red chiles, stemmed but not seeded

4 shallots, quartered

1 red onion, cut into eighths

4 garlic cloves, quartered

1 piece lemongrass, 4 inches long, inner stalk chopped

1/4 cup fresh cilantro leaves

2 kaffir lime leaves, minced

Zest of 2 limes

1 tablespoon toasted coriander seeds

1 teaspoon grated nutmeg

1 teaspoon cumin seeds

1 teaspoon white peppercorns

2 teaspoons shrimp or anchovy paste

1. In the container of a food processor or blender, combine the red chiles, shallots, red onion, garlic, lemongrass, cilantro, lime leaves and zest, coriander seeds, nutmeg, cumin seeds, and white peppercorns. Whirl until all the ingredients are well blended and the mixture is smooth.

2. In a skillet over medium-low heat, dry-roast the shrimp or anchovy paste for 2 to 3 minutes, stirring constantly. Add to the chile mixture and process to blend all the ingredients until smooth. Use the paste at once or place in a container with a tight-fitting lid, cover with vegetable oil, and store in the refrigerator for up to two weeks.

Makes about 1 cup

Curry Powder

Just about every family in India has a curry recipe. Try making the basic recipe below, then adding or subtracting one of the following until you make your own personal curry powder: cumin seeds, turmeric, mace, black peppercorns, fennel seeds, crushed red pepper flakes, coriander, cinnamon, nutmeg, cloves, tamarind, or cardamom seeds.

1/4 cup ground coriander

2 tablespoons ground turmeric

2 teaspoons ground cumin

2 teaspoons ground ginger

2 teaspoons ground allspice

1 teaspoon ground cinnamon

1 teaspoon ground celery seed

1 teaspoon ground black pepper

1/4 teaspoon ground cayenne pepper

1. Combine all the ingredients in an airtight container. Shake until all the spices are well blended.

2. Store in a cool, dark place for up to 6 months.

Makes about 1/2 cup

marinades

Red Wine Marinade

The purpose of any marinade is twofold: An acid (lemon juice, vinegar) breaks down the fibers in tough pieces of meat, and the seasonings infuse the meat with piquant flavor. Try marinating chunks of beef or lamb in this rich-tasting mixture before grilling them on skewers for kabobs. You don't need to buy an expensive packaged marinade.

1/4 cup dry red wine
2 scallions, chopped
2 tablespoons balsamic vinegar
1/2 teaspoon dried rosemary
2 tablespoons olive oil
2 garlic cloves, minced
1/2 teaspoon salt
1/2 teaspoon black pepper

In a small, nonreactive bowl, combine all the ingredients. Stir to blend all the ingredients well. Pour the marinade into a large, self-sealing bag and add the lamb or beef to be marinated. Place the bag in the refrigerator for at least 4 hours or overnight.

Mustard Marinade

Use this tasty mixture to marinate boneless chicken breasts, either for straight grilling or cut into cubes for kabobs. You don't need packaged marinades.

1/3 cup lemon juice
2 scallions, chopped
2 tablespoons soy sauce
2 tablespoons Dijon mustard
2 tablespoons olive oil
1/4 teaspoon hot
   red pepper sauce

1. In a small bowl, combine all the ingredients. Stir to blend well. Pour the marinade into a large, self-sealing bag and add the poultry to be marinated.

2. Place the bag in the refrigerator for at least 4 hours or overnight.

make your own meat tenderizer

Yes, you can buy powdered meat tenderizer, and it won't break your budget, but why buy it when you probably already have several things on hand that will do just as good a job, are healthier, and will add flavor along with the tenderizing action? Almost any acid-based liquid will work.

Beer: Surprise! Place the meat in a nonmetallic dish (glass or enameled), pour a can of beer over it, place it in the refrigerator, and let it sit for 1 hour. For even more tenderizing action, leave the meat sitting in the beer overnight, turning once or twice. If you're slow-cooking the meat (the best cooking method for tough cuts), use beer as part of the cooking liquid.

Buttermilk: This acidy milk makes another great meat tenderizer when used as a marinade.

Lemon juice: If you grow your own lemons, you have a terrific tenderizer for nothing! Lemon juice breaks down tough fibers quickly and easily—and adds a bright citrus taste as well.

Vinegar: Is there anything that vinegar can't do? Soak a tough piece of meat in 1 or 2 cups of vinegar overnight in the refrigerator to tenderize it. Any vinegar will do the job—try different vinegars with different meats to find out which combinations you like the best.

Lemon Herb Marinade
Lovely with lamb chops, this is also great with chicken. It is easy, inexpensive, and delicious.

3 tablespoons vegetable oil

1 teaspoon grated lemon zest

3 tablespoons lemon juice

2 garlic cloves, minced

1 teaspoon dried rosemary, crumbled

1/2 teaspoon dried thyme, crumbled

1/2 teaspoon salt

1/4 teaspoon black pepper

1. In a small, nonreactive bowl, combine all the ingredients. Stir to blend all the ingredients well. Pour the marinade into a large, self-sealing bag and add the lamb, meat, or poultry to be marinated.

2. Place the bag in the refrigerator for at least 4 hours.

Orange Ginger Marinade
Lovely for marinating scallops or lending a sweet, tangy flavor to shrimp or fish, this easy-to-make mixture rivals any prepared marinade.

1/4 cup soy sauce

2 scallions, chopped

1/3 cup orange juice

2 teaspoons grated fresh ginger

2 tablespoons olive oil

2 tablespoons grated orange zest

1 garlic clove, minced

1. In a small, nonreactive bowl, combine all the ingredients. Stir to blend all the ingredients well. Pour the marinade into a large, self-sealing bag and add the seafood to be marinated.

2. Place the bag in the refrigerator for 30 minutes to 1 hour.

Asian Marinade
Sensational with shrimp, this marinade is also good with chicken or flank steak. Compare your own version with bottled ones and you'll be glad you saved the money. If salt is an issue, use low-sodium soy sauce.

1/4 cup lemon juice

1/2 teaspoon salt

2 tablespoons dark sesame oil

1 large garlic clove, minced

1 tablespoon soy sauce

1. In a small, nonreactive bowl, combine all the ingredients. Stir to blend all the ingredients well. Pour the marinade into a self-sealing bag and add the seafood, meat, or poultry to be marinated.

2. Place the bag in the refrigerator for at least 1 hour.

cooking stocks

Beef Stock

At the heart of every great soup, there is a great stock. Although canned broth is convenient, it is really not as flavorful as your own stock. Plus, when you make your own, you have the satisfaction of knowing exactly what goes into it—and what doesn't. When you buy the beef for this rich-tasting stock, ask the butcher to break up the bones into pieces small enough to fit into your stockpot or Dutch oven. This will be cheaper, tastier, and far less salty than most canned broths.

- 4 pounds meaty beef bones, including marrow and shinbones, or knucklebones
- 2 yellow onions, thickly sliced
- 2 carrots, thickly sliced
- 2 stalks celery with leaves, sliced
- 6 sprigs fresh parsley
- 2 small bay leaves
- 1 sprig fresh thyme or 1/2 teaspoon dried thyme, crumbled
- 10 black peppercorns
- 1 tablespoons salt

1. Preheat the oven to 400°F. Place the beef bones, onions, and carrots in a roasting pan and roast until the bones turn a rich brown, for 30 to 45 minutes.

2. Transfer the mixture to a large stockpot or Dutch oven. Add the celery, parsley, bay leaves, thyme, peppercorns, and salt. Add enough water to cover the bone mixture (about 5 quarts).

3. Add a little water to the roasting pan and stir to scrape up the browned bits. Pour the liquid and bits into the stockpot.

4. Place the stockpot over moderately high heat, and slowly bring the mixture to a boil, using a slotted spoon to skim off and discard any fat or scum that rises to the surface. Reduce the heat, partly cover the stockpot, and simmer gently for 3 to 4 hours.

5. Line a fine sieve with cheesecloth and set it over a large bowl. Slowly pour the stock through the sieve; discard the solids. Let the stock cool to room temperature. Pour the stock into serving-size, airtight containers; cover, label, and date. Store the stock in the refrigerator for a week or the freeze for up to 6 months. If fat congeals on top of the stock while refrigerated or frozen, remove and discard before using the stock.

Makes 3 quarts

Helpful Hint | **Make Your Own Bouillon Cubes**

No one can deny the convenience of bouillon cubes, but you don't have to spend your hard-earned money to have them on hand. When cooking a pot of stock, occasionally cook the liquid down to 2 cups—it will be thick and intense in both flavor and color. Let the reduced stock cool completely, then pour it into ice-cube trays and place the trays in the freezer. When the stock cubes are solid, remove them from the ice-cube trays, wrap each in foil, and store the cubes in a labeled and dated self-sealing freezer bag. Each cube will make 1 cup of soup.

Chicken Stock

You can use the same technique to make turkey stock with your leftover holiday bird.

5 1/2-pound stewing hen or 2 pounds chicken wing tips, necks, and backs

3 stalks celery, sliced

1 large carrot, sliced

1 large onion, quartered

1 leek, sliced

6 sprigs fresh parsley

1/2 teaspoon dried thyme

1 bay leaf

1 teaspoon salt

1/2 teaspoon black peppercorns

1. In a large saucepan or Dutch oven, combine all the ingredients. Add enough water to cover the chicken mixture (about 10 to 12 cups). Over moderately low heat, bring the mixture slowly to a boil, using a slotted spoon to skim off and discard any fat or scum that rises to the surface.

2. Reduce the heat, partly cover the saucepan, and simmer gently until the stock is well flavored, about 3 hours. The longer you simmer the stock, the richer the flavor.

3. Line a fine sieve with cheesecloth and set it over a large bowl. Slowly pour the stock through the sieve; discard the solids. Let the stock cool to room temperature. Pour the stock into serving-size, airtight containers; cover, label, and date. Store the stock in the refrigerator for a week or freeze for up to 6 months. If fat congeals on top of the stock while refrigerated or frozen, remove and discard before using the stock.

Makes 2 quarts

Fish Stock

An elegant base for seafood soups and stews, this delicately flavored stock can also be used as a poaching liquid for whole fish. Be careful not to overcook fish stock; too much cooking can destroy the complex flavor. After making the stock, use the cooked fish in salads or spreads.

1 1/2 pounds whole white-fleshed fish, such as cod, snapper, or scrod, cleaned and scaled

1-2 stalks celery, sliced

1 small onion, sliced

1 cup white wine or juice of 1 lemon

6-8 cups cold water

3 sprigs fresh parsley

1 sprig fresh thyme or 1/2 teaspoon dried thyme, crumbled

1 small bay leaf

1/2 teaspoon salt

1/2 teaspoon black peppercorns

1. Cut off the fish head, slit open the fish, and remove the bones. In a large saucepan, combine the fish fillets, head, and bones. Add the celery, onion, wine or lemon juice, water, parsley, thyme, bay leaf, salt, and peppercorns. Over moderately high heat, bring the mixture to a boil, using a slotted spoon to skim off and discard any fat or scum that rises to the surface.

2. Reduce the heat to very low and barely simmer the stock, uncovered, until the fish fillets are just cooked, about 5 minutes. Using a slotted spoon, lift out the fish fillets and set them aside to drain.

3. Continue to simmer the broth for 15 minutes longer.

4. Line a fine sieve with cheesecloth and set it over a large bowl. Slowly pour the stock through the sieve; discard the solids. Let the stock cool to room temperature. Pour the stock into serving-size, airtight containers; cover, label, and date. Store in the refrigerator for a week or the freezer for up to six months.

Makes 1 1/2 quarts

clarifying stock

To have stock that is beautifully clear and tantalizing, you must clarify it after cooking. There are two methods for clarifying stock: The first will yield fairly clear results; the second method will be very clear.

Straining: Line a fine sieve with cheesecloth and pour the stock through; this will remove any small solids in the stock.

Egg-white method: Separate 2 eggs and whisk together the whites; crush the eggshells. Add the whites and shells to the stock and slowly bring to a simmer, uncovered. When the whites begin to set, pour the stock through a cheesecloth-lined sieve or colander; any particles will be trapped in the egg whites. Discard whites and shells.

Vegetable Stock

A creative way to use vegetable peelings, leftover vegetables, or the parts full of nutrition but not generally served with the vegetables, such as mushroom stems, broccoli and cauliflower stalks, and celery tops. That makes homemade vegetable stock very economical and much better than vegetable cubes.

- 1/4 cup (1/2 stick) unsalted butter
- 5 onions, peeled and chopped
- 2 leeks, halved lengthwise, cleaned, and sliced
- 2 whole garlic cloves
- 4 carrots, chopped
- 4 stalks celery with leaves, chopped
- 6-8 dried mushrooms
- 1 small bunch fresh parsley
- 1 sprig fresh thyme or 1/2 teaspoon dried thyme, crumbled
- 1 tablespoon salt
- 1/2 teaspoon ground allspice
- Pinch nutmeg or mace
- 4 quarts cold water
- 1 tablespoon red wine vinegar *(optional)*
- 1 fresh red chile, halved and seeded *(optional)*; wear gloves when handling; they burn

1. In a large saucepan or Dutch oven over moderate heat, melt the butter. Add the onions, leeks, and garlic, and cook, stirring, until the onions are golden, 5 to 8 minutes. Add the carrots, celery, mushrooms, parsley, thyme, salt, allspice, nutmeg or mace, and cold water.

2. Bring the mixture slowly to a boil, using a slotted spoon to skim off and discard any fat or scum that rises to the surface. Reduce the heat, partly cover the saucepan, and simmer gently for 2 hours, adding more water as needed to maintain the level at about 3 quarts. If using, add the red wine vinegar and red chile, and simmer for 30 minutes longer.

3. Line a fine sieve with cheesecloth and set it over a large bowl. Slowly pour the stock through the sieve, gently pressing with a wooden spoon to squeeze all the liquid from the solids; discard the solids and the red chile. If desired, clarify the stock (see Clarifying Stock, above). If a thicker stock is desired, do not discard the solids when straining; puree about 1/2 cup of the cooked vegetables and stir the puree back into the stock. Let the stock cool to room temperature. Pour the stock into serving-size, airtight containers; cover, label, and date. Store the stock in the refrigerator for a week or the freezer for up to 6 months.

Makes about 3 quarts

sauces

Barbecue Sauce
Great with beef, chicken, or pork, this homemade sauce is not only cheaper than bottled ones, but you can customize it to your own family's tastes.

1 medium onion, chopped

1/4 cup vegetable oil

1 cup ketchup

3/4 cup water

2 tablespoons Worcestershire sauce

2 tablespoons sugar

1/4 cup cider vinegar

2 tablespoons mustard

1 teaspoon salt

1/2 teaspoon ground black pepper

1. In a medium, nonreactive saucepan over low heat, combine all the ingredients. Simmer, uncovered, for 20 minutes; remove the saucepan from the heat and let the sauce cool.

2. Store in an airtight container in the refrigerator for up to 1 week, or frozen for up to 6 months.

Makes about 2 1/2 cups

Pan Gravy
This is the finishing touch for any roast. Real pan gravy is made using the drippings from roasted meat or poultry, but you can also used homemade stock or canned broth (the flavor will be less intense, but it will work). Authentic gravy doesn't come in a can or a packet.

1/4 cup pan drippings from roast meat or poultry

Melted butter, as needed

2 cups Beef Stock (page 49) or Chicken Stock (page 50), or canned beef or chicken broth

1/4 cup all-purpose flour

Salt and freshly ground pepper, to taste

1. In a 1-cup measure, pour the pan drippings to equal 1/4 cup. If needed, add melted butter to reach the desired amount. Pour the drippings into a large skillet and set aside.

2. Place the roasting pan with the remaining drippings over moderate heat. Stir in the stock or broth and simmer, stirring to loosen any browned bits on the pan, about 1 minute.

3. Place the skillet over moderate heat and heat the drippings for 1 minute. Blend in the flour and cook, whisking, until the flour is a nutty brown, for 1 to 2 minutes. Gradually add the stock, whisking constantly, and cook until the mixture boils and thickens.

4. Reduce the heat to moderately low and simmer, stirring occasionally, for 2 to 3 minutes longer. Add salt and pepper. If the gravy is lumpier than desired, strain through a sieve. Transfer the gravy to a heated gravy boat and serve immediately.

Makes 2 cups

Demiglaze Sauce

This is a beautiful homemade sauce for meats like lean pork that don't produce enough drippings of their own to make gravy. Far better than canned or packaged gravy mixes, it's cheaper too.

1/4 cup unsalted butter
2 ounces Black Forest or Virginia ham, chopped
1 medium onion, chopped
1 carrot, thinly sliced
1/4 cup all-purpose flour
4 cups Beef Stock (page 49) or canned beef broth
1 1/2 cups Chicken Stock (page 50) or canned broth
2 tablespoons tomato paste
1/2 teaspoon salt
1/4 teaspoon dried thyme
1/4 teaspoon ground black pepper
1/2 cup dry red wine

1. In a large, heavy saucepan over moderate heat, melt the butter or margarine. Add the ham and cook, stirring frequently, until lightly golden, abut 8 minutes. Add the onion and cook, stirring frequently, until it is soft, about 5 minutes. Add the carrot and cook until it is tender, about 5 minutes.

2. Sprinkle the flour over the vegetable mixture and stir until it is blended. Gradually add 3 cups of the beef stock, the chicken stock, tomato paste, salt, thyme, and pepper, stirring constantly. Cook, stirring frequently and skimming off any scum that rises to the surface, until the sauce thickens and thickly coats the back of a spoon, about 30 minutes. Strain the sauce through a sieve and discard the solids.

3. Stir in the remaining cup of beef stock and the red wine and cook, uncovered, until the sauce reduces to 3 1/2 cups.

Makes 3 1/2 cups

Espagnole Sauce

Simple, yet rich, this is another brown sauce for lean meats that don't produce drippings. Homemade is tastier, less salty, and cheaper than canned or packaged brown gravy

1/4 cup unsalted butter
2 ounces Black Forest or Virginia ham, chopped
1 medium onion, chopped
1 carrot, thinly sliced
1/4 cup all-purpose flour
3 cups Beef Stock (page 49) or canned beef broth
1 1/2 cups Chicken Stock (page 50) or canned broth
2 tablespoons tomato paste
1/2 teaspoon salt
1/4 teaspoon dried thyme
1/4 teaspoon black pepper

1. In a large, heavy saucepan over moderate heat, melt the butter or margarine. Add the ham and cook, stirring frequently, until lightly golden, abut 8 minutes. Add the onion and cook, stirring frequently, until it is soft, about 5 minutes. Add the carrot and cook until it is tender, about 5 minutes.

2. Sprinkle the flour over the vegetable mixture and stir until it is blended. Gradually add the beef and chicken stocks, tomato paste, salt, thyme, and pepper, stirring constantly. Cook, stirring frequently and skimming off any scum that rises to the surface, until the sauce thickens and thickly coats the back of a spoon, about 30 minutes. Strain the sauce through a sieve and discard the solids.

Makes 3 cups

Mushroom Wine Sauce

Many a steak lover considers this sauce ambrosia, but it is equally good with veal or chicken. Store-bought mushroom gravies just don't come close in taste or economy.

1/4 cup (1/2 stick) unsalted butter or margarine

2 ounces Black Forest or Virginia ham, chopped

1 medium onion, chopped

1 carrot, thinly sliced

1/4 cup all-purpose flour

3 cups Beef Stock (page 49) or canned beef broth

1 1/2 cups Chicken Stock (page 50) or canned chicken broth

2 tablespoons tomato paste

1/2 teaspoon salt

1/4 teaspoon dried thyme, crumbled

1/4 teaspoon black pepper

3 tablespoons butter

2 shallots, minced

8 ounces button, shiitake, or portobello mushrooms, thinly sliced

2/3 cup dry red wine

1. In a large, heavy saucepan over moderate heat, melt the butter or margarine. Add the ham and cook, stirring frequently, until lightly golden, abut 8 minutes. Add the onion and cook, stirring frequently, until it is soft, about 5 minutes. Add the carrot and cook until it is tender, about 5 minutes.

2. Sprinkle the flour over the vegetable mixture and stir until it is blended. Gradually add the beef and chicken stocks, tomato paste, salt, thyme, and pepper, stirring constantly. Cook, stirring frequently and skimming off any scum that rises to the surface, until the sauce thickens and thickly coats the back of a spoon, about 30 minutes. Strain the sauce through a sieve and discard the solids.

3. In a large skillet over moderate heat, melt the butter. Add the shallots and cook until soft. Add the mushrooms and cook until tender. Add the red wine, increase the heat, and boil, uncovered, until the mixture is reduced by half.

4. Add the mushroom mixture to the sauce, stirring until the ingredients are well blended.

Makes 3 1/2 cups

how to clarify butter

Clarified butter is essential to making certain sauces, such as hollandaise, and for dipping artichoke leaves or steamed lobster. By clarifying butter, you are removing the milk solids, leaving a clear, golden, rich oil.

In a small saucepan over very low heat, melt a stick (1/2 cup) of butter. When the butter has completely liquefied but not yet begun to cook, remove the saucepan from the heat and let the butter stand until the white milk solids sink to the bottom. Place a piece of cheesecloth over a small glass bowl. Carefully pour the golden-yellow liquid butter into the bowl through the cheesecloth; be careful to stop pouring when the white solids begin to move. Remove the cheesecloth and store the clarified butter, covered, in the refrigerator until ready to use.

Béarnaise Sauce

Adding immediate elegance to almost any meal, egg sauces, notably this Béarnaise sauce and the Hollandaise Sauce that follows, are among the most refined. Once made with either raw eggs or eggs only lightly cooked in a double boiler, these recipes cook the eggs enough to remove any fear of salmonella contamination. Slow and steady is the rule when cooking egg sauces—or you may scramble your culinary plans. Béarnaise is a sauce served with filet mignon in the finest restaurants for the finest prices. Jars sold in specialty food stores just don't measure up.

1/3 cup chopped fresh tarragon

2 tablespoons white wine vinegar

1 tablespoon minced shallot

2 egg yolks

2 tablespoons water

1/4 teaspoon salt

6 tablespoons clarified unsalted butter (see How to Clarify Butter, opposite), liquid but not hot

1/8 teaspoon white pepper

1. In a small saucepan over moderately high heat, combine the tarragon, white wine vinegar, and shallot, and cook for 1 to 2 minutes. Remove the saucepan from the heat and let cool.

2. In a 1-quart saucepan over moderately high heat, combine the egg yolks, water, salt, and tarragon mixture, and bring to a boil, whisking constantly.

3. Remove the saucepan from the heat. The mixture will begin to curdle, but continue whisking until the mixture becomes smooth. Stir in the clarified butter, 1 tablespoon at a time. Add the pepper and stir until the mixture is smooth and well blended.

Makes 1 cup

Hollandaise Sauce

Try hollandaise drizzled over fresh, steamed asparagus, broccoli, or cauliflower, or over delicate poached fish. It is a must for eggs Benedict or Florentine. Homemade simply tastes best; it also costs less.

2 egg yolks

2 tablespoons water

1/4 teaspoon salt

1 tablespoon lemon juice

6 tablespoons clarified unsalted butter (see How to Clarify Butter, opposite), liquid but not hot

1/8 teaspoon white pepper

1. In a 1-quart saucepan over moderately high heat, combine the egg yolks, water, salt, and lemon juice, and bring to a boil, whisking constantly.

2. Remove the saucepan from the heat. The mixture will begin to curdle, but continue whisking until the mixture becomes smooth. Stir in the clarified butter, 1 tablespoon at a time. Add the pepper and stir until the mixture is smooth and well blended.

Makes 1 cup

Replacements for Pantry Staples   **469**

Basic White Sauce

Thin, medium, or thick, white sauce is the most versatile of all sauces and can be adapted to suit many a dish. Thin white sauce serves as a base for creamy soups or stews; medium white sauce is added to casseroles and creamed vegetable mixtures, or used as a base for other sauces; thick white sauce works as a binder or a base for dishes like soufflés or croquettes. Making your own white sauce, starting with this basic white sauce, allows you to make all kinds of other recipes, such as the three that follow.

- 1 tablespoon butter or margarine
- 1 tablespoon all-purpose flour
- 1 cup hot milk
- 1/4 teaspoon salt
- 1/8 teaspoon white or black ground pepper

1. In a small heavy saucepan over low heat, melt the butter. Add the flour and cook, whisking constantly, until the mixture is smooth, 2 to 3 minutes; do not let the flour brown. Gradually stir in the milk.

2. Increase the heat to moderate and cook, stirring constantly, until the sauce is thickened and smooth, and no raw flour taste remains, about 3 to 5 minutes. Remove the saucepan from the heat and stir in the salt and pepper.

3. To store, lay plastic wrap directly on the surface of the sauce to prevent a skin from forming. Let the sauce cool to room temperature, then refrigerate until needed. Reheat the sauce in the top of a double boiler.

Makes 1 cup

Cheese Sauce

Remember that you can choose the kind of cheese to use for this homemade sauce. Cheddar is classic, but there are many other possibilities. Pour over potatoes or steamed vegetables for a starter.

- 1 tablespoon butter or margarine
- 1 tablespoon all-purpose flour
- 1/2 teaspoon dry mustard
- 1 cup hot milk
- 1/2-3/4 cup shredded sharp cheddar cheese
- 1/4 teaspoon salt
- 1/8 teaspoon white or black ground pepper

1. In a small heavy saucepan over low heat, melt the butter. Add the flour and dry mustard, and cook, whisking constantly, until the mixture is smooth, 2 to 3 minutes; do not let the flour brown. Gradually stir in the milk.

2. Increase the heat to moderate and cook, stirring constantly, until the sauce is thickened and smooth, and no raw flour taste remains, about 3 to 5 minutes. Remove the saucepan from the heat and stir in the cheese, salt, and pepper.

3. To store, lay plastic wrap directly on the surface of the sauce to prevent a skin from forming. Let the sauce cool to room temperature, then refrigerate until needed. Reheat the sauce in the top of a double boiler.

Makes 1 1/4 cups

Dijon Mustard Sauce
This is wonderful with ham or poached or grilled fish.

1 tablespoon butter or margarine

1 tablespoon all-purpose flour

1 cup hot milk

2 tablespoons Dijon mustard

1 teaspoon white wine vinegar

1/4 teaspoon salt

1/8 teaspoon white or black ground pepper

1. In a small heavy saucepan over low heat, melt the butter. Add the flour and cook, whisking constantly, until the mixture is smooth, 2 to 3 minutes; do not let the flour brown. Gradually stir in the milk.

2. Increase the heat to moderate and cook, stirring constantly, until the sauce is thickened and smooth, and no raw flour taste remains, about 3 to 5 minutes. Remove the saucepan from the heat and stir in the mustard, vinegar, salt, and pepper.

3. To store, lay plastic wrap directly on the surface of the sauce to prevent a skin from forming. Let the sauce cool to room temperature, then refrigerate until needed. Reheat the sauce in the top of a double boiler.

Makes 1 cup

Mushroom Sauce
Serve this creamy mushroom sauce with roast meat or poultry, or use in casseroles. It is a far cry from canned mushroom soup or sauces.

3 tablespoons butter or margarine

1 tablespoon all-purpose flour

1 cup hot milk or Beef Stock (page 49)

1/2 cup chopped mushrooms

1/4 teaspoon salt

1/8 teaspoon white or black ground pepper

1. In a small heavy saucepan over low heat, melt 1 tablespoon of the butter. Add the flour and cook, whisking constantly, until the mixture is smooth, 2 to 3 minutes; do not let the flour brown. Gradually stir in the milk or, if a darker sauce is desired, the beef stock.

2. In a small skillet over moderate heat, melt the remaining 2 tablespoons of butter. Add the mushrooms and cook, stirring, for 3 minutes.

3. Increase the heat to moderate and cook, stirring constantly, until the sauce is thickened and smooth, and no raw flour taste remains, about 3 to 5 minutes. Remove the saucepan from the heat and stir in the mushrooms, salt, and pepper.

4. To store, lay plastic wrap directly on the surface of the sauce to prevent a skin from forming. Let the sauce cool to room temperature, then refrigerate until needed. Reheat the sauce in the top of a double boiler.

Makes 1 cup

dessert sauces

Blueberry Syrup
This fresh homemade syrup is mouthwatering over bread pudding, pound cake, ice cream, or pancakes.

4 cups blueberries, fresh or frozen

2 thin strips (1 x 3 inches) lemon zest

3 cups water

3 cups sugar

1 tablespoon lemon juice

1. In a large saucepan, using a wooden spoon, crush the berries. Add the lemon zest and 1 cup of the water and, over moderate heat, bring the mixture to a simmer. Reduce the heat to low and cook, uncovered, for 5 minutes without simmering.

2. Line a colander or large sieve with cheesecloth and set it over a large bowl. Pour the berry mixture through the colander, squeezing the cheesecloth to extract all of the juice; there should be about 2 cups of blueberry juice. Discard the solids.

3. In a saucepan over moderately high heat, combine 2 cups of water and the sugar, and bring to a boil, stirring until the sugar is dissolved. Continue boiling, without stirring, until a candy thermometer reads 260°F.

4. Add the blueberry mixture. Boil, uncovered, for 1 minute. Remove from heat and let cool. Stir in lemon juice. Store in an airtight container in the refrigerator for up to 1 month.

Makes 3 1/2 cups

Raspberry Sauce
Simple and sensational, this quick, inexpensive sauce will quickly become a kitchen staple to serve over other fruits, sherbets, or ice cream.

1/2 cup sugar

1/2 cup water

2 tablespoons Grand Marnier or other orange-flavored liqueur

2 cups fresh raspberries or dry-pack frozen raspberries

1. In a small saucepan over high heat, bring the sugar and water to a boil. Remove the pan and let the syrup cool.

2. Add the Grand Marnier and raspberries, and stir gently; let stand for 2 minutes. Pour through a sieve into a bowl, pressing to remove the seeds; discard solids.

Makes about 3/4 cup

Mango and Passion Fruit Sauce
This sauce uses fresh fruit and can't be matched by a prepared sauce in a can or a freezer package.

1 large mango, peeled and cut up

1/2 cup (6-8 fruits) passion fruit pulp

1. In a food processor or blender, combine the mango and passion fruit pulp. Whirl until the mixture is a smooth puree.

2. Place in the refrigerator to chill before serving.

Makes 1 cup

Custard Sauce
No packaged vanilla pudding or custard mix can create this classic, creamy, vanilla-tinged sauce also known as crème anglaise.

1 1/2 cups milk
1/4 cup sugar
1/8 teaspoon salt
3 egg yolks, lightly beaten
3/4 teaspoon vanilla

1. In a medium saucepan over low heat, combine the milk, sugar, and salt, and heat just until small bubbles appear on the surface. In a medium bowl, whisk 1/4 cup of the milk mixture into the egg yolks, then stir back into the pan. Cook over low heat, whisking constantly, until the mixture coats the back of a spoon, about 10 minutes.

2. Remove the saucepan from the heat and strain the mixture through a sieve into a medium bowl. Stir in the vanilla. Let the sauce cool to room temperature and refrigerate, covered, until ready to serve.

Makes about 1 1/2 cups

Fruit Coulis
Here is a versatile sauce that can take advantage of berries in season—or less costly frozen ones the rest of the year. You can use raspberries, blueberries, blackberries, and of course, strawberries. You can also use fresh peaches or apricots—just lightly poach them before pureeing.

1/2 pint fresh berries or 1 package (8 ounces) frozen berries
Sugar, to taste

1. Rinse and drain the berries thoroughly (frozen berries do not require rinsing). In the bowl of a food processor or blender, whirl the berries until they form a smooth puree. If desired, add a little sugar while pureeing.

2. Press the mixture through a sieve and discard any solids or seeds. Taste and add additional sugar, if desired.

3. Place the sauce in the refrigerator to chill before serving. Store in an airtight container in the refrigerator for up to 2 days.

Makes about 1 cup

Butterscotch Sauce
Of course, you can buy butterscotch sauce. Try this versatile version warm over ice cream in summer or over hot gingerbread in the fall and you'll always make it yourself.

3/4 cup (1 1/2 sticks) unsalted butter
1 1/2 cups firmly packed brown sugar
1/8 teaspoon salt
1 cup heavy cream
1 teaspoon vanilla extract

1. In a small saucepan over low heat, melt the butter. Add the sugar, salt, and cream, and stir until the sugar has dissolved. Simmer for 8 to 10 minutes over low heat, stirring continuously so that the sugar doesn't crystallize. Remove the saucepan from the heat and stir in the vanilla.

2. Serve warm or cold. Can be refrigerated in a covered container for up to a week.

Makes about 2 1/2 cups

Replacements for Pantry Staples   **473**

Chocolate Sauce

Swiss dark and semisweet chocolate, and Dutch cocoa, combine in a rich triple-chocolate knockout that can't be matched at any price.

2 tablespoons Dutch processed cocoa

3 tablespoons cold water

1/2 cup (1 stick) unsalted butter

6 ounces Swiss dark chocolate

4 ounces semisweet chocolate

1 cup boiling water

1 cup firmly packed light brown sugar

3/4 cup granulated sugar

1/2 cup light corn syrup

1/4 teaspoon salt

1 teaspoon vanilla

1. In a glass measuring cup, combine the processed cocoa and water, and stir until completely dissolved. In the top of a double boiler over low heat, melt the butter. Add the cocoa, and the dark and semisweet chocolate, then stir in the boiling water, brown and granulated sugars, corn syrup, and salt.

2. Set the top of the double boiler over moderate heat, and bring the mixture to a boil; boil, uncovered, for 5 minutes (7 minutes for a thicker sauce that will harden when it comes into contact with ice cream). Remove the saucepan from the heat and let the sauce cool to room temperature, then stir in the vanilla.

Makes about 2 1/2 cups

Hot Chocolate Sauce

This irresistible sauce should be made at the last minute and served piping hot over ice cream or frozen yogurt.

1/3 cup milk

1/2 cup heavy cream

1/4 cup sugar

7 ounces bittersweet chocolate, broken up

1. In a small saucepan over low heat, stir together the milk, cream, and sugar.

2. Add the chocolate, stirring until it is melted and a smooth consistency. Serve at once or keep chilled. Reheat slowly before serving.

Chocolate Toffee Sauce

This sauce is like a liquid Heath Bar poured over your ice cream—divine! But also as good as it gets. You can't buy an indulgence like this.

3 ounces semisweet chocolate

1/2 cup heavy cream

1/2 cup toffee candy

In a microwave-safe bowl, microwave the chocolate following the manufacturer's directions until it is melted. Or place the chocolate in a bowl set over simmering water and stir until melted. Stir in the heavy cream and the toffee candy until melted and well blended. Serve warm.

Makes 1 cup

dry mixes

Biscuit and Pancake Mix
This mix will quickly make many favorite breakfast treats—not only biscuits and pancakes but also scones and waffles (pages 141, 142).

6 cups all-purpose flour (or
   3 cups all-purpose flour and
   3 cups whole wheat flour)

3 1/2 tablespoons baking
   powder

1 cup instant nonfat dry milk

1 tablespoon salt

1 cup vegetable shortening

1. In a large bowl, combine the flour, baking powder, powdered milk, and salt, and stir until well mixed. Using a pastry blender or 2 knives, cut in the shortening until the biscuit mix resembles coarse meal.

2. Put the mix into a self-sealing bag, label, date, and refrigerate for up to 6 weeks.

Makes about 8 cups

Basic Cake Mix
Don't purchase cake mix—make your own. This basic mix can be stored for 10 to 12 weeks and makes about 16 cups. To test this mix, we suggest that you use it to create the delectable Chocolate Cake (page 117) and Spice Cake (page 116) recipes. It's so flexible that you'll quickly develop your own recipes to fill your family's needs.

8 cups all-purpose flour

6 cups sugar

1/4 cup baking powder

1 1/2 teaspoons salt

2 1/4 cups (1-pound can)
   vegetable shortening

1. In a large bowl, sift together the flour, sugar, baking powder, and salt. Stir until all the ingredients are well blended.

2. Add the vegetable shortening and, using a pastry blender or two knives, cut the shortening into the flour mixture until it resembles very coarse crumbs.

3. Place the mix in a large, airtight container or a self-sealing plastic bag. Label and date, and store the mix in a cool, dry place or in the refrigerator for 10 to 12 weeks.

Makes about 16 cups

Helpful Hint | Make Your Own Real Vanilla Extract

Every kitchen needs a bottle of vanilla extract—one of the most used flavorings—but as you know, it is not an inexpensive purchase. While imitation vanilla is less expensive, you pay a big price in the loss of that real vanilla flavor. What to do? Make your own.

Place a vanilla bean in a small, clean jar. Pour 3 tablespoons of plain vodka over the vanilla bean. Close the lid tightly and let the mixture stand for four weeks. Remove and discard the vanilla bean before using the extract.

pasta

Egg Pasta #1

Fresh pasta is actually quite easy to make, cooks more quickly than dried pasta, and tastes amazingly light and delicious. There are three steps to making pasta: (1) mixing together a dough, (2) rolling it out and cutting it, and (3) cooking it. You can mix the dough by hand or in a food processor. This is the simplest recipe: The eggs give enough moisture to form a dough.

3 eggs
2 cups all-purpose flour

1. In a large bowl, beat the eggs. Sift in the flour, stirring constantly, until a soft dough forms.
2. On a lightly floured surface, knead the dough until it is smooth and elastic.
3. Roll out and cut the dough by hand or with a pasta machine (see Rolling and Cutting Fresh Pasta, opposite).
4. To cook, bring a large pot of lightly salted water to a boil. Add the pasta. Fresh pasta cooks *very* quickly—thin strands may be cooked by the time they float to the surface of the water; other varieties will cook in about 1 to 2 minutes, ravioli in 6 minutes.

Makes 4 to 6 servings of spaghetti or linguini or enough for a large lasagna

Egg Pasta #2

A little easier to handle, this dough adds olive oil, water, and salt.

2 cups all-purpose flour
2 large eggs
2 teaspoons olive oil
2 tablespoons water
1/2 teaspoon salt

1. On a lightly floured surface, pour the flour in a mound. Using your hands, make a well in the center of the flour mound.
2. In a small bowl, stir together the eggs, olive oil, and water. Slowly pour the egg mixture into the flour well; sprinkle with the salt.
3. Carefully push the flour from around the edges into the well, stirring with your fingers to form a batter. Continue adding flour to the well until the mixture forms a soft dough.
4. Knead the dough for at least 5 minutes or until it is smooth and elastic. Cover the dough with an inverted bowl or plastic wrap, and let it rest for 1 hour before rolling.
5. Roll out and cut the dough by hand or with a pasta machine (see Rolling and Cutting Fresh Pasta, opposite).
6. To cook, bring a large pot of lightly salted water to a boil. Add the pasta. Fresh pasta cooks *very* quickly—thin strands may be cooked by the time they float to the surface of the water; other varieties will cook in about 1 to 2 minutes, ravioli in 6 minutes.

Makes 4 to 6 servings of spaghetti or linguini or enough for a large lasagna

rolling and cutting fresh pasta

By hand: On a lightly floured surface using a long, thin rolling pin, roll out one piece of dough into a thin (1/16 inch thick) 20 x 14-inch rectangle. Lightly flour the top of the dough to prevent sticking. Fold the rectangle of dough in half lengthwise, then fold it again; you should have a 5 x 14-inch rec-

tangle—do not press the dough together. Using a very sharp knife or pastry wheel and a ruler or straightedge if needed, cut the sheet of dough into strips, making them as narrow or as wide as you like. Carefully unfold the strips and either hang them gently on a drying rack or lay them flat on dish towels. Let dry for 1 to 2 hours. Fresh pasta must air-dry before cooking or it becomes gluey when boiled.

Using a pasta machine: Following the manufacturer's directions, pass the dough several times through the machine's rollers to knead it and make it elastic. Adjust the rollers closer and closer together as you roll the dough until it is thin enough to cut. Set the machine to cut the desired shapes, and cut. Let the pasta dry on a drying rack or flat on dish towels for 1 to 2 hours.

Processor Dough Pasta *You can make quick work of mixing the dough if you use your food processor instead of your fingers.*

2 1/4 cups all-purpose flour
2 eggs
1/4 cup water
1 tablespoon olive oil
1 teaspoon salt

1. Fit a food processor with a plastic dough blade or a metal chopping blade. Combine all the ingredients in the food processor container. Process until the dough rides up in the center, about 20 to 30 seconds.

2. On a lightly floured surface, knead the dough for about 5 minutes or until it is smooth and elastic. Cover the dough with plastic wrap and let it sit for 30 minutes before rolling.

3. Roll out and cut the dough by hand or with a pasta machine (see Rolling and Cutting Fresh Pasta above).

4. To cook, bring a large pot of lightly salted water to a boil. Add the pasta. Fresh pasta cooks *very* quickly—thin strands may be cooked by the time they float to the surface of the water; other varieties will cook in about 1 to 2 minutes, ravioli in 6 minutes.

Makes 4 to 6 servings of spaghetti or linguini or enough for a large lasagna

storing fresh pasta

Let the pasta dry for several hours or until it is dry but not brittle. For long strands of pasta (fettuccine or linguine, for example), when the dough has dried slightly but is still pliable, gently wrap a loose bunch around your fingers to form a "nest." Set the nest to dry completely. For large lasagna rectangles, allow each to dry completely. Then stack the pieces between sheets of wax paper. Store cut pasta in self-sealing plastic bags or airtight containers in the refrigerator for up to 1 week or in the freezer for up to 1 month.

chapter 2

Pickled, Preserved and
Frozen Foods

Fewer and fewer of us grow our own fruits and vegetables anymore, but the waning days of summer still present us with an embarrassment of riches as

an avalanche of tomatoes, peppers, cukes, corn, peaches, and other fresh produce flood fruit stands, roadside stalls, and even supermarket shelves. The flavor of this sun-ripened produce is at its peak, and following the simple law of supply and demand, the price is at its lowest. Indeed, you can often get a bushel of tomatoes or peaches for what you would pay for a handful at a less bounteous time of year. The same lower-price, better-taste principle applies to those fruits and vegetables that have different peak seasons—such as strawberries and asparagus in late spring and pumpkins and hard squash in late fall.

The purpose of the recipes in this chapter is to help you take advantage of nature's largess. If you buy fresh vegetables and fruits at their peak and when their prices are most reasonable, you can freeze them and have your "five a day" out of the freezer all winter long—at summer prices and with that unmatchable summer taste. All the instructions you need are in this chapter. Freezing is incredibly simple. With only a bit more effort, you can make your own unbelievably tasty pickles, relishes, and chutneys. And if you also make your own jellies and jams, you will not only save money but also have ready-made presents for hostesses and new neighbors as well.

pickles and relishes

Dill Pickles—Fermentation Method
Dills are the wonderful pickles for which delis are famous. You can easily make your own for lots less. Buy unwaxed cucumbers and try both the fermentation method in this recipe and the fresh-pack method in the next recipe to see which is easier for you and which tastes better to you.

1 gallon water

2/3 cup salt

1 cup white vinegar

4 pounds small to medium (4-5 inches long) pickling cucumbers, unpeeled and scrubbed

15 sprigs fresh dill

30 peppercorns

15 garlic cloves *(optional)*

1. Prepare the brine: In a large, nonreactive bowl, combine 1/2 gallon of the water, 1/3 cup of the salt, and 1/2 cup of the vinegar.

2. Sprinkle half the dill, 15 of the peppercorns, and if using, half the garlic cloves over the bottom of a clean, 1-gallon stone crock. Place the cucumbers on top of the dill-spice mixture, then layer the remaining dill and spices over the cucumbers. Pour the brine over the cucumber mixture to cover. Place a heavy plate on top of the cucumbers and weight it down to keep it below the level of the brine.

3. Set the crock in a moderate (68°F to 72°F), dark place and let the pickles ferment for 1 to 3 weeks. Skim off and discard any scum that forms on top of the brine daily. The pickles are ready when the scum stops forming, the mixture no longer bubbles, and the pickles are olive-green in color with no white spots.

4. Prepare fresh brine: In a large, nonreactive saucepan, combine the remaining 1/2 gallon of water, 1/3 cup of salt, 1/2 cup of vinegar. Drain the pickles; remove and discard the garlic cloves, if used. Divide and ladle the pickles into sterilized 1-quart canning jars. Pour the fresh brine over the pickles in the jars, dividing it equally. Wipe the rims, cover, and process for 15 minutes in boiling water (see Safe Canning with a Hot-Water Bath, page 72). Cool and test for airtight seals. Label, date, and store in a cool, dark place for 4 to 6 weeks. Once a jar has been opened, store the pickles in the refrigerator.

Makes 4 to 6 quarts

Dill Pickles—Fresh-Pack Method

1/3 cup salt

1/2 gallon hot water

4 pounds small to medium
(4-5 inches long) pickling
cucumbers, unpeeled and
scrubbed

4 garlic cloves

8 sprigs fresh dill

4 teaspoons mustard seed

3 tablespoons salt

1 tablespoon sugar

1 1/2 cups vinegar

3 cups water

1. Prepare the brine: In a large, nonreactive bowl, combine
1/3 cup salt and 1/2 gallon hot water. Stir until the salt has
completely dissolved. Add the cucumbers to the brine;
let stand overnight to pickle.

2. Drain the pickles and discard the soaking brine. Place the pickles,
divided equally, into 2 sterilized 1-quart canning jars, packing
the pickles so that they are standing on end. Place 2 garlic cloves,
4 dill sprigs, and 2 teaspoons of mustard seed in each jar.

3. In a large, nonreactive saucepan, combine 3 tablespoons salt,
1 tablespoon sugar, 1 1/2 cups vinegar, and 3 cups water. Bring
the mixture to a boil. Pour the hot brine over the pickles in the
jars, dividing it equally. Wipe the rims, cover, and process for
20 minutes in boiling water (see Safe Canning with a Hot-Water
Bath, page 72). Cool and test for airtight seals. Label, date, and
store in a cool, dark place for 4 to 6 weeks. Once a jar has been
opened, store the pickles in the refrigerator.

Makes 2 quarts

Bread-and-Butter Pickles
These are the sweet pickles that go so well with meat sandwiches. Once you get the hang of putting them up, you'll never spend your money on store-bought pickles again.

30 small to medium
(4-5 inches long) pickling
cucumbers, unpeeled,
sliced 1/4-inch thick

8 large yellow onions,
halved lengthwise and cut
crosswise into thin slices

1 medium red bell pepper,
cored, seeded, and chopped

1/2 cup pickling salt

4 cups crushed ice

4 cups white vinegar

4 1/2 cups sugar

2 tablespoons mustard seed

2 teaspoons celery seed

1 tablespoon ground
turmeric

1 teaspoon ground ginger

1 teaspoon black
peppercorns

1. In a very large colander set over a larger bowl or Dutch oven,
combine the cucumber slices, onions, and red bell pepper.
Sprinkle the vegetable mixture with the pickling or kosher salt
and toss well. Cover the vegetables with a 2-inch layer of
crushed ice. Refrigerate for 3 to 4 hours, adding ice as needed.

2. In a large, heavy, nonreactive saucepan or Dutch oven over
moderate heat, combine the vinegar, sugar, mustard seed, celery
seed, turmeric, ginger, and peppercorns; bring the mixture to a
boil and boil for 10 minutes. Stir in the cucumber mixture and
return just to a boil.

3. Ladle the vegetables and liquid into sterilized 1-pint canning
jars, leaving 1/4 inch of space between the top of the mixture
and the rim of the jars (see Safe Canning with a Hot-Water
Bath, page 72). Run a long, thin spatula around the inside of
the jars to release any trapped air bubbles. Wipe the rims, cover,
and process for 10 minutes in boiling water. Cool and test for
airtight seals. Label, date, and store in a cool, dark place for 4 to
6 weeks. Once opened, store the pickles in the refrigerator.

Makes 8 pints

Pickled Gherkins
These are the tiny pickles that are served with pâtés and terrines.

10 dozen French gherkins or tiny pickling cucumbers, well scrubbed

1 1/2 cups pickling or kosher salt

30 peppercorns, white, green, or multicolored

6 small bay leaves

18 sprigs fresh tarragon

4-6 cups white wine vinegar

4 1/2 cups sugar

1-2 tablespoons pickling or kosher salt, to taste

1. In a large, nonreactive bowl, place the gherkins or cucumbers and sprinkle with salt. Loosely cover and let stand 24 hours.

2. Drain the pickles and discard the brine. Pack the pickles, standing on end, into 6 sterilized 1-pint canning jars; leave a 1/4-inch space at the top of the jar. Add 5 peppercorns, 1 bay leaf, and 2 sprigs of tarragon to each jar.

3. Meanwhile, in a large, heavy, nonreactive saucepan or Dutch oven, combine the vinegar and sugar with the remaining 6 sprigs of tarragon. Over high heat, bring the mixture to a boil. Pour the mixture over the pickles in each jar to cover. Cover the jars and let stand overnight; the pickles will lose their color.

4. Drain and reserve the vinegar from the jars into a large, nonreactive saucepan. Stir in the salt, and over high heat, bring the mixture to a boil. Remove the pan from the heat and let the brine cool. Pour the cooled brine back over the pickles in the jar, dividing it evenly; the pickles should recover their color.

5. Wipe the rims, cover, and process for 15 minutes in boiling water (see Safe Canning with a Hot-Water Bath, page 72). Cool and test for airtight seals. Label, date, and store in a cool, dark place for 4 to 6 weeks. Once a jar has been opened, store the pickles in the refrigerator.

Makes about 6 half-pints

Pickled Baby Corn
These bright yellow mini corns add crunch to cold meat platters.

1/2 cup sugar

2 cups cider vinegar

1 1/2 cups water

1 teaspoon kosher salt

1 teaspoon mixed whole pickling spices

3 cans (14 ounces each) baby corn, drained

1. In a nonreactive saucepan, combine the sugar, cider vinegar, water, and salt. Cut a square of cheesecloth. Place the pickling spices in the cloth, bring the corners together to make a bag, and secure with string. Add the bag to the brine. Bring the brine to a boil, stirring to dissolve the sugar; cook for 4 to 5 minutes. Remove and discard the spice bag.

2. Place the corn, divided equally, into 3 sterilized 1-pint canning jars, packing the corn so that they are standing on end; pour the hot brine over the corn, leaving a 1/4-inch space between the top of the liquid and the rim of the jar. Wipe the rims, cover, and process for 15 minutes in boiling water (see Safe Canning with a Hot-Water Bath, page 72). Cool and test for airtight seals. Label, date, and store in a cool, dark place for 4 to 6 weeks; the corn will be ready to eat in 1 week. Once a jar has been opened, store the corn in the refrigerator.

Makes 3 pints

Pickle Relish

The word "relish" says it all—savor the flavor—and put it on your hot dog or a ham sandwich. This luscious recipe is most inexpensive, and jars of pickle relish make fine gifts.

4 medium cucumbers,
   unpeeled and finely
   chopped

2 large red bell peppers,
   cored, seeded, and chopped

2 large green bell peppers,
   cored, seeded, and chopped

1 medium yellow onion,
   chopped

1 tablespoon ground
   turmeric

1/2 cup kosher salt

6 cups water

2 cinnamon sticks,
   broken in half

1 tablespoon mustard seed

2 teaspoons whole allspice

1 teaspoon whole cloves

2 cups sugar

2 cups cider vinegar

1. In a large, heavy, nonreactive saucepan or Dutch oven, combine the cucumbers, red and green bell peppers, and onion; sprinkle the turmeric over all the vegetables. In a large bowl, dissolve the salt in the water to make a brine. Pour the brine over the vegetables, loosely cover the saucepan, and let stand for 6 to 8 hours. Drain the vegetables, rinse well several times, and return the vegetables to the saucepan.

2. Cut a 4-inch square of cheesecloth. Place the cinnamon sticks, mustard seed, allspice, and cloves in the center of the cloth, bring the corners together to make a bag, and secure with kitchen string, Add the spice bag to the saucepan along with the sugar and cider vinegar. Over high heat, bring the mixture to a rolling boil and cook until the sugar is completely dissolved. Reduce the heat to moderate and boil gently, uncovered, for 10 minutes. Remove and discard the spice bag.

3. Spoon the relish into 8 warm, sterilized jars, leaving a 1/4-inch space between the top of the relish and the rim of the jar. Wipe the rims, cover, and process for 10 minutes in boiling water (see Safe Canning with a Hot-Water Bath, page 72). Cool and test for airtight seals. Label, date, and store in a cool, dark place for 4 to 6 weeks. Once a jar has been opened, store the relish in the refrigerator.

Makes 8 half-pints

Helpful Hint

In Canning, Acid Content Is a Crucial Factor

Jams, jellies, marmalades, chutneys, pickles—basically any fruit or mixture with a high enough acid content to inhibit the growth of microorganisms—can be safely canned with a hot-water bath. Low-acid vegetables—every type other than tomatoes, which are botanically a fruit—should be frozen for storage or canned with a pressure cooker unless you are pickling them. Pickling adds enough acidity to allow for safe hot-water processing.

Pickled Cauliflower Florets *This is a traditional part of an antipasto plate.*

1 large head cauliflower, cut into florets, about 7 to 8 cups

White vinegar

1 tablespoon salt

1 tablespoon white peppercorns

1 tablespoon light brown sugar

1 medium red bell pepper, seed and finely sliced

6 small dried red chile peppers

1. In a large, nonreactive saucepan or Dutch oven, place the cauliflower florets and pour in enough vinegar to cover. Add the salt, peppercorns, and sugar.

2. Over high heat, bring the brine to a boil. Add the red bell pepper strips, and boil for 1 minute. Using a slotted spoon, transfer the vegetables to 2 warm, sterilized 1-quart jars with wide mouths. Pack the vegetables firmly, dividing the pepper strips evenly between the jars. Tuck 3 chile peppers into each jar.

3. Pour the hot brine over the vegetables in the jars until the cauliflower is completely covered, leaving a 1/4-inch space between the top of the brine and the rim of the jars. Wipe the rims, cover, and process for 20 minutes in boiling water (see Safe Canning with a Hot-Water Bath, page 72). Cool and test for airtight seals. Label, date, and store in a cool, dark place for 4 to 6 weeks; the cauliflower will be ready for eating in 2 weeks. Once a jar has been opened, store the cauliflower in the refrigerator.

Makes about 2 quarts

Pickled Onions *These yummy onions fit many a bill.*

Water to cover the onions

4 pounds small white pickling onions

1/2 cup salt

8 peppercorns

4 fresh red chiles (wear gloves when handling; they burn)

4 bay leaves

4 cups cider vinegar

1. In a large saucepan, bring water to a boil. Place the onions in a large, nonreactive bowl. Pour the hot water over the onions in the bowl and let stand for 5 minutes; drain. Trim the root end and the crowns; the peels should slip off easily. Do not remove too many layers of the onions.

2. Place the peeled onions in a large bowl and cover them with cold water. Add the salt and mix well. Let stand overnight.

3. Drain the onions. Using a large slotted spoon, transfer the onions to 4 warm, sterilized 1-pint jars with wide mouths. To each jar, add 2 peppercorns, 1 red chile, and 1 bay leaf.

4. In a large, nonreactive saucepan over high heat, bring the cider vinegar to a boil. Immediately pour the hot vinegar over the onions in the jars to cover them, leaving a 1/8-inch space between the top of the vinegar and the rim of the jars. Wipe the rims, cover, and process for 10 minutes in boiling water (see Safe Canning with a Hot-Water Bath, page 72). Cool and test for airtight seals. Label, date, and store in a cool, dark place; the onions will be ready to eat in 4 weeks. Once a jar has been opened, store the onions in the refrigerator.

Makes about 4 pints

Red Onion Relish

A noteworthy accompaniment to almost any variety of cheese, this red onion treat is cheaper and better made at home.

- 3 tablespoons olive oil
- 2 pounds red onions, peeled and sliced
- 1/2 cup sugar
- 1 teaspoon kosher salt
- 1/2 teaspoon black pepper, freshly ground
- 4 tablespoons balsamic or sherry vinegar
- 1 cup red wine

1. In a large, nonreactive saucepan over moderate heat, heat the olive oil. Add the onion slices and cook about 20 minutes, stirring occasionally.

2. Stir the sugar, salt, and pepper into the onion mixture. Reduce the heat to low, cover the saucepan, and cook very gently for 10 minutes; if the heat is too high, use a heat diffuser.

3. Add vinegar and the wine, and cook, uncovered, stirring at regular intervals, until the mixture has the consistency of chutney, about 20 to 30 minutes. Skim off and discard any scum that forms during cooking.

4. Ladle the onion relish into two hot, sterilized half-pint jars, leaving a 1/4-inch space between the top of the relish and the rim of the jar. Wipe the rims, cover, and process for 10 minutes in boiling water (see Safe Canning with a Hot-Water Bath, page 72). Cool and test for airtight seals. Label, date, and store in a cool, dark place; the onion relish will be ready to eat in 4 weeks. Once a jar has been opened, store the onion relish in the refrigerator.

Makes 2 half-pints

Pickled Spiced Plums

Enjoy the enticing spices of the Orient with these aromatic plums—the perfect partner to roast pork or lamb.

- 1 2/3 cups sugar
- 2 2/3 cups water
- 1 cup cider vinegar
- 4 cinnamon sticks, broken
- 1 tablespoon whole cloves
- 1 tablespoon black peppercorns
- 2-3 strips orange zest
- 2 pounds small, firm, ripe red or purple plums, well scrubbed

1. In a medium saucepan over moderately high heat, combine the sugar and water, and bring the mixture to a boil, stirring to dissolve the sugar. Reduce the heat and simmer for 10 minutes.

2. Add the cider vinegar, cinnamon sticks, cloves, peppercorns, and orange zest; stir to combine. Cover the pan and simmer the mixture gently for 15 minutes.

3. Using a sterilized skewer or ice pick, prick each plum in several places. Divide the plums equally between two 1-quart, warm, sterilized jars with wide mouths. Pour the hot spiced syrup over the plums to cover them, leaving a 1/4-inch space between the top of the syrup and the rim of the jars. Wipe the rims of the jars, cover, and process for 25 minutes in boiling water (see Safe Canning with a Hot-Water Bath, page 72). Cool and test for airtight seals. Label, date, and store in a cool, dark place; the plums will be ready to eat in 4 weeks. Once a jar has been opened, store the plums in the refrigerator.

Makes about 2 quarts

safe canning with a hot-water bath

Learning to process your canned foods in a hot-water bath will remove any concerns about bacterial contamination. Safe canning includes processing foods at a high enough temperature for a long enough time—you'll find the recommended processing times in each recipe. You can purchase a hot-water bath set or put one together yourself out of things you probably already have or can purchase easily and cheaply (check out yard sales and resale stores for the best bargains).

You will need:

1 very large, deep, heavy, nonreactive saucepan or Dutch oven with a tight-fitting lid

1 wire rack or 1 basket to fit the saucepan

Glass canning jars and lids (the jars and metal screw bands to hold the lids in place can be reused; new lids must be used every time you can)

Canning tongs (these are designed to transfer jars)

Additional wire racks for cooling the jars

Here is how to proceed:

1. Start by sterilizing all the jars. Wash them in hot, soapy water, rinse thoroughly, and set in a saucepan of boiling water that covers the jars by 1 inch; boil for 10 minutes. Remove the saucepan from the heat but let the jars sit in the hot water until ready to use.

2. Prepare the lids following the manufacturer's directions.

3. Once the food is cooked, remove the cooking saucepan from the heat. Carefully remove the jars from the hot water. Ladle the food into the warm, clean jars, leaving a space between the top of the food and the rim of the jar as specified in the recipe (usually between 1/8 inch and 1/4 inch). Run a sterilized spatula around the inside of the jar to remove any large air bubbles.

4. Using a clean, damp cloth, wipe off the rims of each jar. Following the manufacturer's directions, apply the lids and screw bands.

5. Place the rack in the processing saucepan and fill halfway with hot water. Place the filled jars on the rack, then add boiling water (pour around the jars, not directly on the jars) until the jars are covered by at least 1 inch of boiling water.

Cover the saucepan. Set the saucepan over high heat and bring the water to a boil; begin timing when the water comes to a rolling boil. Process for the time specified in the recipe; at high altitudes, increase the boiling time by 1 minute for each 1,000 feet above sea level.

6. When the processing time has been reached, use the tongs to transfer the jars from the saucepan to a second wire rack and let the jars cool completely; be sure to leave space between the jars on the rack. Let the jars stand for 12 to 24 hours.

7. Gently press the center of each lid: if the depression in the center holds, the seal is good and you can remove the screw band and store the jar; if the depression does not hold, the seal is not good and you should store the jar in the refrigerator and use the food immediately.

8. Label and date each jar. Store canned foods in a cool (40°F to 60°F), dark storage space; check the seals periodically and just before opening. Any jar that leaks, or food that smells or looks questionable when opened, should be discarded. *Never* taste food to check for freshness.

Roasted Red Bell Peppers in Oil
Colorful and luscious, these are a must for any antipasto platter and make a superb snack on crusty bread.

4 pounds (about 8 medium) firm red bell peppers

2 tablespoons coriander seed

1 tablespoon peppercorns

5 garlic cloves

5 bay leaves

1-2 cups virgin olive oil

1. Arrange the red bell peppers on a broiler pan or heavy-duty baking sheet. Set the pan 2 to 3 inches from a preheated broiler and broil 8 to 10 minutes, turning the peppers every few minutes so their skins blacken evenly. Transfer the peppers to a large heatproof bowl, cover with plastic wrap, and cool until safe to handle, about 10 minutes. The skins will loosen and slip right off the peppers. Cut the roasted peppers in thick slices, discarding the stalks and seeds.

2. Transfer the roasted peppers to 3 warm, sterilized half-pint jars, dividing the peppers evenly. Add some of the coriander seed, peppercorns, garlic, and bay leaves to each jar, dividing equally and arranging the peppers and spices attractively.

3. Pour olive oil into each jar to cover the peppers, leaving a 1/4-inch space between the top of the oil and the rim of the jars. Using a sterilized skewer, expel any air bubbles from the oil. Wipe the rims of the jars, cover, and store in the refrigerator for up to 1 month; the red peppers will be ready to eat within a few days.

Makes 3 half-pints

Oven-Dried Tomatoes
Oven drying is an easy, relatively quick way to preserve garden-fresh tomatoes.

2 pounds ripe Italian plum or large cherry tomatoes, halved

1/4 cup kosher salt

1/4 teaspoon freshly ground pepper

2 tablespoons dried marjoram, crumbled

Olive oil, to cover

1. Preheat the oven to just below 200°F (warm).

2. Using a teaspoon, remove the seeds but not the fibrous tissue from the tomato halves. Line a baking sheet with foil. Place the tomatoes, cut side up, on the baking sheet and sprinkle them with salt, pepper, and marjoram. Place the baking sheet in the oven and bake for 12 to 24 hours; check periodically to be sure the tomatoes are drying, not cooking. If they are drying too quickly, prop open the oven door slightly. Drying tomatoes will slowly darken and wrinkle. Small tomatoes may take only 12 hours to dry; large tomatoes may take as long as 24 hours.

3. Spoon the tomatoes into 2 warm, sterilized, half-pint jars. Pour olive oil over the tomatoes, leaving a 1/4-inch space between the top of the oil and the rim of the jar. Wipe the rims of the jars, cover, and allow to cool. Label and date the jars, and store in the refrigerator for up to 1 month. Keep the tomatoes refrigerated once the jars are opened.

Makes 2 half-pints

chutneys

Mango Chutney
The pungent flavor of fresh ginger and the heat of red pepper lend dramatic appeal to this classic companion to spicy curries.

5 pounds green mangoes, peeled and chopped

1 teaspoon kosher salt

1 1/4 cups cider vinegar

1 1/4 cups apple cider

1 tablespoon chopped fresh ginger

2 teaspoons ground red pepper

1 large onion, chopped

1 1/2 cups firmly packed dark brown sugar

1. In a large, nonmetallic bowl, place the mangoes and sprinkle them with salt. Set aside the mangoes for 24 hours.

2. Rinse the mangoes under cold running water and drain them thoroughly. In a large, nonreactive saucepan, combine the mangoes, cider vinegar, apple cider, ginger, red pepper, onion, and sugar. Over low heat, simmer the mixture, uncovered, for 30 to 40 minutes.

3. Spoon the chutney into warm, sterilized jars, leaving a 1/4-inch space between the top of the chutney and the rim of the jar. Wipe the rims, cover, and process for 10 minutes in boiling water (see Safe Canning with a Hot-Water Bath, page 72). Place the jars of chutney in a cool, dark place to season; the chutney will be ready to eat in 4 weeks. Once a jar has been opened, store the chutney in the refrigerator.

Makes about 6 half-pint jars

Spicy Tomato Chutney
Turmeric, cumin, mustard seeds and powder, and red pepper all lend spicy notes to this intense chutney that is easy to make and a nice gift for kind neighbors. Stir a dollop into curry as it is cooking to add even more flavor, then serve the chutney alongside for a real eye-opener.

5 pounds ripe red tomatoes, quartered

5 medium yellow onions, chopped

3 garlic cloves, minced

2 tablespoons dry mustard

1 tablespoon salt

1 tablespoon chopped fresh ginger

1 tablespoon cumin seed

2 teaspoons ground turmeric

1 teaspoon mustard seed

1 teaspoon ground red pepper

1 cup cider vinegar

1. In a large, nonreactive saucepan, combine the tomatoes, onions, garlic, dry mustard, salt, ginger, cumin, turmeric, mustard seed, red pepper, and cider vinegar. Over moderately high heat, bring the mixture to a boil; reduce the heat to low and simmer gently, uncovered, stirring occasionally, until the chutney has thickened, about 50 to 60 minutes.

2. Spoon the chutney into warm, sterilized jars, leaving a 1/4-inch space between the top of the chutney and the rim of the jar. Wipe the rims, cover, and process for 10 minutes in boiling water (see Safe Canning with a Hot-Water Bath, page 72). Place the jars of chutney in a cool, dark place to season; the chutney will be ready to eat in 4 weeks. Once a jar has been opened, store the chutney in the refrigerator.

Makes about 8 half-pint jars

Green Tomato Chutney

Don't know how to use your tomato bonanza? Harvest some before they ripen and whip up some jars of this savory side dish. Give some as lovely, inexpensive house gifts.

4 pounds green tomatoes, chopped

2 medium onions, peeled and chopped

1 large green apple, peeled, cored, and chopped

3/4 cup golden raisins

1 teaspoon salt

1 teaspoon ground allspice

1 teaspoon curry powder

1/2 teaspoon ground red pepper

1 cup firmly packed brown sugar

2 cups cider vinegar

1. In a large, nonreactive saucepan, combine the tomatoes, onions, apple, raisins, salt, allspice, curry powder, red pepper, brown sugar, and cider vinegar. Over low heat, bring the mixture to a simmer, uncovered, and cook gently until the chutney has thickened, about 45 minutes. Stir occasionally to prevent the chutney from burning. Stop cooking if the chutney begins to dry out.

2. Spoon the chutney into warm, sterilized jars, leaving a 1/4-inch space between the top of the chutney and the rim of the jar. Wipe the rims, cover, and process for 10 minutes in boiling water (see Safe Canning with a Hot-Water Bath, page 72). Place the jars of chutney in a cool, dark place to season; the chutney will be ready to eat in 4 weeks. Once a jar has been opened, store the chutney in the refrigerator.

Makes about 6 half-pint jars

Lemon Lime Chutney

This citrus sensation is superb with mildly spiced couscous and lamb dishes. An expensive luxury from stores, it is easy to make at home.

4 large lemons

2 limes

2 medium yellow onions, chopped

1 teaspoon salt

2 1/2 cups cider vinegar

3/4 cup golden raisins

1 tablespoon mustard seed

1 teaspoon ground ginger

1/2 teaspoon ground red pepper

2 cups sugar

1. Wash and wipe the unpeeled lemons and limes. Chop them finely, removing any seeds. In a large bowl, combine the chopped lemons, limes, and onions. Sprinkle the mixture with the salt, and set aside for 12 hours.

2. Pour the lemon-lime mixture with the juices into a large, nonreactive saucepan. Bring the mixture to a simmer and cook gently, uncovered, until the fruit is soft. Stir in the cider vinegar, raisins, mustard seed, ginger, red pepper, and sugar. Increase the heat and bring the mixture to a boil; reduce the heat and simmer, uncovered, until the chutney thickens, about 45 minutes.

3. Spoon the chutney into warm, sterilized jars, leaving a 1/4-inch space between the top of the chutney and the rim of the jar. Wipe the rims, cover, and process for 10 minutes in boiling water (see Safe Canning with a Hot-Water Bath, page 72). Place the jars of chutney in a cool, dark place to season; the chutney will be ready to eat in 4 weeks. Once a jar has been opened, store the chutney in the refrigerator.

Makes about 5 half-pint jars

jams, jellies, and marmalades

Dried-Apricot Jam

Buy dried apricots in bulk at health food stores or look for them on sale and stock up. The dried apricots intensify the apricot flavor, giving you a superior jam at a reasonable price.

16 ounces dried apricots

3 1/2 cups orange juice

3/4 cup sugar

1 tablespoon lemon juice

1/2 teaspoon ground cinnamon

1/4 teaspoon ground ginger

1. In a large, nonreactive saucepan or Dutch oven, combine the apricots, orange juice, and sugar. Over moderately high heat, bring the mixture to a boil; reduce the heat, cover the saucepan, and simmer for 30 minutes.

2. Stir in the lemon juice, cinnamon, and ginger. Remove the saucepan from the heat and let the mixture cool to room temperature.

3. Transfer the mixture to the bowl of a food processor or blender. Whirl until the mixture is pureed. Spoon the puree into 4 widemouthed, warm, sterilized half-pint jars, leaving a 1/4-inch space between the top of the jam and the rim of the jar (see Safe Canning with a Hot-Water Bath, page 72). Wipe the rims, cover, label, and date. Store the jam in the refrigerator for up to 3 weeks or in the freezer for up to 1 year.

Makes 4 half-pint jars

the trio of good jamming ingredients

To make a great jam, jelly, or marmalade, you need three components to work in harmony: acid, pectin, and sugar. If the proportions of each or any one of these is off, you may not be happy with the results.

Acid: Added to the mixture as citrus juice (usually lemon) or tartaric acid, this improves both the taste and appearance of the finished product, and in conjunction with pectin, it helps the mixture to jell.

Pectin: Most fruits contain some amount of pectin naturally, and it is released when the fruit is boiled, but not all fruits are created equal. Apples are known for their pectin, and so are sometimes added in one form or another to fruits that are lower in pectin to help them jell. Currants and red plums are also high-pectin fruits; moderate-pectin fruits include apricots, blueberries, peaches, and raspberries. Pectin is also found in peels (particularly citrus) and seeds, so these are sometimes included in part of a recipe to release their pectin during cooking. Pectin is also available in liquid and powdered forms (check out health food stores and larger supermarkets). If you do canning regularly, it is prudent to keep some on hand, just in case your jam or marmalade or jelly is being uncooperative. Follow the manufacturer's directions carefully.

Sugar: Another factor in jelling, sugar (either beet or cane) also helps to preserve the fruit and really brings out its flavor in addition to adding sweetness and countering any bitter taste, such as lemon.

Lemony Fig Jam

The tartness of the lemons sets off the sweetness of the figs. Here is an unusual jam that makes a lovely gift and keeps you out of the expensive food specialty store.

1 pound dried figs

4 cups water

3 cups sugar

Zest and juice of 2 lemons

1/2 cup pine nuts, lightly toasted

1. Wash and roughly chop the figs. In a small bowl, combine the figs and the water. Cover the bowl and let stand for 12 hours or overnight.

2. In a heavy, nonreactive saucepan, combine the figs and soaking water. Over high heat, bring the mixture to a boil; reduce the heat to low and simmer for 35 minutes.

3. Add the sugar and the lemon zest and juice. Stir until the sugar is dissolved. Return the mixture to a boil; reduce the heat slightly, and cook until the jam thickens, for 10 to 15 minutes. Using a slotted spoon, skim off and discard any foam that rises to the surface. Add the pine nuts and stir until they are well incorporated.

4. Remove the saucepan from the heat and stir to distribute the fruit and nuts evenly. Spoon the hot jam into 3 widemouthed, warm, sterilized 1/2-pint jars, leaving a 1/4-inch space between the top of the jam and the rim of the jar. Wipe the rims, cover, and process for 10 minutes in boiling water (see Safe Canning with a Hot-Water Bath, page 72). Dry, label, and date. Store the jars of jam in a cool, dark place; the jam will be ready to eat in 2 weeks. Once a jar has been opened, store the jam in the refrigerator.

Makes about 3 half-pint jars

Pear Jam

Spiced up with cinnamon and cloves, this jam does not require pectin to thicken. It is a spicy jam that you can make for very little money without splurging at a gourmet shop.

8 cups (about 5 1/2 pounds) chopped or coarsely ground peeled, cored pears

4 cups sugar

1 teaspoon ground cinnamon

1/4 teaspoon ground cloves

1. In a large, nonreactive saucepan or Dutch oven, combine the pears, sugar, cinnamon, and cloves. Over moderately low heat, simmer the mixture, uncovered, until it becomes thick, about 1 1/2 to 2 hours. Stir the mixture occasionally while it cooks, and increase the frequency of stirring as the mixture thickens.

2. Remove the saucepan from the heat; skim off and discard any foam that rises to the surface. Spoon the hot jam into 6 widemouthed, warm, sterilized 1/2-pint jars, leaving a 1/4-inch space between the top of the jam and the rim of the jar. Wipe the rims, cover, and process for 10 minutes in boiling water (see Safe Canning with a Hot-Water Bath, page 72). Dry, label, and date. Store the jars of jam in a cool, dark place. Once a jar has been opened, store the jam in the refrigerator.

Makes about 6 half-pint jars

Quince Jam
Available in late winter, quinces have yellow skin and flesh, and are quite tart. They have a high pectin content, so they are perfect for jam.

5 pounds (about 5-7) firm
  quinces

8 cups water

Juice of 3 lemons

8 cups sugar

1. Wash and peel the quinces, then core and roughly chop them.

2. In a large, heavy saucepan, combine the quinces with the water. Bring to a boil; reduce the heat and simmer until the fruit is soft and pale pink, about 35 to 45 minutes.

3. Add the lemon juice and sugar, and stir until the sugar is dissolved. Increase the heat and bring to a boil again; boil rapidly until the jam thickens, about 10 minutes. Using a slotted spoon, skim off and discard any foam that rises to the surface.

4. Remove the saucepan from the heat. Spoon the hot jam into 8 widemouthed, warm, sterilized 1/2-pint jars, leaving a 1/4-inch space between the top of the jam and the rim of the jar. Wipe the rims, cover, and process for 10 minutes in boiling water (see Safe Canning with a Hot-Water Bath, page 72). Dry, label, and date. Store the jars of jam in a cool, dark place; the jam will be ready to eat in 2 weeks. Once a jar has been opened, store the jam in the refrigerator.

Makes about 8 half-pint jars

Peach Jam
The natural sweetness of peaches make this jam a low-sugar-added preserve. Plan to put up a slew when peaches are in season during the summer.

8-10 cups water

2 1/2 pounds ripe peaches

3 strips (1/2 x 2 inches)
  orange zest

2/3 cups fresh orange juice

2/3 cup unsweetened
  white grape juice

2/3 cup firmly packed light
  brown sugar

1 tablespoon fresh
  lemon juice

1/4 teaspoon ground ginger

1. In a large, heavy saucepan or Dutch oven over moderately high heat, bring water to a boil. Add the peaches, 2 or 3 at a time, and boil for 30 seconds. Using a slotted spoon, transfer the peaches to a colander and rinse with cold water; the peels should slide off easily. Peel, pit, and coarsely chop the peaches.

2. In a large, heavy saucepan or Dutch oven, combine the chopped peaches, orange zest and juice, grape juice, brown sugar, lemon juice, and ginger. Over moderate heat, slowly bring the mixture to a boil. Boil, stirring frequently, until the jam thickens, about 30 minutes.

3. Remove the saucepan from the heat and stir to distribute the fruit evenly; skim off and discard any foam that rises to the surface, and remove and discard the orange zest. Spoon the hot jam into 6 widemouthed, warm, sterilized 1/2-pint jars, leaving a 1/4-inch space between the top of the jam and the rim of the jar (see Safe Canning with a Hot-Water Bath, page 72). Wipe the rims, cover, label, and date. Store the jars of jam in the refrigerator for up to 2 months.

Makes about 6 half-pint jars

Strawberry Jam

Go strawberry wild in the early summer when the price of this dainty fruit goes way down. Look for the ripest, reddest berries for the greatest flavor. Making your own will be a bargain.

2 quarts fully ripe
  strawberries

1/4 cup lemon juice

7 cups sugar

3 ounces liquid fruit pectin

1. Wash and hull the strawberries, and place them in a medium bowl. Using a potato masher, crush the berries. You should have 4 cups of crushed berries.

2. In a heavy 6- or 9-quart, nonreactive saucepan or Dutch oven, combine the crushed berries, lemon juice, and sugar. Over high heat, bring the mixture to a boil, stirring constantly; boil, stirring, for 1 minute.

3. Add the liquid pectin; boil and stir for 1 minute longer. Remove the saucepan from the heat. Using a slotted spoon, skim off and discard any foam that rises to the surface.

4. Spoon the hot jam into 8 widemouthed, warm, sterilized 1/2-pint jars, leaving a 1/4-inch space between the top of the jam and the rim of the jar. Wipe the rims, cover, and process for 10 minutes in boiling water (see Safe Canning with a Hot-Water Bath, page 72). Dry, label, and date. Store the jars of jam in a cool, dark place; the jam will be ready to eat in 2 weeks. Once a jar has been opened, store the jam in the refrigerator.

Makes about 8 half-pints

Tri-Berry Jam

Make the most of berries in season with this salute to summer. Homemade will be better and cheaper than store-bought.

4 cups fresh or frozen
  blueberries

2 1/2 cups fresh of frozen
  red raspberries

2 1/2 cups fresh or frozen
  strawberries

1/4 cup lemon juice

2 packages (1 3/4 ounces
  each) powdered fruit pectin

11 cups sugar

1. In a large, nonreactive saucepan or Dutch oven, combine the blueberries, raspberries, strawberries, and lemon juice; using the back of a wooden spoon, slightly crush the fruit. Stir in the pectin. Over high heat, bring the mixture to a boil, stirring constantly.

2. Add the sugar and return the mixture to a boil; boil for 1 minute, stirring constantly. Remove the saucepan from the heat; skim off and discard any foam that rises to the surface.

3. Spoon the hot jam into 6 widemouthed, warm, sterilized 1-pint jars, leaving a 1/4-inch space between the top of the jam and the rim of the jar. Wipe the rims, cover, and process for 15 minutes in boiling water (see Safe Canning with a Hot-Water Bath, page 72). Dry, label, and date. Store the jars of jam in a cool, dark place. Once a jar has been opened, store the jam in the refrigerator.

Makes about 6 pint jars

Apple Ginger Jelly

Although you remove the solids later, the naturally rich pectin in the apple seeds negates the need to add pectin to this glowing orange-red jelly.

5 pounds (8-10) green apples

1/2 cup lemon juice

1 piece (1 inch) fresh ginger, peeled and bruised

6 cups water

3/4 cup sugar for every 1 cup juice

1. Wash and roughly chop the apples (do not peel or core). In a heavy, nonreactive saucepan or Dutch oven, combine the apples, lemon juice, ginger, and water. Over moderate heat, bring the mixture to a simmer; simmer until the fruit is very soft, about 25 to 30 minutes.

2. Strain the apple mixture through a wet jelly bag overnight (see A Bag to Give You Perfectly Clear Jelly, page 82).

3. Measure the juice left after the straining; this will determine how much sugar to add. In a large, nonreactive saucepan over moderately high heat, bring the apple juice to a boil; add the appropriate amount of sugar and stir until the sugar has dissolved. Slightly reduce the heat and gently boil the mixture until the jelly reaches the jelling point (see Has It Jelled Yet? below), about 5 to 10 minutes. Using a slotted spoon, skim off and discard any foam that rises to the surface.

4. Remove the saucepan from the heat. Spoon the hot jelly into 5 widemouthed, warm, sterilized 1/2-pint jars, leaving a 1/4-inch space between the top of the jelly and the rim of the jar. Wipe the rims, cover, and process for 10 minutes in boiling water (see Safe Canning with a Hot-Water Bath, page 72). Dry, label, and date. Store the jars of jelly in a cool, dark place; the jelly will be ready to eat in 2 weeks. Once a jar has been opened, store the jelly in the refrigerator.

Makes about 5 half-pint jars

has it jelled yet?

The crucial moment in jam- and jelly-making is the temperature at which the mixture jells and no longer needs to be cooked. To determine that "jelling point," most cooking experts highly recommend that you use a candy thermometer, but the plate test works pretty well too.

Thermometer: Determine the jelling point for your altitude. Hold a candy thermometer vertically in a pot of boiling water. Read the temperature at eye level and add 8°F for the jelling point. From sea level to about 1,000 feet above, the boiling point should be 212°F and the jelling point is 220°F.

Plate method: At the point indicated in the recipe, remove the saucepan from the heat and drop a teaspoonful of the jam or jelly onto a small, cold plate. Lightly press the jam or jelly with a fingertip—the surface should wrinkle, indicating that it has begun to jell. If the jam or jelly is still too liquid or does not pass the press test, return the saucepan to the heat and cook a few minutes longer, then retest.

Grape Jelly
Peanut butter's best friend, grape jelly is a childhood favorite. Look for Concord grapes in season (September and October).

3 pounds Concord grapes

3 1/4 cups water

3/4 cup sugar for every
  1 cup juice

1. Wash the grapes and remove them from the stems. In a heavy, nonreactive saucepan, combine the grapes and water. Using a potato masher, crush the grapes. Over moderately high heat, bring the mixture to a boil; cover the saucepan, and cook for 10 to 15 minutes. Remove the saucepan from the heat and let the mixture cool to room temperature.

2. Strain the grape mixture through a wet jelly bag overnight (see A Bag to Give You Perfectly Clear Jelly, page 82).

3. Measure the juice left after the straining; this will determine how much sugar to add. In a large, nonreactive saucepan over moderately high heat, bring the grape juice to a boil; add the appropriate amount of sugar and stir until the sugar has dissolved. Increase the heat and boil rapidly until the jelly reaches the jelling point (see Has It Jelled Yet? opposite), about 12 to 16 minutes. Using a slotted spoon, skim off and discard any foam that rises to the surface.

4. Remove the saucepan from the heat. Spoon the hot jelly into 4 widemouthed, warm, sterilized 1/2-pint jars, leaving a 1/4-inch space between the top of the jelly and the rim of the jar. Wipe the rims, cover, and process for 10 minutes in boiling water (see Safe Canning with a Hot-Water Bath, page 72). Dry, label, and date. Store the jars of jelly in a cool, dark place; the jelly will be ready to eat in 2 weeks. Once a jar has been opened, store the jelly in the refrigerator.

Makes about 4 half-pint jars

a brief history of the concord grape

In 1849 Ephraim Wales Bull developed the Concord grape—after planting over 20,000 seedlings to get there. Descended from a wild grape native to the forbidding New England soil, the Concord grape ripens early (essential in a region of early killing frosts), is hardy, and boasts a rich, full, fruity flavor. It is named for the town in which Bull lived and worked. In 1853 Bull finally debuted this new grape—and won first prize at the Boston Horticultural Society Exhibition.

In 1869 a New Jersey dentist, with his wife and son, harvested 40 pounds of Concord grapes, cooked them, then squeezed the juice through cloth bags to remove the skins. They then decanted the juice into twelve 1-quart bottles, sealed them with wax, and processed them in a hot-water bath. This prevented fermentation into wine, and preserved the grape juice (which was used for Communion at the local Methodist church). The dentist's name: Dr. Thomas Welch. And Welch's Grape Juice is still making folks happy today. Nowadays more than 336,000 tons of Concord grapes are harvested every year.

Mint Jelly

The classic, emerald-green accompaniment to lamb, this jelly makes an eye-catching gift. You can make your own very inexpensively, particularly if you have a mint patch.

1 cup tightly packed fresh mint leaves

1 cup water

1/2 cup cider vinegar

3 1/2 cups sugar

5 drops green food coloring

3 ounces liquid pectin

1. Wash the mint, remove the stems, and coarsely chop the leaves. In a large, nonreactive saucepan, combine the mint, water, cider vinegar, and sugar. Over high heat, bring the mixture to a boil, stirring constantly. Remove the saucepan from the heat, and add the food coloring and pectin. Return the saucepan to the heat and return to a boil; boil for 30 seconds. Remove the saucepan from the heat, and strain the mixture through 2 layers of cheesecloth.

2. Spoon the hot jelly into 3 to 4 widemouthed, warm, sterilized 1/2-pint jars, leaving a 1/4-inch space between the top of the jelly and the rim of the jar. Wipe the rims, cover, and process for 10 minutes in boiling water (see Safe Canning with a Hot-Water Bath, page 72). Dry, label, and date. Store the jars of jelly in a cool, dark place. Once a jar has been opened, store the jelly in the refrigerator.

Makes about 3 to 4 half-pint jars

Helpful Hint

A Bag to Give You Perfectly Clear Jelly

Jelly is meant to be crystal clear, unlike jams and marmalades, so removing even the tiniest solid particles is crucial to achieving perfect results. Fortunately, there is equipment to facilitate the desired finished product: a jelly bag.

Cone-shaped with a hanging handle, a jelly bag forces the solids out of the jelly mixture over a period of time (generally 12 hours or overnight). After boiling the fruit with the liquid, dampen the jelly bag and hang it over a large, nonreactive bowl or saucepan. Pour the boiled fruit and liquid through and let stand for the specified amount of time. The weight of the fruit solids will press down and push out the liquid; don't squeeze the bag to extrude more liquid or you may make the jelly cloudy.

Seville Orange Marmalade

This is what most people think of when they hear the word "marmalade." If Seville oranges are difficult to find, substitute any firm, thin-skinned oranges, such as Valencias. Your homemade marmalade will cost less than store-bought and make you very proud.

2 pounds (4-6) Seville oranges

4 cups water

Juice of 3 lemons

8 cups sugar

1/4 cup Scotch whisky
 (optional)

1. Wash the oranges and, using a sharp knife, cut them crosswise into thin slices, catching any juice and reserving the seeds. In a large bowl, combine the oranges with their juice and add the water. Tie the reserved seeds up in a bag of cheesecloth and add it to the bowl. Cover the bowl and let the orange mixture stand in a cool place for 18 hours.

2. In a heavy, nonreactive saucepan, combine the orange mixture and the lemon juice. Over moderately low heat, simmer the mixture, uncovered, until the orange rind is tender, about 20 to 30 minutes.

3. Add the sugar; stir until the sugar has dissolved. Bring the mixture to a boil and cook until the marmalade has reached the jelling point (see Has It Jelled Yet? page 80), about 30 to 40 minutes. Using a slotted spoon, skim off and discard any foam that rises to the surface.

4. Remove the saucepan from the heat; stir to distribute the fruit evenly. Spoon the hot marmalade into 8 widemouthed, warm, sterilized 1/2-pint jars, leaving a 1/4-inch space between the top of the marmalade and the rim of the jar. Wipe the rims, cover, and process for 10 minutes in boiling water (see Safe Canning with a Hot-Water Bath, page 72). Dry, label, and date. Store the jars of marmalade in a cool, dark place; the marmalade will be ready to eat in 2 weeks. Once a jar has been opened, store the marmalade in the refrigerator.

Makes about 8 half-pint jars

Helpful Hint

How to Make Marmalade

A dose of patience and careful attention to stirring are the two qualities needed to make marmalade—the first so you don't try to hurry the process, and the second to avoid scorching the fruit or syrup and tainting the finished taste. Unlike clear jelly, or thicker jam with pureed or chunks of fruit, marmalade is a thick syrup with bits of fruit cooked until they are almost translucent.

Citrus Marmalade

Popularity and tradition marry in this bright marmalade, composed of grapefruit, orange, and lemon. Be sure to plan ahead to make this gourmet treat: It requires two 12-hour (or overnight) standing times for the flavors to develop.

1 large grapefruit
1 large orange
1 large lemon
3 cups water
12 cups sugar

1. Wash the grapefruit, orange, and lemon. Using a sharp knife, cut each citrus fruit crosswise into thin slices, then cut each slice into quarters. Remove and tie the seeds up in a bag of cheesecloth.

2. In a heavy, nonreactive saucepan, combine the grapefruit, orange, and lemon pieces, water, and seeds. Bring the mixture to a boil and cook for 10 minutes. Remove the saucepan from the heat, cover, and let stand in a cool place for 12 hours.

3. Over high heat, return the mixture to a boil; reduce the heat to moderate and cook until the rinds are tender, about 40 minutes. Remove the pan from the heat, cover, and let stand in a cool place for 12 hours longer.

4. Over moderate heat, reheat the mixture and add the sugar; stir until the sugar has dissolved. Return the mixture to a boil and cook until the marmalade has reached the jelling point (see Has It Jelled Yet? page 80), about 20 to 30 minutes. Using a slotted spoon, skim off and discard any foam that rises to the surface.

5. Remove the saucepan from the heat; stir to distribute the fruit evenly. Spoon the hot marmalade into 8 widemouthed, warm, sterilized 1/2-pint jars, leaving a 1/4-inch space between the top of the marmalade and the rim of the jar. Wipe the rims, cover, and process for 10 minutes in boiling water (see Safe Canning with a Hot-Water Bath, page 72). Dry, label, and date. Store the jars of marmalade in a cool, dark place; the marmalade will be ready to eat in 2 weeks. Once a jar has been opened, store the marmalade in the refrigerator.

Makes about 8 half-pint jars

frozen vegetables

Freeze vegetables in self-sealing freezer bags that you have labeled and dated with a permanent marker; be sure to press out any excess air from the bag before sealing. Once the vegetable has thawed, do not refreeze.

Asparagus

2 1/2-3 pounds fresh yields 4 cups frozen

Wash, trim, and cut into 2-inch pieces. Sort asparagus according to the thickness of the stalks; water-blanch thin stalks for 2 minutes, thick stalks for 4 minutes. Rinse briefly under cold water and drain thoroughly. Pack, seal, label, date, and freeze.

Beets

2 1/2-3 pounds fresh yields 4 cups frozen

Wash and trim, leaving 1-inch stems (be careful not to pierce the skins). Sort according to size and cook small beets in boiling water for 25 to 30 minutes, large for 45 to 50 minutes or until tender when pierced with a fork. Drain and cool. Peel off the skins and slice or cube, as desired. Pack, seal, label, date, and freeze.

Bell Peppers

3 pounds fresh yields 4 cups frozen

Wipe firm bell peppers. Cut out stems and remove any seeds. Cut in halves, slices, or rings. Blanch halves for 2 minutes, slices and rings for 1 minute. Cool quickly and drain thoroughly. Pack, seal, label, date, and freeze.

Broad and Lima Beans

2 1/2 pounds fresh yields 4 cups frozen

Shell young, tender beans and discard any damaged ones. Water-blanch small beans for 1 minute, medium beans for 2 minutes, and large beans for 3 minutes. Cool quickly and drain thoroughly. Pack, seal, label, date, and freeze.

Broccoli and Cauliflower

2-2 1/2 pounds fresh yields 4 cups frozen

Wash and peel stalks if woody. Cut stalks and florets into 1 1/2-inch pieces. Steam-blanch for 5 minutes. Cool quickly and drain thoroughly. Pack, seal, label, date, and freeze.

Brussels Sprouts

2-2 1/2 pounds fresh yields
4 cups frozen

Trim off coarse leaves and stems and sort by size. Water-blanch small sprouts for 3 minutes, large sprouts for 5 minutes. Cool quickly and drain thoroughly. Pack, seal, label, date, and freeze.

Carrots

2 1/2-3 pounds fresh yields
4 cups frozen

Wash, trim, and cut into 2-inch pieces or 2-inch-thick slices, if desired. Blanch whole carrots 5 minutes, slices for 2 minutes. Rinse briefly under cold water and drain thoroughly. Pack, seal, label, date, and freeze.

Corn

2 1/2 pounds fresh kernels
yields 4 cups frozen

Ears: Use young cobs only. Remove the husks and silks. Water-blanch for 4 minutes. Cool quickly and drain well. Wrap each ear individually, airtight in freezer paper or foil, molding it to the shape of the ear. Pack several together in a freezer bag, expelling as much air as possible.

Kernels: Blanch the ears as above and cool completely. Using a very sharp knife, cut the kernels off the cobs and separate into meal-size portions. Pack, seal, label, date, and freeze.

Green Beans

1 1/2-2 1/2 pounds fresh
yields 4 cups frozen

Wash and trim off ends and any blemishes. Small green beans may be water-blanched whole, but cut larger beans into 2-inch pieces. Blanch whole beans for 3 minutes; pieces for 2 minutes. Cool quickly and drain thoroughly. Pack, seal, label, date, and freeze.

Mushrooms

1-2 1/2 pounds fresh yields
4 cups frozen

Wipe with a damp cloth to remove any dirt; do not peel or rinse.
Button varieties: Spread whole, raw mushrooms on a baking tray and place in the freezer. When hard, pack, seal, label, date, and freeze.

Wild mushrooms (portobello, shiitake): Slice and sauté in butter. Pour the mushrooms with the cooking liquid into individual bags. Seal, label, date, and freeze.

Peas

> 2 1/2 pounds fresh yields
> 4 cups frozen

Sweet peas: Shell sweet peas, discarding any damaged ones. Water-blanch for 1 1/2 minutes. Cool quickly and drain thoroughly. Pack, seal, label, date, and freeze.

Sugar snap or snow peas: De-string pods and water-blanch for 2 minutes. Cool quickly and drain thoroughly. Pack, seal, label, date, and freeze.

Pumpkin and Other Hard Squash

> 3 pounds fresh yields 4 cups
> frozen puree

Wash, peel, and cut in half; remove any seeds and strings. Cut into slices or cubes. Steam-blanch until tender. Mash and let cool completely. Pack in plastic dishes (leaving a 1/2-inch space at the top), seal, label, date, and freeze.

Spinach and Other Dark Leafy Greens

> 2 1/2 pounds fresh yields
> 4 cups frozen

Wash leaves thoroughly; remove any thick stems and imperfect leaves. Water-blanch for 30 to 60 seconds, or until just wilted. Cool quickly by running cold water over the leaves. Drain thoroughly, pressing out excess moisture. Pack, seal, label, date, and freeze.

Mixed Vegetables

Chop larger vegetables or cut them into bite-size pieces. Blanch according to directions for each individual vegetable, remembering that a shorter blanching time may be required to compensate for the smaller piece size. When they are cool, mix your choice of vegetables and pack in plastic freezer bags in meal-size quantities. Seal, label, date, and freeze.

how to blanch vegetables

You can blanch vegetables with either boiling water or steam. Which method you use—and the time required to do it—depends on the vegetable involved.
Water-blanching: Bring at least 12 cups of water to a boil in a large saucepan. Place 1 pound prepared vegetable pieces in a wire-mesh basket and plunge into the boiling water. When the water returns to a boil, cook the vegetables for the time required. Lift the basket and place it into a large bowl of cold or ice water to cool; change the water as needed or add ice to keep the water cold. Drain completely.
Steam-blanching: Place prepared vegetables in a single layer inside a steamer basket in a large saucepan containing 2 inches of boiling water. Cover, and steam the vegetables for the time required. Cool, but don't rinse the vegetables.

frozen fruits

Use only unblemished fruit and keep the handling time to a minimum (fruit tends to brown when handled). Be sure to press out any excess air before sealing the freezer bags. Thaw frozen fruit in the bag in the refrigerator for several hours or place the bag in a bowl of cool water 30 minutes.

Apples

2 1/2-3 pounds fresh yields
4 cups prepared

Peel, core, and slice the apples. Dip and drain the slices thoroughly. Arrange in a single layer on a rimmed tray and freeze until just firm. Pack, seal, label, date, and freeze.

Apricots

1 1/4-1 1/2 pounds yields
4 cups prepared

Pit and slice or halve the apricots. Dip and drain the slices or halves thoroughly. Arrange in a single layer on a rimmed tray and freeze until just firm. Pack, seal, label, date, and freeze.

Blueberries

1-1 1/2 pound fresh yields
4 cups prepared

Remove any stems. Dip and drain the blueberries thoroughly. Arrange in a single layer on a rimmed tray and freeze until just firm. Pack, seal, label, date, and freeze.

Cherries

2-3 pounds fresh yields
4 cups prepared

Stem and pit the cherries. Dip and drain thoroughly. Arrange in a single layer on a rimmed tray and freeze until just firm. Pack, seal, label, date, and freeze.

Mangoes

2 1/2-3 pounds fresh yields
4 cups prepared

Pit and slice or halve the mangoes. Dip and drain the slices or halves thoroughly. Arrange in a single layer on a rimmed tray and freeze until just firm. Pack, seal, label, date, and freeze.

Peaches and Plums

2-3 pounds fresh yields
4 cups prepared

Pit and slice or halve the peaches or apricots. Dip and drain the slices or halves thoroughly. Arrange in a single layer on a rimmed tray and freeze until just firm. Pack, seal, label, date, and freeze.

Raspberries

1 pound fresh yields 4 cups
prepared

Remove stems and leaves from the raspberries. Dip and drain the berries thoroughly. Arrange in a single layer on a rimmed tray and freeze until just firm. Pack, seal, label, date, and freeze.

Strawberries

1 1/4 pounds fresh yields
4 cups frozen

Remove leaves and hull strawberries. Strawberries can be sliced or left whole. Dip and drain the berries thoroughly. Arrange in a single layer on a rimmed tray and freeze until just firm. Pack, seal, label, date, and freeze.

how to dip fruits for freezing

While working, keep fresh fruit in a bowl of acidulated water (about 8 cups water with 1 1/2 tablespoons of lemon juice or mild vinegar added). This keeps the cut fruit from browning and is commonly refered to as dipping. After dipping, drain the fruit on paper towels to remove as much moisture as possible. This helps prevent ice from forming around the pieces and keeps them from sticking together.

chapter 3

Baked Goods
You Can Make

Nothing can compare to the aroma—or taste—of freshly baked bread. But with the demise of the neighborhood bakery, it is not a pleasure that we

encounter very often these days, except maybe when it is artificially piped into the baked goods section of a fancy supermarket to whet your appetite and open your wallet. The sad truth of the matter is that most of those packaged and wrapped breads, rolls, muffins, cakes, pies, and cookies that you find in the typical supermarket are made from bleached flour—flour that has been stripped of most its healthful nutrients and fiber. And they have often been replaced with taste-diminishing additives and preservatives to give the product a longer shelf life.

If your baking has been limited to the occasional pie, birthday cake, or holiday cookies, you will be pleasantly surprised at how easy, fast, and economical it is to make your own everyday baked goods such as bread, rolls, and muffins. You will discover not only how much better and fresher they taste but also the enormous variety of both savory and sweet baked bread products you can serve up, fresh and additive-free, to your family. The same is true of the really sweet baked goodies—there's an ample selection of cakes, pies, and cookies on the following pages. Some of the cakes can be made in almost no time using the cake mix from Chapter 1, and handmade piecrust is flaky, with a rich flavor that complements any filling.

quick breads

Beer Bread
Use a light lager for a lighter taste or be bold with a stout for a richer, darker flavor—the beer's the limit! If you can find this savory bread at a grocery or bakery, it will cost at least twice as much.

2 1/2 cups all-purpose flour

2 tablespoons sugar

2 teaspoons baking powder

1 teaspoon salt

1 cup beer

1/4 cup plus 2 tablespoons butter, melted

1. Preheat the oven to 350°F. Lightly grease an 8 x 4-inch loaf pan and line the pan with baking paper.

2. In a large bowl, sift together the flour, sugar, baking powder, and salt. Add the beer and the 1/4 cup of melted butter, and stir until a soft dough forms.

3. Spoon the dough into the prepared pan and pour the remaining 2 tablespoons of melted butter over the top of the loaf. Bake until the loaf is golden brown and sounds hollow when tapped, 40 to 45 minutes. Remove the loaf from the pan to a wire rack to cool.

Makes 1 loaf

Cheese and Parsley Bread
Golden, crusty, savory—this loaf is essentially a big scone and totally irresistible. You may have trouble finding such a bread at the supermarket at any price. Luckily, you don't need to.

2 cups whole wheat flour

1 teaspoon baking powder

1 teaspoon baking soda

3/4 cup shredded cheddar or 1/4 cup grated Parmesan cheese

1/4 cup fresh parsley

1 teaspoon salt

3/4 cup milk or buttermilk

1. Preheat the oven to 450°F. In the bowl of a food processor, place the flour, baking powder, baking soda, all but 1 table-spoon of the cheese, parsley, and salt. Whirl until the cheese crumbles into the flour and the parsley is finely chopped.

2. Add the milk or buttermilk all at once, and whirl just until a soft dough forms, about 5 seconds.

3. Lightly flour a work surface and a baking sheet. Turn out the dough onto the work surface and knead gently. Transfer the dough to the baking sheet and form into a round loaf. Using a sharp knife, cut the dough almost through into 8 wedge-shaped pieces. Sprinkle the wedges with the remaining tablespoon of cheese.

4. Bake in the center of the oven until the loaf is puffed and brown, 20 to 25 minutes. Remove the loaf from the oven, wrap it in a lint-free towel, and let it cool slightly. Cut through the marked wedges of the bread to serve.

Makes 1 loaf (8 wedges)

Corn Bread *As tasty to the eye as to the palate, this beautiful yellow bread is a wholesome welcome addition to any meal.*

1 1/2 cups all-purpose flour

1 1/4 cups yellow cornmeal

4 teaspoons baking powder

2 tablespoons sugar

1 teaspoon salt

1 egg

1 1/4 cups cold milk

1/4 cup vegetable oil

1. Preheat the oven to 400°F. Lightly grease an 8-inch square baking pan.

2. In a large bowl, sift together the dry ingredients. In a smaller bowl, combine the egg, milk, and oil; beat until the ingredients are well blended. Make a well in the center of the dry ingredients; pour in the milk mixture all at once and, using a fork, stir just until the wet and dry ingredients are blended—do not overmix.

3. Pour the batter into the prepared pan and bake until the bread pulls away slightly from the sides of the pan and is slightly browned, 20 to 25 minutes.

4. Remove the pan to a wire rack and let the bread cool for 10 minutes. Cut into large squares and serve warm.

Makes 1 loaf (about 9 squares)

variation:

Corn Muffins: Prepare the batter as above, but pour into well-greased or paper-lined muffin cups. Bake until the muffins are lightly browned and springy to the touch, 17 to 20 minutes.

Zucchini and Cheese Bread *Use this recipe to make a loaf or muffins—either is a splendid backdrop to cream cheese, smoked salmon, and a few capers. Toasted, slices of this bread are delicious with a hearty soup.*

2 cups all-purpose flour

1 teaspoon baking powder

1 tablespoon sugar

1 teaspoon salt

6 tablespoons butter, cut up

1 cup shredded sharp cheddar cheese

1 cup milk

1 large egg

1 cup grated zucchini, squeezed dry in a towel to remove excess moisture

1 tablespoon grated onion

1 teaspoon Dijon mustard

1. Preheat the oven to 375°F. Lightly grease an 8 x 4-inch loaf pan.

2. In a large bowl, sift together the flour, baking powder, sugar, and salt. Using a pastry blender or 2 knives, cut in the butter until the mixture resembles coarse bread crumbs. Stir in the cheese.

3. In a medium bowl, combine the milk and egg, and beat until they are well blended. Stir in the zucchini, onion, and mustard. Add the milk mixture to the dry ingredients. Using a fork, stir just until all the ingredients are moistened and the dough holds together; do not overmix or the bread may be too heavy.

4. Spoon the dough into the prepared pan. Bake until the bread is well risen and brown, and a tester inserted into the center of the loaf comes out clean, 40 to 45 minutes.

5. Remove to a wire rack to cool in the pan 10 minutes, then remove the bread from the pan and let it cool completely.

Makes 1 loaf

Baked Goods You Can Make   **507**

Irish Soda Bread

St. Patrick's Day wouldn't be complete without a loaf of this traditional Irish bread, but don't wait until it's offered in the stores. This easy-to-make bread can be topped with a sprinkling of seeds or oatmeal, and is a wonderful accompaniment to stews and hearty soups.

4 cups all-purpose flour

3 tablespoons sugar

3 teaspoons baking powder

1 teaspoon salt

3/4 teaspoon baking soda

6 tablespoons cold butter or margarine

1 1/2 cups currants or raisins

1 tablespoon caraway seed

2 eggs, lightly beaten

1 1/2 cups low-fat buttermilk

1. In a large bowl, sift together the flour, sugar, baking powder, salt, and baking soda. Using a pastry blender or 2 knives, cut in butter until the mixture resembles coarse crumbs. Stir in the currants or raisins and caraway seed.

2. Set aside 1 tablespoon of the beaten egg. In a medium bowl, combine the buttermilk and remaining eggs, and stir until they are well blended. Make a well in the center of the flour mixture. Pour the buttermilk mixture into the well and stir just until the flour is moistened and a sticky dough forms.

3. Flour a work surface well. Turn out the dough onto the work surface and, using well-floured hands, knead the dough about 10 times. Shape the dough into a round loaf.

4. Lightly grease a 9-inch round baking pan. Place the loaf in the prepared pan. Using a sharp knife, cut a cross, 1/4-inch deep, in the top center of the loaf. Brush the loaf with the reserved egg.

5. Bake at 350°F until a toothpick inserted near the center of the loaf comes out clean, about 1 hour and 20 minutes. If the loaf top browns too quickly, tent loosely with foil for the final 20 minutes of baking time. Remove to a wire rack and cool in the pan for 10 minutes before removing the loaf from the pan to the rack to cool completely.

Makes 1 loaf

One-Minute Substitute

If You Run Out of Buttermilk

If a recipe calls for 1 cup buttermilk and you don't have any on hand, pour 1 tablespoon white vinegar or lemon juice in a 1-cup measure and add enough regular milk to make 1 cup. Or simply substitute 1 cup plain yogurt.

Olive and Sun-Dried Tomato Bread

You can almost taste the Mediterranean when you bite into this peasant-style bread, with its strong flavors and chewy texture. This recipe will save you money and add excitement to a bowl of soup.

2 eggs

2/3 cup milk

2 cups all-purpose flour

2 teaspoons baking powder

1 teaspoon kosher salt

3 tablespoons oil drained from sun-dried tomatoes or olive oil

1/2 cup black olives in oil, drained, pitted, and slivered

1/2 cup sun-dried tomatoes packed in oil, drained and sliced

1 tablespoon fresh minced basil or marjoram

1. Preheat the oven to 400°F. Lightly grease an 8-inch springform pan.

2. In the bowl of a food processor or blender, combine the eggs and milk. Whirl just until the ingredients are combined. Sift together the flour and baking powder, and add to the milk mixture. Whirl for 2 minutes; add the salt and oil, and whirl for 1 minute more. Using a spoon, stir in the olives, sun-dried tomatoes, and basil or marjoram.

3. Pour the batter into the prepared pan and bake until a tester inserted into the bread comes out clean, about 30 minutes.

4. Remove the pan to a wire rack and let the bread cool slightly. Remove the outer ring of the pan and serve the bread warm.

Makes 1 loaf

Sesame Pumpkin Bread

Wake up your taste buds with this unusual bread, experiencing autumn in every bite. You may find a similar loaf among the specialty breads at the market, but you can be sure it will be much more costly.

4 cups all-purpose flour

1/4 cup sugar

4 teaspoons baking powder

1 teaspoon salt

1 cup plus 2 tablespoons milk

1 egg

1 cup pumpkin puree

1/3 cup butter, melted

1 tablespoon sesame seed

1. Preheat the oven to 425°F. Lightly grease and flour a baking sheet. In a large bowl, sift together the flour, sugar, baking powder, and salt.

2. In a medium bowl, combine 1 cup of milk and the egg; beat until well blended. Stir in the pumpkin puree and butter. Make a well in the center of the dry ingredients; pour the pumpkin mixture and, using a fork, stir until all the ingredients are well blended.

3. Lightly flour a work surface. Turn out the dough onto the work surface and knead lightly until the dough is smooth, 4 to 5 minutes. Shape the dough into a round loaf and transfer to the prepared baking sheet. Using a sharp knife, cut a cross over the top of the loaf. Brush lightly with the remaining 2 tablespoons milk. Sprinkle with the sesame seeds.

4. Bake the loaf 25 minutes; reduce the heat to 375°F and bake until the loaf sounds hollow when tapped, about 15 minutes longer. Remove the loaf to a wire rack to cool.

Makes 1 loaf

Baked Goods You Can Make   **509**

Banana Nut Bread

Buy bananas in bulk from a price club or when they go on sale at the supermarket, and use some to make this luscious loaf. You can double or triple the recipe and freeze the extra loaves for later. Either way, you will save on a delicious bread for brunches or teatime.

1/2 cup walnuts or pecans

1 3/4 cups all-purpose flour

1 1/2 teaspoons baking powder

1/2 teaspoon baking soda

1/2 teaspoon salt

1/2 teaspoon ground cinnamon

1/4 teaspoon ground allspice

1/2 cup (1 stick) butter, at room temperature

1/3 cup firmly packed light brown sugar

1/2 cup granulated sugar

2 eggs

1 cup mashed ripe bananas

1/3 cup buttermilk

1/4 teaspoon almond extract

1 cup golden seedless raisins

1. Preheat the oven to 350°F. Lightly grease a 9 x 5-inch loaf pan; lightly dust the pan with flour.

2. Spread the walnuts or pecans in a pie plate and toast, uncovered, until the nuts are lightly browned, about 7 minutes. Let the nuts cool, then coarsely chop and set aside.

3. In a medium bowl, combine the flour, baking powder, baking soda, salt, cinnamon, and allspice; stir until all the ingredients are well blended.

4. In a large bowl with an electric mixer on moderate speed, beat the butter until it is creamed. Gradually add the brown and granulated sugars, beating well after each addition. Add the eggs, 1 at a time, beating well after each addition again. Add the flour mixture, a little at a time, beating after each addition only enough to incorporate the flour. The batter will not be smooth.

5. In a small bowl, combine the mashed bananas, buttermilk, and almond extract; stir until the ingredients are blended. Pour the banana mixture into the batter, stir, then fold in the raisins and reserved toasted nuts.

6. Pour and scrape the batter into the prepared pan. Bake the bread on the middle rack of the oven until a toothpick inserted into the center of the loaf comes out clean, 50 to 55 minutes. Remove the pan to a wire rack and let the bread cool in the pan for 10 minutes. Using a knife or spatula, loosen the edges of the bread from the sides of the pan and carefully remove the bread from the pan. Let the bread cool completely on the rack.

Makes 1 loaf

One-Minute Substitute

If You Run Out of Baking Powder

If a recipe calls for 1 teaspoon baking powder and you don't have any on hand, combine 1/4 teaspoon baking soda with 1/2 teaspoon cream of tartar.

Carrot Bread
Spicy goodness that will bring to mind carrot cake, without the high price. Serve with tea or coffee or as dessert.

1 3/4 cups all-purpose flour

2 1/2 teaspoons baking powder

1/2 teaspoon salt

1/4 teaspoon ground cardamom

1/4 teaspoon ground ginger

1/4 teaspoon ground allspice

1/2 cup (1 stick) butter, at room temperature

2/3 cup sugar

2 eggs

1 1/2 cups peeled shredded carrots

1/2 cup orange juice

1. Preheat the oven to 350°F. Lightly grease a 9 x 5-inch loaf pan; lightly dust the pan with flour.

2. In a medium bowl, combine the flour, baking powder, baking powder, salt, cardamom, ginger, and allspice; stir until all the ingredients are well blended.

3. In a large bowl with an electric mixer on moderate speed, beat the butter until it is creamed. Gradually add the sugar, beating well after each addition. Add the eggs, 1 at a time, beating well after each addition again. Add the flour mixture, a little at a time, beating after each addition only enough to incorporate the flour. The batter will not be smooth.

4. In a small bowl, combine the carrots and orange juice; stir until blended. Pour the carrot mixture into the batter and stir until all the ingredients are well blended.

5. Pour and scrape the batter into the prepared pan. Bake the bread on the middle rack of the oven until a toothpick inserted into the center of the loaf comes out clean, about 1 hour. Remove the pan to a wire rack and let the bread cool in the pan for 10 minutes. Using a knife or spatula, loosen the edges of the bread from the sides of the pan and carefully remove the bread from the pan. Let the bread cool completely on the rack.

Makes 1 loaf

Pecan Bread
Slice and serve this nutty Southern bread with fruit and soft cheeses. You can buy it, but you will pay much, much more.

2 cups all-purpose flour

2 teaspoons baking powder

1 teaspoon salt

3/4 cup coarsely chopped pecans

1/3 cup firmly packed light brown sugar

1 cup milk

1 egg

3 tablespoons butter, melted

1. Preheat the oven to 350°F. Lightly grease an 8 x 4-inch loaf pan.

2. In a large bowl, sift together the flour, baking powder, and salt. Stir in the pecans and brown sugar. In a medium bowl, combine the milk and egg, and beat well. Stir the melted butter into the milk mixture.

3. Make a well in the center of the flour mixture. Pour the milk mixture into the well and, using a fork, stir the ingredients just until they are all moistened and the dough holds together; do not overmix.

4. Spoon the dough into the prepared pan. Bake the bread until a tester inserted into the center of the loaf comes out clean, 45 to 50 minutes.

5. Remove the pan to a wire rack and let the bread cool 10 minutes, then remove the bread from the pan and let it cool completely.

Makes 1 loaf

Zucchini Bread

Every gardener we know always has excess zucchini during the summer— this is the delectable way to use it up while saving money on the cookies and desserts that zucchini bread replaces. You can make several loaves and freeze the extras.

1 cup chopped pecans

1 3/4 cups all-purpose flour

1 1/2 teaspoons baking powder

1/2 teaspoon baking soda

1/2 teaspoon salt

1 teaspoon ground cinnamon

1/2 cup (1 stick) butter, at room temperature

3/4 cup sugar

2 eggs

1 1/2 cups shredded zucchini, squeezed to remove excess moisture

1/3 cup buttermilk

1/4 teaspoon almond extract

1. Preheat the oven to 350°F. Lightly grease a 9 x 5-inch loaf pan; lightly dust the pan with flour.

2. Spread the pecans in a pie plate and toast, uncovered, until the nuts are lightly browned, about 7 minutes. Let the nuts cool, then coarsely chop and set aside.

3. In a medium bowl, combine the flour, baking powder, baking soda, salt, and cinnamon; stir until all the ingredients are well blended.

4. In a large bowl with an electric mixer on moderate speed, beat the butter until it is creamed. Gradually add the sugar, beating well after each addition. Add the eggs, 1 at a time, beating well after each addition again. Add the flour mixture, a little at a time, beating after each addition only enough to incorporate the flour. The batter will not be smooth.

5. In a small bowl, combine the zucchini, buttermilk, and almond extract; stir until blended. Pour the zucchini mixture into the batter, stir, then fold in the reserved toasted nuts.

6. Pour and scrape the batter into the prepared pan. Bake the bread on the middle rack of the oven until a toothpick inserted into the center of the loaf comes out clean, about 1 hour. Remove the pan to a wire rack and let the bread cool in the pan 10 minutes. Using a knife or spatula, loosen the edges of the bread from the sides of the pan and carefully remove the bread from the pan. Let the bread cool completely on the rack.

Makes 1 loaf

yeast breads

French Bread

Many meals are finished off with a loaf of French bread to sop up the gravy, hold the cheese, or complement the salad. Nothing is better, but unfortunately, nothing gets stale quicker, so making your own not only saves money but also ensures a fresh, crusty loaf. Surprisingly, this recipe doesn't require kneading.

1 package (1/4 ounce) active dry yeast

1 1/2 cups warm water (110°F-115°F), divided

1 tablespoon sugar

2 teaspoons salt

1 tablespoon butter, melted

4 cups all-purpose flour

Cornmeal

1. In a large bowl, combine the yeast with 1/2 cup of the water and stir until the yeast is dissolved.

2. Add the sugar, salt, butter, and remaining 1 cup water. Stir until all the ingredients are well blended and the powdered ingredients are dissolved. Add the flour and stir until the dough is smooth; do not knead. Cover the bowl and let the dough rise in a warm place until it is doubled in size, about 1 hour.

3. Lightly flour a work surface. Divide the dough in half; let the dough halves rest for 10 minutes. Using a lightly floured rolling pin, roll one dough half into a 10 x 8-inch rectangle. Beginning on a long side, roll up the dough, jelly-roll-fashion; pinch the edges to seal the loaf. Repeat with the remaining dough half.

4. Lightly grease a baking sheet and sprinkle it with cornmeal. Place the loaves, seam side down, on the prepared baking sheet; sprinkle the tops of the loaves with additional cornmeal. Cover the loaves and let rise until doubled in size, about 45 minutes.

5. Preheat the oven to 400°F. Using a sharp knife, make five diagonal cuts across the top of each loaf. Bake the loaves until they are lightly browned, 20 to 30 minutes. Remove the loaves to wire racks to cool.

Makes 2 loaves

Helpful Hint | **Yeast Breads Are Easier to Make Than You Think**
One of the absolute best aromas in the world—fresh baking bread. You may have shied away from yeast breads in the past, thinking the yeast would be difficult to work with. Not at all. Follow the directions and you'll be turning out perfect loaves in no time at all. If you enjoy the aroma and the price of homemade bread and time is a factor, you may want to invest in a bread machine. Most recipes can be converted for a machine.

Multigrain Bread

Whole wheat flour, rye flour, stone-ground cornmeal, wheat bran and germ, and buttermilk form a hearty, wholesome bread your family will rave about. So will your pocketbook.

2 teaspoons sugar

1/2 cup lukewarm water
(105°F-115°F)

2 packets (1/4 ounce each)
active dry yeast

1 1/4-1 1/2 cups
all-purpose flour

1 cup whole wheat flour

1 cup rye flour

1/3 cup sifted stone-ground
yellow or white cornmeal

1/4 cup wheat bran

1/4 cup wheat germ, plain,
toasted, or honey crunch

1 cup buttermilk

3 tablespoons butter, melted

1 1/2 teaspoons salt

1. In a large bowl, combine the sugar, water, and yeast. Stir until the solids are dissolved. Let stand until the mixture is bubbly, about 10 minutes.

2. In another large bowl, combine 1 1/4 cups of the all-purpose flour, the whole wheat and rye flours, cornmeal, wheat bran, and wheat germ.

3. In a small saucepan over low heat, combine the buttermilk, butter, and salt, and cook until the mixture is lukewarm.

4. Pour the buttermilk mixture into the yeast mixture. Using a wooden spoon or an electric mixer with the dough hook attached, beat at moderate speed, adding the flour mixture 1 cup at a time, until the dough is soft but manageable; beat in the remaining 1/4 cup of all-purpose flour, if needed to reach the desired consistency. Continue to beat until the dough is smooth and elastic, 7 to 8 minutes. If mixing by hand, knead on a floured work surface for 8 to 10 minutes.

5. Butter a 5-quart bowl well. Shape the dough into a ball and place the ball in the prepared bowl, turning it until the dough surface is completely coated. Cover the bowl with a cloth and set in a warm, draft-free place until the dough is doubled in size, 1 1/2 to 2 hours.

6. Lightly grease a 9 x 5 x 3-inch loaf pan; lightly flour a work surface. Punch down the dough and turn out onto the work surface. Knead gently for 2 minutes. Shape the dough into a loaf, place it in the prepared pan, cover, and let rise until doubled in size, about 1 hour.

7. Preheat the oven to 375°F. Bake until the loaf is golden brown and sounds hollow when tapped, 40 to 45 minutes. Remove the pan to a wire rack and let the bread cool for 10 minutes. Using a knife, loose the edges of the bread from the sides of the pan, turn out the bread, and set it on the wire rack to cool completely.

Makes 1 loaf

Oatmeal Bread

The old-fashioned goodness of this nutty, crunchy bread makes it the ideal base for sandwiches, but try it toasted with homemade jam or apple butter too. Cooking the oats before using them to make bread results in a lighter, finer texture. Again, by making your own oatmeal bread, you will save money as well as benefit from the aroma of baking bread.

1 1/2 cups milk

1/4 cup (1/2 stick) butter or margarine plus
1 tablespoon, melted

1 cup plus 2 tablespoons quick-cooking oats

5 teaspoons firmly packed light brown sugar

1/4 cup lukewarm water (105°F–115°F)

2 packets (1/4 ounce each) active dry yeast

1 egg, beaten

2 teaspoons salt

1 cup whole wheat flour

2 1/2–3 cups all-purpose flour

Glaze

1 egg beaten with 1 tablespoon water

1. In a small saucepan over moderate heat, combine the milk and 1/4 cup of butter until the mixture is steaming. Add 1 cup oats and stir until the oats are evenly moistened, about 1 minute. Remove the saucepan from the heat and let cool to room temperature, 25 to 30 minutes.

2. In a large bowl, combine 1 teaspoon brown sugar, the water, and the yeast. Stir until the solids are dissolved. Let stand until the mixture is bubbly, about 10 minutes. Using a wooden spoon or an electric mixer with a dough hook attached, beat in the cooled oatmeal mixture, the remaining 4 teaspoons brown sugar, the egg, salt, whole wheat flour, and 2 1/2 cups all-purpose flour. Continue beating at moderate speed, until the dough is soft, but manageable, adding the remaining 1/4 to 1/2 cup flour as needed, 7 to 8 minutes. If mixing by hand, knead on a floured work surface 8 to 10 minutes.

3. Butter a 5-quart bowl well. Shape the dough into a ball and place the ball in the prepared bowl, turning it until the dough surface is completely coated. Cover the bowl with a cloth and set in a warm, draft-free place until the dough is doubled in size, about 1 hour.

4. Lightly grease a 9 x 5 x 3-inch loaf pan and sprinkle the bottom and sides of the pan with 1 tablespoon of the remaining oats; lightly flour a work surface. Punch down the dough, turn out onto the work surface, and knead gently for 2 minutes (the dough will be soft). Shape the dough into a loaf, place it in the prepared pan, cover, and let rise until doubled in size, 1 to 1 1/2 hours.

5. Preheat the oven to 375°F. Lightly brush the top of the loaf with the glaze, then sprinkle with the remaining tablespoon of oats. Bake until the loaf is golden brown and sounds hollow when tapped, 40 to 45 minutes. Remove the pan to a wire rack and let the bread cool 10 minutes. Using a knife, loosen the edges of the bread from the sides of the pan, turn out the bread, and set it on the wire rack to cool completely.

Makes 1 loaf

Focaccia

Thick and chewy, this Italian bread can be topped with grilled or marinated vegetables, grilled meats, cold cuts, cheese—or just drizzled with a little extra-virgin olive oil and enjoyed on its own. It has become popular, but you will find that homemade is better and cheaper than store-bought.

1 packet (1/4 ounce) active dry yeast

1/4 teaspoon sugar

2 cups warm water (105°F-110°F)

4 1/2-5 1/2 cups bread flour or all-purpose flour

1/4 cup olive oil plus additional

1 tablespoon salt

Tiny sprigs fresh rosemary

Kosher salt

1. In a small bowl, combine the yeast, sugar, and water. Stir rapidly to dissolve the solids. Set the bowl in a warm place until the mixture is activated and frothy, about 20 minutes.

2. In a large bowl, pour 4 1/2 cups flour and make a well in the center. Pour the yeast mixture, 1/4 cup oil, and salt into the well, then stir until the ingredients are well blended. Add additional flour as needed to reach the desired consistency.

3. Lightly flour a work surface and lightly coat a large bowl with olive oil. Turn the dough out onto the work surface, and knead until the dough is smooth, about 10 minutes. Place the dough in the prepared bowl, turning it once to coat the entire ball with oil. Cover the bowl with lightly oiled plastic wrap, and set to rise in a warm place for 1 hour.

4. Lightly grease 2 baking sheets. Divide the dough in half, and spread each half on a prepared baking sheet; with fingers, press down and out until each half is a round loaf about 1/2-inch thick. Cover the loaves with lightly oiled plastic wrap and let rise for 10 to 20 minutes.

5. With fingers, press the loaves down and out again. Recover and let the loaves rise for 30 minutes.

6. Preheat the oven to 425°F. With fingers, indent the loaves all over. Press a sprig of rosemary into each dent, drizzle the whole with oil, then sprinkle with salt. Bake until the loaves are firm and golden, about 25 minutes. Serve warm.

Makes 2 loaves

Make It a Gift

Take a Mix-and-Match Approach to Gift Baskets

When pondering gift giving with your own homemade items, take a tip from those high-end catalogs and pair natural partners in an attractive package—breads with jams, jellies, or marmalades; pasta with homemade sauces; cookies with hot cocoa, coffee or tea blends; granola with fresh-baked muffins; canned fruit with a dessert sauce; soup with hearty rolls; pita breads with hummus. Whenever you browse through a yard or rummage sale, look for baskets, saucepans, ceramic or porcelain bowls, and other fun packaging for personalized gifts.

Challah

The traditional bread of the Jewish Sabbath, this attractive loaf is braided and given a shiny coating of egg wash. Scrumptious the day it's baked, and you can use leftovers (if any) to make the best French toast you'll ever taste!

2 packages (1/4 ounce each) active dry yeast

1 cup warm water (110°F–115°F)

1/2 cup vegetable oil

1/3 cup sugar

1 tablespoon salt

5 eggs

6–6 1/2 cups all-purpose flour

1 teaspoon cold water

1 tablespoon sesame or poppy seed *(optional)*

1. In a large bowl, combine the yeast with the warm water and stir until the yeast is dissolved. Add the oil, sugar, salt, 4 eggs, and 4 cups flour. Beat until all the ingredients are well blended and the consistency is smooth. Stir in enough of the remaining flour to form a firm dough.

2. Lightly flour a work surface. Turn out the dough onto the work surface and knead until the dough is firm and elastic, 6 to 8 minutes. Lightly grease a bowl with butter or oil, place the dough in the bowl, and turn it once to coat the entire ball. Cover the bowl and let the dough rise in a warm place until it is doubled in size, about 1 hour.

3. Punch down the dough, turn in onto another floured work surface, and divide the dough in half. Divide each portion into thirds. Roll each piece into a 15-inch-long rope.

4. Lightly grease a baking sheet. Place 3 dough ropes on the sheet, pinching them together at one end. Braid the ropes together and pinch the opposite ends to seal them, then tuck the pinched ends under at both ends. Repeat with the remaining dough ropes to make a second loaf. Cover the loaves with a cloth and let rise until doubled in size, about 1 hour.

5. Preheat the oven to 350°F. In a small bowl, beat the remaining egg with the cold water. Brush the egg mixture over the loaves. If desired, sprinkle the loaves with the sesame or poppy seed. Bake the loaves until they are golden brown, 30 to 35 minutes. Remove the loaves from the baking sheet to wire racks and let cool completely.

Makes 2 loaves

Cinnamon-Raisin Swirl Bread

The ultimate morning treat, this beautiful bread, spiraled with cinnamon, thick with raisins, and drizzled with sugar icing, is a treat for all the senses. And store-bought doesn't fill your house with the same aroma!

6 teaspoons sugar

1 cup lukewarm whole or 2% milk (105°F-115°F)

2 packets (1/4 ounce each) active dry yeast

2 1/4 cups lukewarm water (105°F-115°F)

5 tablespoons butter or margarine, melted

2 teaspoons salt

6-6 1/2 cups all-purpose flour

1 cup dark seedless raisins, soaked in hot water 15-30 minutes, drained well

Cinnamon Swirl Filling

3 tablespoons butter or margarine, melted

1/2 cup sugar

1 tablespoon ground cinnamon

Icing

2 cups sifted confectioners' sugar

2 tablespoons water

1. In a large bowl, combine 1 teaspoon sugar with the milk and yeast, and stir until the solids are dissolved. Let stand until the mixture bubbles, 5 to 10 minutes. In a medium bowl, combine 1 1/4 cups warm water, 4 tablespoons butter, the salt, and the remaining 5 teaspoons sugar. Stir the butter mixture into the yeast mixture.

2. Using a wooden spoon or an electric mixer with a dough hook attached, beat in the flour, 1 cup at a time, until a soft dough forms. Continue to beat at moderate speed until the dough is elastic, 7 to 8 minutes. If mixing by hand, knead on a floured work surface for 8 to 10 minutes.

3. Pour the final 1 tablespoon butter into a 5-quart bowl. Shape the dough into a ball and place the ball in the prepared bowl, turning it until the dough surface is completely coated. Cover the bowl with a cloth and set in a warm, draft-free place until the dough is doubled in size, about 1 hour.

4. Lightly butter two 9 x 5 x 3-inch loaf pans. Lightly flour a work surface. Punch down the dough and turn out onto the work surface. Knead the dough gently for 2 minutes. Divide the dough in half, cover, and let rest for 5 to 10 minutes. Working with a half at a time and using a rolling pin, roll the dough into a 9 x 15-inch rectangle. Sprinkle 1/2 cup of the raisins over each portion of the dough and gently knead until the raisins are evenly distributed. Cover the dough and let rest for 10 minutes.

5. Prepare the filling: In a small bowl, combine 2 tablespoons butter, the sugar, and cinnamon; stir until the ingredients are well blended. Using a rolling pin on a floured surface, again roll each dough half into a 9 x 15-inch rectangle. Spread each half with half of the filling. Beginning on a short side, roll up the dough, jelly-roll-fashion, to make a loaf; repeat with the remaining half. Place each loaf, seam side down, in a prepared pan, cover with a cloth, and let rise for 1 hour.

6. Preheat the oven to 400°F. Brush the tops of the loaves with the remaining tablespoon of butter. Bake until the bread is brown and sounds hollow when tapped, 35 to 40 minutes. Remove the pans to wire racks and let the bread cool for 10 minutes. Using a knife, loosen the edges of the bread from the sides of the pans, turn out the bread, and set on wire racks to cool.

7. Prepare the icing: In a small bowl, combine the confectioners' sugar and water, and stir until the icing is smooth. Brush, pour or drizzle over the cooled loaves.

Makes 2 loaves

Pita Bread
This popular staple of Middle Eastern and Mediterranean cuisine is a wonderfully versatile bread. You can stuff the pockets with almost anything you can think of to make a sandwich; slice the bread into triangles, toast, and serve with any dip; even top with tomato paste, marinated vegetables, and mozzarella cheese for a variation on pizza. Fresh pita is better and cheaper than store-bought.

1 1/2 cups warm water (105°F-110°F)

1 teaspoon dry yeast

1 teaspoon sugar

3 cups bread flour or all-purpose flour

1 heaping teaspoon salt

1 1/2 teaspoons olive oil plus additional

1/4 cup minced fresh herbs, such as thyme, rosemary, cilantro, or parsley *(optional)*

1. In a large bowl, combine the water and yeast. Using a fork, stir rapidly to dissolve the yeast. Add the sugar and 1 1/2 cups flour. Using the paddle attachment of an electric mixer, stir until all the ingredients are well blended. Cover the bowl with lightly oiled plastic wrap and let stand in a warm place until the dough has doubled in size, about 2 hours.

2. Add the salt, 1 1/2 teaspoons oil, and the remaining 1 1/2 cups flour. Again using the paddle attachment, beat the mixture until it is smooth and elastic, 5 to 10 minutes.

3. Lightly flour a work surface and lightly oil a large bowl. Turn out the dough onto the work surface and knead until the dough is smooth and elastic, 10 to 12 minutes. Place the dough in the bowl and turn it until it is completely coated in the oil. Cover the bowl with lightly oiled plastic wrap and set in a warm place to let the dough rise, about 1 1/2 hours.

4. Preheat the oven to 475°F. Line a baking sheet with parchment paper or foil.

5. Lightly flour the work surface again and turn out the dough onto the surface. Divide the dough into 4 balls. Using a rolling pin, roll each ball into a 1/2-inch thick, 6-inch-diameter circle. Place the dough circles on the prepared baking sheet. Lightly brush each circle with oil and, if desired, sprinkle with herbs. Bake until the pita breads are golden, about 8 minutes. Remove the pita breads to wire racks to cool.

Makes 4 pita breads

Sourdough Bread

The starter, a combination of flour, sugar, and water left in a warm place to attract airborne yeast, is essential to the chewy texture and signature flavor of sourdough bread. Once you have a starter, you use some for each loaf you bake, but feed the starter to keep it going—an endless supply for a sensational bread. Our version uses a commercial yeast, so it takes less time to prepare, but developing your own starter is well worth the time. Yes, homemade is cheaper.

Starter

2 cups lukewarm water (105°F–115°F)

1 packet (1/4 ounce) active dry yeast

1 1/2 cups bread flour

Dough

1 1/2 cups starter

1 cup water

2 tablespoons sugar

1 tablespoon salt

5–6 cups bread flour

4 tablespoons (1/2 stick) butter, melted

1. Prepare the starter: In a medium glass or ceramic bowl, combine the ingredients and whisk until well blended. Cover the bowl loosely with wax paper and set in a warm, draft-free place for 12 hours or overnight.

2. Prepare the dough: In a large bowl, combine the starter, water, sugar, salt, and 2 1/2 cups flour. Using a wooden spoon or the paddle attachment of an electric mixer, beat the dough at moderate speed until it is smooth, about 15 seconds.

3. If using an electric mixer, remove the paddle and attach a dough hook. Add 3 tablespoons butter and 2 1/2 cups of the remaining flour, 1/2 cup at a time. Continue beating about 10 minutes, adding an extra 1/2 to 1 cup of flour, if necessary, to make a smooth and elastic dough. (If mixing by hand, you will probably have to knead in the last of the flour.)

4. Butter a 5-quart bowl well. Using your hands, shape the dough into a ball and place in the prepared bowl, turning it to completely coat the surface of the dough with butter. Cover the bowl with a cloth and set in a warm, draft-free place to rise until doubled in size, 1 to 1 1/2 hours. Punch down the dough, cover again, and let rise 1 1/2 hours longer.

5. Lightly flour a work surface and lightly grease two 8-inch-round cake or springform pans. Punch down the dough again and turn out onto the work surface. Knead lightly until the dough is smooth, 2 to 3 minutes. Divide the dough in half and roll each half into a ball. Place each ball into a prepared pan, cover both with a cloth, and let rise until the dough is doubled in size, 45 minutes to 1 hour. Preheat the oven to 350°F.

6. Brush the loaves with the remaining 1 tablespoon of melted butter. Using a sharp knife, cut a diagonal slash across the top of each loaf. Bake until the loaves are richly golden and sound hollow when tapped, 45 to 50 minutes. Remove the loaves to a wire rack to cool.

Makes 2 loaves

muffins

Cranberry Cheddar Muffins
Surprise your family and friends the next time you serve roast poultry and have a basket of these delectable homemade muffins on the table—we guarantee no leftovers!

- 2 cups all-purpose flour
- 2/3 cup firmly packed light brown sugar
- 1/2 cup finely shredded cheddar cheese
- 2 1/2 teaspoons baking powder
- 1/2 teaspoon baking soda
- 12 teaspoon salt
- 1/4 teaspoon ground allspice
- 1/8 teaspoon ground cayenne pepper
- 1 1/4 cups buttermilk
- 1/4 cup (1/2 stick) butter, melted
- 1 egg, separated
- 1 cup washed fresh or frozen cranberries (unthawed)

1. Preheat the oven to 400°F. Lightly grease or insert paper baking cups into 12 (2 1/2-inch) muffin cups.

2. In a large bowl, combine the first eight ingredients and whisk until well blended.

3. In a small bowl, combine the buttermilk, butter, and egg yolk and whisk until well blended. In a separate small bowl, beat the egg white until soft peaks form.

4. Make a well in the center of the dry ingredients. Pour the buttermilk mixture into the well and, using a fork, stir just until all the ingredients are blended; do not overmix. Fold in the egg white and the cranberries.

5. Spoon the muffin batter into the prepared muffin cups, filling each 3/4 full. Bake until a toothpick inserted in a muffin comes out clean, about 20 minutes. Remove the pan to a wire rack and let the muffins cool for 5 minutes. Using a knife, loosen the edges of each muffin from the sides of the cup, and turn out the muffins.

Makes 12 muffins

Helpful Hint

Muffins Are Not Just for Breakfast
Savory muffins—like the cranberry cheddar and the herb bacon ones here—are made to go with lunch and dinner. Try adding other herbs, cheeses, meats, and such to a muffin recipe to make a striking side for grilled meats, poultry, or seafood. Sweet muffins, on the other hand, are a toothsome treat anytime you serve them. They make a marvelous beginning to any day, a welcome addition to a brunch buffet, a comforting classic with afternoon tea. Either type is fresher, tastier, and cheaper when homemade.

Herb Bacon Muffins

You can add whatever herbs you fancy to this muffin recipe—fresh thyme, basil, or marjoram would be superb. You will be glad you made them yourself.

1 3/4 cups all-purpose flour

2 teaspoons baking powder

1/2 teaspoon salt

1/4 cup chopped fresh herbs

1/4 cups grated
Parmesan cheese

1 tablespoon sugar

1/3 cup cooked, crumbled
bacon

1 egg, beaten

1 cup milk

1/4 cup (1/2 stick) butter,
melted

1. Preheat the oven to 400°F. Lightly grease or insert paper baking cups into 12 (2 1/2-inch) muffin cups or 24 miniature muffin cups.

2. In a large bowl, sift together the flour, baking powder, and salt. Add the herbs, cheese, sugar, and bacon, and stir until the ingredients are well blended.

3. In a small bowl, combine the egg, milk, and butter. Stir until the ingredients are well blended. Make a well in the center of the dry ingredients. Pour the milk mixture into the well and, using a fork, stir just until the dry ingredients are moistened. Do not overmix; the batter should be lumpy.

4. Spoon the batter into the prepared muffin cups, filling them 2/3 full. Bake until the muffins are browned: 15 to 20 minutes for regular muffins, 12 to 15 minutes for mini muffins. Remove the pan to a wire rack and let the muffins cool for 5 minutes. Using a knife, loosen the edges of each muffin from the sides of the cup, and turn out the muffins. Serve the muffins warm.

Makes 12 regular muffins or 24 mini muffins

Apple and Raisin Muffins

Grated apple is the sweetener to these muffins, reducing the need for added sugar and letting flavor stand out.

2 cups all-purpose flour

3 teaspoons baking powder

1 teaspoon salt

1/2 teaspoon ground cinnamon

1/4 teaspoon ground nutmeg

3/4 cup peeled, grated apple

1/3 cup golden seedless raisins

2/3 cup firmly packed light
brown sugar

1/4 cup chopped walnuts or
pecans

2 eggs, well beaten

2/3 cups milk

1/4 cup vegetable oil

1 cup corn, bran, or
wheat flakes cereal

1. Preheat the oven to 400°F. Lightly grease or insert paper baking cups into 12 (2 1/2-inch) muffin cups.

2. In a large bowl, combine the flour, baking powder, salt, cinnamon, and nutmeg. Add the apple, raisins, sugar, and nuts. Stir until the dry ingredients are blended.

3. In a small bowl, combine the eggs, milk, and oil, and stir to blend them well. Make a well in the center of the dry ingredients. Pour the milk mixture into the well and, using a fork, stir just until the dry ingredients are moistened. Do not overmix; the batter should be lumpy. Fold in the cereal.

4. Spoon the batter into the prepared muffin cups, filling them 2/3 full. Bake until the muffins are puffed and browned, 15 to 20 minutes. Remove the pan to a wire rack and let the muffins cool for 5 minutes. Using a knife, loosen the edges of each muffin from the sides of the cup, and turn out the muffins. Serve the muffins warm.

Makes 12 muffins

Blueberry Muffins *When blueberries are in season, the flavor is out of this world!*

1 1/2 cups blueberries, fresh or thawed frozen

3 cups all-purpose flour

1 tablespoon baking powder

1/2 teaspoon baking soda

1 teaspoon salt

3/4 cup plus 2 tablespoons sugar

3 tablespoons butter, melted

2 eggs, lightly beaten

1 cup buttermilk

1 1/2 teaspoons vanilla extract

1. Preheat the oven to 400°F. Lightly grease or insert paper baking cups into 12 (2 1/2-inch) muffin cups. Rinse the blueberries and pat dry. In a bowl, combine the blueberries with 2 tablespoons flour, and toss to coat them.

2. In a large bowl, combine the remaining flour, baking powder, baking soda, salt, and 3/4 cup sugar. Stir to blend.

3. In a small bowl, combine the butter, eggs, buttermilk, and vanilla, and stir to blend them well. Make a well in the center of the dry ingredients. Pour the milk mixture into the well and, using a fork, stir just until the dry ingredients are moistened. Do not overmix; the batter should be lumpy. Fold in the blueberries.

4. Spoon the batter into the prepared muffin cups, filling them 2/3 full; sprinkle the muffin tops with 2 tablespoons sugar. Bake the muffins in the center of the oven until the muffins are golden, 20 to 25 minutes. Remove the pan to a wire rack and let the muffins cool for 5 minutes. Using a knife, loosen the edges of each muffin from the cup, and turn out the muffins.

Makes 12 muffins

Bran Muffins *Low in fat and high in fiber—plus an absolutely heavenly flavor when you make them yourself.*

1 cup raisins

1 1/4 cups all-purpose flour

1 tablespoon baking powder

1/3 cup sugar

1 teaspoon cinnamon

1/2 teaspoon salt

1 cup bran cereal (not flakes)

1 cup milk

1 egg

1/4 cup vegetable oil

1. Preheat the oven to 400°F. Lightly grease or insert paper baking cups into 12 (2 1/2-inch) muffin cups. In a small bowl, combine the raisins with 2 tablespoons flour, and toss to coat the raisins completely.

2. In a medium bowl, combine the remaining flour, baking powder, sugar, cinnamon, and salt. Stir until the dry ingredients are well blended.

3. In a large bowl, combine the bran cereal and milk; let the mixture stand 2 minutes. Add the egg and the oil, and stir until the bran mixture is well blended. Add the dry ingredients to the bran mixture and, using a fork, stir just until the dry ingredients are moistened; do not overmix. Fold in the raisins.

4. Spoon the batter into the prepared muffin cups, filling them 2/3 full. Bake until the muffins are golden brown, 18 to 20 minutes. Remove the pan to a wire rack and let the muffins cool for 5 minutes. Using a knife, loosen the edges of each muffin from the sides of the cup, and turn out the muffins.

Makes 12 muffins

Baked Goods You Can Make   **523**

rolls

Parker House Rolls
These classic homemade rolls will melt in your mouth. The secret may be the potato.

2 tablespoons sugar

1/2 cup lukewarm water
(105°F–115°F)

2 packets (1/4 ounce each)
active dry yeast

1 cup milk

1 cup water

2 teaspoons salt

1/2 cup (1 stick) plus
3 tablespoons butter,
melted

1 large all-purpose potato,
peeled, diced, boiled,
and riced

6 1/2–7 cups
all-purpose flour

1 egg, lightly beaten

1. In a small bowl, combine the sugar, water, and yeast; stir until the solids are completely dissolved. Let the yeast mixture stand until it is bubbly, about 10 minutes.

2. In a small saucepan over moderately high heat, combine the milk and water, and bring to a boil. Pour the hot liquid into a large bowl. Add the salt and 3 tablespoons butter, stir to blend, and let cool 10 minutes. Using a wooden spoon or electric mixer with a paddle at moderate speed, add the potato, 2 cups flour, and the egg, beating for 1 minute after each addition. Add the yeast mixture and beat 1 minute longer.

3. If using the mixer, remove the paddle and attach a dough hook. Add 4 1/2 cups flour and beat 3 to 5 minutes or until a soft, manageable dough forms, adding 1/4 to 1/2 cup of flour as needed to reach the desired consistency.

4. Butter a 5-quart bowl well. Using your hands, shape the dough into a ball and place in the prepared bowl, turning it to completely coat the surface of the dough with butter. Cover the bowl with a cloth and set in a warm, draft-free place to rise until doubled in size, about 50 minutes.

5. Lightly flour a work surface and lightly grease 6 baking sheets. Punch down the dough and turn out onto the work surface. Divide the dough into 4 equal portions, working with 1 portion at a time. Using a rolling pin, roll the dough portion into a 1/4-inch thick, 8 x 10-inch rectangle. Using a floured 2 1/2-inch biscuit cutter, cut the dough into 12 rounds. Gather the scraps together, and reroll; cut 4 more rounds.

6. Brush each dough round with melted butter. Using the blunt side of a knife, crease each circle along the diameter and fold, stretching the top half so it covers the bottom half. Pinch the edges to seal. Repeat with the remaining 3 portions of dough.

7. Arrange the rolls on the prepared baking sheets and brush the tops with the remaining butter. Cover the rolls with a cloth and let rise for 30 minutes. Preheat the oven to 350°F.

8. Bake until the rolls are golden brown, about 30 minutes. Serve immediately or cool on wire racks.

Makes 64 rolls

variations:

Cloverleaf Rolls: After the dough rises, on a floured work surface, pinch off 72 walnut-size pieces of dough and roll each into a 1-inch-diameter ball. Lightly grease muffin pan cups; place 3 dough balls in each cup to make a cloverleaf shape. Cover, let rise, and bake as above.

Fantans: Roll out the risen dough and cut all the rounds with a 2-inch biscuit cutter. Spread butter on top of 1 round, and place another on top; repeat to make a roll with 5 round layers with butter between each layer. Take one layered roll, slightly fold it up, and tuck it into a greased muffin pan cup so the folds are facing up. Cover, let rise, and bake as above.

Soda Bread Rolls

Sprinkle a little oatmeal or some caraway seeds over the tops of these rolls that are hard to find in stores after St. Patrick's Day. Make them yourself anytime.

2 cups all-purpose flour

2 teaspoons baking soda

1 1/2 teaspoons salt

1/3 cup vegetable shortening or margarine

2 cups whole wheat flour

1 2/3 cups buttermilk

1. Preheat the oven to 400°F. Lightly grease a baking sheet.

2. In a large bowl, sift together the all-purpose flour, baking soda, and salt. With a pastry blender or two knives, cut in the shortening until the mixture resembles coarse bread crumbs. Stir in the whole wheat flour. Add the buttermilk and stir to blend thoroughly and to form a soft dough.

3. Lightly flour a work surface. Turn out the dough onto the work surface and knead until the dough is smooth, 4 to 5 minutes. Divide the dough into 8 pieces and roll each into a ball. Place the dough balls, evenly spaced 2 to 3 inches apart, on the prepared baking sheet. Using a sharp knife, cut a cross in the top of each ball.

4. Bake until the rolls are crusty brown and sound hollow when tapped, about 20 minutes. Remove the rolls to a wire rack to cool slightly; serve the rolls warm.

Makes 8 rolls

Crescent Rolls

Don't spend your money on store-bought tubes. These homemade crescent rolls taste much better, have incredible texture, and are not at all difficult to prepare.

1 package (1/4 ounce) active dry yeast

1/4 cup warm water (110°F-115°F)

1 tablespoon plus 1/2 cup sugar

3/4 cup warm milk (110°F-115°F)

3 eggs, lightly beaten

1/2 cup (1 stick) butter or margarine, softened

1 teaspoon salt

5-5 1/2 cups all-purpose flour

Additional butter or margarine, melted

1. In a large bowl, combine the yeast and water, and stir until the yeast is dissolved. Add 1 tablespoon sugar, and let the mixture stand until bubbly, about 5 minutes.

2. Add the milk, eggs, butter or margarine, salt, and 1/2 cup sugar. Stir until all the ingredients are well blended. Add 5 cups flour, 1 cup at a time, stirring after each addition until the mixture forms a stiff dough; add as much of the remaining 1/2 cup of flour as you need to reach the desired consistency.

3. Butter a large bowl well; lightly flour a work surface. Turn out the dough onto the work surface and knead until the dough is smooth and elastic, 6 to 8 minutes. Using your hands, shape the dough into a ball and place in the prepared bowl, turning it to completely coat the surface of the dough with butter. Cover the bowl with a cloth and set in a warm, draft-free place to rise until doubled in size, about 1 1/2 hours.

4. Reflour the work surface and lightly grease 2 baking sheets. Punch down the dough and divide it into thirds; work with one portion at a time. Place 1 dough portion on the work surface. Using a rolling pin, roll out the dough into a 12-inch-diameter circle. Using a sharp knife or pizza cutter, cut the circle into 8 wedges. Brush the wedges with some melted butter. Starting at the wide end, roll up each wedge. Place each wedge on the baking sheet, 2 inches apart, with the small point tucked underneath and slightly bend the wedge to form a crescent shape. Repeat with the remaining dough. Cover the crescents with a cloth and let rise in a warm place until doubled in size, about 30 minutes.

5. Preheat the oven to 375°F. Bake until the crescents are golden brown, 10 to 12 minutes. Remove the crescents to wire racks and cool slightly.

Makes 24 rolls

Cinnamon Rolls

Your whole house will be infused with the aroma of these sweet delicacies as they're baking. Store-bought rolls can't do that. Cream cheese frosting is the perfect finishing touch.

1 package (1/4 ounce)
  active dry yeast

1 cup warm milk
  (110°F-115°F)

1/2 cup sugar

1/3 cup butter, melted

2 eggs

1 teaspoon salt

4-4 1/2 cups
  all-purpose flour

Cinnamon Filling

3/4 cup firmly packed
  brown sugar

2 tablespoons ground
  cinnamon

1/4 cup (1/2 stick) butter,
  melted

Cream Cheese Frosting

1/2 cup (1/2 stick) butter,
  softened

1 1/2 cups
  confectioners' sugar

1/4 cup cream cheese,
  softened

1/2 teaspoon vanilla extract

1/8 teaspoon salt

1. In a large bowl, combine the yeast and the milk; stir until the yeast is completely dissolved. Add the sugar, 1/3 cup butter, eggs, salt, and 2 cups flour. Beat until the ingredients are smooth. Stir in enough remaining flour to form a soft, sticky dough.

2. Lightly flour a work surface; lightly grease a large bowl. Turn out the dough onto the work surface and knead until the dough is smooth and elastic, 6 to 8 minutes. Place in the prepared bowl, turning it to completely coat the surface of the dough with butter. Cover the bowl with a cloth and set in a warm, draft-free place to rise until doubled in size, about 1 hour.

3. Prepare the filling: In a small bowl, combine the brown sugar and cinnamon until they are well blended. Lightly grease two 13 x 9 x 2-inch baking pans; reflour the work surface.

4. Punch down the dough and turn out onto the work surface. Divide the dough in half. Using a rolling pin, roll each half into an 11 x 8-inch rectangle. Brush each rectangle with some of the melted butter. Sprinkle half the filling over each rectangle, leaving a 1/2-inch border around all the edges. Starting from a long side, roll up each rectangle, jelly-roll-fashion, and pinch the seams together to seal. Using a sharp knife, cut each roll into 8 slices. Place the slices, cut side down, in the prepared baking pans. Cover the pans and let rise until doubled in size, about 1 hour.

5. Preheat the oven to 350°F. Bake the rolls until they are golden brown, 20 to 25 minutes. Remove the pans to wire racks and let the rolls cool for 5 to 10 minutes.

6. Prepare the frosting: In a small bowl, combine the ingredients and beat until the frosting is smooth. Frost the warm cinnamon rolls and serve immediately.

Makes 16 rolls

Hot Cross Buns

A traditional Easter morning bun, just sweet enough and loaded with dried fruit. Homemade hot cross buns can be had any time of year.

2 packages (1/4 ounce each) active dry yeast

2 cups warm milk (110°F–115°F)

1/3 cup butter or margarine, softened

2 eggs, lightly beaten

1/4 cup sugar

1 1/2 teaspoons salt

6-7 cups all-purpose flour

1/2 cup raisins

1/2 cup dried currants

1 teaspoon ground cinnamon

1/4 teaspoon ground allspice

2 tablespoons water

1 egg yolk

Icing

2 cups sifted confectioners' sugar

2 tablespoons water

1. In a large bowl, combine the yeast and milk and stir to dissolve the yeast. Add the butter, eggs, sugar, and salt; stir until the ingredients are well blended.

2. In a medium bowl, combine 3 cups flour, the raisins, currants, cinnamon, and allspice. Add the flour mixture to the yeast mixture, and stir until well blended. Add enough of the remaining flour to form a soft dough.

3. Lightly flour a work surface; butter a large bowl well. Turn out the dough onto the work surface and knead until the dough is smooth and elastic, 6 to 8 minutes. Place the dough in the prepared bowl, turning it to completely coat the surface of the dough with butter. Cover the bowl with a cloth and set in a warm, draft-free place to rise until doubled in size, about 1 hour.

4. Lightly grease 3 baking sheets. Punch down the dough. Pinch off enough to form a 1 1/2-inch to 2-inch-diameter ball. Repeat with the remaining dough, placing the dough balls 2 inches apart on the prepared baking sheets. Using a sharp knife, cut a cross on top of each dough ball. Cover the buns with a cloth and let rise until doubled in size, about 30 minutes.

5. Preheat the oven to 375°F. Meanwhile, combine the 2 tablespoons water with the yolk and whisk until they are well blended. Brush the egg-yolk mixture over the risen buns. Then bake until the buns are golden brown, 15 to 20 minutes. Remove the buns to wire racks to cool.

6. Prepare the icing: In a small bowl, combine the confectioners' sugar and water, and stir until the icing is smooth. Place the icing in a pastry bag or self-sealing plastic bag and snip off one corner. Pipe a cross in the cuts on top of each bun.

Makes 30 buns

Sticky Buns *A nutty variation on the cinnamon roll, these gooey, sticky, sensational treats will have them banging down the kitchen door for more.*

2 tablespoons sugar

1/2 cup lukewarm water
  (105°F-115°F)

2 packets (1/4 ounce each)
  active dry yeast

1 cup milk

1 cup water

2 teaspoons salt

1/2 cup (1 stick) plus
  3 tablespoons butter,
  melted

1 large all-purpose potato,
  peeled, diced, boiled, and
  riced

6 1/2-7 cups
  all-purpose flour

1 egg, lightly beaten

Filling

1/2 cup firmly packed light
  brown sugar

1/2 cup light corn syrup

2 teaspoons ground
  cinnamon

1 cup (2 sticks) softened
  butter

Additional melted butter

2 cups chopped pecans

1. In a small bowl, combine the sugar, warm water, and yeast; stir until the solids are completely dissolved. Let the yeast mixture stand until it is bubbly, about 10 minutes.

2. In a small saucepan over moderately high heat, combine the milk and water, and bring to a boil. Pour the hot liquid into a large bowl. Add the salt and 3 tablespoons of the melted butter, stir to blend, and let cool for 10 minutes. Using a wooden spoon or electric mixer with a paddle attached at moderate speed, add the potato, 2 cups of the flour, and the egg, beating for 1 minute after each addition. Add the yeast mixture to the flour mixture and beat for 1 minute longer.

3. If using the mixer, remove the paddle and attach a dough hook. Add 4 1/2 cups of the remaining flour and beat for 3 to 5 minutes or until a soft, manageable dough forms, adding 1/4 to 1/2 cup of flour as needed to reach the desired consistency.

4. Butter a 5-quart bowl well. Using your hands, shape the dough into a ball and place in the prepared bowl, turning it to completely coat the surface of the dough with butter. Cover the bowl with a cloth and set in a warm, draft-free place to rise until doubled in size, about 50 minutes.

5. Lightly flour a work surface and lightly grease 6 baking sheets. Punch down the dough and turn out onto the work surface. Divide the dough in half. Using a rolling pin, roll each dough half into a 1/4-inch thick, 15 x 12-inch rectangle.

6. Prepare the filling: In a small bowl, combine the brown sugar, corn syrup, cinnamon, and 1 cup of softened butter. Stir until the filling is well blended. Lightly grease a 15 x 10-inch jelly-roll pan.

7. Spread half of the filling over each rectangle, leaving a 1/2-inch-wide border around all the edges. Sprinkle each rectangle with 1 cup of the pecans. Starting from a long side, roll up each rectangle, jelly-roll-fashion, and pinch the seams together to seal; place seam side down. Using a sharp knife, cut each roll into fifteen 1-inch-thick slices. Arrange the slices, not touching, in the prepared jelly-roll pan. Cover the pan with a cloth and let rise about 20 minutes.

8. Preheat the oven to 350°F. Bake until the buns are golden brown, about 40 minutes; brush the buns with a little melted butter and bake for 5 minutes longer.

Makes 30 buns

Baked Goods You Can Make   **529**

cakes

Spice Cake
Inviting on its own, this spice-filled cake is also wonderful with Buttercream Frosting (page 119). Much less expensive than a bakery sheet cake, it is also tastier. This cake and the chocolate cake recipe that follows are also outstanding examples of what you can do with the Basic Cake Mix from Chapter 1.

5 cups Basic Cake Mix
(page 61)

1 1/4 teaspoons ground
nutmeg

1 1/4 teaspoons ground
cinnamon

1/2 teaspoon ground cloves

1 cup water

1/4 cup butter or margarine

1/2 cup sour cream or plain
nonfat yogurt

2 eggs, lightly beaten

1. Preheat the oven to 375°F. Generously grease a 13 x 9 x 2-inch baking pan.

2. In a large bowl, combine the cake mix, nutmeg, cinnamon, and cloves; stir to distribute the spices evenly.

3. In a small saucepan over moderately high heat, combine the water and butter or margarine. Bring the mixture to a boil. Remove the saucepan from the heat and pour the butter mixture into the bowl. Using a wooden spoon or an electric mixer, beat the batter until all the ingredients are well blended. Stir in the sour cream or yogurt and the eggs; beat until they are incorporated and no streaks of white remain.

4. Pour the batter into the prepared baking pan. Bake until a toothpick inserted into the center of the cake comes out clean and the top of the cake springs back when lightly touched, about 40 minutes. Remove the baking pan to a wire rack and let the cake cool completely.

Makes one 13 x 9 x 2-inch sheet cake

Chocolate Cake
If you like chocolate, this cake is guaranteed to please your guests and your pocketbook.

3 1/3 cups Basic Cake Mix (page 61)

9 tablespoons cocoa powder

1 cup milk

2 eggs, lightly beaten

3 tablespoons butter or margarine, melted

1. Preheat the oven to 375°F. Lightly grease and flour two 8-inch round cake pans.

2. In a large bowl, combine the cake mix and cocoa. Add 1/2 cup of the milk. Using an electric mixer on medium speed, beat the batter for 2 minutes. Add the remaining 1/2 cup milk, the eggs, and butter or margarine; beat for 2 minutes longer.

3. Pour the batter into the prepared cake pans, dividing it equally. Bake the cake until a toothpick inserted into the center comes out clean and the top of the cake springs back after you touch it, about 25 minutes.

4. Remove the cake pans to wire racks and let stand for 10 minutes to cool slightly. Run a knife around the edges of the cake layers to loosen them from the sides of the pans, invert the pan and remove the cake layers. Set the cake layers on the wire racks and let them cool completely. Fill and frost as desired.

Makes 1 layer cake or 12 servings

Devil's Food Cake
This is a one-bowl cake—meant to be beaten with an electric mixer so all the ingredients are in an order to prevent overmixing. Devil's food cake has a beguiling, bitter chocolate flavor that is moister and more distinctive in homemade versions.

1 tablespoon unsweetened cocoa powder

2 cups sifted cake flour

1 1/2 teaspoons baking soda

1 teaspoon salt

1/2 teaspoon baking powder

1 1/2 cups sugar

1 cup buttermilk, at room temperature

1/2 cup (1 stick) butter or margarine, softened

1 teaspoon vanilla extract

3 eggs, at room temperature

3 ounces semisweet chocolate, melted

1. Preheat the oven to 350°F. Lightly grease two 8-inch round cake pans, dust with the cocoa, divided equally; tap out any excess powder.

2. In a large bowl, combine the flour, baking soda, salt, baking powder, sugar, buttermilk, butter, vanilla, eggs, and chocolate, being careful to add the ingredients in the order listed. Using an electric mixer at low speed, beat all the ingredients for 1 minute, using a spatula to scrape down the sides of the bowl occasionally. Increase the speed to medium-high, and beat for 2 minutes longer, scraping the sides of the bowl twice.

3. Pour the batter into the prepared cake pans. Bake until a toothpick inserted into the center of the cake layers comes out clean, about 30 minutes. Remove the pans to wire racks and let the cake layers cool for 10 minutes. Turn each layer out of its cake pan, then set the layers back on the wire racks to cool completely. Fill and frost as desired.

Makes 1 layer cake or 12 servings

White Cake

Try this sheet cake, topped with Broiled Brown Sugar-Coconut Icing (below) for a terrific offering at a potluck picnic or barbecue. Or make it as a layer cake with Buttercream Frosting (opposite). Either way, it's a fresh, delectable cake for half the price.

2 1/2 cups sifted cake flour

3 teaspoons baking powder

1/2 teaspoon salt

2/3 cup butter or margarine, at room temperature

1 1/2 cups granulated sugar

1 teaspoon vanilla extract

1/2 teaspoon almond extract

3/4 cup milk

4 egg whites, at room temperature

1. Preheat the oven to 375°F. Grease and flour a 13 x 9 x 2-inch baking pan.

2. In a small bowl, sift together the flour, baking powder, and salt. In a large bowl, using an electric mixer at moderately high speed, beat the butter or margarine until it is light. Gradually add 1 1/4 cups of the flour, beating constantly until the mixture is fluffy. Reduce the mixer speed to low, and beat in the vanilla and almond extracts. Add the flour mixture to the bowl, alternating with the milk, beginning and ending with the flour mixture, and adding about 1/3 of the ingredients at a time.

3. In a medium bowl with the electric mixer with clean beaters attached, beat the egg whites until they are frothy. Begin adding the remaining 1/4 cup of sugar, a little at a time, until the mixture forms soft peaks. Fold the egg-white mixture into the batter just until the ingredients are blended and no white streaks remain.

4. Spoon the batter into the prepared pan and, using a spatula, smooth the top. Bake until the cake is lightly browned and springs back when lightly touched, 25 to 30 minutes. Remove the pan to a wire rack and let stand for 5 minutes. Frost as desired.

Makes 20 servings

Broiled Brown Sugar-Coconut Icing

2/3 cup firmly packed brown sugar

1/4 cup softened butter or margarine

1/4 cup heavy cream

1/2 cup flaked coconut

1. Preheat the broiler. In a large bowl using a wooden spoon, combine all the ingredients and beat until well blended.

2. Spread the icing over a warm cake and broil 5 inches from the heat source until the icing bubbles and browns slightly, 3 to 4 minutes. Remove the pan to the wire rack again, and cool the cake slightly before serving.

Makes enough to frost one 13 x 9 x 2-inch sheet cake

Buttercream Frosting
This classic cake frosting is easy and cheap to make and luscious to eat.

1/3 cup butter or margarine, softened

1 box (16 ounces) confectioners' sugar, sifted

1/4 cup light cream

2 teaspoons vanilla extract

1-2 drops food coloring *(optional)*

1. In a medium bowl with an electric mixer on moderately high speed, beat the butter or margarine until it is light and fluffy.

2. Reduce the speed to medium, and alternately add the sugar and the cream, a little at a time and beating constantly. Add the vanilla and beat until the frosting is creamy. If desired, add food coloring to tint the frosting.

Makes enough to fill and frost one 8- or 9-inch layer cake, 24 cupcakes, or one 13 x 9 x 2-inch sheet cake

Chocolate Buttercream Frosting
This is the icing that kids like to lick out of the bowl. Inexpensive and easy to make, it is delicious.

1/3 cup butter or margarine, softened

1 box (16 ounces) confectioners' sugar, sifted

1/4 cup light cream

2 teaspoons vanilla extract

3 ounces semisweet chocolate, melted, or 1/2 cup sifted unsweetened cocoa powder

1. In a medium bowl with an electric mixer on moderately high speed, beat the butter or margarine until it is light and fluffy.

2. Reduce the speed to medium, and alternately add the sugar and the cream, a little at a time and beating constantly. Add the vanilla and melted chocolate or cocoa powder; beat until the frosting is creamy.

Makes enough to fill and frost one 8- or 9-inch layer cake, 24 cupcakes, or one 13 x 9 x 2-inch sheet cake

Orange Buttercream Frosting
Lightly flavored with orange juice and zest, this homemade icing would be particularly tempting on a spice cake. Make it fresh and save money.

1/3 cup butter or margarine, softened

1 box (16 ounces) confectioners' sugar, sifted

1/4 cup fresh orange juice, strained

2 teaspoons vanilla extract

1 tablespoon grated orange zest

1-2 drops orange food coloring *(optional)*

1. In a medium bowl with an electric mixer on moderately high speed, beat the butter or margarine until it is light and fluffy.

2. Reduce the speed to medium, and alternately add the sugar and the orange juice, a little at a time and beating constantly. Add the vanilla and orange zest, and beat until the frosting is creamy. If desired, add orange food coloring to tint the frosting.

Makes enough to fill and frost one 8- or 9-inch layer cake, 24 cupcakes, or one 13 x 9 x 2-inch sheet cake

Baked Goods You Can Make **533**

Angel Cake

Aptly named indeed, this cake is so light and airy that you'll swear it'll float away if you don't eat it quickly. It's also free of any fat, and can be the base for many a light, luscious dessert. It is not hard to make yourself, and the homemade one will be even lighter and airier.

1 1/2 cups egg whites (about 15 eggs)

1 1/2 teaspoons cream of tartar

1/4 teaspoon salt

1 1/2 cups sugar

1 cup sifted cake flour

2 teaspoons vanilla extract

1/4 teaspoon almond extract

1. Place the oven rack at the lowest possible position. Preheat the oven to 325°F; set out a 10-inch tube pan.

2. In a large bowl with an electric mixer at medium speed, combine the egg whites, cream of tartar, and salt, and beat until the mixture is frothy. Gradually add the sugar, 2 tablespoons at a time, beating constantly. Increase the speed to high and continue beating until the mixture forms very soft peaks.

3. Fold the flour, 1/4 cup at a time, into the egg whites, then fold in the vanilla and almond extracts.

4. Spoon the cake batter into the ungreased tube pan and gently smooth the top with a spatula. Cut the spatula through the batter once to break and release any large air bubbles.

5. Bake the cake until the top springs back when lightly touched, 50 to 60 minutes. Invert the tube pan with the central tube over the neck of a large bottle; let the cake cool completely. Using a knife, loosen the edges of the cake from the sides of the pan, and turn out the cake onto a cake plate.

Makes 12 servings

Cheesecake with Strawberry Glaze

You can substitute raspberries, blackberries, or blueberries in this recipe. Whatever you choose, you will have a dessert to rival very expensive bakery or deli cheesecake.

Crust

1 1/4 cups crumbled purchased or homemade Graham Crackers (page 132)

5 tablespoons butter or margarine, melted

1/4 cup sugar

Filling

3 packages (8 ounces each) cream cheese

1 cup sugar

3 eggs

1 cup sour cream

Strawberry Glaze

1/4 cup strawberry jelly

1 tablespoon water

1 pint fresh strawberries, hulled and thinly sliced

1. Prepare the crust: Preheat the oven to 325°F. In a medium bowl, using a fork, toss the crumbs, butter, and sugar until well blended. Press the crust mixture firmly over the bottom of a 9-inch springform pan.

2. Prepare the filling: In the bowl of a food processor or blender, combine the cream cheese and sugar, and pulse until they are well blended and smooth. With the motor running, add the eggs 1 at a time. Scrape down the sides of the bowl, add the sour cream, and whirl until the filling is smooth and well blended.

3. Pour the filling into the prepared pan and bake until the filling is only slightly loose in the center of the cheesecake, about 50 minutes. Transfer the pan to a wire rack and let the cheesecake cool to room temperature. Remove the sides of the pan before glazing the cheesecake.

4. Prepare the glaze: In a small saucepan over moderately high heat, combine the jelly and water, and bring the mixture to a boil. Remove the pan from the heat and let the glaze cool slightly. Brush the cheesecake with about 1/3 of the glaze. Beginning along an outside edge of the cake top, arrange the sliced strawberries in overlapping concentric circles. Brush the remaining glaze lightly over the strawberries.

Makes one 9-inch cheesecake or 6 to 8 servings

Chocolate Cheesecake

You love chocolate; you love cheesecake—now you can have your cheesecake and your chocolate too!

Crust

1 1/4 cups chocolate wafer cookie crumbs

5 tablespoons butter melted

1/4 cup sugar

Filling

3 packages (8 ounces each) cream cheese

1 cup sugar

3 eggs

1/4 cup unsweetened Dutch-process cocoa powder

1/4 cup boiling water

1 cup sour cream

Chocolate curls and/or chocolate-dipped nuts *(optional)*

1. Prepare the crust: Preheat the oven to 325°F. In a medium bowl using a fork, toss the crumbs, butter, and sugar until well blended. Press the crust mixture firmly over the bottom of a 9-inch springform pan.

2. Prepare the filling: In the bowl of a food processor or blender, combine the cream cheese and sugar, and pulse until they are well blended and smooth. With the motor running, add the eggs 1 at a time. Scrape down the sides of the bowl. In a small bowl or cup, combine the cocoa with the boiling water, stirring until the cocoa has completely dissolved. Add the liquid cocoa and the sour cream to the cream-cheese mixture, and whirl until the filling is smooth and well blended.

3. Pour the filling into the prepared pan and bake until the filling is only slightly loose in the center of the cheesecake, about 50 minutes. Transfer the pan to a wire rack and let the cheesecake cool to room temperature. Remove the sides of the pan before glazing the cheesecake and, if desired, garnish with chocolate curls and chocolate-dipped nuts before serving.

Makes one 9-inch cheesecake or 6 to 8 servings

Pumpkin Cheesecake

Surprise your family and friends this Thanksgiving with this spicy pumpkin cheesecake instead of the traditional pumpkin pie. It will be an inexpensive treat that they will think came from the bakery.

Crust

1 1/4 cups crumbled Gingersnaps (page 131)

5 tablespoons butter melted

1/4 cup sugar

Filling

3 packages (8 ounces each) cream cheese

1 1/2 cups firmly packed light brown sugar

3 eggs

1 can (29 ounces) unsweetened pumpkin puree

1/4 teaspoon ground cinnamon

1/4 teaspoon ground cloves

1/4 teaspoon ground nutmeg

1. Prepare the crust: Preheat the oven to 325°F. In a medium bowl, using a fork, toss the crumbs, butter, and sugar until well blended. Press the crust mixture firmly over the bottom of a 9-inch springform pan.

2. Prepare the filling: In the bowl of a food processor or blender, combine the cream cheese and sugar, and pulse until they are well blended and smooth. With the motor running, add the eggs 1 at a time. Scrape down the sides of the bowl. Add the pumpkin puree, cinnamon, cloves, and nutmeg, and whirl until the filling is smooth and well blended.

3. Pour the filling into the prepared pan and bake until the filling is only slightly loose in the center of the cheesecake, about 50 minutes. Transfer the pan to a wire rack and let the cheesecake cool to room temperature. Remove the sides of the pan before glazing the cheesecake.

Makes one 9-inch cheesecake or 6 to 8 servings

pies and meringues

Basic Double Crust Pie Pastry

Both savory (meat, cheese, and such) and sweet, pies are among the most popular items in the frozen food section of any grocery store. And sweet pies are featured in every bakery section. (You'll find recipes for main-dish pies starting on page 172 and ones for sweet pies on page 124.) When you have made your own, you will understand why homemade is best even before you add up your savings. Don't waste your cash on pre-made piecrust. Piecrust is easy to make, doesn't take very long, and if you know a few tricks, it will turn out light and flaky every time. Here is the basic recipe for a pie that has a top crust as well as a bottom one.

2 1/4 cups all-purpose flour
1/2 teaspoon salt
1/2 cup (1 stick) cold butter, cut up
1/4 cup vegetable shortening
5-6 tablespoons ice water

1. In a large bowl, sift together the flour and salt. Using a pastry blender or 2 knives, cut in the butter and shortening until the mixture resembles coarse bread crumbs.

2. Add the ice water, 1 tablespoon at a time, stirring the mixture with a fork to incorporate the water into the dough. Add water only until the dough begins to hold together. Handling the dough as little as possible, divide it in half, shape each half into a ball, and wrap each ball in plastic wrap. Chill the dough balls for at least 1 hour before using.

3. For the bottom crust, place 1 ball of dough on a lightly floured board or pastry cloth. Flatten the ball slightly; then, using a lightly floured or covered rolling pin, roll from the center of the ball outward in all directions. Make the dough circle large enough to cover the bottom and sides of a pie plate plus about 1 inch more.

4. For top crust, place the remaining ball of dough on the lightly floured surface and flatten slightly. Roll the dough from the center outward in all directions until the circle is large enough to cover the pie plate plus about a 1/2-inch margin.

Makes enough for a 8- or 9-inch double crust pie

Basic Single Crust Pie Pastry
Use this recipe when you are making an open-face pie or one with a meringue or crumb topping.

1 1/2 cups all-purpose flour

1/4 teaspoon salt

6 tablespoons cold butter, cut up

3 tablespoons vegetable shortening

3-4 tablespoons ice water

1. In a large bowl, sift together the flour and salt. Using a pastry blender or two knives, cut in the butter and shortening until the mixture resembles coarse bread crumbs.

2. Add the ice water, 1 tablespoon at a time, stirring the mixture with a fork to incorporate the water into the dough. Add water only until the dough begins to hold together. Handling the dough as little as possible, shape it into a ball, and wrap it in plastic wrap. Chill the dough ball for at least 1 hour before using.

3. Place the dough on a lightly floured board or pastry cloth. Flatten the ball slightly; then, using a lightly floured or covered rolling pin, roll from the center of the ball outward in all directions. Make the dough circle large enough to cover the bottom and sides of a pie plate plus about 1 inch more. Drape carefully over a pie plate and fold over the outer edge and crimp it with your fingers to make a decorative edge. Fill and bake according to the pie recipe.

4. For a prebaked pie shell, preheat the oven to 375°F. Place the pie shell on a baking sheet and prick the bottom. Line the bottom with two layers of foil and add dried beans or pastry beads to weight it down; otherwise the bottom will puff up during cooking. Bake 10 to 15 minutes or until golden brown.

Makes enough for a 8- or 9-inch single crust pie

Pecan Pie
Each bite is a bit of heaven in your mouth. And your pocketbook will be heavier for not having bought this easy-to-make delicacy.

Basic Single Crust Pie Pastry (above)

3 large eggs

1 cup light corn syrup

1/8 teaspoon salt

2/3 cups chopped pecans

1/3 cup melted butter

1 teaspoon vanilla extract

1 cup white or brown sugar (or half each)

10-20 large perfect pecan halves

1. Preheat the oven to 450°F. Line a 9-inch pie plate with the piecrust; turn under the edges of the dough and, if desired, form a decorative edge around the piecrust.

2. In a large bowl, beat the eggs slightly. Add the corn syrup, salt, chopped pecans, butter, vanilla, and sugar. Stir until all the ingredients are well blended. Pour the syrup mixture into the prepared piecrust. Arrange the pecan halves over the top of the pie, spacing them evenly, in concentric circles or as desired.

3. Bake the pie for 10 minutes; reduce the heat to 350°F and bake until a knife inserted in the center comes out clean, 45 to 55 minutes more. Do not open the oven door during the baking time. Let the pie cool for at least 20 minutes before serving.

Makes 6 to 8 servings

Perfect Apple Pie
You will win kudos for this pie, and you will never enjoy a store-bought apple pie again after you have tasted it.

Basic Double Crust Pie
   Pastry (page 123)

1 large egg, separated

4 tart apples, such as Granny
   Smith, Jonathan,
   Winesaps, or Northern Spy

4 sweet apples, such as
   Golden Delicious,
   Gravenstein, McIntosh, or
   York Imperial

2 tablespoons lemon juice

1/2 cup firmly packed light
   brown sugar

1/2 cup granulated sugar

1/3 cup sifted
   all-purpose flour

1/4 teaspoon ground cinnamon

1/8 teaspoon ground allspice

1/8 teaspoon grated nutmeg

2 tablespoons butter

1 tablespoon cold water

1. Preheat the oven to 425°F. Line a 9-inch pie plate with the bottom piecrust, letting the edges hang over about 1 inch. In a cup, whisk the egg white until frothy and brush over the bottom crust; reserve the egg yolk for the top crust glaze. Roll out the remaining piecrust. Cover the top crust with plastic wrap until ready to use.

2. Peel, core, and slice all the apples about 1/4-inch thick, placing them in a large bowl. Sprinkle the apple slices with the lemon juice as you work to prevent browning. In a small bowl, combine the sugars, flour, cinnamon, allspice, and nutmeg. Sprinkle the sugar mixture over the apple slices, tossing as you work to coat all the slices. Spoon the apple slices into the prepared bottom piecrust, mounding the slices higher in the center. Cut the butter into small pieces and scatter the pieces throughout the apple slices.

3. Using a pastry brush, moisten the edges of the bottom piecrust with a little water. Carefully transfer the top crust to cover the pie filling. Fold the top edges of the pastry over and under the bottom crust edges; pinch the edges together to seal. Cut slits or make decorative vents. If desired, form a decorative edge around the piecrust. In a small bowl, whisk together the reserved egg yolk and cold water. Brush the glaze over the top of the pie, avoiding the slits or decorative vents.

4. Bake the pie 15 minutes; reduce the temperature to 375°F and bake until the filling is bubbly and the piecrust is golden brown, about 35 minutes more. If the crust edges are browning too quickly, cover them with pieces of foil. Place the pie on a rack to cool for at least 20 minutes before serving.

Makes 8 servings

Custard Pie *This creamy pie is never so good from a store as it is from your kitchen.*

Basic Single Crust Pie
  Pastry (page 124)
4 eggs
2 1/2 cups milk
1/2 cup sugar
1 teaspoon vanilla extract
1 teaspoon almond extract
1 teaspoon salt
1 teaspoon ground nutmeg

1. Preheat the oven to 400°F. Line a 9-inch pie plate with the piecrust; turn under the edges of the dough and, if desired, form a decorative edge around the piecrust. Prick the bottom of the crust and bake it for 10 minutes.

2. Meanwhile, in a large bowl, beat the eggs. Add the remaining ingredients and stir to blend well. Pour the egg mixture into the piecrust. Cover the edges of the crust with pieces of foil and bake until a knife inserted near the center comes out clean, 20 to 25 minutes. Let the pie cool completely before serving; store in the refrigerator.

Makes 6 to 8 servings

Meringue Shells *Since these are cooked through, it is safe to use fresh egg whites. The finished appearance should be dry and crisp, but not browned.*

1 cup egg whites (10 large
  eggs)
3/4 cup granulated sugar
1/2 cup sifted confectioners'
  sugar

1. Preheat the oven to 250°F. Line a baking sheet with parchment paper.

2. In a large bowl with an electric mixer on low, slowly beat the egg whites until they are frothy. Continuing to beat on low, gradually add 1/2 cup of the granulated sugar until the egg whites are silvery in appearance. Increase the mixer speed to moderate, and slowly add the remaining 1/4 cup of granulated sugar, beating just until the egg whites form stiff peaks. Using a spatula, fold in the confectioners' sugar.

3. Fit a pastry bag with a number 6 star tip, and fill the bag with the meringue.

4. Pipe 6 coiled circles of meringue onto the prepared baking sheet. Pipe a second-tier ring of meringue along the outer edge of each of the first circles. Or, spoon 6 mounds of meringue onto the baking sheet and, using the back of the spoon, press a hollow in the center of each mound to make a shell.

5. Bake the meringues for 1 hour; turn off the oven but do not open the oven door. Let the meringues stand in the warm oven for 1 hour longer. Remove the meringues to wire racks to cool.

Makes 6 individual meringues or 1 meringue pie shell

Serving example:

Meringue Shells with Raspberry Sauce: Sweetly tart raspberries are the perfect foil for crispy sweet meringue shells. Make 3/4 cup Raspberry Sauce (page 58). Place each meringue shell on an individual serving plate or shallow bowl. Spoon some of the raspberry sauce into each shell and serve immediately.

Strawberry Pavlova

Legend has it that this resplendent sweet was concocted in honor of the celebrated ballerina Anna Pavlova. You can honor your own heroine or hero with this heart-shaped delicacy.

1/2 recipe Meringue Shells (opposite)

Filling

2 cups whipping cream

2 tablespoons sugar

1 quart fresh strawberries, trimmed and sliced

1. Preheat the oven to 250°F. Line a 14-inch pizza pan with parchment paper. Spoon the meringue onto the prepared pan, forming a 12-inch heart shape with slightly built-up edges. Bake the meringue shell for 1 hour; turn off the oven but do not open the oven door. Let the meringue shell stand in the warm oven for 1 hour longer. Remove the meringue shell to a wire rack to cool.

2. Prepare the filling: In a large bowl with an electric mixer on moderately high, beat the whipping cream until it forms soft peaks. Gradually add the sugar, beating constantly, until stiff peaks form.

3. Spoon the whipped cream into the meringue shell, mounding it decoratively. Arrange the strawberry slices on top of the whipped cream and serve immediately.

Makes 12 servings

cookies

Chocolate Chip Cookies

This American classic has been loved for generations and has never really been improved upon. Homemade are just better and less expensive.

1 cup butter or margarine, softened

3/4 cup sugar

3/4 cup firmly packed brown sugar

2 eggs

1 teaspoon vanilla extract

2 1/4 cups all-purpose flour

1 teaspoon salt

1 teaspoon baking soda

1 cups (6 ounces) semisweet chocolate chips

1 cup chopped walnuts or pecans *(optional)*

1. Preheat the oven to 350°F; lightly grease 2 or more baking sheets. In a medium bowl, combine the butter and sugars; beat until the mixture is well creamed. Add the eggs one at a time, beating well after each addition. Add the vanilla and stir until all the ingredients are well blended.

2. In a small bowl, combine the flour, salt, and baking soda. Add the flour mixture to the creamed mixture, stirring until all the ingredients are well blended. Add the chocolate chips and, if desired, the nuts, and stir until they are evenly distributed.

3. Using a tablespoon, drop the cookie dough onto the prepared sheets, spacing the cookies about 2 inches apart. Bake until the cookies are golden brown, about 10 minutes. Transfer the cookies to wire racks to cool.

Makes about 3 1/2 dozen

Baked Goods You Can Make

Oatmeal Cookies
Wholesome and wholly appealing, this is the cookie that says "home." Homemade are tastier and cheaper.

1 cup raisins

1 cup boiling water

3/4 cup shortening

1 cup firmly packed light brown sugar

1/2 cup granulated sugar

2 eggs

1 teaspoon vanilla extract

2 1/2 cups all-purpose flour

1 teaspoon baking soda

1 teaspoon salt

1 teaspoon ground cinnamon

1/2 teaspoon baking powder

1/4 teaspoon ground cloves

2 cups quick-cooking oats

1. Preheat the oven to 375°F; set out 2 or more baking sheets.

2. In a small bowl, combine the raisins and the boiling water. Let stand until the raisins are plump, about 15 minutes. Drain the raisins, reserving the liquid. Add enough water to the raisin liquid to equal 1/2 cup.

3. In a large bowl, combine the shortening, sugars, eggs, and vanilla, and beat until the mixture is well creamed. Stir in the raisin liquid. Add the flour, baking soda, salt, cinnamon, baking powder, and cloves, and stir until all the ingredients are well blended. Stir in the raisins and the oats.

4. Using a teaspoon, drop the dough onto the prepared sheets, spacing the cookies about 2 inches apart. Bake until the cookies are light brown, 10 to 12 minutes. Transfer the cookies to wire racks to cool completely.

Makes 5 dozen cookies

Peanut Butter Cookies
One of America's favorite flavors in one of its favorite cookies is a perfect home-bake success. It is easy and delectable.

1/2 cup butter or margarine, softened

1/2 cup granulated sugar

1/2 cup firmly packed brown sugar

1/2 cup Peanut Butter (page 33)

1 egg

1/2 teaspoon vanilla extract

1 1/4 cups all-purpose flour

1/2 teaspoon baking soda

1/2 teaspoon baking powder

Additional granulated sugar

1. In a large bowl, combine the butter or margarine and the sugars; beat until the mixture is well creamed. Add the peanut butter, egg, and vanilla; beat until the mixture is smooth.

2. In a small bowl, combine the flour, baking soda, and baking powder. Add the flour mixture to the creamed mixture, and beat until all the ingredients are well blended. Cover the bowl with plastic wrap and place in the refrigerator until the dough is chilled, about 1 hour.

3. Preheat the oven to 375°F; set out 2 or more baking sheets.

4. Pinch off a walnut-size portion of the chilled dough. Using your hands, roll the dough into a 1-inch-diameter ball and place the ball on one of the baking sheets. Repeat with the remaining dough, spacing the cookies about 2 inches apart. Using a fork dipped in granulated sugar, flatten each dough ball by pressing the tines in a crisscross pattern on each cookie.

5. Bake until the cookies are set and the bottoms are lightly browned, 10 to 12 minutes. Transfer the cookies to wire racks to cool completely.

Makes about 4 dozen cookies

Brownies

This recipe is studded with nuts, but you can substitute chocolate chips or just make a plain brownie. Bought ones are no match for warm brownies out of your oven, filling the air with the smell of chocolate and costing half as much.

5 squares (1 ounce each) unsweetened chocolate, coarsely chopped

1 1/2 cups all-purpose flour

1 teaspoon baking powder

1/2 teaspoon salt

3/4 cup (1 1/2 sticks) butter or margarine, softened

1 1/2 cups sugar

4 eggs

2 teaspoons vanilla extract

2 cups coarsely chopped walnuts or pecans

1. Preheat the oven to 350°F. Line a 13 x 9 x 2-inch baking pan with foil. Lightly grease and flour the foil, and set aside the pan.

2. In a small, heavy saucepan over the lowest heat, melt the chocolate, stirring occasionally. Remove the saucepan from the heat and let the chocolate cool.

3. In a small bowl or on a sheet of wax paper, combine the flour, baking powder, and salt.

4. In a large bowl with an electric mixer on medium speed, cream the butter or margarine for 2 minutes. Add the sugar and beat for 2 minutes longer. Add the eggs, 1 at a time, beating well after each addition. Beat in the vanilla and the cooled chocolate.

5. Using a wooden spoon, add the flour mixture to the chocolate mixture and stir until all the ingredients are well blended. Stir in the nuts. Pour the batter into the prepared pan. Bake the brownies until a toothpick inserted in the center comes out clean, about 35 minutes. Remove the baking pan to a wire rack and let the brownies cool before cutting.

Makes 24 (2 1/2-inch-square) brownies

One-Minute Substitute

If You Run Out of Chocolate

Unsweetened chocolate: If a recipe calls for 1 square (1 ounce) unsweetened chocolate and you don't have any on hand, combine 3 tablespoons unsweetened cocoa powder with 1 tablespoon butter, margarine, or vegetable shortening.

Semisweet chocolate: If 1 ounce semisweet chocolate is called for, combine 3 tablespoons unsweetened cocoa powder with 1 tablespoon butter, margarine, or vegetable shortening and 1 tablespoon sugar.

Blondies

The yin to brownies' yang, blondies are sold at many stores for a pretty penny, but they are not the same as fresh ones out of your oven.

3/4 cup butter, softened

1 1/2 cups sugar

3 eggs

2 teaspoons vanilla extract

1 3/4 cups all-purpose flour

1 teaspoon baking powder

1/2 teaspoon salt

2 cups coarsely chopped walnuts or pecans

1. Preheat the oven to 350°F. Line a 13 x 9 x 2-inch baking pan with foil. Lightly grease and flour the foil.

2. In a large bowl with an electric mixer on medium speed, cream the butter for 2 minutes. Add the sugar and beat for 2 minutes longer. Add the eggs and beat well; beat in the vanilla.

3. Using a wooden spoon, gradually add the flour, baking powder, and salt to the creamed mixture and stir until all the ingredients are well blended. Stir in the nuts. Pour the batter into the prepared pan. Bake the blondies until a toothpick inserted in the center comes out clean, about 35 minutes. Remove the baking pan to a wire rack and let the blondies cool before cutting.

Makes 24 (2 1/2-inch-square) blondies

Chocolate Sandwich Cookies

Try making your own version of this popular store-bought cookie. For a flavor sensation, replace the vanilla in the filling with 1/4 teaspoon peppermint extract.

3/4 cup butter, softened

1 cup sugar

1 egg

1/2 teaspoon vanilla extract

2 cups all-purpose flour

3/4 cup cocoa powder

1 teaspoon baking powder

1/2 teaspoon baking soda

1/2 teaspoon salt

1/4 cup milk

Filling

3 tablespoons butter, softened

1 1/2 cups confectioners' sugar

1 tablespoon milk

1 teaspoon vanilla extract

1. In a large bowl, combine the butter and sugar, and beat until they are well creamed. Add the egg and vanilla, and beat until all the ingredients are well blended.

2. In a small bowl, combine the flour, cocoa powder, baking powder, baking soda, and salt. Add the flour mixture and the milk, alternating, to the creamed mixture, and beat until each addition is well blended.

3. Divide the dough in half. Shape each dough half into a 10 1/2-inch-long roll. Wrap each dough roll in plastic wrap and refrigerate 12 hours or overnight.

4. Preheat the oven to 325°F; lightly grease 2 or more baking sheets. Unwrap 1 dough roll and, using a sharp knife, cut the dough into 1/8-inch-thick slices. Arrange the dough slices on the prepared cookie sheets, spacing them 2 inches apart. Bake until the edges of the cookies are set, 9 to 11 minutes. Transfer the cookies to wire racks to cool completely.

5. Prepare the filling: In a medium bowl, combine all the ingredients and, using an electric mixer, beat until smooth.

6. Using a knife or spatula, spread about 1 teaspoon of the filling on 1 cookie; top with a second cookie. Repeat with the remaining cookies and filling.

Makes 5 dozen sandwich cookies

Coconut Macaroons

Look in health food stores or the natural-foods section of your supermarket for desiccated coconut—it makes for a particularly delectable macaroon, which you can make better and more inexpensively than any manufacturer.

3 egg whites

1 cup sugar

2 1/2 cups desiccated coconut

1 cup macadamia nuts or almonds, finely chopped

1. Preheat the oven to 350°F; lightly grease 2 baking sheets.

2. In a medium bowl with an electric mixer on high, beat the egg whites until soft peaks form. Gradually add the sugar, beating after each addition, until stiff, glossy peaks form. Add the coconut and nuts, and fold until the ingredients are well blended.

3. Using a tablespoon, scoop out a portion of the dough. Using damp hands, roll the dough into a ball and place the ball on the prepared baking sheet. Repeat with the remaining dough.

4. Bake until the macaroons are lightly golden, 20 to 25 minutes. Transfer the macaroons to wire racks to cool completely. Store in an airtight container for 2 to 3 days.

Makes about 35 cookies.

Gingersnaps

The bright tang of ginger infuses each bite of these old-fashioned favorites. The spicy aroma of their baking will warm the kitchen and make you glad you are making your own for less cost and more taste.

3/4 cup shortening

1/2 cup sugar

1/2 cup firmly packed brown sugar

1 egg

1/4 cup molasses

2 cups all-purpose flour

2 teaspoons baking soda

1 1/2 teaspoons ground ginger

1 teaspoon ground cinnamon

1/2 teaspoon salt

Additional granulated sugar

1. Preheat the oven to 350°F; lightly grease 2 or more baking sheets.

2. In a large bowl, combine shortening and sugars and beat until well creamed. Add the egg and molasses, and beat until the ingredients are well blended.

3. In a small bowl, combine the flour, baking soda, ginger, cinnamon, and salt. Gradually add the flour mixture to the creamed mixture, beating after each addition, until the ingredients are well blended.

4. Place the additional granulated sugar in a small bowl. Pinch off a walnut-size portion of the dough. Using your hands, roll the portion into a ball, then roll the ball in the sugar and place it on the prepared baking sheet. Repeat with the remaining dough, spacing the cookies about 2 inches apart.

5. Bake until the cookies are lightly browned and crinkly, 12 to 15 minutes.

Makes 3 to 4 dozen cookies

Baked Goods You Can Make   **545**

Graham Crackers

Store-bought just won't taste the same after you enjoy your home-made graham crackers.

1 cup all-purpose flour

1 1/4 cups whole wheat flour plus additional

5 tablespoons sugar

1 teaspoon baking powder

1/2 teaspoon salt

1/2 teaspoon baking soda

1/4 teaspoon ground cinnamon

3 tablespoons chilled butter or margarine, cut into small pieces

1/4 cup solid vegetable shortening

2 tablespoons honey

1 tablespoon molasses

1/4 cup water

1 teaspoon vanilla extract

1. In a medium bowl, combine the flours, sugar, baking powder, salt, baking soda, and cinnamon. Using a pastry blender or 2 knives, cut in the butter and shortening until the mixture resembles coarse crumbs.

2. In a small bowl, combine the honey, molasses, water, and vanilla, and stir until well blended. Using a fork, gradually add the honey mixture to the flour mixture, tossing the ingredients together until they are well blended. Form the dough into a ball; the mixture may be crumbly, but do not add water. Cover the dough with plastic wrap and place in the refrigerator until the dough is chilled, for several hours.

3. Place the oven rack in the center of the oven and preheat to 350°F; set out 2 large baking sheets. Divide the dough in half and let it stand at room temperature for 15 minutes.

4. Spread wax paper over a work surface. Lightly sprinkle whole wheat flour over the wax paper. Place 1 dough half on the paper, and flatten the dough with a rolling pin. Sprinkle the dough with more whole wheat flour, and cover it with a second piece of wax paper. Using the rolling pin, roll out the dough to form a 7 x 15-inch rectangle; if the dough breaks, pinch the pieces together before continuing to roll.

5. Peel off the top piece of wax paper. Using a fork, mark dotted lines at 1/2- to 1-inch intervals, breaking the dough into 2 1/2-inch squares. Using a spatula, transfer the dough to a baking sheet, placing the squares close together. Repeat with the remaining dough and second baking sheet. Gather the scraps and reroll until all the dough is made into squares.

6. Bake until the crackers are lightly browned on the edges, about 15 minutes. Transfer the crackers to wire racks to cool. Store the graham crackers in an airtight container at room temperature for 1 month, or freeze the crackers in a freezer-safe container for up to 6 months.

Makes 24 to 28 crackers

Sugar Cookies

We include a recipe for frosting, but these sugar cookies are buttery tender and tasty on their own. These are the cookies you bake in holiday shapes with the children, and there is no store-bought equivalent to that.

1 1/2 cups sugar

1 1/2 cups butter, softened

2 eggs

2 tablespoons vanilla extract

4 cups all-purpose flour

1 teaspoon salt

1 teaspoon baking soda

1 teaspoon cream of tartar

Frosting

1 1/2 cups
   confectioners' sugar

3 tablespoons butter,
   softened

1 tablespoon vanilla extract

1 tablespoon milk

Food coloring, as desired

Colored sugar, as desired

1. In a large bowl, combine the sugar and butter, and beat until the mixture is well creamed. Add the eggs and vanilla, and beat until the mixture is smooth

2. In a small bowl, combine the flour, salt, baking soda, and cream of tartar. Add the flour mixture to the cream mixture, and beat until all the ingredients are well blended. Cover the bowl with plastic wrap and place in the refrigerator until the dough is chilled, about 30 minutes.

3. Preheat the oven to 350°F, set out 2 or more baking sheets, and lightly flour a work surface.

4. Turn out the dough onto the prepared work surface. Using a rolling pin, roll the dough out to a 1/4-inch thickness. Using cookie cutters dipped in flour, cut out as many cookies as possible. Carefully transfer the cookies to the ungreased baking sheets. Collect the dough scraps, reroll, and cut out additional cookies until there is no more dough left.

5. Bake until the cookies are just lightly browned on the edges, 10 to 12 minutes. Transfer the cookies to wire racks to cool completely.

6. Prepare the frosting: In a medium bowl, combine the ingredients and beat until creamy. Add a little additional milk as needed to reach the desired consistency. Add a few drops of food coloring as desired. Spread the frosting over the cooled cookies and sprinkle with colored sugar.

Makes 7 dozen cookies

Snacks, Nibbles and Drinks

When it comes to satisfying the afternoon munchies, the recipes in this chapter provide healthful alternatives to greasy fast food and those

bags of salty goodies from the vending machine. You'll find real honest-to-goodness homemade potato chips, pretzels, and French fries, even pizza. And when you taste them, you'll finally realize why these foods became so popular in the first place. You may even spoil yourself and never be able to settle for the commercial versions again. Your own pizza dough, you'll discover, is yeasty and delicious, inviting new and interesting toppings.

You'll also find recipes for those breakfast treats that we often go out for—or buy frozen and pay too much for. Homemade French toast, made quickly with day-old bread, costs about two-thirds less than heated frozen French toast—and with no preservatives or additives, it tastes a lot fresher and sweeter. In addition, there are recipes here that can be real money savers when you entertain. You'll discover how easy it is to make your own finger foods and dips, instead of hiring a caterer or buying out the local deli. These savory treats include an antipasto platter, pâté, and rich cheesy nibbles as well as several delicious easy-to-make dips.

And for that insatiable thirst or caffeine craving, the recipes here provide not only some pleasing summer quenchers but also some delightful and economical substitutes to the pricey products at your local coffee boutique.

fast foods and snacks

Potato Chips
We are a nation of snackers, so we might as well make our own and be sure they are as healthy as we can make them.

Vegetable oil or shortening for deep-fat frying (about 2 quarts)

1 pound Idaho potatoes, peeled

Salt to taste

1. Pour the oil or melt the shortening in a deep-fat fryer or large, heavy saucepan to a depth of 3 inches. Insert a deep-fat thermometer and heat the oil to 375°F.

2. Meanwhile, slice the potatoes into 1/8-inch-thick rounds. As you work, drop the rounds into ice water. When ready to fry, lift the rounds from the water and pat dry on paper towels.

3. Place the potato slices in the fryer in small batches to avoid affecting the temperature of the oil; fry until crisp and golden, 3 to 5 minutes per batch. Using a slotted spoon or fryer basket, transfer the chips to paper towels to drain. Allow the oil to reheat to the correct temperature before frying the next batch.

4. Lightly sprinkle the chips with salt.

Makes 4 Servings

Pretzels
Big, chewy, and oh, so satisfying! You may never get to taste these pretzels—if your family gets to them first!

1 1/2 teaspoons active dry yeast

3/4 cup warm (110°F-115°F) water

1 1/2 teaspoons sugar

3/4 teaspoon salt

1 1/2 cups all-purpose flour

2 tablespoons butter, melted

Coarse or kosher salt

1. In a large mixing bowl, combine the yeast and warm water, and stir to dissolve the yeast. Stir in the sugar and the salt. Add the flour, 1/2 cup at a time, to form a soft dough.

2. On a lightly floured surface, turn out the dough and knead until the dough is soft and elastic, about 5 minutes (the dough will be slightly sticky). Place the dough in a lightly oiled bowl, turning once to coat the top of the dough ball with oil. Cover the bowl and let the dough rise in a warm (70°F to 80°F) place until it is doubled in size, about 1 hour.

3. Preheat the oven to 425°F. Punch down the dough and divide it into 6 equal portions. On a lightly floured surface, roll 1 dough portion into a 14-inch-long rope; twist the rope into a pretzel shape—an oval with overlapping ends in the middle. Place the pretzel on a lightly greased baking sheet. Repeat with the remaining dough portions. Brush each pretzel with the melted butter and sprinkle with salt.

4. Bake the pretzels until they are golden brown, 15 to 20 minutes. Transfer the pretzels to wire racks to cool slightly.

Makes 6 pretzels

French Fries

Who can resist those hot, crisp-on-the-outside, creamy-on-the-inside potato delights! The good news is that you can make them easily yourself, and because you control the frying and can do it right, very little fat will remain on the fries—making them a whole lot healthier than the fast-food variety. Vegetable oil or vegetable shortening will both work for deep-fat frying.

2 quarts (about) vegetable oil or shortening

1 pound Idaho potatoes, peeled

Salt to taste

1. Pour the oil or melt the shortening in a deep-fat fryer or large, heavy saucepan to a depth of 3 inches. Insert a deep-fat thermometer and heat the oil to 375°F.

2. Meanwhile, cut the potatoes into 2 x 1/4 x 1/4-inch strips. As you work, drop the strips into a bowl of ice water. When ready to fry, lift the strips from the water and pat them completely dry on paper towels.

3. Place the potato strips in the fryer in small batches to avoid lowering the temperature of the oil; fry until brown and crisp, about 5 minutes per batch. Using a slotted spoon or fryer basket, transfer the fries to paper towels to drain. Keep warm on a hot tray or in a 200°F oven. Allow the oil in the fryer to reheat to the correct temperature before frying the next batch.

4. Sprinkle the fries with salt and serve hot.

Makes 4 servings

Oven-Baked French Fries

A healthier alternative to the perennial favorite, these fries are loaded with flavor but low in fat and contain no cholesterol.

2 tablespoons cornstarch

4 cups water

2 tablespoon reduced-sodium soy sauce

4 medium potatoes, peeled and cut into strips

4 teaspoons olive oil

1/4 teaspoon salt

1. In a large bowl, combine the cornstarch, water, and soy sauce, and whisk until well blended and smooth. Add the potatoes to the bowl; cover and refrigerate for 1 hour.

2. Preheat the oven to 375°F. Drain the potatoes and place on paper towels to drain; pat dry. In a large bowl, toss the potatoes with the olive oil and sprinkle with the salt. Coat a baking sheet with nonstick cooking spray. Arrange the potato strips in a single layer over the baking sheet. Bake for 15 minutes; turn the strips over and bake for 15 to 20 minutes longer or until the fries are tender and golden brown.

Makes 4 servings

Pizza

Making your own pizza is not only thrifty but an easy way to please everyone—let each family member choose the topping for his or her part of the finished pie. It will be easier if you have a baking stone or baking tiles for the bottom of the oven and a baker's paddle to put the pizza in and take it out of the oven. This recipe makes enough dough for a single family-size pizza, or you can divide it into four pieces to make individual pizzas—everyone can top his or her own!

Dough

1/4 cup warm (110°-115°F) water

1 packet (1/4 ounce) active dry yeast

1 1/2 cups unsifted all-purpose flour

1/4 cup water at room temperature

3 tablespoons olive oil

1/2 teaspoon salt

Topping

Cornmeal

1/2 cup tomato sauce or paste

Toppings as desired: shredded mozzarella cheese, sliced pepperoni, sliced mushrooms, bell pepper strips, sautéed Italian sausage, sliced olives, thinly sliced onions, Canadian bacon, pineapple, anchovies

1. In a small bowl, combine the warm water, yeast, and 1/4 cup of the flour. Stir to combine; this will form a sponge. Cover the bowl and let rise for 30 minutes.

2. Stir down the sponge; add the room-temperature water, the remaining 1 1/4 cups flour, olive oil, and salt. On a lightly floured surface, turn out the dough and knead for 10 minutes (or use the dough hook of an electric mixer and knead for 5 minutes). The dough is now ready to use.

3. For use within 1 day, wrap the dough tightly in plastic wrap and store in the refrigerator. Let it sit at room temperature for 1 to 2 hours before using. For future use, wrap the dough tightly in plastic wrap and place in a self-sealing freezer-safe plastic bag; squeeze out all the air before sealing. Freeze for up to 3 months. Thaw in the plastic wrap in the refrigerator for several hours, then bring the dough to room temperature before using.

4. Remove the oven racks and place a baking stone on the bottom of the oven. Preheat the oven to 450°F for about 20 minutes; it should be very hot. Dust a heavy upside-down baking sheet or a wooden baker's paddle with cornmeal. On a lightly floured surface using a lightly floured rolling pin, roll the dough into a 12-inch circle. Flop the dough over the rolling pin and unroll onto the cornmeal-covered baking sheet or paddle. (You can also sprinkle cornmeal on a regular baking pan and cook the pizza on an oven rack, but the crust may be soggier.)

5. Spread the tomato sauce or paste (or a mix of 1/4 cup of each) over the pizza dough, leaving a 1-inch margin. Scatter the toppings as desired.

6. Gently shake the pizza off the baking sheet or paddle onto the baking stone. Bake until the crust is golden brown, about 20 minutes. Serve immediately.

Makes a 12-inch pizza

Chicken Nuggets
For many parents, these morsels are a life- and time-saver, but the cost of buying them can really eat away at your budget.

1 1/2 pounds boneless skinless chicken breasts

2 large eggs

2 tablespoons water

1/2 cup Seasoned Coating Mix (page 44)

2 cups plain dry bread crumbs

1. Cut each chicken breast into 1-inch cubes. In a self-sealing bag, place the coating mix. In a pie plate, whisk together the eggs and water until frothy. In a large, shallow dish, place the bread crumbs.

2. Drop the chicken cubes, a few pieces at a time, into the bag of coating mix; seal and shake until the strips are well coated. Shake off any excess coating mix. Dip each cube into the beaten egg, then into the bread crumbs, gently pressing the crumbs onto the chicken until they stick. Arrange the coated cubes on a large, nonstick baking sheet. Once all the cubes are coated and on the baking sheet, place the sheet in the refrigerator to chill for 30 minutes.

3. Preheat the oven to 400°F. Bake the chicken nuggets until they are golden brown and crisp, about 15 minutes, turning them once or twice during the cooking time. Serve hot or at room temperature.

Makes about 6 servings

breakfast treats

Griddle French Toast
There are two methods for making French toast—this recipe is a quick fix in the morning; the following recipe can be prepared the night before for baking while the coffee brews.

4 eggs

1 cup milk

1 teaspoon vanilla

1/8 teaspoon ground nutmeg

1/8 teaspoon ground cinnamon

8 slices bread

1. In a medium bowl, lightly beat the eggs and the milk. Stir in the vanilla, nutmeg, and cinnamon. Pour the mixture into a large, shallow dish with a flat bottom.

2. Spray a griddle or large, flat skillet with nonstick baking spray. Heat the griddle to hot but not smoking. Dip each piece of bread into the egg mixture, completely soaking it, then place the slice on the griddle. Cook until the bread is brown on one side, flip it over, and grill the other side of the bread. Serve immediately or keep warm briefly in a 200°F oven.

Makes 4 servings

Baked French Toast

You can make this the night before, then pop it into the oven in the morning.

3 eggs

1 1/2 cups milk

2 tablespoons unsalted butter or margarine, melted

3 tablespoons light or dark brown sugar

1/2 teaspoon finely grated lemon zest

1/8 teaspoon ground nutmeg

1/8 teaspoon ground cinnamon

14 slices French bread (about 3/4-inch thick)

1 tablespoon confectioners' sugar

1. In a medium bowl, beat the eggs, milk, butter, brown sugar, lemon zest, nutmeg, and cinnamon. Pour half the mixture into a greased 17 x 11 1/2 x 3-inch baking dish. Lay the bread slices on top in a single layer, pressing them as close together as possible. Pour the remaining mixture over the bread slices and cover the pan with aluminum foil. Refrigerate overnight or at least 2 hours.

2. Preheat the oven to 350°F. Bake, uncovered, until the toast is puffy and golden brown, 50 to 60 minutes. Sprinkle with the confectioners' sugar. Serve hot with maple or blueberry syrup, honey, or fresh fruit, nuts, and yogurt.

Makes 4 servings

Drop Biscuits

To add extra flavor, stir 1 teaspoon of your favorite herb into the dough.

2 cups Biscuit and Pancake Mix (page 61)

1/2 cup nonfat or 1% milk

1. Preheat the oven to 450°F. In a medium bowl, combine the mix and milk, and stir until just moistened.

2. Coat a baking sheet lightly with nonstick cooking spray. Drop the mixture by heaping tablespoons onto the baking sheet. Bake until lightly browned, 8 to 10 minutes.

Makes about 20 biscuits

Cutout Biscuits

For a savory addition, stir 1/2 cup finely shredded cheddar or grated Parmesan cheese into the dough.

2 cups Biscuit and Pancake Mix (page 61)

1/2 cup nonfat or 1% milk

1. Preheat the oven to 450°F. In a medium bowl, combine the mix and milk, and stir until just moistened.

2. On a lightly floured surface, turn out the dough and gently knead 10 times. Using a floured rolling pin, roll the dough out to a 1/2-inch thickness and, using a 2 1/2-inch floured cutter, cut out biscuit rounds. Reroll the scraps and cut out more biscuit rounds. Place the rounds on an ungreased baking sheet.

3. Bake the biscuits until they are lightly browned, 10 to 12 minutes.

Makes about 10 biscuits

Pancakes

Sliced bananas and strawberries, whole blueberries, or even chocolate chips can be added to pancake batter before cooking for a luscious breakfast treat.

2 cups Biscuit and Pancake
  Mix (page 61)

2 large eggs, lightly beaten

1 cup nonfat or 1% milk

1. In a large bowl, combine the mix with the eggs and milk. Stir until the batter is just blended. Don't overmix—the batter should be slightly lumpy.

2. Coat a griddle or large, flat skillet with nonstick cooking spray. Over moderate heat, bring the griddle or skillet to hot but not smoking. Spoon the batter onto the griddle, using about 1/4 cup per pancake, and cook until bubbles form across the top, about 2 minutes. Flip the pancakes and cook about 2 minutes more. Serve immediately or keep warm in a 200°F oven.

Makes about 10 to 12 pancakes

Scones

This treat from Scotland is essentially a sweet biscuit. You can add all sorts of things to scones, including currants, chopped dried apricots, or mini chocolate chips—experiment with gusto!

2 cups Biscuit and Pancake
  Mix (page 61)

1 tablespoon sugar

2 eggs

1/2 cup heavy cream

1 teaspoon vanilla extract

1. Preheat the oven to 425°F. In a large bowl, stir together the mix and sugar.

2. In a medium bowl, beat the eggs with the cream and the vanilla until well blended. Pour the egg mixture into the mix and stir until a soft dough forms.

3. On a lightly floured surface, turn out the dough and gently knead 5 to 6 times. Using a lightly floured rolling pin, roll out the dough to a 1/2-inch thickness and, using a floured 3-inch cutter, cut out scone rounds. Reroll the scraps as necessary (do not knead again).

4. Place the scones 2 inches apart on an ungreased baking sheet and bake until golden brown, 10 to 15 minutes.

Makes about 8 scones

variation:

Scone Wedges: Follow the above recipe through Step 2. Turn the dough onto a lightly greased baking sheet and pat into a large round (like a soda bread loaf). If desired, brush the top with additional cream and sprinkle with additional sugar or a combination of sugar and cinnamon. Using a floured knife, cut the dough round into 8 wedges, but don't separate the pieces. Bake in the preheated oven for about 12 minutes or until golden brown. Carefully separate the scone wedges and serve immediately.

Waffles
A classic breakfast or brunch dish for special occasions, waffles give maple syrup a good name, but also go deliciously with fresh fruit toppings.

2 large eggs, separated

1 3/4 cups Biscuit and Pancake Mix (page 61)

1 cup nonfat or 1% milk

3 tablespoons butter or margarine, melted

1 teaspoon vanilla extract (optional)

1. Following the manufacturer's directions, preheat a waffle iron.

2. In a large bowl, lightly beat the egg yolks. Add the mix, milk, melted butter or margarine, and vanilla, if desired; stir until the mixture is just moistened. In a medium bowl, beat the egg whites with an electric mixer until soft peaks form. Using a rubber spatula, gently fold the egg whites into the batter until no white streaks remain.

3. Cook the waffles following the manufacturer's directions.

Makes about 5 (4 x 8-inch) waffles

the origin of waffles

Surprisingly, waffles have been enjoyed for centuries. From the time of the ancient Greeks through the Middle Ages, flat cakes were baked between two metal plates. These were known as obleios, and were popular into the 13th century. At that time, an enterprising craftsman forged decorative plates to resemble honeycombs. The name "waffle" is derived from the Dutch *wafel,* which first appeared in print in 1620. And the Pilgrims, who took refuge in Holland before immigrating to America, introduced waffles to this country. Thomas Jefferson brought a waffle iron back with him after his years in Paris, and within a century, you could buy waffles from vendors on the streets. In the 20th century, an electric waffle iron made these breakfast treats even more popular and easy to make, and in 1953, Frank Dorsa debuted his Eggo waffles—the height of convenience.

appetizing nibbles

Antipasto Platter
The star of the buffet table is an antipasto ("before the meal") platter, which most people have catered by an Italian restaurant for a hefty price. This classic appetizer has colorful marinated vegetables, cheese, and sausage in an eye-catching arrangement. Accentuate the drama by placing contrasting colors or shapes next to each other—straight or diagonal patterns on a rectangular plate or concentric circles on a round or oval platter.

1 pound small new potatoes, quartered

3 tablespoons olive oil

1 teaspoon dried rosemary

1 teaspoon salt

1 large red bell pepper, cut into 1-inch strips

1 large green bell pepper, cut into 1-inch strips

1 medium zucchini, cut into 1-inch slices

1 medium summer squash, cut into 1-inch slices

2 small red onions, cut into thin wedges

8 ounces button mushrooms

2 garlic cloves, minced

8 ounces fresh mozzarella, sliced

1/2 pound prosciutto, sliced

1 cup oil-cured Greek black or green olives

Sprigs of rosemary or thyme

Marinade

3 tablespoons balsamic vinegar

1 tablespoon extra-virgin olive oil

1 tablespoon chopped parsley

1/4 teaspoon dried thyme

2 teaspoons Dijon mustard

1 small garlic clove, minced

1 teaspoon lemon zest

1/2 teaspoon salt

1/4 teaspoon ground pepper

1. Preheat the oven to 450°F. In a large, shallow baking pan, combine the potatoes with the olive oil, rosemary, and salt. Toss to coat the potatoes well. Bake the potatoes, uncovered, 15 minutes.

2. Add the red and green bell peppers, zucchini, summer squash, red onions, and mushrooms to the baking pan. Sprinkle the minced garlic over all the vegetables. Bake, uncovered, until the vegetables are lightly browned and tender, 35 to 45 minutes.

3. Meanwhile, prepare the marinade: In a small bowl, combine the ingredients and whisk until well blended and the marinade is a smooth consistency.

4. Pour the marinade over the cooked vegetables in the baking pan, and stir gently until they are thoroughly coated. Let the vegetables cool to room temperature.

5. Arrange the marinated vegetables, mozzarella cheese, prosciutto, and olives in an attractive pattern on a large serving platter. Garnish with rosemary or thyme.

Makes 6 to 8 servings

Chicken Liver Pâté

This smooth, rich paste is easy to make at home for your fanciest occasions. Serve it with toast points or water crackers.

2 tablespoons butter

1/2 pound chicken livers, cleaned, trimmed, and halved

1 package (3 ounces) cream cheese, softened to room temperature

1-2 tablespoons brandy

1 teaspoon salt

1/8 teaspoon ground pepper

1/2 teaspoon dried thyme

1/8 teaspoon ground nutmeg

1. In a heavy skillet over moderately high heat, melt the butter. Add the chicken livers and cook until they are lightly browned, 4 to 5 minutes.

2. Transfer the livers to the bowl of a food processor or blender. Pour in the pan drippings, scraping up the browned bits in the skillet and adding them to the bowl. Add the cream cheese, brandy, salt, pepper, thyme, and nutmeg. Whirl until the mixture forms a smooth paste, 20 to 30 seconds. Taste and adjust the seasonings as desired.

3. Using a spatula, scrape the paste into a crock or serving bowl, smoothing the top. Cover the crock and refrigerate overnight.

Makes 4 servings

Ham, Pork, and Veal Terrine

A simple, classic baked terrine is perfect for a picnic in summer or sampling by a roaring fire in winter with pumpernickel or crusty French bread.

1 pound diced cooked ham

1 pound minced pork

1 pound minced veal

1 garlic clove, minced

1 teaspoon dried thyme

1/2 teaspoon dried marjoram

1/4 teaspoon ground nutmeg

1 teaspoon salt

1/8 teaspoon ground pepper

1/2 cup dry white wine

4 small bay leaves

6-8 slices bacon

1/4 pound fresh chicken livers, cleaned, trimmed, and halved

1. Preheat the oven to 300°F. In a large, nonreactive bowl, combine the ham, pork, and veal. Add the garlic, thyme, marjoram, nutmeg or mace, salt, and pepper. Using clean, damp hands, mix the ingredients until they are well blended. Mix in the wine, cover, and refrigerate for 1 hour.

2. On the bottom of a 9 x 5-inch loaf pan, arrange the bay leaves. Line the sides of the pan crosswise with half of the bacon slices, allowing the ends to hang over the edges of the pan. Pack half of the meat mixture into the loaf pan. Arrange the chicken livers along the center of the meat, then add the remaining meat mixture. Cover the meat loaf with the remaining bacon slices, tucking in the ends and folding the ends of the bottom slices over the top of the loaf.

3. Set the loaf pan in a baking dish. Add enough warm water to come halfway up the sides of the loaf pan. Bake the terrine until the loaf pulls away from the sides of the pan and the juices run clear when the loaf is pierced with a clean skewer or toothpick, 2 to 2 1/2 hours.

4. Set the loaf pan on a wire rack and let the terrine cool. Pour off any liquid. When the terrine is completely cool, turn in out onto a plate, cover with plastic wrap, and refrigerate overnight.

Makes about 10 servings

Country Pork Sausages

Needing no casings, these hearty and delicious homemade sausages are ready to star at your next brunch. Because you make them, you know what's in them and you can adjust the seasonings to suit your own tastes.

2 pounds lean pork, trimmed

1/4 pound uncooked pork fat

1 1/2 teaspoons kosher salt

1 1/2 teaspoons dried sage, crumbled

1/2 teaspoon dried thyme, crumbled

1/4 teaspoon crushed black peppercorns

1 small onion, finely chopped

1. Cut the pork and pork fat into 1/2-inch cubes. Place the cubes in a large bowl, cover, and refrigerate until the meat is chilled.

2. In a small bowl, combine the salt, sage, thyme, and peppercorns. Sprinkle the seasoning mixture over the meat, add the onion, and, using your hands, mix all the ingredients together thoroughly.

3. In the bowl of a food processor or blender, place half the sausage mixture. Whirl until the mixture is a medium-coarse consistency. Scrape the pureed mixture to another large bowl, and repeat with the second half of the sausage mixture. Cover the bowl and refrigerate 12 hours or overnight to let the texture firm up and the flavors develop fully.

4. Using damp hands, divide the sausage mixture into 10 to 12 equal portions, and roll each portion into a ball. Form each ball into a small sausage patty. Either cook immediately, or place the sausages on foil, with pieces of foil between any layers. Wrap the entire package of sausages in additional foil or a self-sealing plastic bag. Refrigerate the uncooked sausages for up to 2 days; store in the freezer for up to 3 weeks.

5. To cook: Preheat a large, heavy skillet over moderate heat. Add the sausages and cook, turning often, until they are browned on all sides and cooked through, 13 to 15 minutes. Drain off any fat as it accumulates, and transfer the cooked sausages to paper towels to drain completely before serving.

Makes 10 to 12 sausage patties

Deviled Eggs

Contrary to popular terminology, eggs should never actually be boiled; they should be "hard cooked" as in the recipe below. Although you can cook the eggs up to one day ahead, to avoid contamination they should not be stuffed until shortly before serving.

12 eggs

1/2 cup regular or reduced-fat mayonnaise

4 teaspoons yellow mustard

4 teaspoons white wine vinegar

1 teaspoon salt

1 teaspoon sugar

1 teaspoon ground white pepper

1/2 cup finely chopped celery

Paprika *(optional)*

1. In a large saucepan, place the eggs in a single layer. Add enough cold water to cover the eggs by 1 inch. Set the saucepan over high heat and bring to a full boil; immediately remove the saucepan from the heat, cover, and let stand for 15 minutes.

2. Drain the eggs and crack the wide end of each, then plunge into a large bowl of ice water. To peel, crack each shell all over by tapping it on a countertop. Hold each egg under cold running water while removing the shell. Set each shelled egg on a paper towel to drain as you peel them.

3. Using a small, sharp knife, cut each egg in half lengthwise. Using a small spoon, scoop out the yolks and put them in a sieve set over a medium bowl. Arrange the egg-white halves on a plate and refrigerate. Using the back of a spoon, press the egg yolks through the sieve into the bowl.

4. Add the mayonnaise, mustard, vinegar, salt, sugar, pepper, and celery to the sieved yolks. Using a fork, stir gently to combine all the ingredients well.

5. Using a small spoon or a pastry bag fitted with a number 6 star tip, fill each egg-white half with about 1 tablespoon of the egg-yolk mixture. If desired, sprinkle the eggs with a little paprika before serving.

Makes 12 servings

variations:

Caper-Dill Eggs: To the 1/2 cup mayonnaise, add 3 tablespoons drained and chopped capers, 3 tablespoons minced fresh dill, and 1/2 teaspoon ground white pepper.

Chili Eggs: To the 1/2 cup mayonnaise, add 4 teaspoons chili powder and 1 teaspoon ground cumin.

Curried Eggs: To the 1/2 cup mayonnaise, add 4 teaspoons curry powder and 3 tablespoons chopped chutney.

Spicy Eggs: To the 1/2 cup mayonnaise, add 1/4 cup prepared horseradish and 2 tablespoons minced fresh parsley.

Globe Artichokes in Olive Oil

End of winter, around February or March, is the time to find small, tender baby artichokes in the market. Use these seasoned artichokes in salads, serve them with strong-flavored cheeses, or just enjoy them on their own.

2 pounds (about 6 small) fresh young globe artichokes

1 large lemon, halved

4 cups white wine vinegar

1 tablespoon kosher salt

1 tablespoon dill seed

1 tablespoon black peppercorns

2 bay leaves

2 sprigs fresh herbs such as rosemary, dill, or marjoram

2 garlic cloves, sliced

2 small fresh red chiles

3-4 cups extra-virgin olive oil

1. Using scissors, cut off the outer, tough leaves of each artichoke; trim off the pointed tip of each remaining leaf. Using a sharp knife, cut each artichoke in half lengthwise and rub the cut halves with the lemon halves to prevent browning. Fill a medium bowl with cold water and place the artichoke halves in the bowl with any remaining juice in the lemons. Let stand for 1 hour.

2. In a large, nonreactive saucepan over moderately high heat, combine the vinegar, salt, dill seed, peppercorns, and bay leaves; bring the mixture to a boil.

3. Drain the artichokes and add them to the saucepan; reduce the heat to moderately low and simmer for 10 minutes.

4. Drain the artichokes again and let them dry; discard the cooking liquid. Transfer the artichokes to 2 warm, sterilized, wide-mouthed quart jars, dividing them equally (see Safe Canning with a Hot-Water Bath, page 72). Add 1 herb sprig, half the garlic slices, and 1 chile pepper to each jar. Pour the olive oil over the artichokes, leaving a 1/4-inch space between the top of the oil and the rim of the jar. Wipe the rims, cover, and store in the refrigerator for up to 1 month. The artichokes will be ready for eating in a few days.

Makes 2 quarts

Marinated Goat Cheese

How do you make a good thing even better? In the case of goat cheese, you marinate it yourself in herb-infused olive oil. You can buy marinated goat cheese, but this is easy and made to your own taste.

1 goat cheese (3-4 ounces)

1/4 teaspoon mixed pepper-corns (black, white, green)

1/8 teaspoon coriander seed, crushed

Fresh thyme sprigs

Fresh rosemary sprigs

Fresh fennel sprigs

1 bay leaf

1 small red chile pepper

1 garlic clove

1/2 cup olive oil

1. In a warm, sterilized widemouthed jar, center the goat cheese. Tuck the peppercorns, coriander seed, thyme, rosemary and fennel sprigs, bay leaf, chile pepper, and garlic around the cheese.

2. Pour in the olive oil until the top of the oil is 1/4 inch from the rim of the jar. Wipe the rim, cover the jar, and label and date it. Store the cheese in the refrigerator for up to 1 month; the cheese will be ready for eating in 1 week.

Makes 1 cheese

Spinach-Feta Phyllo Triangles

It's true that phyllo, the multilayered Greek dough, is difficult and time-consuming to make. Purchased phyllo dough, however, is a wonderful base for appetizers, desserts, or other dishes that are very expensive to buy finished. Follow the package directions to thaw frozen dough; once opened, the dough will keep in the refrigerator for about 1 week.

4 tablespoons butter or margarine plus 2 teaspoons melted butter or margarine

1 small yellow onion, finely chopped

1 package (10 ounces) frozen chopped spinach, thawed and squeezed dry

1 tablespoon minced fresh dill or 1/4 teaspoon dried dill, crumbled

1/2 cup (4 ounces) crumbled feta cheese

1 egg, lightly beaten

6 sheets frozen phyllo pastry, thawed

1. Preheat the oven to 350°F. In a large skillet over moderate heat, melt the 4 tablespoons butter or margarine. Add the onion and sauté until translucent, 3 to 5 minutes. Add the spinach and cook for 2 minutes longer. Stir in the dill. Transfer the spinach mixture to a large bowl. Add the feta cheese and the egg, and stir until the mixture is well blended.

2. Lay 1 sheet of the phyllo pastry on a work surface and brush lightly with 1 teaspoon of the melted butter. Top with a second sheet of phyllo, brush with butter, repeat with a third sheet of phyllo.

3. Using a sharp knife or pizza cutter, and a ruler if you like, cut the stack of buttered phyllo sheets lengthwise into six 1 3/4-inch-wide strips. Cut the strips in half to make 12 strips. Place 1/2 teaspoon of the spinach-feta mixture at the end of each strip. Fold the end of each strip diagonally over the filling to form a triangle. Continue folding diagonally along the entire strip, alternating directions (like folding a flag), and ending with a triangle. When each triangle is complete, brush the top with some of the butter.

4. Repeat, using the remaining phyllo sheets, butter, and spinach-feta filling to make another 12 triangles.

5. Line a baking sheet with parchment paper. Arrange the filled triangles over the paper-lined sheet, and bake until the triangles are golden brown, about 25 minutes.

Makes 24 triangles

Quesadillas
You can serve a quesadilla as a lunch dish or use a pizza cutter to cut it into small triangles and arrange on a plate with sour cream and guacamole as an appetizer.

4 eight-inch flour tortillas

1 cup (4 ounces) shredded Monterey Jack cheese

1 large red bell pepper, cored, seeded, and cut into 1/4-inch slices

1/4 cup cooked fresh or thawed frozen corn kernels

3 scallions with tops, thinly sliced

1/4 cup chopped fresh cilantro

1/4 cup fresh or prepared salsa

Sour cream, plain yogurt, or guacamole *(optional)*

1. Preheat the oven to 425°F. Place each tortilla on a 12-inch square of foil. Sprinkle each tortilla with the cheese, bell pepper, corn, scallions, cilantro, and salsa, dividing the toppings equally. Moisten the edges of 1 tortilla and fold in half, encasing the toppings; press the edges together. Repeat with the remaining tortillas.

2. Move a folded tortilla so it is centered on the top half of the foil square. Fold in each side edge of the foil over the quesadilla. Fold the bottom half of the foil up and over the quesadilla until the top and bottom foil edges are even; fold the edges together twice to make a packet. Repeat with the remaining quesadillas. Arrange the foil-wrapped quesadillas on a baking sheet.

3. Bake the quesadillas until the cheese melts, about 7 minutes. Remove the baking sheet from the oven, unwrap each quesadilla, and arrange it on a plate or serving platter. If desired, garnish with a dollop of sour cream, plain yogurt, or guacamole.

Makes 4 servings

Zucchini Strips
Because it cooks quickly, zucchini is an ideal choice for batter frying.

2 quarts (about) vegetable oil or shortening for deep-fat frying

1 cup all-purpose flour

1/2 cup cold water or stale beer

1 pound firm, bright green zucchini, cut into 2 x 1/4 x 1/4-inch strips

Balsamic vinegar

1. Pour the oil or melt the shortening in a deep-fat fryer or large, heavy saucepan to a depth of 3 inches. Insert a deep-fat thermometer and heat the oil to 375°F.

2. Meanwhile, in a medium bowl, combine 1/2 cup of the flour and the water or beer. Whisk until the mixture is smooth and well blended. Pour the remaining 1/2 cup of flour into a shallow dish. Working in small batches, dredge the zucchini strips in the flour, shaking off any excess, then toss the coated strips in the batter, separating any that cling together.

3. Place the zucchini strips in the fryer in small batches to avoid affecting the temperature of the oil; fry until brown and crisp, about 5 minutes per batch. Using a slotted spoon or fryer basket, transfer the strips to paper towels to drain. Allow the oil in the fryer to reheat to the correct temperature before frying the next batch.

4. Lightly drizzle the zucchini strips with the balsamic vinegar before serving.

Makes 4 servings

dips

Baba Ghanoush
Much loved in the Middle East, this smoky favorite, available in super-markets and delis for $4 to $5 for 4 ounces, gets its smoky flavor from charring the eggplant first. You can make this delicious dip yourself and serve it with pita triangles.

1 large (1 1/4 pounds) eggplant

1/4 cup lemon juice

1 tablespoon extra-virgin olive oil

2 garlic cloves, quartered

1/4 cup tahini (sesame paste)

Salt and ground black pepper, to taste

1. Preheat the broiler. Using a sharp fork or skewer, prick the eggplant all over. Place the eggplant in the broiler 6 inches from the heat source. Broil, turning every 5 minutes, until the skin is blackened and the eggplant is soft, about 20 minutes. Remove the eggplant and let stand until it is cool to the touch.

2. Using a sharp knife, remove the peel from the eggplant; discard the peel. Place the eggplant flesh in the bowl of a food processor or blender, cutting as needed to fit. Add the lemon juice, olive oil, garlic, and tahini. Pulse until the mixture is well blended and is a spreadable consistency. Taste and season as desired with the salt and pepper.

3. Scrape the baba ghanoush into a bowl, cover, and refrigerate for at least 2 hours before serving to allow the flavors to develop.

Makes about 2 cups

Guacamole
One of the greatest recipes ever, this creamy blend of avocados, tomato, red onion, and cilantro is a divine dip for chips, crudités, pretzels, and more. It can also be a memorable addition to taco salads, grilled poultry, or fish, and is a must for wraps. At $4 for 4 ounces at the grocery, it pays you to make your own, which also tastes fresher and better.

2 ripe Hass avocados, halved and pitted (reserve 1 pit)

1 medium tomato, cored, seeded, and finely chopped

1/2 cup finely chopped red onion

1/3 cup chopped fresh cilantro

2 tablespoons lime juice

3/4 teaspoon salt

3/4 teaspoon ground cumin *(optional)*

3/4 teaspoon jalapeño pepper sauce *(optional)*

1. Using a spoon, scoop out the avocado flesh into a medium, nonreactive bowl. Using a fork, mash the avocado until it is not quite smooth (there should be small chunks of avocado flesh).

2. Add the tomato, onion, cilantro, and lime juice, and stir with the fork until the ingredients are well blended but the consistency is still slightly rough. If desired, stir in the cumin and jalapeño sauce to add more heat to the guacamole.

3. Spoon the guacamole into a serving bowl and push the reserved pit down into the dip. The pit helps keep the guacamole from turning brown. Serve immediately or cover the bowl with plastic wrap and refrigerate until ready to serve.

Makes 2 1/2 cups

Green Goddess Dip

Making your own is not only easy and cheaper, you can lower the calories and fat of this delectable dip by using low- or nonfat sour cream and low- or nonfat mayonnaise.

- 1 cup sour cream
- 1 cup mayonnaise
- 1 small ripe avocado, peeled, pitted, and cut into chunks
- 2 large scallions, trimmed and sliced
- 1/3 cup fresh parsley leaves
- 2 tablespoons lemon juice
- 2 teaspoons anchovy paste
- 1 garlic clove
- 1 teaspoon dried tarragon, crumbled
- 1/2 teaspoon ground black pepper
- 1/4 teaspoon salt

Working in batches if necessary, in the bowl of a food processor or blender, whirl all the ingredients until they are blended and the dip is a smooth consistency, scraping down the bowl sides as needed. Serve with raw vegetables or chips.

Makes 3 1/2 cups

Hummus

Another staple of Middle Eastern cooking, hummus is excellent with pita triangles, crudités, or bagel chips, but it can be used as a spread in sandwiches too. Buying it from delis or specialty stores can cost $1 an ounce or more.

- 2 cups cooked chickpeas or 1 can (19 ounces) chickpeas, drained and rinsed
- 1 tablespoon extra-virgin olive oil
- 2 garlic cloves, quartered
- 1/2 teaspoon ground cumin
- 1/4 cup tahini (sesame paste)
- 1/4-1/2 cup freshly squeezed lemon juice
- Salt and freshly ground pepper, to taste
- Minced fresh parsley or paprika

1. In the bowl of a food processor or blender, combine the chickpeas, olive oil, garlic, cumin, and tahini. Whirl until the mixture is a rough consistency.
2. With the motor running, slowly pour in the lemon juice a little at a time until the desired consistency is reached. Taste the hummus and season with the salt and pepper. Before serving, sprinkle with fresh parsley or paprika.

Makes 1 1/2 cups

Skordalia

A mouthwatering blend of garlic roasted to nutty perfection, walnuts, and lemon juice, this dip has an unusual base: mashed potatoes. This is a Greek garlic sauce that you might buy in a Greek grocery. Use it with beet salad or as a dip for raw vegetables.

14 unpeeled garlic cloves

5 slices firm-textured white bread, preferably stale

1 1/2 cups mashed potatoes

1/2 cup shelled walnuts

1/4 cup fresh lemon juice

3/4 teaspoon salt

3/4 teaspoon ground black pepper

2/3 cup extra-virgin olive oil

Fresh parsley sprigs or lemon zest *(optional)*

1. Preheat the oven to 350°F. Place the garlic cloves on a large piece of foil. Bring the long edges together and fold under twice; fold each short end over twice to form a packet. Fill a small baking dish with 1/4 inch water and place the foil packet in the baking dish. Bake until the garlic is tender, about 45 minutes. Remove the garlic from the oven and let cool to the touch.

2. Meanwhile, in a large, shallow baking dish, arrange the bread slices in a single layer. Pour in enough water to cover the bread and let stand for 5 to 10 minutes.

3. Gently squeeze the bread to remove most of the water. In the bowl of a food processor or blender, place the bread. Squeeze each clove of garlic to extract the flesh and add it to the bowl; discard the peels. Add the mashed potatoes, walnuts, lemon juice, salt, and pepper. Pulse until the ingredients are just combined. With the motor running, slowly drizzle in the olive oil and continue whirling until the dip is well blended and smooth.

4. Spoon the dip into a serving bowl and, if desired, garnish with parsley sprigs or lemon zest.

Makes about 3 cups

Helpful Hint | **Dips Are Not Just for Dipping**

So much more than something to plunge crackers, chips, or crudités into, dips are a versatile performer in your culinary productions. Many can be used as condiments, toppings for various dishes, fillings for omelets, or spreads for sandwiches. Experiment!

Tapenade
Not for the faint of palate, this rich spread combines the heady taste of Mediterranean or Greek olives, anchovies, capers, and garlic. Available in more and more specialty departments of supermarkets, it is a pricey treat. Make your own and enjoy it on toasted slices of Italian bread, drizzled with extra-virgin olive oil. Tapenade also makes an exceptional spread for an Italian hard sausage sandwich.

1 cup oil-cured Mediterranean or Greek black olives, pitted

6-8 anchovy fillets

1/4 cup capers, drained

2 garlic cloves, halved

2 teaspoons lemon juice

3-4 tablespoons extra-virgin olive oil

Freshly ground black pepper, to taste

1. In the bowl of a food processor or blender, combine the olives, anchovy fillets, capers, garlic, and lemon juice. Whirl until the mixture is finely chopped.

2. Add 3 tablespoons of the olive oil, pulsing on and off, until the mixture is a spreadable, grainy paste; add additional olive oil as needed to reach the desired consistency. Taste the tapenade and season with the pepper.

Makes about 1 cup

Tzatziki
A creamy cucumber concoction to cool the fires of the spiciest dish, this quintessential Greek dip is a natural in summer, when cucumbers are plentiful. You can buy it in specialty shops, but it is easy to make your own. Serve it with crudités, chips, or pita triangles, as a dressing for Greek salad, or as a side for grilled kabobs or fish.

1 medium cucumber, peeled, sliced lengthwise, and seeded

2 cups plain, nonfat yogurt

1 garlic clove, minced

1 tablespoon minced fresh mint

2 tablespoons olive oil

Kosher salt and freshly ground black pepper, to taste

Additional olive oil

1. Cut the cucumber into small dice and place the pieces between layers of paper towels to dry well.

2. In a medium bowl, combine the yogurt, cucumber pieces, garlic, mint, and olive oil, and stir until all the ingredients are well blended. Taste the tzatziki and season with salt and pepper.

3. Spoon the tzatziki into a serving bowl and drizzle olive oil over the top.

Makes about 2 1/2 cups

cold drinks

Classic Iced Tea
An American original, iced tea made its debut at the St. Louis World's Fair in 1904—in reaction to muggy weather and the need for a cool pick-me-up. Always best when it is freshly made, iced tea is an economical thirst quencher.

1 quart cold water

2 tablespoons loose tea leaves or 6 regular-sized tea bags

Sugar Syrup (opposite) to taste

Lemon wedges or small fresh mint sprigs *(optional)*

1. In a large saucepan or teakettle over high heat, bring 2 cups of the cold water to a full, rolling boil.

2. Rinse a teapot with boiling water and discard the water. Place the tea in the pot and slowly pour the 2 cups of boiling water over the tea, cover the teapot, and let the tea steep for 3 to 5 minutes.

3. Stir the tea once, strain the tea leaves or remove and discard the tea bags. Pour the tea into a large pitcher, add the remaining 2 cups of cold water and sweeten to taste with the sugar syrup.

4. To serve, fill glasses with ice cubes and pour the cold tea over the ice; if desired, garnish each serving with a lemon wedge or sprig of fresh mint.

Makes 4 servings

Cranberry Iced Tea
A fruity twist on the American classic, this red tea is perfect for a special occasion. The fresh tea makes it delicious and economical.

2 cups cold water

4 tablespoons loose tea leaves or 6 regular-sized tea bags

2 cups cranberry juice cocktail

Sugar Syrup (opposite) to taste

Fresh or frozen whole cranberries or lime slices *(optional)*

1. In a large saucepan or teakettle over high heat, bring 2 cups of the cold water to a full, rolling boil.

2. Rinse a teapot with boiling water and discard the water. Place the tea in the pot and slowly pour the 2 cups of boiling water over the tea, cover the teapot, and let the tea steep for 3 to 5 minutes.

3. Stir the tea once, strain the tea leaves or remove and discard the tea bags. Pour the tea into a large pitcher, add the 2 cups of cranberry cocktail, and sweeten to taste with the sugar syrup.

4. To serve, fill glasses with ice cubes and pour the cold tea over the ice; if desired, garnish each serving with a few whole cranberries or a lime wedge.

Makes 4 servings

Helpful Hint

Make the Perfect Sweetener: Sugar Syrup

Keep a jar of this sugar syrup in your refrigerator to sweeten iced teas and coffees. Because the sugar is already dissolved, you'll get the ideal sweetness without any graininess added. Here's how to make it:

In a small saucepan over moderate heat, combine 2 cups sugar and 2 1/2 cups water. Cook, stirring frequently, until the mixture boils and the sugar has dissolved completely. Remove the saucepan from the heat, cover, and let stand for 1 to 2 minutes to allow the steam to dissolve any unmelted crystals on the sides of the saucepan. Pour the cooled syrup into a 1-quart jar, cover tightly, and store in the refrigerator.

Makes 3 cups

Raspberry Iced Tea

Raspberries are sweet-tart, so they are a good foil for tea in this popular variation of homemade iced tea, a rare treat for a reasonable price.

- 4 quarts water
- 1 1/2 cups sugar
- 1 package (12 ounces) frozen unsweetened raspberries
- 10 individual tea bags
- 1/4 cup lemon juice

1. In a large, nonreactive saucepan or Dutch oven over moderately high heat, combine the water and sugar; bring the mixture to a boil. Remove the saucepan from the heat and stir until the sugar has completely dissolved.
2. Add the raspberries, tea bags, and lemon juice to the saucepan. Cover the saucepan and steep the tea for 3 minutes. Set a large sieve over a heatproof pitcher. Pour the tea mixture through, straining and discarding the solids. Place the pitcher in the refrigerator until the tea is completely chilled. Serve the tea over ice.

Makes 4 quarts (about 16 servings)

Frosty Caramel Cappuccino

A gourmet-style coffee concoction that you can whip up for pennies without leaving home or standing in line.

- 1 cup half-and-half
- 1 cup 2% milk
- 3 tablespoons plus 2 teaspoons caramel sauce
- 2 teaspoons instant espresso powder
- 8-10 ice cubes
- 4 tablespoons whipped cream (fresh or canned)

1. In the bowl of a food processor or blender, combine the half-and-half, milk, 3 tablespoons of the caramel sauce, espresso powder, and ice cubes. Cover and whirl until the mixture is smooth.
2. Pour the cappuccino into two chilled glasses. Top with whipped cream and drizzle with the remaining 2 teaspoons of caramel sauce. Serve immediately.

Makes 2 servings

Iced Coffee Slush

Ah, iced coffee without diluted flavor—because you freeze the coffee itself. This chilly delight will take the heat out of summer without making a hole in your purse or requiring a trip to a coffee emporium.

3 cups hot strong brewed coffee

1/2-1 cup sugar

4 cups milk

2 cups half-and-half

1 1/2 teaspoons vanilla extract

1. In a freezer-safe bowl, combine the coffee and the amount of sugar desired. Stir until the sugar has completely dissolved. Cover the bowl and refrigerate until the coffee mixture is thoroughly chilled. Stir in the milk, half-and-half, and vanilla. Re-cover the bowl and place in the freezer until the coffee mixture is solid.

2. Transfer the bowl from the freezer to the refrigerator several hours before serving. Using a mallet, break up the coffee mixture. Transfer the mixture to the bowl of a food processor or blender, and whirl until the coffee mixture is slushy. Serve immediately.

Makes 2 1/4 quarts (about 12 servings)

Lemonade Syrup

Whip up a batch of this syrup whenever you see lemons on sale, then keep it on hand to make the best homemade lemonade you've ever tasted—in a flash! This makes a much less expensive and better-tasting lemonade than anything you can buy.

3 cups sugar

1 cup boiling water

3 cups fresh lemon juice (about 16 lemons)

2 tablespoons grated lemon zest

1. In a 1 1/2-quart, heatproof container, place the sugar. Add the boiling water, stirring constantly, until the sugar has completely dissolved. Let the sugar mixture stand until it is cool.

2. Add the lemon juice and zest, and stir until all the ingredients are well blended. Cover the container, and store in the refrigerator for up to 1 week.

Makes 5 1/2 cups syrup

variation:

Limeade Syrup: Substitute 3 cups fresh lime juice and 2 tablespoons grated lime zest and proceed as above.

Lemonade
Tart, sweet, and oh, so refreshing, this syrup-based lemonade is quick, delicious, and cheap.

1/4-1/3 cups Lemonade Syrup (opposite)

3/4 cup cold water

Ice cubes

Lemon wedge or fresh mint sprig (optional)

In a tall glass, combine the desired amount of syrup and cold water, and stir until they are well blended. Add ice cubes and, if desired, garnish with a lemon wedge or mint sprig.

Makes 1 glass

Lemon Squash
This is the fizzy version of economical lemonade, loaded with bright lemon taste and bubbles.

4 strips (3 inches each) lemon zest, cut into thin slices

1 cup Lemonade Syrup (opposite)

3 cups chilled club soda, seltzer, or sparkling water

Lemon slices or small fresh mint sprigs (optional)

1. In a 2-quart pitcher, combine the lemon zest, and syrup to taste. Stir until all the ingredients are well blended.
2. Just before serving, pour in the club soda, seltzer, or sparkling water; stir gently to blend the ingredients. Fill glasses with ice cubes, pour the lemon squash over the ice, and if desired, garnish each serving with a lemon wedge or small sprig of fresh mint.

Makes 4 servings

variation:

Lime Squash: Prepare as directed above, substituting lime zest and Limeade Syrup (opposite) for the lemon zest and Lemonade Syrup or to taste. Garnish with lime wedges or fresh strawberries.

Orange Blossom
For a nonalcoholic version of this festive drink, substitute sparkling water for the gin and add it after shaking the orange juice and sugar. This is a popular cocktail that is easy and inexpensive to make at home.

1 large piece orange zest

1 teaspoon superfine sugar plus small saucer for dipping

2 ounces gin

1 ounce orange juice

1 orange slice

1. Rub the orange zest around the rim of a chilled martini glass. Dip the rim into the saucer of sugar.
2. In a cocktail shaker, combine the remaining superfine sugar, gin, and orange juice. Cover and shake until the mixture is well blended. Place a strainer over the glass, and pour the mixture through. Garnish with the orange slice.

Makes 1 serving

Berry Orange Shrub
Wonderfully fizzy and full of taste, this drink can be its own dessert, a soda fountain kind of concoction that would cost a fortune at an ice-cream store.

1 quart cran-raspberry juice

1/2 cup sugar

Zest of 1 orange, cut into thin strips

2/3 cup orange juice

4 cups club soda

Orange sherbet

1. In a medium, nonreactive saucepan over low heat, combine the cran-raspberry juice, sugar, and orange zest; slowly bring the mixture to a boil. Reduce the heat and simmer, stirring occasionally, 10 minutes. Remove the saucepan from the heat.

2. Stir in the orange juice and let the mixture cool to room temperature. Pour the mixture into a 2-quart pitcher, cover, and refrigerate until the mixture is chilled.

3. Before serving, remove and discard the orange zest. Pour 1/2 cup of the shrub mixture into punch cups or glasses, add 1/2 cup of the club soda, and top with a scoop of the orange sherbet.

Makes 8 servings

Sparkling Fruit Bowl
Beautifully colored, with essence of raspberries, strawberries, and oranges, this is a spicy, fizzy fruit punch for parties.

1 package (10 ounces) dry-pack frozen raspberries

1 package (10 ounces) dry-pack frozen strawberries

6 cups water

1 1/2 cups sugar

10 whole cloves

1/2 teaspoon ground cardamom

6 strips (3 x 1/2 inch each) orange zest

1 vanilla bean, split

2 cups orange juice

2 cups club soda

1. In a large, nonreactive saucepan or Dutch oven over moderately high heat, combine the first eight ingredients and bring to a boil. Reduce the heat to moderately low and simmer, uncovered, stirring occasionally, about 10 minutes.

2. Place a large sieve over a large pitcher. Pour the berry mixture through, straining out the solids; do not press the solids. Let the berry mixture cool to room temperature. Stir in the orange juice.

3. Just before serving, stir in the club soda. Serve the punch over ice.

Makes 10 servings

Fruit Juice Spritzer

Here is a lovely, light, and fizzy cooler that you can customize to suit your taste and your menu—try cran-raspberry juice, pineapple juice, Concord grape juice, pink grapefruit juice, tangerine juice, or anything else that tickles your fancy. If you don't use wine, you can blend 2 juices instead. A wonderful start to a summer party that won't break the bank.

- 3 cups chilled dry white wine or fruit juice of choice
- 1 1/2 cups chilled fruit juice of choice or complementary juice
- 1 1/2 cups chilled carbonated beverage (soda, seltzer, or ginger ale)
- Fresh mint leaves or citrus wedges *(optional)*

1. In a 2-quart pitcher, combine the wine or fruit juice, additional or complementary juice, and carbonated beverage.
2. Serve straight or over ice cubes. If desired, garnish individual glasses with mint leaves or citrus wedges.

Makes 8 servings

Bloody Mary Mix

Keep this mix ready to go in the refrigerator and you can whip up fantastic Bloody Marys in a flash—or just serve it over ice as a spicy tomato juice treat. You can buy Bloody Mary mixes, but the homemade version is livelier and much, much cheaper.

- 2 1/4 cups tomato juice
- 1/4 cup lemon juice
- 1/2 teaspoon black pepper
- 1/2 teaspoon salt
- 1/2 teaspoon celery seed
- 1 teaspoon Worcestershire sauce
- 1/2 teaspoon hot red pepper sauce

In a 1-quart jar with a tight-fitting lid, combine the ingredients. Cover the jar tightly and shake to blend well. Refrigerate for up to 1 week; shake well before using.

Makes 2 1/2 cups

Bloody Mary

An eye-opener for breakfast or brunch, this spicy drink stands up to even the most flavorful foods. Homemade with your own mix, it's a treat without being a threat to your pocketbook.

- 1/2 cup cracked ice
- 2 1/2 ounces vodka
- 5 ounces Bloody Mary Mix (above)
- 1 celery stalk

In a tall glass, place the cracked ice. Pour the vodka and Bloody Mary mix over the ice. Garnish with the celery stalk.

Makes 1 serving

Sangria

The color of garnets, full of fruit, and always welcome regardless of the season, sangria is an easy-to-make, delightful wine punch that is served at Spanish restaurants. Homemade is fresher-tasting and a lot less pricey.

2 oranges, sliced

2 lemons, sliced

2 cinnamon sticks

3/4 cup brandy

1 bottle (750 milliliters) red wine of choice

1 bottle (750 milliliters) sparkling cider, chilled

Ice cubes

1. In a large punch bowl or glass pitcher, combine the first four ingredients.

2. Pour the red wine and sparkling cider over the fruit mixture, gently stirring until the punch is well blended. Just before serving, add ice cubes as desired.

Makes about 1 3/4 quarts

hot drinks

Caffe Latte

Why pay $3 to $5 for a cup of special coffee when you can so easily make it yourself—and at a fraction of the price?

1 1/2 cups skim or low-fat milk

2/3 cup freshly brewed espresso

Ground cinnamon or sweetened cocoa powder *(optional)*

1. In a small saucepan over low heat, cook the milk just until tiny bubbles begin to form around the edges of the saucepan, 10 to 15 minutes; do not let the milk come to a boil. If a skin forms on the surface of the milk, remove it with a spoon and discard.

2. Divide the espresso between two 8-ounce cups. Add 1/3 cup of the hot milk to each cup.

3. Using an electric mixer or wire whisk, beat the remaining hot milk until it is frothy. Spoon the milk froth into the coffee cups, dividing it equally. If desired, sprinkle a little cinnamon or sweetened cocoa powder over the foam before serving.

Makes 2 servings

variations:

Chocolate Mint Latte: Prepare as directed above, adding a finely chopped 1/2-ounce chocolate-covered peppermint patty to each cup along with the espresso.

Caffe Latte à l'Orange: Prepare as directed above, adding 1 tablespoon Grand Marnier or other orange-flavored liqueur to each cup along with the espresso.

Cappuccino Mix

Love the convenience of instant special coffees to keep at the office or to brew a fast cup for an afternoon pick-me-up? Make your own and you'll save a bundle.

1 cup instant coffee creamer

1 cup instant chocolate milk powder

2/3 cup instant coffee crystals or espresso powder

1/2 cup sugar

1/2 teaspoon ground cinnamon

1/4 teaspoon ground nutmeg

In an airtight container, combine the ingredients. Cover and shake until they are well blended. For 1 cup of instant cappuccino, place 3 tablespoons in a mug or coffee cup. Add 6 ounces boiling water and stir until the mix has completely dissolved.

Makes 3 cups dry mix

Cocoa

On a cold, blustery day, there's nothing quite like cocoa made the good, old-fashioned way.

2 tablespoons sugar

1 tablespoon unsweetened cocoa

1/4 cup water

3/4 cup 1% milk

Miniature marshmallows *(optional)*

1 cinnamon stick, 4 inches long *(optional)*

1. In a small saucepan, combine the sugar and cocoa. Add the water. Over moderate heat, bring the mixture to a boil, stirring constantly until the sugar has dissolved. Lower the heat and simmer 2 minutes, whisking constantly.

2. Stir in the milk. Increase the heat to moderate and cook until the cocoa is heated through; do not allow the mixture to boil.

3. To serve, pour the cocoa into a mug or cup. If desired, top with several marshmallows and use the cinnamon stick as a stirrer.

Makes 1 serving

Hot Chocolate Viennese

Chocolate, coffee, and hot milk—triple yum! This is a coffeehouse treat that you can enjoy for much less at home.

1/3 cup unsweetened cocoa powder

1/3 cup sugar

2 1/2 cups milk

1 1/2 cups freshly brewed strong coffee or espresso

1. In a medium saucepan, combine the cocoa powder and sugar, pressing out any lumps. Stirring constantly, pour in enough of the milk to moisten the dry mixture, about 1/2 cup; whisk in the coffee and the remaining 2 cups milk.

2. Over moderately low heat, cook, stirring occasionally, until the mixture steams but does not boil, 8 to 10 minutes. Pour the hot chocolate into mugs or coffee cups and serve.

Makes 4 servings

Chai

The spicy, creamy tea drink that has shot up in popularity, chai is a lovely afternoon soother or stimulator. It is convenient and economical to make your own.

2 cups water

2 individual tea bags

1 cinnamon stick

6 cardamom pods, crushed

1 whole clove

1/4 teaspoon ground ginger

2 1/2 cups milk

1/3 cup sugar

Whipped cream, ground cinnamon, and cinnamon sticks *(optional)*

1. In a small saucepan over moderately high heat, combine the first six ingredients; bring the mixture to a boil. Reduce the heat, cover the saucepan, and simmer 5 minutes.

2. Stir in the milk. Increase the heat and return the mixture to a boil; boil 1 minute. Remove the saucepan from the heat, place a sieve over a warmed teapot, and pour the mixture through; discard the solids. Add the sugar and stir until dissolved.

3. To serve, pour into 4 mugs or cups and, if desired, top with a dollop of whipped cream, sprinkle with cinnamon, and tuck a cinnamon stick along the side.

Makes 4 servings

Hot Spiced Tea

Give extra zest to hot tea with this inviting spice mixture—it will make your kitchen smell fabulous while it warms you to your toes. No mix can match this hot spiced tea at any price. It's the perfect drink for a winter afternoon.

2 cinnamon sticks

6-12 whole allspice

1 teaspoon whole cloves

12 cups water

12 individual tea bags

1 cup packed brown sugar

1 cup cranberry juice

1/2 cup orange juice

1/4 cup lemon juice

1. Cut a 4-inch square of double-thickness cheesecloth. Combine the cinnamon sticks, allspice, and cloves in the center. Bring together the corners of the cheesecloth to form a bag; secure with a piece of kitchen string.

2. In a large, nonreactive saucepan or Dutch oven over high heat, combine the water and the spice bag; bring the water to a boil. Remove the saucepan from the heat and add the tea bags; cover the saucepan and let the tea steep 5 minutes. Remove and discard the tea bags and spice bag.

3. Stir in the brown sugar until it has completely dissolved. Add the juices, stirring until the ingredients are well blended. Return the saucepan to low heat, and gently heat the spiced tea through.

Makes 3 quarts

Hot Mulled Cider

One of the best warm-me-ups, this cider has some surprises in its spice. You don't have to go to a ski lodge to enjoy it.

4 cups apple cider
10 whole cloves
10 black peppercorns
4 strips (3 x 1/2 inch each) orange zest
1 cinnamon stick, cracked
1 vanilla bean, split

1. In a medium saucepan over moderate heat, combine the ingredients; bring the mixture to a boil. Remove the saucepan from the heat and let stand 30 minutes to steep. Remove and discard the spices.

2. Return the saucepan to low heat and slowly cook until the cider begins to steam. Ladle the cider into mugs, wait 3 to 5 minutes, and serve.

Makes 4 servings

Holiday Wassail

A traditional holiday punch served warm or cool, this wassail is festive for parties and quite economical when you make it up fresh.

1 quart hot brewed tea
1 cup sugar
1 bottle (32 ounces) cranberry juice
1 bottle (32 ounces) apple juice
2 cups orange juice
3/4 cup lemon juice
24 whole cloves
2 cinnamon sticks
1 orange, sliced

1. In a large, nonreactive saucepan or Dutch oven over moderately high heat, combine the hot tea and sugar, stirring until the sugar has dissolved. Add the juices, 12 cloves, and the cinnamon sticks. Bring the mixture to a boil and boil 2 minutes.

2. Remove the saucepan from the heat. Pour the wassail into a heatproof punch bowl. Insert the remaining cloves into the orange slices and float them on the wassail as garnish. Serve the wassail warm or cooled to room temperature.

Makes 12 to 16 servings

chapter 5

Make Your Own
Take-Out Food

Have you ever noticed how the prepared-food sections are taking up more and more of your supermarket? That's because we are quickly becoming a nation

addicted to ready-made dishes, and the supermarket is only responding to the demand. The only problem is that those eat-as-they-are or pop-in-the-microwave dishes carry an enormous price premium for the little extra convenience that they provide. This chapter is dedicated to the true convenience foods that you can make fresh in your own kitchen. Most make minimal demands on your time. And many are foods that you can make ahead—or leave simmering in a slow cooker—for a meal later.

On the following pages, you'll find tasty meat, egg, and bean dishes and satisfying savory pies of the type that you might pick up at the deli counter or from the freezer case. A homemade turkey potpie is great way to use up leftover Thanksgiving meat. You'll also find a nice selection of delicious easy-to-make pasta dishes. (For a special treat, try them with fresh pastas from Chapter 1.) There are hearty soups that will fill your kitchen with good smells, delight your family, and use up leftovers. And unlike the bland canned versions, homemade soups can provide more flavor with less salt. There is also a wide selection of deli-style salads that you can make without a lot of fuss, ranging from sides like coleslaw to main dishes like Cobb salad—and, unlike some deli salads, they will never have too much mayonnaise.

deli-style dishes

Savory Meat Mix

The base for many a dish, this can be made with either ground beef or ground turkey. Two recipes that use this mix follow, and there is another at the beginning of the Pasta Dishes section (page 175).

2 tablespoons olive or canola oil

2 medium onions, chopped

2 garlic cloves, minced

1 celery stalk, chopped

2 carrots, chopped

2 1/2 pounds lean ground beef or turkey

2 teaspoons dried basil

1 teaspoon dried oregano

1 teaspoon salt

1/2 teaspoon ground pepper

Large pinch sugar

1 tablespoon Worcestershire sauce

1 can (14 1/2 ounces) diced tomatoes in sauce

1. In a large, deep skillet or Dutch oven over moderate heat, heat the oil. Add the onions, garlic, celery, and carrots to the skillet and sauté until softened, about 5 minutes, stirring occasionally. Crumble the beef or turkey into the skillet, breaking it up with a large spoon; cook, stirring occasionally, until the meat is no longer pink. Drain off as much fat as possible

2. Add the basil, oregano, salt, pepper, sugar, Worcestershire sauce, and the tomatoes with their sauce; stir until all the ingredients are well mixed. Reduce the heat, cover the skillet, and simmer 20 to 25 minutes.

3. Remove the skillet from the heat and let the mixture cool completely. Spoon off any visible fat and then divide the mixture among 3 to 4 (1 pint) self-sealing, freezer-safe plastic bags. Seal, label, date, and freeze. The mix will keep up to three months in the freezer.

Makes 3 1/2 to 4 pints of mix

Skillet Noodle Supper

This is a favorite family dinner that takes only 20 minutes or so to bring to the table.

1 package (10 ounces) frozen mixed vegetables

1 pint Savory Meat Mix (above), thawed

2 cups cooked egg noodles

1 can (8 ounces) tomato sauce

1 cup shredded cheddar cheese

1. Cook the vegetables following the package directions on the stovetop or in the microwave.

2. In a large skillet over moderate heat, combine the vegetables, meat mix, noodles, and tomato sauce, and gently stir to combine the ingredients. Cover the skillet and cook about 10 minutes, stirring occasionally; add a few sprinkles of water as needed to prevent the mixture from sticking.

3. Sprinkle the cheese over the top of the mixture in the skillet; do *not* stir. Cover the skillet again and heat just until the cheese is melted. Serve from the skillet.

Makes 4 to 6 servings

Chili Con Carne *This will be the fastest chili you ever put together with fresh meat.*

1 pint Savory Meat Mix (opposite), thawed

2 teaspoons to 1 tablespoon or more chili powder

1 teaspoon cumin

2 cans (15 1/2 ounces each) red kidney beans, drained and rinsed

Hot pepper sauce, to taste

Hot cooked rice, tortilla chips, shredded cheddar or Monterey Jack cheese, sour cream or plain yogurt *(optional)*

1. In a medium saucepan, combine the meat mix, chili powder, cumin, and kidney beans. Cover and cook over moderately high heat until the chili is heated through, about 10 minutes. Add hot pepper sauce to the desired level of spiciness.

2. Serve the chili over rice or with tortilla chips, if desired. Sprinkle a little cheese over each serving or top with a dollop of sour cream or yogurt, if desired.

Makes 6 servings

Tomato Herb Tarts *Frozen puff pastry makes these individual tarts easy to whip up in a jiffy. Tarts you buy at the grocery are never as fresh-tasting or as inexpensive.*

1 sheet frozen puff pastry

1/2 cup finely shredded cheddar cheese

2 tablespoons grated Parmesan cheese

1 pound ripe tomatoes, peeled and sliced

2 tablespoons minced fresh parsley

2 tablespoons minced fresh basil

2 tablespoons minced fresh thyme

1 tablespoon virgin olive oil

Freshly ground black pepper

1. Preheat the oven to 400°F.

2. Place the sheet of puff pastry on a work surface. Using a large, round cutter, cut 4 to 6 circles from the pastry. Place the pastry circles on a baking sheet, and bake until puffed and golden brown, 10 to 12 minutes. Remove baking sheet; do not turn off the oven.

3. Sprinkle some of the cheddar and Parmesan cheeses, divided equally, over each pastry circle, leaving a small border around the edges. Layer tomato slices, divided equally, on top of the cheese on each circle. Sprinkle some of the parsley, basil, and thyme over the tomatoes. Drizzle each circle with some of the olive oil, then sprinkle pepper as desired.

4. Return the baking sheet to the oven and bake until the cheeses are completely melted, about 5 minutes. Turn off the oven and let the tarts stand for a few minutes before removing them from the oven. Serve immediately or at room temperature.

Makes 4 to 6 tarts

Texas-Style Barbecue Sauce

Meant for spareribs (see Barbecued Spareribs, below), this tangy taste of the Lone Star State can also be used on chicken. Again, you can adjust ingredients to your own taste and save money at the same time.

1 1/2 cups ketchup

1 cup cider vinegar

2/3 cup peanut or safflower oil

1/3 cup Worcestershire sauce

1/2 cup firmly packed dark brown sugar

3 tablespoons mild yellow mustard

1/2 teaspoon freshly ground black pepper

Juice of 1 large lemon

1-2 fresh red chile peppers, minced *(optional)*; wear gloves when handling; they burn

In a medium saucepan over moderate heat, combine the ingredients. Bring the mixture to a boil; immediately reduce the heat to low, cover, and simmer until the sugar has completely dissolved and the sauce has thickened slightly, about 20 minutes.

Makes about 3 cups

One-Minute Substitute

If You Run Out of Brown Sugar

If a recipe calls for 1/2 cup brown sugar and you don't have any on hand, stir 1 tablespoon molasses into 1/2 cup regular granulated sugar.

Barbecued Spareribs

You get the best results when you make your own ribs; you also save money.

5 pounds pork spareribs in slab of 6-8 ribs

3 cups Texas-Style Barbecue Sauce (above)

1. Place the ribs in a large self-sealing bag, glass baking dish, or nonreactive bowl. Pour 2 cups of the barbecue sauce over the ribs, cover, and refrigerate overnight.

2. On a covered kettle-style grill, following the manufacturer's directions, prepare the coals for the indirect method of cooking. Add the ribs and cook 1 to 1 1/2 hours, basting frequently with the marinating sauce. In a small saucepan over low heat, warm the reserved barbecue sauce and serve on the side with the ribs.

Makes 6 servings

Baked Beans
A staple of the Puritans, baked beans solved a religious dilemma for these hardworking people. The tenets of their faith forbade working on the Sabbath, including cooking. Beans could be baked slowly on Saturday, then reheated or served cold for Sunday breakfast or lunch.

- 1 pound dried peas or navy beans, sorted and rinsed
- 1/3 cup molasses
- 1 teaspoon dry mustard
- 1 teaspoon salt
- 1/2 teaspoon ground black pepper
- 1/4 pound salt pork
- 1 medium onion, peeled

1. Place the beans in a 4-quart Dutch oven and add enough water to cover plus 2 inches. Bring the water to a boil and boil 2 minutes. Remove the saucepan from the heat, cover, and let stand 1 hour.

2. Add more water to cover the beans and return the pan to the heat. Bring to a boil, reduce the heat, and simmer until the beans are tender, about 1 hour, adding more water as necessary to keep the beans covered. Drain the beans, reserving the cooking liquid.

3. Place the drained beans in a 2-quart bean pot or casserole dish. In a bowl, combine the molasses, mustard, salt, and pepper, and pour the mixture over the beans. Cut the pork into 1/2-inch slices up to but not through the rind. Add the pork and the onion to the bean mixture, pressing them down until they are buried. If needed, add the reserved cooking liquid until the beans are completely covered.

4. Place the bean pot or casserole in a 250°F oven and cook, covered, 5 hours, adding additional reserved cooking liquid or water to prevent the bean mixture from drying out. Remove the cover for the last hour of cooking time.

Makes 6 servings

Helpful Hint | **Always Have Beans on Hand**
Any pantry should be well stocked with a variety of beans. Dried will cost less but must be soaked before cooking. Canned beans don't always hold their shape and are often very high in salt. Always rinse canned beans under cold running water to reduce the sodium content by as much as 40 percent before using them. Many bean dishes are simple, delicious, filling, and very nutritious, but the best ones are made at home.

Classic Refried Beans

One of the mainstays of Mexican cooking, refried beans can be used in dips, tacos, tortillas, burritos—and just about any other dish too! They are traditionally served as a side dish with rice and are very mild in flavor, although you can spice them up easily.

- 1 pound (approximately 2 cups) dried pinto or red kidney beans, sorted and rinsed
- 1 large yellow onion, quartered
- 3 garlic cloves, unpeeled
- 1/2 teaspoon ground cumin
- 3-4 drops hot pepper sauce
- 1/4 cup vegetable shortening, lard, vegetable oil, or bacon drippings
- Chopped fresh cilantro leaves, shredded cheddar or Monterey Jack cheese, or homemade Spicy Tomato Salsa (page 31)

1. In a 4-quart Dutch oven, place the beans and the onion, and add water to cover plus 2 inches. Bring the mixture to a boil and boil 2 minutes. Remove the saucepan from the heat, cover, and let stand for 1 hour. Drain the beans and discard the soaking liquid.

2. Return the beans to the saucepan and add enough water to cover. Add the onion and garlic, and bring the mixture to a boil. Reduce the heat to low, cover the saucepan, and simmer until the beans are very tender, about 2 hours, adding water as needed to keep the beans covered. Remove and discard the onion and garlic.

3. Using a potato masher, mash the beans to the desired consistency. Stir in the cumin and hot pepper sauce.

4. To fry: In a heavy skillet over moderate heat, melt the shortening or lard, or heat the oil or bacon drippings. Add the mashed bean mixture and cook, stirring occasionally, until the mixture forms a smooth paste and begins to pull away from the sides of the pan, 5 to 10 minutes. Continue to cook, scraping the mixture from the bottom of the pan and turning it over until the bean mixture is thick and has a creamy texture.

5. Serve the beans with sprinkled cilantro, cheese, or salsa on top.

Makes about 9 servings

Refritos Rapido

Still want homemade refried beans but crunched for time? That's not a problem with this recipe.

- 2 tablespoons vegetable oil
- 1 large onion, chopped
- 2 cans (15 ounces each) pinto, kidney, or black beans, drained and rinsed
- 1 teaspoon ground cumin
- Salt, to taste
- Chili powder, to taste (optional)

1. In a large, heavy skillet over moderate heat, heat the oil. Add the onion and sauté until just softened. Add the beans, cumin, salt, and chili powder, if desired. Cook, stirring, until heated through, 5 to 10 minutes. Remove the pan from the heat.

2. Using a potato masher, mash the bean mixture to the desired consistency. Return the skillet to moderate heat and cook until the mixture is thick and creamy in texture, about 15 minutes.

Makes 4 to 6 servings

Basic Rice Pilaf

Once you learn how to make pilaf (seasoned rice or other grains), you have the base for an almost infinite variety of dishes. Try using brown rice, wild rice, bulgur, or barley instead of white rice; stir in cooked meats, seafood, or vegetables; add a handful of toasted pine nuts, pistachios, or pecans—you've got a gourmet meal in minutes.

1 tablespoon virgin olive oil or vegetable oil

1 cup long-grain white rice

2 cups Chicken Stock (page 50)

1. In a medium, heavy saucepan over moderately high heat, heat the oil until it is very hot. Add the rice; cook, stirring constantly, until the oil is absorbed and the rice is translucent, about 5 minutes.

2. Add the stock, raise the heat to high, and bring the mixture to a boil. Stir once, lower the heat, and cover the pan tightly. Simmer until the broth is absorbed and the rice is tender, 15 to 20 minutes.

Makes about 3 cups (4 to 6 servings)

Curry with Rice

Flavorful, economical, and easy to prepare, curry is one of the most adaptable recipes you'll ever make. It's a fast and easy way to use up leftovers. Meat, poultry, seafood, vegetables—just about anything can be used to make curry.

1/4 cup all-purpose flour

1/2 teaspoon salt

1/4 teaspoon ground black pepper

1 1/2 pounds skinless, boneless chicken or turkey breasts or thighs, or lamb, cut into 1-inch cubes

3 tablespoons vegetable oil

1 large yellow onion, chopped

2 garlic cloves, minced

2 small celery stalks, chopped

1-2 tablespoons Curry Powder (page 46)

1 3/4 cups Chicken Stock (page 50) or reduced-sodium canned chicken broth

4 medium carrots, peeled and cut crosswise into 1/2-inch slices

2 cups cauliflower florets (about 1/2 head medium cauliflower)

1 1/4 cups basmati rice

1. In a large, self-sealing bag, combine the flour, salt, and pepper. Working in small batches, add the chicken, turkey, or lamb to the bag, seal, and shake to coat the meat with the flour mixture.

2. In a large skillet with a tight-fitting lid over moderately high heat, heat the oil 1 minute. Divide the meat into 2 batches. Add one batch to the skillet and sauté until lightly brown, about 5 minutes. Remove the meat to paper towels to drain. Repeat with the remaining meat.

3. In the drippings left in the skillet, sauté the onion, garlic, and celery, stirring occasionally, until soft, about 5 minutes. Add the curry powder, stock, carrots, cauliflower, and reserved meat to the skillet. Reduce the heat to low, cover, and simmer until the cauliflower is just tender, 20 to 30 minutes.

4. Meanwhile, in a large saucepan over high heat, cook the basmati rice following the package directions. Transfer the cooked rice to a large, heated serving bowl. Spoon the curry over the rice and serve immediately.

Makes 4 servings

main-dish pies

Classic Chicken Potpie

Frozen chicken potpies can't hold a candle to this lovely dish that uses up the leftovers from Sunday's roast chicken. The pie can be made ahead and frozen, tightly covered with freezer-safe foil, for up to 3 months.

1 cup chopped peeled potatoes

1 cup sliced carrots

1/3 cup chopped yellow onion

1/2 cup butter or margarine

1/2 cup all-purpose flour

3/4 teaspoon salt

1/2 teaspoon dried thyme, crumbled

1/2 teaspoon ground black pepper

1 1/2 cups Chicken Stock (page 50) or reduced-sodium canned chicken broth

3/4 cup milk

2 cups chopped cooked chicken

1/2 cup frozen peas

1/2 cup frozen corn

Basic Double Crust Pie Pastry (page 123)

1. In a large saucepan, combine the potatoes and carrots, and cover them with water. Bring the water to a boil; reduce the heat, cover, and simmer until crisp-tender, 8 to 10 minutes. Drain the potato-carrot mixture and set aside.

2. In a large skillet over moderate heat, sauté the onion in the butter or margarine until tender. Stir in the flour, salt, thyme, and pepper until well blended. Gradually add the stock and milk, stirring constantly. Bring the mixture to a boil; cook, stirring constantly, until the mixture is thickened. Stir in the chicken, peas, corn, and the potato-carrot mixture. Remove the skillet from the heat.

3. Preheat the oven to 425°F. Line a 9-inch pie plate with the bottom piecrust; trim the edges of the dough even with the edges of the plate. Spoon the pie filling into the bottom crust. Roll out the remaining piecrust; cut slits or decorative vents in the crust. Carefully transfer the crust to cover the pie filling. Fold the top edges of the pastry over and under the bottom crust edges; pinch the edges together to seal. If desired, form a decorative edge around the piecrust with a fork or with your fingers.

4. Bake the pie until the crust is golden brown, 35 to 40 minutes. Let the pie stand for 15 minutes before serving. To bake a frozen pie, cover the edges with pieces of foil and set on a baking sheet. Bake in a 425°F oven 30 minutes. Reduce the heat to 350°F and bake for an additional 70 to 80 minutes or until the crust is golden brown.

Makes 6 servings

Turkey Potpie

This is a very tasty way to use up Thanksgiving leftovers. If you don't want turkey again so soon, make the pie and freeze it in freezer-safe foil for up to 3 months.

1/4 cup chopped yellow onion

1 tablespoon butter or margarine

2 cans (10 3/4 ounces each) condensed cream soup (chicken, mushroom, asparagus)

3 cups chopped cooked turkey

1 large unpeeled tart apple, chopped

1/3 cup golden raisins

1 teaspoon lemon juice

1/4 teaspoon ground nutmeg

Basic Single Crust Pie Pastry (page 124)

1. In a large saucepan over moderate heat, sauté the onion in the butter or margarine until tender. Stir in the soup, turkey, apple, raisins, lemon juice, and nutmeg. Spoon the turkey mixture into an ungreased 11 x 7 x 2-inch baking dish.

2. Preheat the oven to 425°F. On a lightly floured surface with a lightly floured rolling pin, roll out the pastry to fit the top of the baking dish. Carefully transfer the crust to cover the pie filling; press the edges of the crust to the edges of the baking dish to seal, and flute the crust edges. Cut slits in the piecrust.

3. Bake the pie until the crust is golden brown and the filling is bubbly, 25 to 30 minutes.

Makes 6 servings

Savory Beef Pie

A toothsome array of spices makes this potpie a spicy and delicious meal.

2 medium potatoes, peeled and quartered

1 pound lean ground beef

3/4 cup sliced scallions

1 large carrot, finely chopped

1 garlic clove, minced

1/2 teaspoon dried thyme

1/2 teaspoon dried sage

1/2 teaspoon salt

1/2 teaspoon black pepper

1/4 teaspoon celery salt

Pinch ground cinnamon

1/4 cup minced fresh parsley

1/4 cup prepared chili sauce

Basic Double Crust Pie Pastry (page 123)

1 tablespoon Dijon mustard

1 tablespoon milk

1. In a large saucepan over high heat, cook the potatoes in boiling water until tender. Drain and mash the potatoes; set aside.

2. Meanwhile, in a large skillet over moderate heat, brown the beef until no pink remains; drain the liquid from the skillet and return the pan to the heat. Stir in the scallions, carrot, garlic, thyme, sage, salt, pepper, celery salt, and cinnamon. Simmer the mixture 4 to 5 minutes. Stir in the reserved potatoes, parsley, and chili sauce. Remove the skillet from the heat.

3. Preheat the oven to 450°F. Line a 9-inch pie plate with the bottom piecrust; trim the edges of the dough even with the edges of the plate. Brush the bottom crust with the mustard. Spoon the pie filling into the bottom crust. Roll out the remaining piecrust; cut slits or decorative vents in the crust. Carefully transfer the crust to cover the pie filling. Fold the top edges of the pastry over and under the bottom crust edges; pinch the edges together to seal. If desired, form a decorative edge around the piecrust. Brush the top of the crust with the milk.

4. Bake the pie 10 minutes. Reduce the heat to 350°F and bake until the crust is golden brown, about 25 minutes.

Makes 6 servings

Quiche Lorraine

One of the best-known quiches, this yummy custard pie takes its name from the Lorraine region in France. It was originally made just from cream and bacon, but now includes cheese—either a good Gruyère or other Swiss cheese. You can buy a quiche from the grocery for $8 to $12, but it will never taste as good as your own fresh out of the oven.

Basic Single Crust Pie Pastry (page 124)

6 slices good-quality bacon, diced and lightly fried

1 1/2 cups shredded Gruyère cheese

1 1/2 cups light cream

4 eggs

1/2 teaspoon salt

Small pinch ground red pepper

Small pinch ground nutmeg

1. Preheat the oven to 400°F.

2. Line a 9-inch pie plate with the prepared pastry and flute the edges. Place in the refrigerator and chill 15 to 20 minutes. Fill the crust with pie weights or beans and bake 10 minutes. Remove the piecrust and remove the weights or beans; do not turn off the oven.

3. Sprinkle the cooked bacon over the bottom of the piecrust. Sprinkle the cheese over the bacon. In a large bowl, combine the cream, eggs, salt, red pepper, and nutmeg. Beat until the ingredients are well blended. Carefully pour the cream mixture over the cheese and bacon in the piecrust.

4. Bake, uncovered, 15 minutes at 400°F; reduce the heat to 350°F and bake until the filling is set in the center, 15 to 20 minutes longer. Let the quiche stand for 10 minutes before serving to allow the custard to set.

Makes 6 main course or 12 appetizer servings

One-Minute Substitute

If You Run Out of Cream

Heavy cream: If a recipe calls for 1 cup heavy cream (not for whipping) and you don't have any on hand, combine 3/4 cup milk with 1/3 cup melted butter in a 2-cup measure and whisk until the mixture is well blended.

Light cream: If a recipe calls for 1 cup light cream and you don't have any on hand, combine 3/4 cup milk with 1/4 cup melted butter in a 2-cup measure and whisk until the mixture is well blended.

Half-and-half: If a recipe calls for 1 cup half-and-half and you don't have any on hand, combine 7/8 cup milk with 1 1/2 tablespoons melted butter in a 2-cup measure and whisk until the mixture is well blended.

Spinach-Wild Rice Pie *Here is a quiche-like pie that will delight everyone in the family, including the vegetarians.*

Basic Single Crust Pie
   Pastry (page 124)

3 eggs

1 cup half-and-half

1 cup cooked wild rice

1 cup (4 ounces) shredded
   Swiss cheese

1/2 cup frozen chopped
   spinach, thawed

1. Preheat the oven to 450°F. Line a 9-inch pie plate with the piecrust; turn under the edges of the dough and, if desired, form a decorative edge around the piecrust. Line the piecrust with a double thickness of foil. Bake the piecrust 5 minutes; remove the foil and bake 5 minutes more. Remove the piecrust from the oven and reduce the heat to 350°F.

2. In a large bowl, beat the eggs with the half-and-half. Add the wild rice, cheese, and spinach, and blend well. Pour the egg mixture into the piecrust. Cover the edges of the crust with pieces of foil and bake until a knife inserted near the center comes out clean, 30 to 35 minutes.

Makes 6 to 8 servings

pasta dishes

Spaghetti with Meat Sauce *Please a crowd in 30 minutes with this classic spaghetti recipe.*

1 pint Savory Meat Mix
   (page 166), thawed

1 can (14 1/2 ounces) diced
   tomatoes in sauce

1 can (6 ounces)
   tomato paste

1/2 cup dry red wine or
   water

2 teaspoons dried basil,
   crumbled

1 teaspoon dried oregano,
   crumbled

1 package (16 ounces)
   spaghetti or homemade
   spaghetti

Freshly grated
   Parmesan cheese

1. In a large saucepan or Dutch oven over moderate heat, combine the meat mix, tomatoes, tomato paste, wine or water, basil, and oregano. Stir until all the ingredients are well mixed. Bring the mixture to a boil over high heat, reduce the heat to low, and simmer, uncovered, stirring occasionally, about 30 minutes.

2. Meanwhile, cook the spaghetti following the package directions, and drain. Serve the spaghetti topped with the meat sauce and sprinkle Parmesan cheese over each serving.

Makes 6 to 8 servings

Spaghetti with Speedy Tomato Sauce *Never buy bottled sauce again!*

This tasty sauce can be whipped up in no time at all, and all the ingredients can be kept on hand for whenever you wish. During the summer, when fresh tomatoes are plentiful and cheap, substitute 3 pounds fresh, chopped tomatoes for the canned.

1 can (16 ounces) Italian plum tomatoes

1 can (6 ounces) tomato paste

1 teaspoon dried oregano, crumbled

1 teaspoon dried basil, crumbled

1 teaspoon sugar

1/2 teaspoon salt

1/4 teaspoon black pepper

1 batch homemade spaghetti or 1 pound purchased spaghetti

Freshly grated Parmesan cheese

1. In a large saucepan over moderate heat, combine the tomatoes and their liquid, tomato paste, oregano, basil, sugar, salt, and black pepper. Bring the mixture to a boil; reduce the heat and simmer, uncovered, 15 to 20 minutes.

2. Meanwhile, cook the homemade spaghetti until just tender or follow the package directions for commercial spaghetti.

3. Serve the sauce over the spaghetti and sprinkle with Parmesan cheese.

Makes about 6 servings

Pasta with Fresh Tomato Sauce *Incomparable on its own, bursting with the*

flavor of fresh, vine-ripened tomatoes, this classic also forms the base for many other pasta sauces. Overripe tomatoes can be used in this recipe, and impart an especially intense flavor. If tomatoes are not in season, you can substitute canned Italian plum tomatoes. But fresh tomato sauce just can't come in a can.

3 pounds ripe fresh tomatoes or 1 can (35 ounces) Italian plum tomatoes, chopped

2 tablespoons olive oil

3 garlic cloves

2 tablespoons tomato paste

2-3 tablespoons chopped fresh basil leaves, or 2 teaspoons dried basil, crumbled

1 teaspoon sugar

1 teaspoon salt

1/4 teaspoon freshly ground black pepper

1 pound hot cooked pasta, such as spaghetti, vermicelli, or linguine

Freshly grated Parmesan cheese

1. If using fresh tomatoes, in a large, nonreactive saucepan or Dutch oven, bring water to a boil. Place the tomatoes in the boiling water for 1 minute to loosen the skins, then transfer the tomatoes to a bowl of cold water. Using a slotted spoon, transfer the tomatoes to paper towels to drain. Peel the tomatoes, cut them in half, and squeeze gently to expel the seeds; chop the tomato flesh.

2. In a large, heavy, nonreactive saucepan or Dutch oven over moderate heat, heat the oil. Add the garlic and cook 1 minute. Add the tomatoes, tomato paste, basil, and sugar, and bring the mixture to a boil, stirring constantly. Reduce the heat to low and simmer until the sauce thickens, 12 to 15 minutes.

3. Stir in the salt and pepper. Serve over the hot cooked pasta with a little Parmesan cheese sprinkled over all.

Makes 3 cups

Pasta Puttanesca
Put some spice in your tomato sauce with some real Mediterranean ingredients!

- 2 tablespoons olive oil
- 2 garlic cloves, minced
- 1 cup halved, pitted, large black Greek olives
- 1/4 cup drained capers
- 8 chopped anchovies
- 1/8-1/4 teaspoon crushed red pepper flakes
- 3 cups Fresh Tomato Sauce (opposite)
- 1 pound hot cooked pasta

1. In a large skillet over moderately low heat, heat the oil. Add the garlic and sauté, stirring occasionally, until soft, about 2 minutes. Add the olives, capers, anchovies, red pepper flakes to desired spiciness, and tomato sauce.

2. Increase the heat to moderately high. Simmer the sauce, uncovered, 15 minutes, stirring often. Serve over the hot cooked pasta.

Makes 6 servings

One-Minute Substitute

If You Run Out of Tomato Sauce
If a recipe calls for 2 cups tomato sauce and you don't have any on hand, combine 3/4 cup tomato paste and 1 cup water in a 2-cup measure and whisk until the mixture is well blended.

Fettuccine Alfredo
The king of cream sauces, Alfredo has a rich flavor that is entirely dependent on the quality of the cheese, so indulge in the best. You will still pay less than restaurant prices. There is no comparison with prepared Alfredo sauces.

- 3 tablespoons butter
- 1/3 cup minced shallots
- 1 1/4 cups heavy cream
- 1 cup light cream
- 1/2 teaspoon salt
- Pinch ground nutmeg
- 3/4 cup grated Parmesan cheese
- 1 pound fettuccine, cooked and drained

1. In a medium saucepan over moderate heat, melt the butter. Add the shallots and sauté until they are soft, 3 to 4 minutes. Stir in the heavy cream, light cream, salt, and nutmeg. Increase the heat to high and bring the mixture to a boil, stirring constantly. Reduce the heat to low and simmer, uncovered, until the sauce thickens, 4 to 5 minutes. Stir in the Parmesan cheese.

2. Place the fettuccine in a large, heated serving bowl and pour the Alfredo sauce over the pasta. Toss before serving.

Makes 4 servings

Penne with Four-Cheese Sauce
If you love cheese, this sauce is for you— not one, but four intriguing cheeses combine to make a superb pasta sauce. You can buy frozen lasagna made with this sauce for a considerable price that doesn't hold a candle to this savory homemade version.

3 tablespoons butter

2 garlic cloves, minced

2 tablespoons all-purpose flour

1 cup light cream

1 cup milk

1 cup shredded fontina cheese

1 cup shredded provolone cheese

1/2 cup shredded mozzarella cheese

1/2 cup grated Parmesan cheese

1/2 teaspoon salt

1/4 teaspoon ground pepper

1 pound hot cooked penne or other pasta, such as farfalle or rotini

1. In a large, nonstick saucepan over moderate heat, melt the butter. Add the garlic and cook until soft, about 2 minutes. Stir in the flour and cook until bubbly, about 1 minute. Remove the saucepan from the heat and gradually whisk in the cream and milk. Return the saucepan to moderate heat and cook, stirring often, until the sauce just boils and thickens, 3 to 5 minutes.

2. Add the cheeses, salt, and pepper, and cook, stirring constantly, until the cheeses melt and the sauce is smooth, 1 to 2 minutes.

3. Transfer the pasta to a heated serving bowl. Pour the cheese sauce over all and toss to mix well.

Makes 4 servings

Linguine with Red Clam Sauce
The secret is to sauté the garlic in the oil very gently so you don't burn the garlic and make it bitter. Properly cooked garlic has a light, nutty flavor that really brings out the flavor of the clams. No canned or frozen sauce can match the freshly made one.

1/4 cup olive oil

1 large yellow onion

3 garlic cloves, minced

1 can (28 ounces) Italian plum tomatoes, drained and chopped

1 teaspoon dried basil, crumbled

1/2 teaspoon sugar

1/4 teaspoon dried thyme

1/4 teaspoon salt

1/8-1/4 teaspoon crushed red pepper flakes

2 cans (6 1/2 ounces each) minced clams, with liquid

1/4 cup minced flat-leaf parsley

1 pound linguine, cooked and drained

1. In a large skillet over moderate heat, heat the oil for 1 minute. Add the onion and garlic, and sauté until soft, about 5 minutes. Add the tomatoes, basil, sugar, thyme, salt, and red pepper flakes. Simmer, uncovered, 3 minutes.

2. Stir in the clams and their liquid, and cook 1 minute more. Stir in the parsley.

3. Place the linguine in a large, hot serving bowl. Pour the clam sauce over the pasta, and toss well.

Makes 4 servings

Linguine with White Clam Sauce *One of the best pasta sauces, and so easy and inexpensive to make from scratch!*

1/4 cup olive oil

1 large yellow onion

3 garlic cloves, minced

1/3 cup dry vermouth or dry white wine

1/2 teaspoon salt

1/8-1/4 teaspoon crushed red pepper flakes

2 cans (6 1/2 ounces each) minced clams, with their liquid

1/4 cup minced flat-leaf parsley

1 pound linguine, cooked and drained

1. In a large skillet over moderate heat, heat the oil for 1 minute. Add the onion and garlic, and sauté until soft, about 5 minutes. Add the vermouth or wine, salt, and red pepper flakes. Simmer, uncovered, 3 minutes.

2. Stir in the clams and their liquid, and cook 1 minute more. Stir in the parsley.

3. Place the linguine in a large, hot serving bowl. Pour the clam sauce over the pasta, and toss well.

Makes 4 servings

Pasta with Classic Basil Pesto *It pays to use extra-virgin olive oil in this sauce, because it is not cooked. The intense flavor of the oil marries beautifully with the basil, garlic, and Parmesan cheese. Homemade is fresher and much tastier than any packaged pesto sauce.*

6 1/2 cups (about 2 bunches) firmly packed fresh basil

2 garlic cloves

1/4 cup extra-virgin olive oil

2 tablespoons butter, softened

1/2 cup grated Parmesan cheese

3/4 cup pine nuts

1/2 teaspoon grated lemon zest

1 teaspoon salt

1/4 teaspoon freshly ground pepper

1 pound hot cooked pasta

1. Pack the basil along with the garlic into the bowl of a food processor or blender. Whirl at high speed until all the leaves are pureed, about 2 minutes, scraping down the sides of the bowl as needed. With the motor still running, pour in the oil in a slow, steady stream.

2. Add the butter, cheese, pine nuts, lemon zest, salt, and pepper. Puree, scraping down the sides of the bowl 2 or 3 times, until the mixture forms a paste, about 3 minutes. Add a tablespoon or two of water if the mixture seems too stiff.

3. While the pasta is still very hot, add the pesto, about 1/2 cup at a time, tossing thoroughly after each addition to evenly distribute the sauce in the pasta; if the pesto is too sticky, add 1 tablespoon hot water to thin it slightly.

Makes 1 1/2 cups or 4 servings

Pesto Is More Than Green Basil Sauce

Pestare means "to pound" in Italian, and that is the technique used to make this simple, classic sauce. Most people are familiar with the green sauce made from pulverized basil leaves, but not all pestos are made from basil—they're not even all green. The technique is what makes it pesto.

Pasta with Mushroom Pesto *An earthy variation on the theme that would be quite costly if you had to buy it.*

2 tablespoons butter

1 garlic clove, minced

10 ounces fresh mushrooms, thinly sliced

2 tablespoons butter, softened

2 tablespoons snipped chives or scallion tops

1/2 cup grated Parmesan cheese

3/4 teaspoon salt

1/4 teaspoon freshly ground black pepper

1 pound hot cooked pasta

1. In a large skillet over moderately high heat, melt the butter. Add the garlic and mushrooms, and sauté until golden, 2 to 3 minutes.

2. Transfer the mushroom mixture to the bowl of a food processor or blender. Add the butter, chives or scallions, cheese, salt, and pepper. Whirl until the mixture is a smooth puree.

3. While the pasta is still very hot, add the mushroom pesto, about 1/2 cup at a time, tossing thoroughly after each addition to evenly distribute the sauce in the pasta; if the pesto is too sticky, add 1 tablespoon of hot water to thin it slightly.

Makes 3/4 cup or 4 servings

Pasta with Sun-Dried Tomato Pesto *Intense tomato flavors are enhanced by walnuts in another pesto that is always better when it is freshly made.*

1 cup tightly packed fresh basil leaves

1/2 cup sun-dried tomatoes in oil, undrained

1/4 cup chopped walnuts, raw or lightly toasted

1 small red chile pepper, seeded and chopped *(optional);* wear gloves when handling; they burn

1/2 cup olive oil

1/3 cup freshly grated Parmesan cheese

1 pound hot cooked pasta

1. Pack the basil into the bowl of a food processor or blender. Whirl at high speed until all the leaves are pureed, about 2 minutes, scraping down the sides of the bowl as needed. Add the tomatoes with their liquid, walnuts, and if using, red chile pepper. Whirl again to puree all the ingredients. With the motor still running, pour in the oil in a slow, steady stream.

2. Scrape the tomato-basil mixture into a large bowl. Fold in the cheese until it is incorporated.

3. While the pasta is still very hot, add the pesto, about 1/2 cup at a time, tossing thoroughly after each addition to evenly distribute the sauce in the pasta; if the pesto is too sticky, add 1 tablespoon of hot water to thin it slightly.

Makes about 1 cup or 4 servings

Ravioli *You can fill these tasty morsels with just about anything you like plus a soft cheese of some kind, such as the ricotta used below.*

1 batch pasta dough

Prosciutto-Ricotta Filling

2 teaspoons olive oil

1 ounce prosciutto, coarsely chopped

3 garlic cloves, minced

1 cup part-skim ricotta cheese

1/2 cup grated Parmesan cheese

1 egg yolk

1/2 cup minced fresh basil

1/2 teaspoon salt

1/4 teaspoon black pepper

Tomato Sauce

2 teaspoons olive oil

1 small yellow onion, chopped

2 garlic cloves, minced

1 can (28 ounces) Italian plum tomatoes, chopped with their juice

1/2 teaspoon salt

Freshly grated or shaved Parmesan cheese

1. Prepare the pasta dough. Cover the dough and let sit for 1 hour.

2. Meanwhile, prepare the prosciutto-ricotta filling: In a large nonstick skillet over moderate heat, heat the oil for 1 minute. Add the prosciutto and garlic and cook until the garlic is soft, about 2 minutes. Transfer the prosciutto mixture to a medium bowl and let cool to room temperature. Add the ricotta and Parmesan cheeses, egg yolk, basil, salt, and pepper, and stir gently to blend; set aside the prosciutto-ricotta filling.

3. Divide the dough into 2 equal portions. Re-cover 1 portion. On a lightly floured surface, roll out the second portion into a 9 x 12-inch rectangle, about 1/16-inch thick. Using a sharp knife or pastry wheel, cut the rectangle into 4 strips 3 inches wide and 9 inches long.

4. On 2 of the dough strips, drop 3 equal mounds of the filling, spacing the mounds about 1 inch apart and leaving a 1/2-inch margin all around the edges of the strip. Using a pastry brush, brush the margins around each mound with water. Carefully place 1 of the remaining dough strips on top of 1 mound-covered strip; repeat. Firmly press the dough along the margins and around each mound to seal the strips firmly. Slice each strip crosswise into 3 ravioli. Repeat with the remaining portion of the dough.

5. Prepare the tomato sauce: In a large, nonstick skillet over moderate heat, heat the oil for 1 minute. Add the onion and sauté, stirring occasionally, until soft, about 5 minutes. Add the garlic and cook 2 minutes more. Add the tomatoes and their juice, and the salt; bring the mixture to a boil over moderate heat; reduce the heat to a bubbling simmer, and cook, uncovered, stirring often, until the sauce thickens slightly, about 10 minutes.

6. Meanwhile, in a large pot of boiling water, cook the ravioli until firm-tender, about 6 minutes. Drain well, divide among 4 heated serving plates, and top with some of the tomato sauce. Serve with Parmesan cheese.

Makes 12 ravioli, about 4 servings

Make Your Own Take-Out Food   **595**

Lasagna

Homemade lasagna is a wonderfully welcoming dish that is better than anything you can buy. And you can make it with just the ingredients you like best. Homemade pasta offers a subtle base to the other ingredients.

1 batch homemade pasta or
   1 pound lasagna noodles,
   cooked until almost tender
   and drained

1/2 cup grated
   Parmesan cheese

1 cup shredded
   mozzarella cheese

Sauce

2 cans (28 ounces each)
   Italian plum tomatoes,
   undrained

1 medium yellow onion,
   finely chopped

4 garlic cloves, minced

1/4 cup chopped fresh basil

1/2 teaspoon dried thyme,
   crumbled

1/2 teaspoon salt

1/2 teaspoon ground
   black pepper

2 tablespoons all-purpose
   flour mixed with 1/4 cup
   cold water

Sausage Filling

1 tablespoon butter or
   olive oil

1 medium yellow onion,
   finely chopped

4 garlic cloves, minced

1 pound bulk Italian sausage,
   mild or spicy as desired

2 tablespoons butter or
   olive oil

10 ounces mushrooms,
   coarsely chopped

1. Prepare the sauce: In a large Dutch oven over moderately high heat, combine the tomatoes and their juice, the onion, garlic, basil, thyme, salt, and pepper; bring the mixture to a boil. Reduce the heat to moderately low, and simmer, uncovered, stirring occasionally to break up the tomatoes, 15 minutes. Slowly whisk in the flour-water paste and simmer, stirring constantly, until the sauce thickens, about 2 minutes.

2. Prepare the sausage filling: In a large skillet over high heat, melt 1 tablespoon butter or heat the oil. Add the onion and garlic, and sauté until the onion is golden, about 3 minutes. Add the sausage and cook, stirring occasionally to break up any lumps, until no pink remains, about 10 minutes. Transfer the sausage mixture to a large bowl.

3. In the same skillet over high heat, melt 2 tablespoons butter or heat the oil. Add the mushrooms and cook until light brown, about 5 minutes. Add the mushrooms to the sausage mixture along with 4 cups of the sauce.

4. Cover the bottom of an ungreased 9 x 13-inch baking dish with 1/2 of the remaining sauce. Top with a single layer of slightly overlapping lasagna noodles, 3 cups of the sausage filling, and 1/4 cup of the Parmesan cheese. Repeat the layers, beginning with the noodles. Scatter the mozzarella cheese over the top of the lasagna.

5. Cover the dish with foil, shiny side down, set the dish on a baking sheet, and bake until bubbly, 45 to 55 minutes. Let the lasagna stand for 10 minutes before serving.

Makes 6 servings

soups

Beef Barley Soup

The culinary use of barley can be traced back to the Stone Age. Pearl barley is the type most often used for soups—it is polished and the bran has been removed. Homemade beef barley soup is filling and delicious, a bargain all around.

1 tablespoon butter

1/2 cup chopped carrot

1/2 cup chopped celery

1/2 cup chopped onion

4 cups Beef Stock (page 49) or reduced-sodium canned beef broth

4 cups water

2 cups chopped cooked roast beef

1 can (14 1/2 ounces) diced tomatoes, undrained

1 cup quick-cooking barley

1 1/2 teaspoons salt

1/2 teaspoon dried basil, crumbled

1/2 teaspoon dried oregano, crumbled

1/2 teaspoon ground pepper

1/2 cup frozen peas

1. In a large saucepan or Dutch oven over moderate heat, melt the butter. Add the carrot, celery, and onion, and sauté until the vegetables are tender, about 5 minutes.

2. Add the stock, water, roast beef, tomatoes and their liquid, barley, salt, basil, oregano, and pepper; bring the mixture to a boil. Reduce the heat, cover the saucepan, and simmer for 20 minutes, stirring occasionally. Stir in the peas. Simmer, uncovered, 5 minutes longer.

Makes 8 servings

Helpful Hint | Make the Most of Soup

One of the all-time, soul-satisfying comfort foods, homemade soup is easy to make, nutritious and very tasty to eat, and usually extremely economical. It is a wonderful way to use up leftovers, from vegetable peelings to pot roast. Best of all, it is a filling meal you can make in a single pot. Add a tossed green salad and crusty bread or rolls, and you're ready to eat!

Black Bean Soup

Southwestern flavor fills every bowl of this stick-to-your-ribs favorite. Black beans are loaded with fiber, are a good source of iron, and contain lots of B vitamins. Homemade black bean soup can feed a crowd for practically pennies. There is no canned or dried equivalent.

1 pound dried black beans, sorted and rinsed

Water, as needed to cover

8 thick slices bacon

2 large yellow onions, chopped

2 celery stalks, chopped

2 medium carrots, chopped

2 garlic cloves, minced

2 bay leaves

1 teaspoon dried thyme, crumbled

8 cups water

1/2 teaspoon hot red pepper sauce

1/4 cup chopped fresh cilantro

2 tablespoons lemon juice

Sour cream or plain yogurt *(optional)*

8 fresh cilantro sprigs *(optional)*

1. Place the black beans in a 5-quart, heavy saucepan or Dutch oven; add enough cold water to cover the beans. Over high heat, bring the mixture to a boil; cook 2 minutes. Remove the saucepan from the heat, cover, and let the beans stand for 1 hour. Drain the beans and discard the cooking liquid; set aside the beans.

2. Using sharp kitchen shears, stack the bacon slices and cut them crosswise into 1/2-inch strips. (Place the bacon in the freezer for 1/2 hour before cutting.) Return the saucepan to moderately high heat and add the bacon strips. Cook, stirring occasionally, until the bacon is crisp, 5 to 8 minutes. Using a slotted spoon, transfer the bacon to paper towels to drain.

3. In the bacon drippings in the saucepan over moderate heat, sauté the onions, celery, carrots, garlic, bay leaves, and thyme, stirring occasionally, until the vegetables are tender, 8 to 10 minutes.

4. Add the water and reserved beans, and return to a boil; reduce the heat to moderately low, cover the saucepan, and simmer 45 minutes. Remove and discard the bay leaves.

5. In the bowl of a food processor or blender, place 1 cup of the black bean mixture and whirl until it is a smooth puree. Pour the bean puree back into the saucepan, add the reserved bacon, hot red pepper sauce, cilantro, and lemon juice, and stir until all the ingredients are well blended. Ladle the soup into individual soup bowls. If desired, garnish each serving with a dollop of sour cream or plain yogurt and a cilantro sprig.

Makes 8 servings

Chicken Noodle Soup

The medicinal mainstay of grandmothers and a childhood favorite of many, this yummy soup is full of vegetables, chunks of chicken, and egg noodles. Homemade is tastier and cheaper than canned or dried, and this version is quick and easy to make.

1 teaspoon butter

1 medium carrot, chopped

1 celery stalk, chopped

1/4 cup chopped onion

6 cups Chicken Stock (page 50) or canned broth

1 1/2 cups chopped cooked chicken

1 teaspoon salt

1/2 teaspoon dried marjoram

1/2 teaspoon dried thyme

1/8 teaspoon ground pepper

1 1/4 cups uncooked medium egg noodles

1 tablespoon minced parsley

1. In a large saucepan or Dutch oven over moderate heat, melt the butter. Add the carrot, celery, and onion, and sauté until the vegetables are tender, 8 to 10 minutes.

2. Add the stock, chicken, salt, marjoram, thyme, and pepper. Bring the mixture to a boil; reduce the heat and stir in the noodles. Cook until the noodles are tender, about 10 minutes. Stir in the parsley.

Makes 6 servings

Manhattan Clam Chowder

Big, bold, tomato taste is the trademark of this clam chowder. This easy home recipe tastes wonderful and costs very little.

2 tablespoons butter

1 large onion, chopped

1 large celery stalk, chopped

2 teaspoons chopped green bell pepper

1 garlic clove, minced

2 cups hot water

1 large potato, cubed

1 can (28 ounces) diced tomatoes, undrained

2 cans (6 1/2 ounces each) minced clams, undrained

1 teaspoon salt

1/2 teaspoon dried thyme

1/4 teaspoon ground pepper

Dash ground cayenne pepper

2 teaspoons minced parsley

1. In a 3-quart saucepan or Dutch oven over low heat, melt the butter. Add the onion, celery, bell pepper, and garlic, and cook, stirring frequently, until the vegetables are very soft, about 20 minutes.

2. Add the water and potato. Increase the heat to moderately high and bring the mixture to a boil; reduce the heat, cover, and simmer until the potato is tender, about 15 minutes.

3. Stir in the tomatoes with their liquid, clams with their liquid, salt, thyme, pepper, and cayenne. Cook until the chowder is heated through; stir in the parsley.

Makes 6 to 8 servings

Make Your Own Take-Out Food   **599**

New England Clam Chowder

This creamy, rich soup is how New Englanders like their clam chowder. You won't find anything like it in a can at any price.

24 cherrystone or chowder clams (about 2 pounds), scrubbed

4 slices turkey bacon, cut into 1/2-inch pieces

1 large onion, chopped

2 tablespoons all-purpose flour

1 pound all-purpose potatoes, peeled and cut into 1/2-inch cubes

2 cups reduced-fat (2%) milk

2 teaspoons fresh thyme leaves

1 bay leaf

Pinch ground red pepper

1/4 cup chopped flat-leaf parsley

1. Bring clams and 2 cups water to boil in a large saucepan over high heat. Reduce heat, cover, and simmer 5 minutes. Uncover and transfer clams with tongs or a slotted spoon to bowl as they open. Strain clam broth, adding enough water to equal 1 1/2 cups; set aside. Wipe out saucepan.

2. Lightly coat saucepan with nonstick cooking spray and set over medium heat. Sauté bacon and onion until onion is golden, about 7 minutes. Sprinkle in flour and cook, stirring constantly, just until bubbling but not browned, about 1 minute.

3. Add potatoes, milk, reserved clam broth, thyme, bay leaf, and pepper. Bring to a simmer over medium heat and cook, stirring occasionally, until potatoes are tender, about 10 minutes (do not boil).

4. Meanwhile, remove clams from shells and cut into bite-size pieces if necessary. Stir in clams and cook until heated through, about 2 minutes longer. Discard bay leaf. Ladle into bowls and sprinkle with parsley.

Makes 4 servings

Cream of Tomato Soup

Pair this with a grilled cheese sandwich and you've got the ultimate comfort meal. If you have eaten canned tomato soup all your life, you are in for a big treat!

2 1/2 cups diced peeled tomatoes, fresh or canned

1/4 cup diced celery

1/4 cup diced onion

1 tablespoon vegetable oil

2 tablespoons all-purpose flour

1 cup cream

1 teaspoon salt *(optional)*

1/8 teaspoon ground black pepper

3 tablespoons sour cream *(optional)*

3 teaspoons minced fresh parsley *(optional)*

1. In a medium saucepan over moderately high heat, combine the tomatoes, celery, and onion, and bring the mixture to a boil. Reduce the heat to low, cover the saucepan, and simmer 15 minutes, stirring often. Remove the saucepan from the heat and let the mixture cool for 10 minutes.

2. Pour the tomato mixture into the bowl of a food processor or blender. Whirl until the tomato mixture is a smooth puree.

3. In a large saucepan over moderate heat, heat the oil. Add the flour and stir until the mixture is smooth. Gradually add the cream, stirring constantly. Bring the cream mixture to a boil and cook for 2 minutes. Gradually add the tomato mixture, stirring constantly. Add the salt, if desired, and the pepper. Continue to cook until the soup is heated through. Ladle the soup into individual bowls and garnish each with a dollop of the sour cream and a sprinkle of the parsley, if desired.

Makes 3 servings

Gumbo

Is it soup or is it stew? We just know it's delicious if you whip it up yourself from scratch. This good Cajun flavor doesn't come in a can.

1/4 cup olive oil

1 pound beef brisket or chuck steak, cut into 1/2-inch chunks

6 ounces baked ham, cut into 1/2-inch chunks

1 large yellow onion, chopped

6 scallions, including green tops, thinly sliced

1 large red bell pepper, cored, seeded, and diced

3 tablespoons all-purpose flour

1 cup thinly sliced fresh okra or 1/2 package (10 ounces) frozen okra

4 cups Chicken Stock (page 50) or reduced-sodium canned chicken broth

8 ounces cabbage, cored and cut into 1/2-inch chunks

4 cups thinly sliced mustard greens

3 cups thinly sliced turnip greens

1/2 teaspoon salt

1/4 teaspoon ground black pepper

1 bay leaf

1/2 teaspoon dried thyme, crumbled

1/2 teaspoon dried marjoram, crumbled

4 whole allspice

2 whole cloves

1/8 teaspoon ground cayenne pepper

6 cups trimmed, washed, and chopped spinach

1 bunch watercress, tough stems removed and leaves chopped

1. In a large saucepan or an 8-quart Dutch oven over moderate heat, heat the olive oil about 2 minutes. Add the brisket or chuck steak and ham, and cook, stirring frequently, until the meat is lightly browned, about 5 minutes. Using a slotted spoon, transfer the meat to a bowl and set aside.

2. Add the onion and scallions to the Dutch oven and cook, stirring frequently, until the vegetables are softened, about 5 minutes. Add the red bell pepper and cook, stirring frequently, until it is crisp-tender, about 4 minutes. Stir in the flour until the vegetables are well coated. Add the okra and cook, stirring constantly, until all the ingredients are well combined. Gradually pour in the stock, stirring until well blended.

3. Add the cabbage, mustard greens, turnip greens, salt, pepper, bay leaf, thyme, marjoram, allspice, cloves, cayenne, and reserved meats. Bring the mixture to a boil, reduce the heat to moderately low, and simmer, stirring occasionally, until the gumbo is thickened and the beef is tender, about 1 1/2 hours.

4. Add the spinach and watercress. Cover the Dutch oven and cook until tender, about 15 minutes longer. Remove and discard the bay leaf.

Makes 4 servings

Lentil Soup
Long a staple of both Indian and Middle Eastern cooking, lentils are an excellent source of fiber, protein, folate, and iron. That's why lentil soup is so good for you. It tastes so good because you made it yourself—a low-cost one-dish dinner.

1 cup dried lentils, sorted and rinsed

6 cups Chicken Stock (page 50) or canned broth

1 tablespoon vegetable oil

2 cups chopped onion

1 garlic clove, minced

2 1/2 cups chopped fresh tomatoes

1 cup sliced carrots

1/2 teaspoon dried thyme

1/4 teaspoon dried marjoram

1. In a large saucepan over moderately high heat, combine the lentils and the stock, and bring the mixture to a boil. Reduce the heat to low and simmer 30 minutes.

2. Meanwhile, in a large skillet over moderately high heat, heat the oil. Add the onions and garlic, and sauté until tender, about 5 minutes. Pour the onion mixture into the saucepan with the lentils.

3. Add the tomatoes, carrots, thyme, and marjoram to the lentil mixture. Cook the mixture until the lentils and vegetables are tender, about 30 minutes.

Makes 8 servings

Minestrone
Italian cooks have no definite rules for what goes into minestrone. It just has to be a hearty mix of vegetables, white beans, and pasta or rice. To make it vegetarian, substitute vegetable broth for the beef broth. Nothing in a can tastes as good as this simple, homemade inexpensive soup.

1 tablespoon olive oil

1 large yellow onion, chopped

2 garlic cloves, minced

3 1/2 cups beef broth

1 can (15 ounces) great northern beans, drained

1 3/4 cups chopped tomatoes or 1 can (14 1/2 ounces) Italian-style tomatoes, undrained, cut up

2 cups coarsely shredded cabbage

2 large carrots, thinly sliced

1 teaspoon dried oregano

1 teaspoon dried basil

1/2 teaspoon salt

1/2 teaspoon ground pepper

2 ounces vermicelli, broken

1 small zucchini, sliced

Grated Parmesan cheese

1. In a large, nonstick saucepan over medium-high heat, heat oil. Add onion and garlic and sauté 5 minutes or until onion is tender. Stir in broth, beans, tomatoes, cabbage, carrots, oregano, basil, salt, and pepper.

2. Bring to a boil and stir in vermicelli. Reduce heat, cover, and simmer, 15 minutes or until vegetables and pasta are tender. Stir in zucchini and cook, uncovered, 3 minutes. Serve with cheese.

Makes 8 servings

Onion Soup

Easier to make than you may think, this classic of French cooking is mostly a matter of slicing onions! Nothing in a can or a packet compares.

- 2 tablespoons butter
- 5 medium yellow onions, thinly sliced
- 2 tablespoons sugar
- 3 1/2 cups Beef Stock (page 49) or canned broth
- 5 cups water
- 1/4 cup brandy *(optional)*
- 1/2 teaspoon salt
- 1/2 teaspoon ground pepper
- 4 slices (1/2-inch thick) French bread, toasted
- 4 tablespoons shredded Gruyère cheese

1. Preheat the oven to 400°F. In a large saucepan or 5-quart Dutch oven over moderately high heat, melt the butter. Add the onions and sugar, increase the heat to high, and sauté until the onions are lightly golden, about 10 minutes. Reduce the heat to moderately low and sauté 10 minutes longer, stirring occasionally.

2. Add the stock and water, increase the heat to high, and bring to a boil; reduce the heat to moderately low and simmer, uncovered, 20 minutes. Add the brandy, if desired, and the salt and pepper, and increase the heat to high; return the soup to a boil.

3. Place four 8-ounce ovenproof ramekins or soup bowls on a heavy-duty baking sheet or ovenproof metal tray. Ladle the soup into the bowls, dividing it equally. Place 1 slice French bread and 1 tablespoon of the cheese on top of each portion of soup.

4. Bake, uncovered, until the cheese is melted, about 5 minutes.

Makes 4 servings

Vegetable Soup

The best vegetable soup is made with the freshest produce, and it doesn't come from a can. You make it yourself from what's ripe in the garden or at the farmers' market.

- 3 tablespoons olive oil
- 1 large red onion, diced
- 5 garlic cloves, minced
- 2 large carrots, thinly sliced
- 4 medium squashes, diced
- 2 medium zucchini, diced
- 1/2 pound green beans, sliced
- 2 pounds tomatoes, peeled and chopped
- 5 cups Vegetable Stock (page 51) or canned broth
- 1 pound new potatoes, diced
- 3/4 teaspoon salt
- 3/4 teaspoon dried marjoram
- 1/2 teaspoon ground pepper

1. In a large saucepan or 5-quart Dutch oven over moderate heat, heat the oil. Add the onion and garlic, and cook until soft, about 5 minutes. Add the carrots and cook, stirring frequently, until the vegetables are soft, about 5 minutes.

2. Add the squashes, zucchini, green beans, tomatoes, stock, potatoes, salt, marjoram, and pepper. Increase the heat to high and bring the mixture to a boil; reduce the heat to moderately low, cover, and simmer until the vegetables are tender, 40 to 50 minutes.

Makes 4 servings

Split Pea Soup
This is a great winter soup to make when you have a ham bone in the house. You can make this soup to feed a crowd for pennies.

1 package (16 ounces) dried green split peas

2 1/2 quarts water, plus additional soaking water

1 ham bone

1 large onion, chopped

1 teaspoon salt

1/2 teaspoon ground black pepper

1/2 teaspoon dried thyme, crumbled

1 bay leaf

1 cup diced carrots

1 cup diced celery

1. In a large saucepan or Dutch oven, combine the split peas and enough water to cover the peas by 2 inches. Over high heat, bring the mixture to a boil; boil for 2 minutes. Remove the pan from the heat, cover, and let stand 1 hour. Drain and rinse the peas, discarding the soaking liquid. Return the peas to the saucepan.

2. Add the 2 1/2 quarts of water, the ham bone, onion, salt, pepper, thyme, and bay leaf to the saucepan. Over high heat, bring the mixture to a boil; reduce the heat to low, cover, and simmer 1 1/2 hours, stirring occasionally.

3. Using a slotted spoon, transfer the ham bone to a cutting board; let cool. Remove the meat from the bone; discard the bone. Cut the meat into dice, and return to the saucepan.

4. Add the carrots and celery to the saucepan. Over moderately low heat, simmer the soup, uncovered, until it reaches the desired consistency and the vegetables are tender, 45 to 60 minutes. Remove and discard the bay leaf before serving.

Makes 10 servings

Gazpacho
A great joy of summer is fresh tomatoes—and this chilled soup is the most refreshing way to use that bounty. Whip up a batch and keep it in the refrigerator in a pitcher for a quick, refreshing snack, lunch, or start to a grilled dinner. It's a treat you can make better than groceries or delis can, adapting it to your own taste.

3 cups chopped tomatoes

2 celery stalks, chopped

1 medium green pepper, chopped

1 medium cucumber, chopped

1/4 cup parsley, minced

1 tablespoon chives, minced

1 scallion, thinly sliced

1 garlic clove, minced

1 can (46 ounces) tomato juice

1/3 cup red wine vinegar

1/4 cup olive oil

1 teaspoon salt

1/2 teaspoon Worcestershire sauce

1/2 teaspoon ground pepper

Seasoned croutons *(optional)*

In a large, nonreactive bowl, combine all the ingredients, except croutons, and stir until well blended. Cover the bowl and refrigerate the soup for several hours or overnight. If desired, top each serving with a few croutons.

Makes 10 servings

salads

Classic Coleslaw
The quintessential side for a perfect picnic, tangy slaw offers crunchy texture and good nutrition. No deli slaw—at any price—can compare with your own.

1 small head green cabbage, shredded and immersed in ice water for 1 hour

3 medium carrots, shredded

1 cup Mayonnaise (page 29)

1/3 cup sugar

1/4 cup cider vinegar

1. Drain the cabbage and transfer it to paper towels. Blot the cabbage with additional towels until it is completely dry. In a large bowl, combine the cabbage and carrots, and toss to mix them thoroughly.

2. In a small bowl, combine the mayonnaise, sugar, and cider vinegar; stir until the mixture is well blended and a smooth consistency.

3. Pour the dressing over the cabbage mixture and toss until all the ingredients are well blended.

Makes 10 to 12 servings

Sweet-and-Sour Coleslaw
A tasty variation on a theme with lots of color—for even more color, substitute red cabbage for the green. Again, you can't match this recipe with one from a grocery or a deli.

8 cups shredded cabbage (about 1 small green cabbage)

2 carrots, peeled and grated

1 red bell pepper, cored, seeded, and finely chopped

1/3 cup corn oil

1 medium red onion, finely chopped

2 tablespoons firmly packed brown sugar

1/3 cup cider vinegar

1 tablespoon sweet pickle relish

1 teaspoon Dijon mustard

1 teaspoon salt

1/4 teaspoon ground black pepper

1. In a large, heatproof bowl, combine the cabbage, carrots, and red bell pepper.

2. In a large skillet over moderately high heat, heat the oil for 1 minute. Add the onion and sauté 2 to 3 minutes. Stir in the sugar and sauté 2 minutes longer. Stir in the vinegar, pickle relish, mustard, salt, and pepper.

3. Pour the hot dressing over the vegetables in the bowl, and toss to combine all the ingredients well. Let the coleslaw cool to room temperature before serving.

Makes 8 servings

Potato Salad

What would a picnic or barbecue be without this stalwart standby adding its creamy goodness and rib-sticking potatoes? Make your own for less money and better flavor. "Waxy" potatoes, such as new potatoes, red new potatoes, and California long whites, are ideal for salad making, since they have a firmer texture when cooked.

1 1/2 pounds potatoes, cut into same-size chunks

1 tablespoon cider vinegar

1 teaspoon sugar

1/2 cup chopped celery

1/2 cup chopped red onion

1/4 cup chopped stuffed olives

1/2 teaspoon salt

1/2 teaspoon celery seed

3/4 cup Mayonnaise (page 29) or salad dressing

2 hard-cooked eggs, chopped

1. In a large, nonreactive saucepan, combine the potatoes with enough water to cover. Over high heat, bring the water to a boil; boil until the potatoes are tender, 20 to 30 minutes. Drain the potatoes and remove the peels. When the potatoes are cool enough to handle, cut them into cubes and place in a medium bowl.

2. Drizzle the cider vinegar over the potatoes, then sprinkle with the sugar. Add the celery, onion, olives, salt, and celery seed. Add the mayonnaise and eggs, and fold gently until all the ingredients are well blended. Cover the bowl and refrigerate for at least 1 hour before serving.

Makes 4 servings

Hot German Potato Salad

A wonderful warm variation, this potato salad uses a cooked vinegar dressing with bacon for an enticing side dish to grilled or roasted meats. Make your own to save money and serve it warm.

4 thick slices bacon, diced

1/2 cup finely chopped yellow onion

1 tablespoon all-purpose flour

1/2 cup Beef Stock (page 49) or reduced-sodium canned beef broth

1/2 cup cider vinegar

2 tablespoons sugar

1 teaspoon salt

1/4 teaspoon ground black pepper

3 pounds small red- or white-skinned new potatoes, boiled, peeled, and cut into 1/4-inch-thick slices

1 cup sliced scallions

1/4 cup minced fresh parsley

1. In a medium skillet over moderately low heat, cook the bacon until it is crisp, about 5 minutes. Transfer the bacon to paper towels to drain completely.

2. Return the skillet to the heat and add the onion; sauté until the onion is soft, about 5 minutes. Stir in the flour until it is well blended; remove the skillet from the heat. Slowly add the stock, stirring constantly; stir in the vinegar, sugar, salt, and pepper. Return the skillet to the heat and bring the mixture to a boil, stirring constantly. Cook the dressing for 1 minute longer, reduce the heat to low, and keep the dressing warm.

3. Place the potatoes in a heatproof serving bowl. Add the scallions, parsley, and reserved bacon. Pour the hot dressing over the potato mixture and toss gently until all the ingredients are well blended.

Makes 6 servings

Pasta Salad

This salad uses roasted bell peppers for a colorful combination, but this basic pasta salad is also a good place to use whatever vegetables are in season—just blanch or sauté the vegetables before adding to the pasta. Made at home, it will be cheaper and tastier.

8 ounces pasta, such as fusilli, farfalle, or penne

1 medium red bell pepper, cored, seeded, and cut into 1/4-inch-thick strips

1 medium yellow bell pepper, cored, seeded, and cut into 1/4-inch-thick strips

2 tablespoons olive oil

2 tablespoons red wine vinegar

1/2 teaspoon salt

1/4 teaspoon ground black pepper

2 tablespoons minced fresh parsley

2 tablespoons minced fresh basil

2 tablespoons drained capers

2 garlic cloves, minced

1/2 cup diced red onion

1 cup peeled, seeded, and chopped tomatoes

1. Cook the pasta following the package directions until it is firm but tender. Drain the pasta and place it in a large serving bowl.

2. Add the remaining ingredients and toss gently until well blended.

3. Let the salad stand at room temperature for 30 minutes for the flavors to develop. Toss gently again before serving.

Makes 4 servings

Egg Salad

Dark pumpernickel or a flavorful rye sets off the creamy texture and taste of this old favorite—cheaper and better when you make it yourself with the ingredients you like best.

4 hard-cooked eggs, chopped

1/4 cup chopped green olives

1/4 cup Mayonnaise (page 29) or salad dressing

In a medium bowl, combine all the ingredients and gently fold until well blended.

Makes 4 servings

Ham Salad

A zesty addition to a picnic or buffet, serve on a crusty roll or with buttery crackers. Again, you can economize and customize by making this salad at home.

1 cup minced ham

1/4 cup Mayonnaise (page 29) or salad dressing

2 tablespoons sweet pickle relish

2 teaspoons mustard

1 teaspoon drained prepared horseradish

In a medium bowl, combine the ingredients and gently fold until well blended.

Makes 4 servings

Creamy Chicken Salad

Serve this old favorite on a bed of lettuce, with fruit, or as a filling for sandwiches. Chicken salad costs $8 a pound and up at the deli and isn't nearly as good as homemade, particularly if you use homemade mayonnaise.

2 cups Mayonnaise (page 29)

3/4 cup chopped celery

1 tablespoon mustard

1 1/4 teaspoons poppy seed

1/2 teaspoon salt

10 cups cubed cooked chicken

Chopped pecans

1. In a large bowl, combine the mayonnaise, celery, mustard, poppy seed, and salt. Stir until the ingredients are well blended.

2. Add the cooked chicken and gently fold to coat. Cover the bowl and place in the refrigerator for 3 to 4 hours until the salad is chilled. Sprinkle with the pecans before serving.

Makes about 12 servings

Curried Chicken Salad

A piquant filling for pita bread, this salad is also sensational served with tropical fruit or cooked rice. It's as good as any you can buy and costs much less.

1/2 cup Mayonnaise (page 29) or salad dressing

1/2 cup chutney

1-3 tablespoons curry powder

6 cups cubed cooked chicken

1. In a large bowl, combine the mayonnaise, chutney, and desired amount of curry powder. Stir until the ingredients are well blended.

2. Add the cooked chicken and gently fold to coat. Cover the bowl and place in the refrigerator for 3 to 4 hours until the salad is chilled and the flavors have developed.

Makes about 12 servings

Turkey Salad

A great way to use up leftover turkey, this recipe will allow you to make wonderful sandwiches for next to nothing. Serve on whole wheat rolls with lettuce.

1 cup finely chopped cooked turkey

1/4 cup Mayonnaise (page 29) or salad dressing

1/4 cup minced celery

1 tablespoon chili sauce

In a medium bowl, combine the ingredients and gently fold until well blended.

Makes 4 servings

Tuna Salad

An ingenious variation on the plain mayonnaise-tuna mixture, this special salad adds capers, red onion, and dill. And you can make it better and cheaper than what you would buy at the deli.

1/4 cup plus 1 tablespoon Mayonnaise (page 29)

3 tablespoons finely chopped red onion

3 tablespoons sweet pickle relish

2 tablespoons chopped celery

2 tablespoons lemon juice

1 tablespoon drained capers

1 tablespoon minced fresh dill

1/4 teaspoon salt

2 cans (6 1/2 ounces each) solid light tuna, drained

1. In a medium bowl, combine the mayonnaise, onion, pickle relish, celery, lemon juice, capers, dill, and salt. Stir until the dressing is well blended and smooth.
2. Add the tuna and gently fold until all the ingredients are well blended.

Makes 4 servings

Crab Salad

Though this salad is fabulous in a sandwich or served on whole-grain crackers, for a eye-catching buffet table, mound it in wedges of fresh papaya and sprinkle with a little chopped fresh parsley. Crab salad is a special treat—always pricey—so put the money into more and better crab and make your own.

1/4 cup Mayonnaise (page 29)

1/4 cup finely chopped celery

1/4 cup minced fresh parsley

2 tablespoons lemon juice

1/4 teaspoon salt

Pinch ground cayenne pepper

1 pound lump crabmeat, chopped

1/4 cup diced red bell pepper

1. In a medium bowl, combine the mayonnaise, celery, parsley, lemon juice, salt, and cayenne pepper. Stir until the dressing is well blended and smooth.
2. Add the crabmeat and red bell pepper, and gently fold until all the ingredients are well blended.

Makes 4 servings

Shrimp Salad

For some reason, shrimp seems to signal a party! This luscious salad is lovely served on a bed of mixed greens, as a filling for soft rolls, or with flatbreads. Make it yourself with shrimp you know are fresh and your own mayonnaise, and your less expensive version will be the best.

1/4 cup Mayonnaise (page 29)

1/4 cup finely chopped celery

2 tablespoons lemon juice

2 tablespoons minced fresh tarragon

1/4 teaspoon salt

Pinch ground cayenne pepper

1 pound diced cooked shrimp or tiny cocktail shrimp

1. In a medium bowl, combine the mayonnaise, celery, lemon juice, tarragon, salt, and cayenne pepper. Stir until the dressing is well blended and smooth.

2. Add the shrimp and gently fold until all the ingredients are well blended.

Makes 4 servings

Cobb Salad

Created at Hollywood's famed Brown Derby restaurant in 1936 by the owner, Robert Cobb, this noteworthy salad always features cooked chicken or turkey, bacon, eggs, avocado, and tomato in an eye-pleasing arrangement. Your own will be less expensive than any restaurant version.

1 large shallot, minced

1 tablespoon Dijon mustard

1 tablespoon red wine vinegar

3 tablespoons olive oil

1 medium head romaine lettuce, but into 2-inch-long pieces

2 hard-cooked eggs, peeled and coarsely chopped

1/2 cup drained, Roasted Bell Peppers in Oil (page 73) or bottled red bell peppers, cut into 2 x 1/4-inch strips

3 plum tomatoes, cut length-wise into 8 wedges

1 peeled, pitted, and sliced avocado

2 cups cooked chicken, cubed

24 niçoise olives

1/2 cup crisp-cooked, crumbled bacon

1/2 cup crumbled blue cheese

1. In a large bowl, combine the shallot, mustard, vinegar, and oil. Whisk until the dressing is well blended. Pour 1/2 of the dressing into a small bowl and set aside.

2. Add the romaine lettuce to the bowl and toss to coat with the remaining dressing. Divide the lettuce equally between 4 individual serving plates.

3. Arrange the eggs, bell pepper strips, tomatoes, avocado slices, chicken, and olives, divided equally, on top of the lettuce on each plate. Drizzle some of the reserved dressing over each salad and sprinkle with 1/8 cup of the bacon and 1/8 cup of the blue cheese.

Makes 4 servings

Salade Niçoise

A gorgeous and appetizing array of tuna, eggs, and vegetables, this great classic from the South of France is a picture-perfect composed salad. Delight your family and friends with your own version— fresh and custom made. No restaurant can match that or your costs.

1 large shallot, minced

1 tablespoon Dijon mustard

1 tablespoon drained capers

1 tablespoon
   red wine vinegar

3 tablespoons olive oil

1 medium head romaine
   lettuce, cut into 2-inch-
   long pieces

2 hard-cooked eggs, peeled
   and halved lengthwise

1/2 cup drained, Roasted
   Bell Peppers in Oil
   (page 73) or bottled
   red bell peppers, cut into
   2 x 1/4-inch strips

3 plum tomatoes, cut
   lengthwise into 8 wedges

2 carrots, peeled, parboiled,
   and thinly sliced

1/2 pound green beans,
   trimmed, blanched, and
   halved crosswise

1 pound small red new
   potatoes, boiled and cut
   into 1/4-inch-thick slices

24 niçoise olives

1 can (6 1/2 ounces)
   oil-packed tuna, drained

1. In a large bowl, combine the shallot, mustard, capers, vinegar, and oil. Whisk until the dressing is well blended. Pour 1/2 of the dressing into a small bowl and set aside.

2. Add the romaine lettuce to the bowl and toss to coat with the remaining dressing. Divide the lettuce equally between 4 individual serving plates.

3. Arrange the egg halves, bell pepper strips, tomatoes, carrots, beans, potatoes, olives, and tuna, divided equally, on top of the lettuce on each plate. Drizzle some of the reserved dressing over each salad or serve the dressing on the side.

Makes 4 servings

chapter 6

Easy-to-Make Sweet Treats

We are a country with a sweet tooth. Collected in this chapter are recipes for all kinds of sweet delicacies—candy, custards, fresh fruit mixtures,

ice creams, frozen yogurts, and ices—that will more than satisfy that yen for sweetness. What all these recipes have in common is that they are made with all-natural ingredients, with none of the fillers, stabilizers, or artificial sweeteners that often give store-bought sweets that faintly sawdust texture and slightly off taste. As a matter of fact, you'll find that sweets such as these are so good when you make them yourself that you may never venture into a candy shop or ice-cream parlor again—and certainly never buy a stale, boxed supermarket sweet again. And the treats you make at home won't cost you nearly as much as those pricey specialty store products do.

Some people may be surprised that you can make your own candies, but our grandparents thought nothing of making them, and it's really no more diffi-cult than making cookies—and sometimes easier. And whether you make dinner mints, lollipops, or peanut brittle, they taste incredibly better than the wrapped products you grew up with. On the following pages, you'll find hot and cold fruit desserts, along with custards and puddings and even a cappuccino mousse. And when summer comes, you have a full assortment of ice creams, frozen yogurts, ices, granitas, sorbets, and sherbets that you can try—topped perhaps with one of the dessert sauces from Chapter 1.

candy

Gumdrops

These chewy goodies can be tailored to the occasion: For Christmas, use red and green food coloring and peppermint extract; for spring, try yellow and orange coloring and lemon or orange extract. Children will want to help make them.

3 envelopes unflavored gelatin

1 1/4 cups water

1 1/2 cups sugar

1/4-1/2 teaspoon flavoring extract of choice

2 food colorings of choice

Additional sugar

1. In a small bowl, sprinkle the gelatin over 1/2 cup of the water; let the mixture stand for 5 minutes.

2. In a small saucepan over moderate heat, combine the sugar and the remaining water; bring the mixture to a boil, stirring constantly. Add the gelatin mixture and reduce the heat. Simmer the mixture, stirring constantly, for 5 minutes. Remove the saucepan from the heat and stir in the flavoring extract.

3. Divide the mixture, placing each half into a small bowl for the desired color; add 2 to 4 drops of the desired color into each bowl and stir until the color is even.

4. Lightly grease two 8 x 4 x 2-inch loaf pans. Pour from 1 bowl into 1 prepared pan; repeat with the remaining bowl and pan. Place the loaf pans in the refrigerator and chill until the mixture is firm, about 3 hours.

5. Lightly coat a work surface with sugar and fill a small saucer with sugar; cover a baking sheet with wax paper. Using a sharp knife, loosen the edges of the gumdrop mixture from the sides of the pans, then turn the mixture out onto the prepared surface. Cut the gumdrops into 1/2-inch cubes. Roll each cube in the sugar in the saucer until the gumdrop is completely coated. Place the gumdrops on the prepared baking sheet and let them stand at room temperature, uncovered, until they are dry on all sides, 3 to 4 hours; turn the gumdrops every hour to allow each side to dry. Cover the gumdrops with plastic wrap and store in the refrigerator until ready to serve.

Makes about 1 pound candy

Helpful Hint

Checking the Candy Thermometer

The one crucial item needed for candy making is a good-quality candy thermometer—which you should test before each use: Bring water to a boil and dip in the thermometer. It should read 212°F. Adjust your recipe temperature up or down based on your test.

Lollipops

Few goodies are as evocative of childhood as these brightly colored sweets on a stick. Flavoring oils can be purchased at health food stores—the flavor is more intense, and since, unlike extracts, they are not alcohol-based, the flavor won't evaporate either.

12 lollipop sticks

1 cup sugar

1/2 cup water

2 tablespoons light corn syrup

4-8 drops food coloring of choice

2-3 drops flavoring oil of choice

1. Line a large baking sheet with foil. Arrange the lollipop sticks on the prepared pan, spacing the sticks 4 inches apart.

2. In a heavy saucepan over moderate heat, combine the sugar, water, and corn syrup; cook, stirring, until the sugar has dissolved. Cover the saucepan, increase the heat to high, and boil the mixture for 1 minute to wash down any sugar crystals. Remove the cover, and boil the syrup until it registers 310°F on a candy thermometer. Immediately remove the saucepan from the heat and set it on a wire rack.

3. Let the syrup cool for 5 minutes, then add the food coloring and flavoring oil of choice; stir until the color is even.

4. Spoon the colored syrup over the top end of each lollipop stick, making a puddle about 2 to 3 inches in diameter. Let the lollipops stand until they are completely cool and the candy has hardened. Wrap each lollipop in plastic wrap and secure below the candy.

Makes about 12 lollipops

Butterscotch

Buttery good, this recipe calls for rum extract to create its distinctive flavor. This homemade candy is rich and delicious and very inexpensive.

1 teaspoon plus 1 cup butter cut into cubes

2 1/2 cups firmly packed light brown sugar

3/4 cup water

1/2 cup light corn syrup

1/4 cup honey

1/2 teaspoon salt

1/2 teaspoon rum extract

1. Use the 1 teaspoon of butter to coat a 15 x 10 x 1-inch baking pan; set aside.

2. In a heavy saucepan over moderate heat, combine the sugar, water, and corn syrup. Cover the saucepan and bring the mixture to a boil; do not stir. Uncover the saucepan and continue to cook the mixture until a candy thermometer reads 270°F (soft-crack stage).

3. Add the honey, salt, and butter cubes. Cook, stirring constantly, until the mixture reaches 300°F (hard-crack stage). Remove the saucepan from the heat. Stir in the rum extract.

4. Pour the butterscotch into the prepared pan without scraping; do not spread. Let the butterscotch cool until the candy is almost set, 1 to 2 minutes. Using a sharp knife, score the butterscotch into 1-inch squares and let the candy cool completely. Break the candy squares along the scored lines. Store the butterscotch in an airtight container.

Makes 1 1/2 pounds candy

Caramels
Chewy, gooey, and irresistible, these candies save money and make great treats for Christmas stockings or birthday favor baskets.

1 cup sugar

1 cup dark corn syrup

1 cup butter or margarine

1 can (14 ounces) sweetened condensed milk

1 teaspoon vanilla extract

1. Line an 8-inch square baking pan with foil and grease the foil with butter; set aside.

2. In a 3-quart saucepan over moderate heat, combine the sugar, corn syrup, and butter or margarine. Bring the mixture to a boil, stirring constantly; reduce the heat slightly and boil slowly for 4 minutes without stirring.

3. Remove the saucepan from the heat and stir in the condensed milk. Return the saucepan to the heat, reducing the heat to moderately low. Cook the mixture until a candy thermometer reads 238°F (soft-ball stage), stirring constantly. Remove the saucepan from the heat and stir in vanilla.

4. Pour the candy into the prepared pan and let stand until the caramels are cool. Remove the caramels from the pan and cut them into 1-inch squares. Wrap each caramel individually in wax paper or plastic wrap, twisting the ends to seal.

Makes 64 caramels

Fudge
Using not one, but three kinds of chocolate, plus pecans and marshmallows, makes this a deep, rich, chocolaty dream of a fudge that will match any you can buy.

3 1/3 cups sugar

1 cup butter or margarine

1 cup firmly packed dark brown sugar

1 can (12 ounces) evaporated milk

32 large Marshmallows, halved (page 207)

2 cups (12 ounces) semisweet chocolate chips

2 milk chocolate candy bars (7 ounces each), broken into pieces

2 squares (1 ounce each) semisweet baking chocolate, chopped

1 teaspoon vanilla extract

2 cups chopped pecans

1. Grease a 15 x 10 x 1-inch baking pan.

2. In a large saucepan over moderate heat, combine the sugar, butter or margarine, brown sugar, and evaporated milk. Cook, stirring, until the sugar has completely dissolved. Increase the heat to high and bring the mixture to a boil; boil for 5 minutes, stirring constantly.

3. Remove the saucepan from the heat and add the marshmallows, stirring until they are melted. Add the chocolate chips and pieces and stir until they are melted. Fold in the vanilla and pecans until the mixture is well blended.

4. Pour the mixture into the prepared baking pan, spreading it evenly. Place the baking pan in the refrigerator and chill the fudge until it is firm. Using a sharp knife, cut the fudge into squares.

Makes 5 1/2 pounds

Peppermint Patties
These patties provide a burst of peppermint in your mouth.

3 3/4 cups confectioners' sugar

3 tablespoons butter, softened

2-3 teaspoons peppermint extract

1/2 teaspoon vanilla extract

1/4 cup evaporated milk

2 cups (12 ounces) semisweet chocolate chips

2 tablespoons shortening

1. In a medium bowl, combine the sugar, butter, peppermint, and vanilla. Pour in the milk and beat until the ingredients are well blended.

2. Cover 2 to 3 baking sheets with wax paper. Pinch off some of the peppermint mixture and roll it into a 1-inch-diameter ball. Place the peppermint ball on the prepared baking sheet and press with the bottom of a glass to flatten the ball into a 1/4-inch-thick patty. Repeat with the remaining peppermint mixture. Cover the patties with plastic wrap and place the baking sheet in the freezer for 30 minutes.

3. In a heavy saucepan over low heat or a microwave-safe bowl following the manufacturer's directions, melt the chocolate chips and shortening; stir until the mixture is smooth.

4. Dip each peppermint patty into the melted chocolate to coat the patty completely. Place the coated patty back on the wax-paper-covered baking sheet. Repeat to coat all the patties with chocolate. Let the coated patties stand at room temperature until the chocolate is set. Store in an airtight container.

Makes 5 dozen patties

Pastel Mint Patties
Pretty confections perfect for a wedding or baby shower buffet.

1/4 cup butter, softened

1/3 cup light corn syrup

4 cups confectioners' sugar

1/2-1 teaspoon peppermint extract

3 food colorings of choice

About 1 cup granulated sugar

1. In a small bowl, combine the butter and corn syrup. Add 2 cups sugar and the peppermint. Beat the mixture until it is well blended. Add another cup of sugar and beat well.

2. Lightly coat a work surface with the remaining sugar. Turn out the mixture onto the surface. Knead until the sugar is completely absorbed and the mixture is smooth.

3. Divide the peppermint mixture into three portions. Set aside one portion to remain white; tint the remaining portions the color desired by adding 1 to 2 drops of food coloring and kneading until the portion is the desired color.

4. Cover a baking sheet with wax paper. Place the granulated sugar in a shallow bowl or saucer. Pinch off a walnut-size piece of mixture. Using your hands, roll the piece into a ball, then roll the ball in the granulated sugar. Place the ball on the prepared baking sheet and, using a fork, flatten into a patty. Repeat with the remaining peppermint mixture and sugar. Let the patties stand, uncovered, at room temperature for 1 day. Store the patties in an airtight container.

Makes about 7 1/2 dozen patties

Easy-to-Make Sweet Treats **617**

Pralines

This Southern confection is loaded with pecans—for the best-tasting pralines, select the freshest, best-quality pecans you can find. Homemade pralines are an easy, inexpensive treat that you can share with friends.

1 cup sugar

1 cup firmly packed brown sugar

1 cup milk

8 large purchased or homemade Marshmallows (page 207)

2 cups coarsely chopped pecans

2 tablespoons butter

1/2 teaspoon vanilla extract

Dash ground cinnamon

1. Lightly grease 2 baking sheets with butter; set aside.

2. In a medium, heavy saucepan over low heat, combine the granulated and brown sugars, milk, and marshmallows. Cook, stirring constantly, until the marshmallows are completely melted. Increase the heat to moderate and cook, stirring occasionally, until a candy thermometer reads 234°F to 240°F (soft-ball stage). Without stirring or scraping, pour the hot mixture into a second heavy saucepan. Add the pecans, butter, vanilla, and cinnamon. Stir rapidly until the mixture is thickened and creamy, about 3 minutes.

3. Using a tablespoon, drop the mixture onto the prepared baking sheets, placing the pralines about 1 inch apart; flatten the pralines slightly. Let stand until the pralines are set. Store in an airtight container.

Makes about 2 dozen pralines

Peanut Brittle

Crunchy with peanuts, melt-in-your-mouth delicious, this is a true classic candy that the whole family can help to make and package as gifts. It's not nearly as much fun to buy it.

2 3/4 cups sugar

1/2 stick unsalted butter

2/3 cup water

1 1/2 cups lightly salted peanuts

1. Grease a 9 x 13-inch baking pan, then line the pan with foil.

2. In a large, heavy saucepan over moderate heat with a wooden spoon, combine the sugar, butter, and water; simmer, stirring occasionally, until the mixture becomes a golden-brown syrup, about 25 minutes. Once the darkened mixture begins to bubble, remove the saucepan from the heat to a cool surface.

3. Add the peanuts to the syrup and stir until the nuts are evenly distributed. Pour the mixture into the prepared pan, spreading it evenly and ensuring that the peanuts are distributed equally.

4. Let the peanut brittle stand until it is cool and set completely, about 30 minutes. Using a knife handle, break the peanut brittle into bite-size pieces; store in an airtight container in a cool, dry place for up to 1 month.

Makes about 45 pieces

Peanut Butter Cups *This is a tantalizing combination of chocolate and peanut butter.*

- 1 milk or dark chocolate candy bar (7 ounces), broken into pieces
- 1/4 cup butter
- 1 tablespoon shortening
- 1/4 cup creamy Peanut Butter (page 33)

1. Line the cups in a miniature muffin pan with paper or foil baking cups.

2. In a heavy saucepan over low heat or in a microwave-safe bowl following the manufacturer's directions, combine the chocolate, butter, and shortening. Stir until the mixture is smooth.

3. In a second heavy saucepan over low heat or in a microwave-safe bowl following the manufacturer's directions, heat the peanut butter until it has melted.

4. Pour 1 tablespoon of the chocolate into each of the prepared cups. Drop 1 tablespoon of peanut butter onto the chocolate in each cup. Pour the remaining chocolate, divided equally, into the cups, covering the peanut butter.

5. Place the muffin pan in the refrigerator until the cups are set, about 30 minutes. Store in airtight container in refrigerator.

Makes 1 dozen cups

Toffee Bars *These candy bars are a crunchy confection sure to delight.*

- 1 tablespoon plus 1 3/4 cups butter, softened
- 2 cups sugar
- 1 tablespoon light corn syrup
- 1 cup chopped pecans
- 1/4 teaspoon salt
- 1 pound milk chocolate candy coating

1. Use the 1 tablespoon of butter to grease a 15 x 10 x 1-inch baking pan; set aside.

2. In a heavy 3-quart saucepan over moderate heat, melt the remaining butter. Add the sugar and corn syrup; cook and stir until a candy thermometer reads 295°F (soft-crack stage). Remove the saucepan from the heat; stir in the pecans and salt.

3. Quickly pour the toffee mixture into the prepared pan. Let the toffee mixture stand for 5 minutes. Using a sharp knife, score the top of the toffee into the desired-size bars. Let the toffee stand at room temperature until cool. Break or cut the toffee into bars along the score lines.

4. Cover 1 or 2 baking sheets with wax paper. In a heavy saucepan over low heat or in a microwave-safe bowl following the manufacturer's directions, melt the chocolate candy coating, stirring often. Dip each toffee bar into the chocolate coating until it is completely covered. Then place the coated bar on the prepared baking sheet. Let the coated bars stand at room temperature until the chocolate has set.

Makes 2 1/4 pounds candy bars

Cow Pies
A silly name for a scrumptious sweet, full of almonds and raisins, with chocolate holding it all together.

2 cups (12 ounces) semisweet or milk chocolate chips

1 tablespoon shortening

1/2 cup raisins

1/2 cup chopped slivered almonds

1. In a heavy saucepan over low heat or a microwave-safe bowl following the manufacturer's directions, combine and melt the chocolate chips and the shortening; stir until the mixture is smooth. Remove the saucepan from the heat and stir in the raisins and almonds.

2. Line 2 baking sheets with wax paper. Using a tablespoon, scoop up the chocolate mixture and drop it onto the prepared sheets. Place the baking sheets in the refrigerator and chill the cow pies until ready to serve.

Makes 2 dozen candies

Fruit and Nut Truffles
Serve these sumptuous sweets with after-dinner espresso.

9 ounces bittersweet chocolate

2 tablespoons heavy cream

2 tablespoons cognac or rum

1 1/4 cups apricots, finely chopped

1/2 cup hazelnuts, finely chopped

2 tablespoons crystallized ginger, minced

2 tablespoons confectioners' sugar, sifted

30 hazelnut halves

1. Line a large baking sheet with baking parchment or foil. Lay a large piece of wax paper on a work surface.

2. In the top of a double boiler over low heat, cook 4 ounces of the chocolate, stirring, until it is melted. Remove the top saucepan from the heat and add the cream and cognac, beating until the mixture is well blended. Add the apricots, hazelnuts, ginger, and sugar, and stir until all the ingredients are well blended. Set the saucepan in the refrigerator and chill the mixture until it is firm enough to handle.

3. Using a spoon, scoop up a walnut-size portion of the mixture. Using your hand, roll the portion into a 1-inch-diameter ball, and place the ball on the prepared work surface. Repeat with the remaining mixture.

4. In the top of the double boiler over low heat, cook the remaining 5 ounces of chocolate, stirring, until it is melted. Remove the double boiler from the heat.

5. Using a fork, spear 1 fruit and nut ball. Dip the ball into the melted chocolate until the ball is completely coated; allow any excess chocolate to run back into the saucepan. Place the coated ball on the prepared baking sheet and top with 1 hazelnut half. Repeat with the remaining fruit and nut balls, chocolate, and hazelnut halves. Place the baking sheet in the refrigerator until the truffles are chilled and the chocolate has set.

6. Store the truffles in an airtight container in the refrigerator for up to 1 month.

Makes 30 truffles

Marshmallows

An electric stand mixer makes these homemade marshmallows quick and easy to whip up. They cost less than the commercial ones, and your children will love the process.

3 tablespoons confectioners' sugar

3 tablespoons cornstarch

1 1/2 tablespoons unflavored gelatin

1/3 cup water

1/2 cup granulated sugar

2/3 cup light corn syrup

1. Line a 13 x 9 x 2-inch baking pan with wax paper. In a small sieve, combine 1 tablespoon of the confectioners' sugar and 1 tablespoon of the cornstarch, and sift the mixture over the prepared pan.

2. In a medium bowl, combine the gelatin and water; let stand until the gelatin has softened, about 5 minutes.

3. Place the bowl in a large saucepan or deep skillet of simmering water. Stir until the gelatin has dissolved. Add the granulated sugar and continue to stir until the sugar has dissolved. Remove the bowl from the water and add the corn syrup. Using an electric mixer, beat the mixture until it is creamy and thick, 10 to 15 minutes. Let the mixture stand until it is cool.

4. Using a wet spatula, spread the mixture in the prepared pan, smoothing the top evenly. Let the mixture sit until it is cool and set, about 20 minutes.

5. Carefully lift the marshmallow mixture onto a cutting board. Following Step 1, lightly dust the marshmallow with 1 tablespoon of the remaining confectioners' sugar and cornstarch. Using a sharp knife, cut the marshmallow into small squares. In a cup, combine the remaining 1 tablespoon of confectioners' sugar and the cornstarch. Dip each marshmallow into the mixture until it is completely coated. Store the marshmallows in an airtight container in a cool, dry place for 1 to 2 weeks.

Makes about 36 marshmallows

One-Minute Substitute

If You Run Out of Corn Syrup

If a recipe calls for 1 cup corn syrup and you don't have any on hand, combine 1 cup regular granulated sugar and 1/4 additional cup of the liquid used in the recipe in a 2-cup measure. Stir until the mixture is blended.

Candied Citrus Peels
Dip these zesty treats in chocolate for an easy confection, or use them for decorations on cakes, ice cream, and other desserts.

3 firm, ripe lemons or
  oranges
1/4 cup granulated sugar
1/2 cup water

1. Using a swivel-bladed vegetable peeler, remove the peel from the citrus fruit, leaving the bitter white pith. Using a sharp knife, cut the peel into strips. For decorations, cut it into matchstick-thin strips; for dipping in chocolate, cut it into larger strips.

2. In a small saucepan, combine the citrus strips and add enough cold water to cover the strips. Over high heat, bring the water to a boil. Immediately drain the strips and rinse them under cold running water.

3. Return the strips to the saucepan; add the sugar and the 1/2 cup of water. Over moderate heat, cook the mixture until the liquid has evaporated and the peel is bright and shiny.

4. Spread a sheet of foil over a work surface. Transfer the candied peel to the foil to cool, keeping the strips separate. Store in an airtight container in the refrigerator for up to 6 months.

Makes about 1 cup

custards, mousses, and puddings

Vanilla Pudding
Marvelously satisfying on its own, vanilla pudding can also be the base for toasted nuts or coconut, miniature chocolate chips, or fresh berries. Or spoon some over Dried Fruit Compote (page 214).

3/4 cup sugar
1 1/2 tablespoons cornstarch
Pinch salt
2 cups milk
1 egg
2 tablespoons butter
1 teaspoon vanilla extract

1. In a medium saucepan, combine the sugar, cornstarch, and salt. Add the milk and stir until the mixture is smooth. Over moderate heat, cook the mixture, stirring constantly, until it boils and thickens; reduce the heat and simmer, stirring constantly, for 2 minutes. Remove the saucepan from the heat.

2. In a medium bowl using an electric mixer, beat the egg until it is foamy. Gradually stir in about 1/2 cup of the hot milk mixture. Stirring constantly, pour the egg mixture back into the remaining hot milk mixture. Cook over low heat, stirring constantly, for 2 minutes longer.

3. Remove the saucepan from the heat, stir in the butter and vanilla. Immediately pour the pudding into a large serving bowl or individual dessert dishes. Let the pudding cool to room temperature, then refrigerate.

Makes 4 to 6 servings

Chocolate Pudding

Like a grilled cheese sandwich, chocolate pudding is pure comfort food. You can make it from a packet or take a few more minutes and make it much better from scratch.

3/4 cup sugar

1 1/2 tablespoons cornstarch

Pinch salt

2 cups milk

2 ounces semisweet chocolate, chopped

1 egg

2 tablespoons butter

1 teaspoon vanilla extract

1. In a medium saucepan, combine the sugar, cornstarch, and salt. Add the milk and stir until the mixture is smooth; add the chocolate. Over moderate heat, cook the mixture, stirring constantly, until it boils and thickens; reduce the heat and simmer, stirring constantly, for 2 minutes. Remove the saucepan from the heat.

2. In a medium bowl using an electric mixer, beat the egg until it is foamy. Gradually stir in about 1/2 cup of the hot milk mixture. Pour the egg mixture back into the remaining hot milk mixture. Cook over low heat, stirring constantly, for 2 minutes longer.

3. Remove the saucepan from the heat, stir in the butter and vanilla. Immediately pour the pudding into a bowl or individual dessert dishes. Let the pudding cool to room temperature, then refrigerate.

Makes 4 to 6 servings

Rice Pudding

This is an old favorite that you can buy at any deli or grocery store. Once you have made your own—with or without raisins—you will save your money for other things.

3 1/2 cups milk

1/2 cup uncooked long-grain rice

1/3 cup sugar

1/2 teaspoon salt *(optional)*

1/2 cup raisins

1 teaspoon vanilla extract

Ground cinnamon *(optional)*

1. Preheat the oven to 325°F; lightly butter a 1 1/2-quart baking dish.

2. In a medium saucepan, combine the milk, rice, sugar, and if desired, the salt. Over moderate heat and stirring constantly, bring the mixture to a boil. Pour the hot mixture into the prepared baking dish, cover, and bake 45 minutes, stirring every 15 minutes.

3. Stir in the raisins and vanilla, re-cover, and bake 15 minutes longer. Remove the baking dish from the oven. If desired, sprinkle the top of the pudding with cinnamon before serving; serve warm or chilled.

Makes about 6 servings

Orange Rice Pudding
A new twist on an old favorite, this pudding uses a custard base for a very creamy rice pudding.

1/2 cup short-grain rice

2/3 cup water

1/8 teaspoon salt

1 cup milk

1 cup heavy cream

1/3 cup sugar

2 eggs

1 teaspoon grated
orange zest

1/8 teaspoon ground nutmeg

1. Preheat oven to 325°F; butter a 6-cup ovenproof dish.

2. In a medium saucepan over moderate heat, combine the rice, water, and salt; bring the mixture to a boil. Reduce the heat, cover the saucepan, and simmer 12 minutes. Remove the saucepan from the heat and add the remaining ingredients. Stir vigorously until well blended.

3. Pour the rice mixture into the prepared baking dish. Bake until the pudding is set, about 50 minutes. Serve warm or chilled.

Makes 6 servings

Crème Brûlée
This classic French custard is as tasty and exotic as its name.

Custard

3 cups milk

3/4 cup sugar

1 vanilla bean, split
lengthwise

4 strips (3 x 1/2 inch each)
orange zest

3 strips (2 x 1/2 inch each)
lemon zest

3 strips (2 x 1/2 inch each)
lime zest

1/4 teaspoon salt

3 eggs plus 3 egg yolks

Topping

3/4 cup firmly packed light
or dark brown sugar

1. Set 8 ungreased 6-ounce flameproof ramekins, spaced apart, on a folded kitchen towel in a large baking pan.

2. Prepare the custard: In a medium nonreactive saucepan over moderate heat, combine the milk, 1/4 cup of the sugar, vanilla bean, orange, lemon, and lime zests, and salt. Bring to a simmer; remove from heat, cover, and let stand for 30 minutes.

3. Preheat the oven to 325°F. In a large bowl using a whisk, combine the eggs and additional yolks and the remaining 1/2 cup sugar; beat until just blended. Set a large sieve over the bowl, and pour the milk mixture through into the egg mixture. Whisk until the ingredients are blended.

4. Spoon the custard into the ramekins. Pour enough water into the baking pan to come halfway up the sides of the ramekins. Bake, uncovered, until a knife inserted into the center of a custard comes out clean, about 45 minutes.

5. Remove the ramekins from the baking pan to wire racks. Preheat the broiler. Sprinkle 1 1/2 teaspoons of the brown sugar over the top of each custard. Place the ramekins in the broiler, 6 to 8 inches from the heat source, and broil until the sugar melts, about 45 seconds.

6. Remove the ramekins to wire racks and let cool to room temperature. Serve at room temperature or slightly chilled; do not refrigerate too long or the crust will begin to soften.

Makes 8 servings

Crème Caramel

You can make this popular restaurant dessert yourself for pennies. To make a lower-fat version, substitute 3 cups evaporated skim milk for the whole milk, 1 1/2 cups egg substitute for the whole eggs and yolks, and reduce the sugar to 2/3 cup.

Caramel

1/2 cup sugar

1/2 cup water

Custard

3 cups milk

3/4 cup sugar

1 vanilla bean, split
   lengthwise

4 strips (3 x 1/2 inch each)
   orange zest

3 strips (2 x 1/2 inch each)
   lemon zest

3 strips (2 x 1/2 inch each)
   lime zest

1/4 teaspoon salt

3 eggs plus 3 egg yolks

1. Prepare the caramel: In a small saucepan over moderately high heat, combine the sugar and water, and bring the mixture to a boil. Continue to boil until the sugar turns amber in color, about 5 minutes. Pour the caramel into the bottoms of 8 ungreased 6-ounce ramekins. Tilt each ramekin to coat the bottom and about 1 inch of the sides. Place the ramekins on a folded kitchen towel in a baking pan large enough to hold them without touching.

2. Prepare the custard: In a medium nonreactive saucepan over moderate heat, combine the milk, 1/4 cup of the sugar, vanilla bean, orange, lemon, and lime zests, and salt. Bring the mixture to a simmer; remove the saucepan from the heat, cover, and let stand for 30 minutes.

3. Preheat the oven to 325°F. In a large bowl using a whisk, combine the eggs and additional yolks and the remaining 1/2 cup sugar; beat until just blended. Set a large sieve over the bowl, and pour the milk mixture through into the egg mixture. Whisk until the ingredients are blended.

4. Spoon the custard into the caramel-coated ramekins. Pour enough water into the baking pan to come halfway up the sides of the ramekins. Bake, uncovered, until a knife inserted into the center of a custard comes out clean, about 45 minutes.

5. Remove the ramekins from the baking pan to wire racks and let the custard cool to room temperature; refrigerate until ready to serve.

6. To serve, run a knife around the edges of the custards to loosen them, then invert the ramekins onto rimmed dessert plates or shallow dessert bowls. Allow the caramel to run down the custards and form a pool around them.

Makes 8 servings

Helpful Hint

Take Extra Care When Making Custard

Although it is surprisingly easy to make, custard requires a bit of cooking know-how: Don't overmix the eggs; more yolks mean smoother texture means slower cooking time; the container used for baking will determine the time, and it's safest to stick to the one specified in the recipe. You can do it, and it will be better than any you buy (and cheaper too).

Easy-to-Make Sweet Treats   **625**

Chocolate Mousse

The ultimate mousse experience—and the higher quality the chocolate you use, the more outstanding the final result. Expensive at a gourmet shop or restaurant, chocolate mousse can be made at home for much less and tastes even better.

8 ounces semisweet chocolate, coarsely chopped

3 eggs, separated

3/4 cup heavy cream

1/2 cup sugar

1/4 cup water

1 teaspoon vanilla extract

1. In the top of a double boiler over simmering water, melt the chocolate. Meanwhile, in a medium bowl with an electric mixer, beat the egg yolks until they are thick. Pour a little of the melted chocolate into the egg yolks, whisking constantly, then whisk all the egg yolk mixture back into the double boiler. Add 1/4 cup of the cream and whisk until well blended. Cook, stirring constantly, until the mixture thickens and reaches 160°F, about 4 minutes. Remove the top of the double boiler and let the chocolate mixture cool to room temperature, whisking often.

2. In a small saucepan over moderate heat, combine the sugar and water, and bring the mixture to a boil. Using a pastry brush dipped in water, brush down the sides of the saucepan, then cook the syrup without stirring until it reaches 238°F on a candy thermometer, about 5 minutes.

3. In a medium heatproof bowl with an electric mixer on medium speed, beat the egg whites until they are frothy. Place the bowl in a larger saucepan of boiling water (double-boiler style). With the mixer on low speed, gradually beat the boiling sugar syrup into the egg whites until the meringue peaks stiffly and a candy thermometer inserted at the center reaches 160°F. Whisk 1/3 cup of the hot meringue into the chocolate mixture, then fold in the remaining meringue.

4. In a small bowl with an electric mixer on high, beat the remaining 1/2 cup of cream until it forms soft peaks; beat in the vanilla. Fold the whipped cream into the chocolate mixture until no white streaks remain. Spoon into individual serving dishes or glasses, cover, and refrigerate for at least 1 hour or until serving time.

Makes 8 servings

Cappuccino Mousse

The aroma and flavor of cappuccino in a mousse is seductive. Make your own cappuccino mousse and serve it with espresso on the side. You'll save money and delight friends.

8 ounces semisweet chocolate, coarsely chopped

1/2 teaspoon ground cinnamon

3 eggs, separated

3/4 cup heavy cream

1/2 cup sugar

1/4 cup freshly brewed espresso

1 teaspoon vanilla extract

1. In the top of a double boiler over simmering water, melt the chocolate; stir in the cinnamon. Meanwhile, in a medium bowl with an electric mixer, beat the egg yolks until they are thick. Pour a little of the melted chocolate into the egg yolks, whisking constantly, then whisk all the egg yolk mixture back into the double boiler. Add 1/4 cup of the cream and whisk until well blended. Cook, stirring constantly, until the mixture thickens and reaches 160°F, about 4 minutes. Remove the top of the double boiler and let the chocolate mixture cool to room temperature, whisking often.

2. In a small saucepan over moderate heat, combine the sugar and espresso, and bring the mixture to a boil. Using a pastry brush dipped in water, brush down the sides of the saucepan, then cook the syrup without stirring until it reaches 238°F on a candy thermometer, about 5 minutes.

3. In a medium heatproof bowl with an electric mixer on medium speed, beat the egg whites until they are frothy. Place the bowl in a larger saucepan of boiling water (double-boiler style). With the mixer on low speed, gradually beat the boiling sugar syrup into the egg whites until the meringue peaks stiffly and a candy thermometer inserted at the center reaches 160°F. Whisk 1/3 cup of the hot meringue into the chocolate mixture, then fold in the remaining meringue.

4. In a small bowl with an electric mixer on high, beat the remaining 1/2 cup of cream until it forms soft peaks; beat in the vanilla. Fold the whipped cream into the chocolate mixture until no white streaks remain. Spoon into individual serving dishes or glasses, cover, and refrigerate for at least 1 hour or until serving time.

Makes 8 servings

fruit desserts

Brandied Peaches
You can buy brandied peaches in jars at gourmet stores, but you can just as easily—and much more cheaply—make your own fresh brandied peaches.

3 cups water

2 cups sugar

1/2 cup brandy

1 tablespoon whole cloves

2 cinnamon sticks

Zest of 1 lemon, slivered

Zest of 1 orange, slivered

4 peaches, peeled, pitted, and halved

1. In a large, heavy saucepan over high heat, combine the first seven ingredients and bring to a strong boil. Reduce the heat to moderate, prick the peach halves several times with the tines of a fork, and add them to the saucepan.

2. Cover the saucepan and reduce the heat to the lowest simmer; poach until the peaches are just cooked but still firm, about 20 minutes. Serve the peaches hot or warm, or chill and serve the peaches cold.

Makes 4 servings

Dried Fruit Compote
Keep ready-to-use self-sealing bags of these dried fruits on hand, then quickly poach them for a fast and fantastic dessert. You can buy dried fruit compotes in specialty stores, but your own will be better.

1 1/4 cups dried pitted prunes

2/3 cup golden raisins

1/2 cup dried figs

1/2 cup dried apricots

1 1/2 cups orange juice

1/3 cup water

1/4 cup sugar

1 cinnamon stick, broken

1/4 teaspoon ground ginger

1/8 teaspoon ground cloves

Pinch black pepper

3/4 teaspoon vanilla extract (optional)

1. In a medium nonreactive saucepan over high heat, combine all the ingredients except the vanilla; bring the mixture to a boil. Reduce the heat to low, cover the saucepan, and simmer until the fruit is tender, 25 to 30 minutes.

2. Remove the saucepan from the heat. Remove and discard the cinnamon stick pieces. Let the mixture stand until it is room temperature. If desired, stir in the vanilla. Serve at room temperature or chilled; store in an airtight container in the refrigerator for up to 3 days.

Makes 6 servings

Hot Curried Tropical Fruit

Intriguing hints of fresh ginger and curry lend pizzazz to mango, pineapple, and papaya. Try sprinkling with a little toasted coconut before serving. This is a take-out favorite that you can make at home for much less cash and much more flavor.

4 cups water

2 cups sugar

1/4 cup thinly sliced
  fresh ginger

1 tablespoon curry powder

1 tablespoon whole cloves

2 cinnamon sticks

Zest of 1 lemon, slivered

Zest of 1 orange, slivered

1 firm, medium mango,
  peeled, pitted, and sliced

1 medium pineapple, peeled,
  cored, and thinly sliced

1 papaya, peeled, seeded,
  and sliced

1. In a large, heavy saucepan over high heat, combine the first eight ingredients and bring to a strong boil. Reduce the heat to moderate, and add the mango, pineapple, and papaya.

2. Cover the saucepan and reduce the heat to the lowest simmer; poach the fruit until it is just cooked but still firm, about 15 minutes. Serve the fruit hot or warm, or chill and serve the fruit cold.

Makes 4 servings

Wine Poached Pears with Strawberries

Since Seckel pears hold up well through cooking, serve them standing with a drizzle of Custard Sauce (page 59). This is a restaurant dessert you can make at home for a modest sum and enjoy extravagantly.

4 cups red wine

1 cup sugar

1/4 cup thinly sliced
  fresh ginger

2 cinnamon sticks

Zest of 1 lemon, slivered

Zest of 1 orange, slivered

4 Seckel pears, peeled and
  cored with stems intact

2 cups strawberries, hulled

1. In a large, heavy saucepan over high heat, combine the first six ingredients and bring the mixture to a strong boil. Reduce the heat to moderate, and add the pears.

2. Cover the saucepan and reduce the heat to the lowest simmer; poach until the pears are just cooked but still firm, about 15 minutes. Remove the saucepan from the heat and let stand to cool for 5 minutes; stir in the strawberries.

3. Using a slotted spoon, remove the pears and strawberries to a serving platter or individual bowls. Return the saucepan to high heat, and bring the poaching liquid to a boil; boil until the liquid is reduced to about 1 1/2 cups. Pour the hot poaching liquid over the pears and strawberries before serving.

Makes 4 servings

ice cream

French Vanilla Ice Cream *This is the real thing—rich, creamy, and full of the strong, wonderful flavor of vanilla.*

1 3/4 cups milk

2 1/2 cups heavy cream

1 cup sugar

1 vanilla bean, split lengthwise

1/4 teaspoon salt

6 egg yolks

1. In a large saucepan over moderate heat, combine the milk and cream, 1/2 cup of the sugar, the vanilla bean, and salt. Scald the mixture just until small bubbles appear.

2. In a medium bowl, combine the egg yolks and remaining 1/2 cup sugar. Whisk until they are well blended. Gradually whisk a little milk mixture into the egg mixture, then pour the combined mixtures into the saucepan. Over low heat, cook, whisking constantly, until the custard mixture coats the back of a spoon, about 15 minutes.

3. Remove the saucepan from the heat and let the custard cool to room temperature. Remove the vanilla bean and scrape the seeds into the custard; discard the pod. Cover the saucepan and refrigerate until the custard is cold, 1 to 2 hours.

4. Transfer the custard to an ice-cream maker and, following the manufacturer's directions, freeze the ice cream.

Makes 1 quart

churn it yourself: ice-cream makers

Few pleasures in life compare with homemade ice cream—or frozen yogurt. But to make it, you will need an ice-cream maker. As a general rule, homemade ice cream costs half as much as commercial. You'll pay for an ice-cream maker in the first 10 to 12 quarts you make. To minimize costs, keep an eye out at yard or rummage sales, at resale or thrift shops, or at discount or oversale stores.

Old-fashioned crank churns: These use a combination of rock salt and ice packed around the churn to freeze the cream mixture. As the handle is cranked, the interior paddles stir the cream mixture while it is freezing. Naturally, the harder the ice cream gets, the harder it is to turn the handle, so you get a good workout before the delicious reward. This machine works particularly well for family gatherings or parties, where folks can trade off on the cranking but everyone enjoys the results.

Electric ice-cream makers: These handy machines are more costly but much easier on you, so you are likely to end up using them more frequently than a hand-churned model. Larger electric makers both freeze and churn for you. A less costly version requires a freezer or for the insert to be frozen ahead of time, but still does the arm-tiring churning for you. Less expensive 1-quart models from major manufacturers can be purchased for $30 to $40. (Most of the recipes here are for 1 quart.)

Blueberry Ice Cream

When blueberries come into season, toward the end of summer, indulge in this glorious concoction served in glass bowls so everyone can admire the color as well as the taste.

2 cups blueberries,
  washed and stemmed

1 1/3 cups sugar

4 strips (2 x 1/2-inch)
  lemon zest

1/2 teaspoon ground
  white pepper

1/2 teaspoon ground ginger

1 3/4 cups milk

2 1/2 cups heavy cream

1 vanilla bean,
  split lengthwise

1/4 teaspoon salt

6 egg yolks

1. In a medium saucepan over moderate heat, combine the blueberries, 1/3 cup of the sugar, and lemon zest. Cook, stirring very frequently, until the blueberries are very soft, 4 to 5 minutes. Place a fine sieve over a medium bowl. Pour the blueberry mixture through the sieve, pressing with the back of a wooden spoon to extract all the juice; discard the solids. Stir in the pepper and ginger. Set aside the blueberry mixture.

2. In a large saucepan over moderate heat, combine the milk and cream, 1/2 cup of the sugar, the vanilla bean, and salt. Scald the mixture just until small bubbles appear.

3. In a medium bowl, combine the egg yolks and remaining 1/2 cup sugar. Whisk until they are well blended. Gradually whisk a little milk mixture into the egg mixture, then pour the combined mixtures into the saucepan. Over low heat, cook, whisking constantly, until the custard mixture coats the back of a spoon, about 15 minutes.

4. Remove the saucepan from the heat and let the custard cool to room temperature. Remove the vanilla bean and scrape the seeds into the custard; discard the pod. Cover the saucepan and refrigerate until the custard is cold, 1 to 2 hours.

5. Pour the reserved blueberry mixture into the custard and stir until all the ingredients are well blended. Transfer the custard to an ice-cream maker and, following the manufacturer's directions, freeze the ice cream.

Makes 1 quart

Helpful Hint | **Lowering the Fat in Homemade Ice Cream**
We love the richness and texture of full-fat ice cream, but our bellies and thighs are not always so appreciative. Fortunately, it is not hard to lower the fat on homemade ice cream, and since it is home-churned as well, you should still have satisfyingly creamy results. The trick is to substitute an equal amount of evaporated skim milk for the whole milk and 3/4 cup egg substitute for the egg yolks when making a 1-quart batch.

Peach Ice Cream

Ripe, juicy peaches are a true taste of summer, so how could they be any better? In a luscious ice cream that you make yourself.

2 large, ripe peaches

1/3 cup firmly packed
   light brown sugar

1 tablespoon lemon juice

1/4 teaspoon ground ginger

1 3/4 cups milk

2 1/2 cups heavy cream

1 cup sugar

1 vanilla bean,
   split lengthwise

1/4 teaspoon salt

6 egg yolks

1. Blanch, peel, and pit the peaches, then finely chop them. In a medium bowl, combine the peach pieces, brown sugar, lemon juice, and ginger. Toss the ingredients together until they are well blended. Set aside the peach mixture.

2. In a large saucepan over moderate heat, combine the milk and cream, 1/2 cup of the sugar, the vanilla bean, and salt. Scald the mixture just until small bubbles appear.

3. In a medium bowl, combine the egg yolks and remaining 1/2 cup sugar. Whisk until they are well blended. Gradually whisk a little milk mixture into the egg mixture, then pour the combined mixtures into the saucepan. Over low heat, cook, whisking constantly, until the custard mixture coats the back of a spoon, about 15 minutes.

4. Remove the saucepan from the heat and let the custard cool to room temperature. Remove the vanilla bean and scrape the seeds into the custard; discard the pod. Cover the saucepan and refrigerate until the custard is cold, 1 to 2 hours.

5. Pour the reserved peach mixture into the custard, and stir until all the ingredients are well blended. Transfer the custard to an ice-cream maker and, following the manufacturer's directions, freeze the ice cream.

Makes 1 quart

Citrus Ice Cream

Tangy citrus combines with cream to create a refreshingly unusual treat, ideal for pairing with fresh fruit salad.

1/2 cup fresh citrus juice of
   choice

1 egg

1 cup sugar

1 cup heavy cream

1 1/2 cups milk

1 tablespoon grated zest of
   citrus fruit of choice

Pinch salt

1. In a heavy saucepan over low heat, combine the citrus juice, egg, and sugar, and cook, whisking constantly, until the sugar has dissolved and the mixture registers 170°F on a candy thermometer. Stir in the cream, milk, zest, and salt.

2. Remove the saucepan from the heat and let the mixture cool to room temperature. Cover the saucepan and refrigerate until the custard is cold, about 1 hour.

3. Transfer the custard to an ice-cream maker and, following the manufacturer's directions, freeze the ice cream.

Makes 5 to 6 cups

Strawberry Ice Cream
Celebrate the beginning of summer with homemade ice cream bursting with fresh strawberries.

1 3/4 cups milk

2 1/2 cups heavy cream

1 1/3 cups sugar

1 vanilla bean,
  split lengthwise

1/4 teaspoon salt

6 egg yolks

4 strips (3 x 1/2-inch)
  orange zest

2 cups strawberries

1. In a large saucepan over moderate heat, combine the milk and cream, 1/2 cup of the sugar, the vanilla bean, and salt. Scald the mixture just until small bubbles appear.

2. In a medium bowl, combine the egg yolks and another 1/2 cup sugar. Whisk until they are well blended. Gradually whisk a little milk mixture into the egg mixture, then pour the combined mixtures into the saucepan; add the orange zest. Over low heat, cook, whisking constantly, until the custard mixture coats the back of a spoon, about 15 minutes.

3. Remove the saucepan from the heat and let the custard cool to room temperature. Remove the vanilla bean and scrape the seeds into the custard; discard the pod. Remove and discard the orange zest. Cover the saucepan and refrigerate until the custard is cold, 1 to 2 hours.

4. Meanwhile, rinse and hull the strawberries. In the bowl of a food processor or blender, combine the strawberries with the remaining 1/3 cup sugar. Whirl until the mixture is pureed to the desired consistency.

5. Remove the saucepan from the refrigerator and stir the strawberries into the custard until they are well blended. Transfer the custard to an ice-cream maker and, following the manufacturer's directions, freeze the ice cream.

Makes 1 quart

Honey Banana Ice Cream
Gingersnaps (page 131) make a perfect partner for this homemade delight.

6 egg yolks

2 cups milk

1/2 cup honey

2 teaspoons vanilla extract

2 cups heavy cream

1 cup (3 ripe) bananas,
  mashed

1. In the top of a double boiler set over simmering water, combine the egg yolks and milk, and whisk until they are well blended. Add the honey and vanilla extract. Over moderate heat, cook, stirring constantly, until the mixture coats the back of a spoon and registers 170°F on a candy thermometer.

2. Pour the mixture into a large bowl, cover, and refrigerate until the mixture is chilled, about 1 hour.

3. Add the cream and mashed bananas to the egg mixture, and stir until the ingredients are well blended. Transfer the custard to an ice-cream maker and, following the manufacturer's directions, freeze the ice cream.

Makes 5 to 6 cups

Hawaiian Ice Cream
A taste of the tropics in every bite, this coconut-pineapple ice cream is rich and cooling and not too extravagant because you make it yourself.

1 1/3 cups milk

3 eggs

1 cup sugar

1/2 cup sweetened, flaked coconut

2 teaspoons vanilla extract

1 can (1 pound) crushed pineapple, drained

1 1/3 cups heavy cream

1. In a small, heavy saucepan over moderately high heat, scald the milk just until tiny bubbles appear.

2. In a medium heavy saucepan over low heat, combine the eggs and sugar. Pour the scalded milk into the egg mixture, whisking constantly. Cook, whisking constantly, until the custard thickens and registers 170°F on a candy thermometer.

3. Set a fine sieve over a large bowl. Pour the custard through the sieve; discard the solids. Add the coconut and vanilla; whisk until well blended. Stir in the pineapple and cream. Cover the bowl and refrigerate until the custard is cold, 1 to 2 hours.

4. Transfer the custard to an ice-cream maker and, following the manufacturer's directions, freeze the ice cream.

Makes about 1 quart

Chocolate Chocolate Chip Ice Cream
What is better than chocolate? More chocolate! Remember, however, that just because homemade is cheaper, it doesn't have fewer calories.

1 3/4 cups milk

2 1/2 cups heavy cream

1 cup firmly packed light brown sugar

1/4 teaspoon salt

6 egg yolks

1/4 cup unsweetened Dutch-process cocoa powder

1 teaspoon vanilla extract

1/2 cup mini chocolate chips

1. In a large saucepan over moderate heat, combine the milk and cream, 1/2 cup of the sugar, and salt. Scald the mixture just until small bubbles appear.

2. In a medium bowl, combine the egg yolks and remaining 1/2 cup sugar. Whisk until they are well blended. Whisk in the cocoa until it is well blended. Gradually whisk a little milk mixture into the egg mixture, then pour the combined mixtures into the saucepan. Over low heat, cook, whisking constantly, until the custard mixture coats the back of a spoon, about 15 minutes.

3. Remove the saucepan from the heat and let the custard cool to room temperature. Whisk in the vanilla. Cover the saucepan and refrigerate until the custard is cold, for 1 to 2 hours.

4. Add the mini chocolate chips and stir until they are evenly distributed. Transfer the custard to an ice-cream maker and, following the manufacturer's directions, freeze the ice cream.

Makes 1 quart

Chocolate Silk Ice Cream
A rich, chocolate custard is the base for this decadent delight.

1 1/4 cups milk

3 eggs

3/4 cup sugar

2 ounces unsweetened chocolate, chopped

2 teaspoons vanilla extract

1/4 teaspoon salt

2 cups heavy cream

1. In a small, heavy saucepan over moderately high heat, scald the milk just until tiny bubbles appear.

2. In a medium heavy saucepan over low heat, combine the eggs and sugar. Pour the scalded milk into the egg mixture, whisking constantly. Cook, whisking constantly, until the custard thickens and registers 170°F on a candy thermometer.

3. Set a fine sieve over a large bowl. Pour the custard through the sieve; discard the solids. Add the chocolate, vanilla, and salt; whisk until well blended. Stir in the cream. Cover the bowl and refrigerate until the custard is cold, 1 to 2 hours.

4. Transfer the custard to an ice-cream maker and, following the manufacturer's directions, freeze the ice cream.

Makes about 1 quart

Rocky Road Ice Cream
Chocolate chips, marshmallows, and pecans make up this popular ice cream flavor. Once you've made your own, you'll wonder how you could have spent so much money on commercial ice cream.

3 cups milk

3 cups half-and-half

9 squares (1 ounce each) semisweet chocolate

2 3/4 cups sugar

3/4 teaspoon salt

6 cups heavy cream

3 cups miniature marshmallows

2 1/4 cups mini chocolate chips

1 1/2 cups chopped pecans

6 teaspoons vanilla extract

1. In a large, heavy saucepan over moderately high heat, combine the milk and half-and-half. Cook, stirring constantly, until the mixture registers 175°F on a candy thermometer. Add the semisweet chocolate, sugar, and salt; stir until the chocolate has melted and the sugar has completely dissolved.

2. Remove the saucepan from the heat and place it in a large bowl of ice water to cool the mixture quickly; stir and chill for 2 minutes. Remove the saucepan and let the mixture cool completely.

3. Pour the mixture into a large bowl. Add the cream, marshmallows, chocolate chips, pecans, and vanilla. Stir until all the ingredients are well blended. Cover the bowl and refrigerate until the mixture is cold, 30 minutes.

4. Working in batches, transfer the mixture to an ice-cream maker and, following the manufacturer's directions, freeze the ice cream. Keep the remaining mixture refrigerated until ready to freeze; stir well before adding to the ice-cream maker.

5. Let stand in the ice-cream maker or place in the freezer to firm for 2 to 4 hours before serving.

Makes about 4 1/2 quarts

Mint Chocolate Chip Ice Cream

Mint and chocolate are a natural combination, and this is a popular flavor for ice cream, which you can make better and cheaper at home.

1 3/4 cups milk

2 1/2 cups heavy cream

1 cup pureed fresh mint leaves

1 cup sugar

1/4 teaspoon salt

6 egg yolks

1 teaspoon vanilla extract

1/2 cup mini chocolate chips

1. In a large saucepan over moderate heat, combine the milk and cream, mint leaves, 1/2 cup of the sugar, and salt. Scald the mixture just until small bubbles appear.

2. In a medium bowl, combine the egg yolks and remaining 1/2 cup sugar. Whisk until they are well blended. Gradually whisk a little milk mixture into the egg mixture, then pour the combined mixtures into the saucepan. Over low heat, cook, whisking constantly, until the custard mixture coats the back of a spoon, about 15 minutes.

3. Remove the saucepan from the heat and let the custard cool to room temperature. Whisk in the vanilla. Cover the saucepan and refrigerate until the custard is cold, 1 to 2 hours.

4. Add the mini chocolate chips and stir until they are evenly distributed. Transfer the custard to an ice-cream maker and, following the manufacturer's directions, freeze the ice cream.

Makes 1 quart

Peppermint Ice Cream

A feast for the eyes, this mouthwatering concoction of crushed peppermint candies in a creamy base is a natural holiday sweet. You can't always find it in the stores, but you can always make it at home—for much less.

4 egg yolks

1 1/2 cups half-and-half

3/4 cup sugar

1/4 teaspoon salt

2 cups heavy cream

4 1/2-6 teaspoons vanilla extract

1-1 1/4 cups crushed peppermint candy

1. In a large, heavy saucepan over low heat, combine the egg yolks, half-and-half, sugar, and salt. Cook, stirring constantly, until the mixture coats the back of a spoon and registers 160°F on a candy thermometer.

2. Remove the saucepan from the heat and place it in a large bowl of ice water to cool the mixture quickly; stir and chill for 2 minutes. Stir in the heavy cream and vanilla. Remove the saucepan and let the mixture cool completely.

3. Cover the saucepan with plastic wrap and refrigerate for several hours or overnight until the mixture is very cold.

4. Stir in the peppermint candy until it is evenly distributed. Transfer the mixture to an ice-cream maker and, following the manufacturer's directions, freeze the ice cream.

5. Let stand in the ice-cream maker or place in the freezer to firm for 2 to 4 hours before serving.

Makes 1 quart

Butter Pecan Ice Cream
Toasting the pecans really brings out their flavor in this old favorite.

3/4 cup chopped pecans

3 tablespoons butter, melted

1/8 teaspoon salt

1/4 cup plus 1 tablespoon sugar

1/2 cup firmly packed brown sugar

2 tablespoons cornstarch

2 eggs, beaten

1/3 cup maple-flavored pancake syrup

2 1/2 cups milk

1 cup heavy cream

2 teaspoons vanilla extract

1. Preheat the oven to 350°F. On a rimmed baking sheet, spread the pecans in a single layer. Drizzle the pecans with the butter and sprinkle with the salt and 1 tablespoon of the sugar; toss to coat the nuts. Toast the pecans for 15 minutes, stir, and toast for 15 minutes longer. Remove the baking sheet from the oven and let the pecans cool completely.

2. In the top of a double boiler set over simmering water, combine the remaining 1/4 cup of sugar, brown sugar, cornstarch, eggs, and pancake syrup. Stir until the ingredients are well blended. Gradually stir in the milk. Increase the heat to high and cook, stirring constantly, until the mixture thickens and coats the back of a spoon.

3. Remove the saucepan from the heat and let the custard cool to room temperature. Cover the saucepan and refrigerate until the custard is cold, for several hours or overnight.

4. Add the toasted pecans, cream, and vanilla, and stir until they are evenly distributed. Transfer the custard to an ice-cream maker and, following the manufacturer's directions, freeze the ice cream.

5. Let stand in the ice-cream maker or place in the freezer to firm for 2 to 4 hours before serving.

Makes about 2 quarts

Ice Cream Cake
This frozen cake is perfect for a summer birthday—or any time you need an easy but sensational dessert. Use whatever combination of ice cream pleases your fancy.

1 1/2 cups crumbled Chocolate Sandwich (page 130) or Oreo cookies

2 tablespoons butter, melted

1 1/2 pints first flavor ice cream, softened

3/4 cup Hot Chocolate Sauce (page 60), cooked then cooled but still liquid

1 1/2 pints second flavor ice cream, softened

1/2 cup grated chocolate or sliced, toasted almonds

1. In a small bowl, combine the cookie crumbs with the butter and toss until well blended. In an 8-inch springform pan, press the cookie mixture over the bottom and halfway up the sides. Place the pan in the freezer for 30 minutes.

2. Spoon the first-flavor ice cream into the prepared springform pan, spreading it in an even layer over the cookie crust. Return the pan to the freezer until the ice cream is firm, about 30 minutes. Pour the chocolate sauce into the pan, spreading it evenly over the ice-cream layer; freeze until firm, about 15 minutes. Spoon the second-flavor ice cream into the pan, spreading it in an even layer over the hardened chocolate sauce. Using a knife or spatula dipped in hot water, smooth the top of the cake, then sprinkle with either the grated chocolate or toasted almond slices. Cover the cake with plastic wrap and return to the freezer for at least 1 hour.

3. To serve, wipe the bottom of the springform pan with a hot, damp cloth, then carefully remove the sides of the pan. Dip a sharp knife in hot water before cutting the cake.

Makes 8 to 10 servings

frozen yogurt

Lemon Frozen Yogurt
Light and refreshing, the lemon flavor really comes through in this homemade frozen yogurt. Try a scoop with fresh berries.

1 carton (32 ounces) nonfat, plain yogurt

1 2/3 cups sugar

1/3 cup lemon juice

1 tablespoon grated lemon zest

4 drops yellow food coloring *(optional)*

1. In a medium bowl, combine the yogurt, sugar, lemon juice and zest. Stir until all the ingredients are well blended. If a brighter yellow color is desired, stir in the food coloring.

2. Transfer the mixture to an ice-cream maker and, following the manufacturer's directions, freeze the yogurt. Let stand in the ice-cream maker or place in the freezer to firm for 2 to 4 hours before serving.

Makes 5 cups

Strawberry Frozen Yogurt
The fresh strawberries add just the right sweet note to this simple, speedy homemade frozen yogurt.

2 cups (16 ounces) nonfat plain yogurt

2 cups pureed fresh strawberries

1 can (14 ounces) fat-free sweetened condensed milk

1 cup nonfat milk

3 teaspoons vanilla extract

1. In a large bowl, combine all the ingredients and stir until well blended.
2. Working in batches if needed, pour the mixture into an ice-cream maker, filling it two-thirds full; store the remaining yogurt in the refrigerator until ready to freeze. Following the manufacturer's directions, freeze the yogurt. Let stand in the ice-cream maker or place in the freezer to firm for 2 to 4 hours before serving. Remove from the freezer 30 to 45 minutes before serving to soften slightly.

Makes 1 1/2 quarts

Mocha Chip Frozen Yogurt
Coffee and chocolate marry divinely in this rich dessert that you can put together quickly and inexpensively for your family's enjoyment.

3 cups regular or low-fat plain yogurt

1 1/2 tablespoons instant espresso powder

3/4 cup sugar

1 cup heavy cream

2 ounces bittersweet chocolate, chopped

1 teaspoon vanilla extract

1. Set a large fine sieve over a large bowl. Add the yogurt and place in the refrigerator for 1 hour to drain.
2. In another large bowl, combine the espresso powder, sugar, and cream; stir until the sugar has completely dissolved. Beat the mixture until it holds soft peaks. Add the drained yogurt, chocolate, and vanilla, stirring until all the ingredients are well blended and no streaks of white remain.
3. Pour the mixture into an ice-cream maker and, following the manufacturer's directions, freeze the yogurt.

Makes 5 to 6 cups

Helpful Hint

Frozen Yogurt: An Alternative to Ice Cream
Once the province of health food aficionados, frozen yogurt has spread widely and grown wildly in popularity. Generally lower in fat and calories (though not always) than ice cream, frozen yogurt combines the slight tanginess associated with yogurt with the cool creaminess of ice cream. For the most healthful results, use nonfat yogurt when making it. It is made much like ice cream, and you need an ice-cream maker to make it.

ices, granitas, sherbets, and sorbets

Orange Ice *This treat requires only five ingredients and no ice-cream maker.*

3 cups water

1 cup sugar

1 can (12 ounces) frozen orange juice concentrate, thawed

2 tablespoons lemon juice

1/2 cup half-and-half

1. In a medium saucepan over high heat, combine 1 cup of the water and the sugar. Boil, stirring frequently, until the sugar has completely dissolved, about 1 minute.

2. Remove the saucepan from the heat and stir in the orange juice concentrate, lemon juice, and the remaining 2 cups of water. Stir until all the ingredients are well blended.

3. Pour the orange mixture into a large, freezer-safe bowl, cover, and freeze until firm.

4. Remove the bowl from the freezer and, using an electric mixer, beat the orange mixture until smooth. Add the half-and-half and beat again until well blended. Re-cover the bowl and return the orange mixture to the freezer.

5. Let the orange ice stand at room temperature for 20 minutes before serving.

Makes 10 to 12 servings

Blood-Orange Champagne Granita *If blood oranges are unavailable, substitute ruby red or pink grapefruit.*

1 1/2 cups sugar

1 cup water

2 cups freshly squeezed blood-orange juice

2 cups champagne

Pinch salt

1. In a medium saucepan over moderate heat, combine the sugar and water, stirring constantly until the sugar has dissolved. Bring the mixture to a boil, reduce the heat, and simmer for 3 minutes. Remove the saucepan from the heat and let stand until the syrup is cool, about 1 hour.

2. In a large bowl, combine the syrup, juice, champagne, and salt. Stir until all the ingredients are well blended.

3. Pour the mixture into ice-cube trays or a large, shallow pan. Cover with plastic wrap and place in the freezer. As the granita freezes, stir it with a fork, every 45 minutes, two or three times, to break up the ice and create an icy, flaky texture. Cover with plastic wrap and freeze for 8 hours or overnight.

4. When ready to serve, place the granita in the refrigerator for 15 minutes to soften; then, using an ice-cream scoop or large spoon, scrape across the top to bring up the granita in thin shavings. Serve in chilled glasses or bowls.

Makes 12 servings

Cappuccino Granita
An Italian specialty, this granita goes well with a few chocolate-covered coffee beans.

1 1/4 cups brewed strong black coffee or espresso

1/4 cup granulated sugar

5 tablespoons Kahlúa or other coffee-flavored liqueur

1 cup heavy cream

1 tablespoon confectioners' sugar

Unsweetened cocoa powder

1. In a small bowl, combine the coffee, sugar, and 3 tablespoons of the Kahlúa.

2. Pour the coffee mixture into ice-cube trays or a large, shallow pan. Cover with plastic wrap and place in the freezer. As the granita freezes, stir it with a fork, every 45 minutes, two or three times, to break up the ice and create an icy, flaky texture. Cover the granita with plastic wrap and freeze 8 hours or overnight.

3. In a medium bowl with an electric mixer, beat the cream with the remaining Kahlúa and confectioners' sugar until soft peaks form.

4. To serve, roughly break up the granita. Using an ice-cream scoop or large spoon, scrape across the top to bring up the granita in thin shavings. Place the granita in individual chilled serving bowls and top each with a dollop of the Kahlúa whipped cream. Sprinkle a dusting of cocoa powder over each serving.

Makes 6 to 8 servings

Kiwi Granita
A lovely green with a lively, tart taste, this homemade granita would be a fitting finale to a rich meal.

1 cup water

2 cups sugar

Juice of 2 lemons

6 large, ripe kiwis, peeled and coarsely chopped

1. In a small saucepan over moderate heat, combine the water, sugar, and half the lemon juice. Cook, stirring constantly, until the sugar has dissolved. Bring the syrup to a boil, reduce the heat, and simmer 3 minutes. Remove the saucepan from the heat and let stand until the syrup is just warm.

2. In the bowl of a food processor or blender, place the kiwis and whirl until they are pureed. Add the remaining lemon juice and whirl to blend. Pour the kiwi puree into the syrup.

3. Pour the kiwi mixture into ice-cube trays or a large, shallow pan. Cover with plastic wrap and place in the freezer. As the granita freezes, stir it with a fork every 45 minutes, two or three times, to break up the ice and create an icy, flaky texture. Cover the granita with plastic wrap and freeze 6 hours or until solid.

4. When ready to serve, place the granita in the refrigerator for 15 minutes to soften; then, using an ice-cream scoop or large spoon, scrape across the top to bring up the granita in thin shavings. Serve in chilled glasses or bowls.

Makes about 4 cups

Peach Granita

An out-of-this-world cooler for a hot summer's day, this granita is an easy home project.

1 cup water

1/2 cup sugar

4 ripe peaches, peeled, pitted and coarsely chopped

1 tablespoon peach schnapps or other fruit liqueur

1. In a small saucepan over moderate heat, combine the water and sugar, and stir until the sugar has completely dissolved. Bring the mixture to a boil, reduce the heat, and simmer 3 minutes. Remove the saucepan from the heat and let stand until the syrup is cool, about 1 hour.

2. In the bowl of a food processor or blender, place the peach pieces and whirl until they are pureed. Add the syrup and schnapps, and whirl until all the ingredients are well blended.

3. Pour the peach mixture into ice-cube trays or a large, shallow pan. Cover with plastic wrap and place in the freezer. As the granita freezes, stir it with a fork every 45 minutes, two or three times, to break up the ice and create an icy, flaky texture. Cover the granita with plastic wrap and freeze 6 hours or until solid.

4. When ready to serve, place the granita in the refrigerator for 15 minutes to soften; then, using an ice-cream scoop or large spoon, scrape across the top to bring up the granita in thin shavings. Serve in chilled glasses or bowls.

Makes about 4 cups

Lime Sherbet

Refreshingly tart, this homemade sherbet is better than any you can buy and costs lots less.

4 1/4 cups sugar

1 1/2 cups lime juice

3 tablespoons lemon juice

2 tablespoons grated lime zest

7 1/2 cups milk

1/2 cup buttermilk

1 drop green food coloring *(optional)*

1. In a large bowl, combine the first four ingredients and stir until well blended. Gradually stir in the milk and buttermilk. If a brighter green color is desired, stir in the green food coloring.

2. Working in batches if needed, pour the lime mixture into an ice-cream maker, filling it two-thirds full; store the remaining mixture in the refrigerator until ready to freeze. Following the manufacturer's directions, freeze the sherbet. Let stand in the ice-cream maker or place in the freezer to firm for 2 to 4 hours before serving. Remove from the freezer 10 minutes before serving to soften slightly.

Makes about 2 1/2 quarts

Strawberry Milk Sherbet
Smooth as ice cream but made with milk for a lighter treat, this sherbet is easy to make at home and an inexpensive treat whenever you want it.

1 pint strawberries, rinsed and hulled
1 cup milk
1 cup sugar

1. In the bowl of a food processor or blender, place the strawberries and whirl until they are pureed and a smooth consistency.
2. In a medium saucepan over high heat, combine the milk and sugar, and bring the mixture to a boil. Remove the saucepan from the heat and let stand until the milk mixture is just warm.
3. In a medium bowl, combine the strawberry puree and milk mixture, and whisk until they are well blended.
4. Pour the strawberry-milk mixture into an ice-cream maker. Following the manufacturer's directions, freeze the sherbet.

Makes 1 pint

Cassis Sorbet
A black-currant liqueur, cassis has a smooth, strong flavor that makes this sorbet particularly delicious as a formal dinner dessert that makes guests and your pocketbook happy.

1 1/2 cups water
1/2 cup sugar
1 cup cassis (black-currant liqueur)

1. In a medium saucepan over high heat, combine the water and sugar, and bring the mixture to a boil, stirring constantly until the sugar has dissolved. Remove the saucepan from the heat and let stand until the syrup is just warm.
2. In a medium bowl, combine the syrup and cassis, and stir until they are well blended.
3. Pour the cassis mixture into an ice-cream maker. Following the manufacturer's directions, freeze the sorbet.

Makes 1 pint

Citrus Sorbet
Oranges, lemons, and limes all lend their distinctive notes to this refreshing sorbet that you make at home for pennies.

1 cup water
1/2 cup sugar
1 1/4 cups orange juice
1/4 cup lemon juice
3 tablespoons lime juice

1. In a medium saucepan over high heat, combine the water and sugar, and bring the mixture to a boil, stirring constantly until the sugar has dissolved. Remove the saucepan from the heat and let stand until the syrup is just warm.
2. In a medium bowl, combine the syrup and the juices, and stir until they are well blended.
3. Pour the citrus mixture into an ice-cream maker. Following the manufacturer's directions, freeze the sorbet.

Makes 1 pint

Honeydew Sorbet

Serve a scoop of this delicate sorbet in a wedge of fresh honeydew. Or try substituting cantaloupe for the honeydew. Either way, you don't have to wait for your ice-cream parlor to feature this delicious flavor once a year.

6 cups honeydew melon cubes

3/4 cup sugar

3 tablespoons Midori or other melon-flavored liqueur

1. In the bowl of a food processor or blender, place all the ingredients. Whirl until the melon is pureed, and the ingredients are blended into a smooth consistency. Place the bowl in the refrigerator until the melon mixture is completely chilled.

2. Pour the melon mixture into an ice-cream maker. Following the manufacturer's directions, freeze the sorbet.

Makes 1 pint

Lemon Sorbet

Wonderfully tart, this classic sorbet works either as a dessert or as a palate cleanser between courses. As a variation, add 1/2 cup fresh mint leaves to the syrup before it cools, then strain before freezing. Make it better and cheaper yourself.

3 cups water

1 1/2 cups sugar

1 1/2 cups lemon juice

1 tablespoon grated lemon zest

1. In a medium saucepan over high heat, combine the water and sugar. Bring the mixture to a boil and cook, stirring constantly, until the sugar has completely dissolved, about 5 minutes. Remove the saucepan from the heat and let the syrup cool.

2. Add the lemon juice and zest to the syrup. Stir until all the ingredients are well blended.

3. Pour the lemon mixture into an ice-cream maker. Following the manufacturer's directions, freeze the sorbet. Let stand in the ice-cream maker or place in the freezer to firm for 2 to 4 hours before serving. Remove from the freezer 10 minutes before serving to soften slightly.

Makes about 1 quart

Raspberry Sorbet

Since it uses frozen raspberries, you can make this sorbet any time of the year. Try drizzling with a little Chocolate Sauce (page 60) before serving. Homemade is cheaper and better.

1 package (10 ounces) frozen raspberries, thawed
1 cup water
1 cup sugar
1 tablespoon lemon juice

1. In the bowl of a food processor or blender, place the raspberries and whirl until they are pureed and a smooth consistency.
2. In a medium saucepan over high heat, combine the water and sugar, and bring the mixture to a boil, stirring constantly until the sugar has dissolved. Remove the saucepan from the heat and let stand until the syrup is just warm.
3. In a medium bowl, combine the syrup, raspberry puree, and lemon juice, and stir until they are well blended.
4. Pour the raspberry mixture into an ice-cream maker. Following the manufacturer's directions, freeze the sorbet.

Makes 1 pint

Strawberry Sorbet

Look for really ripe, firm, red strawberries for extraordinary flavor and ravishing color. This sorbet is another treat you can make better and more frugally at home.

6 cups strawberries
1 3/4 cups sugar
2 cups fresh orange juice, strained
2 tablespoons Grand Marnier or other orange-flavored liqueur

1. Wash and hull the strawberries, drain well, and cut them in half. In a small bowl, combine the strawberry halves, sugar, and orange juice. Let the strawberry mixture stand for 1 hour.
2. In the bowl of a food processor or blender, whirl the strawberry mixture until it is a smooth puree. Add the Grand Marnier and pulse until well blended.
3. Pour the mixture into ice-cube trays or a large, shallow pan and freeze until just firm but not hard, 1 to 2 hours.
4. Spoon the mixture back into the bowl of the food processor and pulse until the mixture becomes slushy. Repeat to refreeze, then break up the sorbet. Return the mixture to the pan and freeze until solid.
5. Before serving, place the pan in the refrigerator and let the sorbet soften slightly, about 15 minutes.

Makes about 1 1/2 pints

frozen pops

Frozen Fruit Pops
Any flavor of gelatin will do to make these cool treats that you can keep in the freezer all summer.

1 package (3 ounces)
   fruit-flavored gelatin

1/2 cup sugar

2 cups boiling water

1 1/2 cups cold water

10-12 frozen pop molds or
   3-ounce paper cups

10-12 frozen pop sticks or
   plastic spoons

1. In a medium bowl, combine the gelatin and sugar. Pour in the boiling water, stirring until the gelatin and sugar are completely dissolved. Stir in the cold water.

2. Pour the gelatin mixture into the frozen pop molds or paper cups, and place in the freezer until the pops are almost firm, about 2 hours. Insert a frozen pop stick or plastic spoon into the center of each pop. Return to the freezer until the pops are firm, 4 to 8 hours. To serve, unmold or tear away the paper cup from the pop.

Makes 10 to 12 pops

Fudge Pops
Cold, chocolaty, and oh, so satisfying, these treats are easy to make at home and taste much better than the commercial ones.

1 package (3.4 ounces)
   cook-and-serve chocolate
   fudge pudding mix

3 cups milk

1/4 cup sugar

1/2 cup whipping cream

12-13 frozen pop molds or
   3-ounce paper cups

12-13 frozen pop sticks or
   plastic spoons

1. In a medium saucepan over moderate heat, combine the pudding mix, milk, and sugar. Bring the mixture to a boil; cook, stirring constantly, for 2 minutes. Remove the saucepan from the heat and let the pudding stand for 30 minutes, stirring the mixture several times, until it is cool.

2. In a small bowl using an electric mixer, whip the cream until soft peaks form. Fold the whipped cream into the pudding mixture until all the ingredients are well blended and no streaks of white remain.

3. Pour the pudding mixture into the frozen pop molds or paper cups, and place in the freezer until the pops are almost firm, about 2 hours. Insert a frozen pop stick or plastic spoon into the center of each pop. Return to the freezer until firm, 3 to 4 hours. To serve, unmold or tear away the paper cup from the pop.

Makes 12 to 13 pops

Orange Cream Pops

Yum! Creamy orange-flavored pops that you make at home go down very well on a hot day.

1 package (3 ounces) orange gelatin

1 cup boiling water

1 cup (8 ounces) low-fat vanilla yogurt

1/2 cup reduced-fat (2%) milk

1/2 teaspoon vanilla extract

10 frozen pop molds or 3-ounce plastic cups

10 frozen pop sticks or plastic spoons

1. In a large bowl, combine the gelatin and boiling water, and stir until the gelatin has completely dissolved. Let stand until the gelatin is room temperature.

2. Add the yogurt, milk, and vanilla, and stir until all the ingredients are well blended.

3. Pour the gelatin mixture into the frozen pop molds or paper cups, and place in the freezer until the pops are almost firm, about 2 hours. Insert a frozen pop stick or plastic spoon into the center of each pop. Return to the freezer until the pops are firm, 4 to 8 hours. To serve, unmold or tear away the paper cup from the pop.

Makes 10 pops

Strawberry Ice Pops

Fresh strawberries make these pops extra special—tasting like the pricey, high-end pops from the ice-cream store.

2 pints fresh strawberries, washed and hulled

1/2 cup apple juice concentrate

8 frozen pop molds or 3-ounce plastic cups

8 frozen pop sticks or plastic spoons

1. In a large bowl, using a potato masher, mash the strawberries roughly, leaving some chunks of strawberry intact. Add the apple juice concentrate and stir until the ingredients are well blended.

2. Spoon or pour the strawberry mixture into the frozen pop molds or paper cups, and place in the freezer until the pops are almost firm, about 2 hours. Insert a frozen pop stick or plastic spoon into the center of each pop. Return to the freezer until the pops are firm, 4 to 8 hours. To serve, unmold or tear away the paper cup from the pop.

Makes 8 pops

Tropical Pops

If you can't be sipping tropical drinks, you can at least keep your cool with these inexpensive, homemade tropical pops.

12 large or 24 small frozen
pop molds or 1-cup or
1/2-cup plastic cups

12-24 frozen pop sticks or
plastic spoons

6 cups fresh tropical fruit,
such as pineapples,
papayas, and/or mangoes,
peeled and cored as
needed, cut into bite-size
pieces, reserving any juices

3 cups mixed tropical
fruit punch or orange or
pineapple juice

1. In a large bowl, combine the fresh fruit with any juices collected during their preparation. Stir the fruits well to distribute them equally.

2. Spoon the fruit mixture into the frozen pop molds or plastic cups, filling each three-quarters full.

3. Pour some of the fruit punch or juice into each mold or cup, leaving room at the top for the liquid to expand. Place in the freezer until the pops are almost firm, about 2 hours. Insert a frozen pop stick or plastic spoon into the center of each pop. Return to the freezer until the pops are firm, 4 to 8 hours. To serve, unmold or tear away the paper cup from the pop.

Makes 12 (1-cup) pops or 24 (1/2-cup) pops

Chocolate-Nut Frozen Bananas

Bananas are one of those fruits that can be frozen and eaten out of hand. But for a special treat, try dipping them in chocolate and nuts!

8 wooden skewers, sharp
ends cut off

8 small bananas

8 ounces dark chocolate

3 tablespoons vegetable
shortening

1 cup coarsely chopped
walnuts, toasted

1 cup coarsely chopped
macadamia nuts, toasted

1. Line a baking sheet with plastic wrap.

2. Insert 1 skewer into each banana, pushing it so the end is about halfway along the length of the fruit. Place each skewered banana on the prepared baking sheet. Cover the baking sheet with plastic wrap and place in the freezer until the bananas are frozen solid, about 8 hours.

3. In a small bowl placed over simmering water, combine the chocolate and shortening, and melt, stirring occasionally. Remove the bowl from the heat. In a shallow plate, combine the walnuts and macadamia nuts, and toss to mix well.

4. Remove the sheet of bananas from the freezer. Holding one banana pop by the stick end over the bowl, spoon chocolate over the banana, coating it completely. Then hold the banana over the nuts and scoop up and sprinkle nuts over the chocolate-covered banana. Return the banana to the baking sheet. Repeat to coat all the bananas with chocolate and nuts. Return the baking sheet to the freezer until the chocolate hardens and is frozen. Wrap each banana separately in plastic wrap, then place them all in a large, self-sealing freezer-safe plastic bag and store in the freezer.

Makes 8 servings

Part 2:

health and
beauty care for
you and yours

Your Own
Beauty Products

Some of the loveliest and most seductive ads on television and in magazines are for cosmetics— makeup, scents, and skin care products in beautiful

packages. They are all very intriguing and inviting until you read the small print and realize that you don't know what all those ingredients are or what they are designed to do. And, although you may feel, as one cosmetics company suggests, that the price doesn't matter because "you're worth it," you just might want to know what is going onto your skin.

Making your own beauty products is neither difficult nor mystifying. These recipes have all been thoroughly reviewed by experts. For not much more than a little time and effort, you can even give yourself spa treatments that will benefit your spirits as well as your skin—with face masks, exfoliants, and wrinkle fighters. Your pocketbook will barely be involved. You might even want to involve friends in the making and using of these recipes for special spa hours.

For everyday use, you can make cleansers, moisturizers, and toners; toothpaste and gargles; shampoos and hair rinses; shaving gels and refreshing splashes—with or without scent. For your bath, you can prepare lovely bath gels from soap slivers, almond rose or cinnamon soap, and several bath scrubs and milk baths. For hands and feet, there are special creams and soaks. There is also a selection of recipes for homemade men's toiletries: shaving soap, aftershaves, a shaving cut lotion, and a muscle rub.

face care products

Anti-Wrinkle Eye Cream

Apply this cream with a gentle touch around the eye, using light, circular strokes. It is especially geared for the soft tissue under and around the eyes—and it works just as well as, if not better than, the pricey versions sold in stores.

2 tablespoons elder flower water (available through mail order)

1/4 cup avocado oil

2 tablespoons almond oil

4 teaspoons wheat germ oil

2 tablespoons lanolin

2 tablespoons glycerin

2 drops geranium essential oil

1 vitamin E capsule, 400 IU

1. Warm the elder flower water in a nonreactive saucepan over low heat.

2. In the top of a double boiler, set over simmering water, warm the avocado, almond, and wheat germ oils. Stir in the lanolin until melted. Remove from heat.

3. Gradually beat in the warmed elder flower water. Stir in the glycerin and geranium essential oil. Pierce the vitamin E capsule with a needle, squeeze out the contents, and stir in.

4. Pour mixture into a clean widemouthed 6-ounce glass jar with a tight-fitting lid. Store in a cool, dark place.

Tired Eye Remedy

Here's a simple soak you can apply to soothe irritated or inflamed eyes. The price is a few rose petals from your garden.

8 ounces boiling water

2-3 rose petals

1. Pour the boiling water over the rose petals into a bowl. Steep for about 10 minutes. Cool and strain the petals out.

2. Soak two large cotton balls in the rose tea and apply over closed eyelids. Rest and relax.

One-Minute Substitute

Fast Relief with Witch Hazel Eye Compresses

We give our eyes a workout reading, watching TV, and staring at the computer screen. Here's a basic eye care remedy that costs no more than a few cents and provides a very valuable service. Just keep a small jar of witch hazel in the refrigerator. Soak two cotton pads in the chilled liquid, lie down, cover both eyelids, and relax for 5 minutes.

Rich Neck Moisturizer

In your beauty regimen, don't forget the neck, which can show the first signs of aging. Products like this often sell at beauty counters for $12 to $25 or more, but you can make it for just a few dollars with all-natural ingredients. This recipe uses oils to keep the skin supple. Use a small amount and massage from the neckline all the way to the chin.

1 teaspoon dried chamomile
1 1/8 cups boiling water
3 tablespoons avocado oil
3 tablespoons almond oil
2 teaspoons jojoba oil
1 ounce shaved or grated beeswax
2 teaspoons glycerin
20 drops lemon essential oil

1. Place the chamomile in a large cup, and add the boiling water. Cover and allow to steep for 15 minutes. Strain the liquid into another cup.

2. In the top of a double boiler, set over simmering water, warm the avocado, almond, and jojoba oils. Add the beeswax. Stir until melted. Remove from heat and beat in 1 ounce (2 tablespoons) of the warmed chamomile infusion, drop by drop until the mixture thickens and cools. Thoroughly mix in the glycerin and lemon essential oil.

3. Spoon into a sterilized, widemouthed, 6-ounce glass or ceramic jar with a tight-fitting lid. Store in a cool, dark place.

know your skin type

To pick the best products for your skin, you need to know your skin type. Most people have a combination of skin types—particularly on the face—where oily areas around the chin, nose, and forehead are different from the normal or dry skin around the eyes and on the cheeks.

There are four basic skin types:

Normal skin is clear, supple, and soft. It is neither too dry nor too oily, and it is not overly sensitive to sun, humidity, or the environment.

Dry skin looks dull, feels tight after washing, and needs sun protection and frequent moisturizing to prevent flaking.

Oily skin feels soft and supple, but it looks shiny and needs cleaning several times a day. Oily skin tends to support large pores and is more prone to pimples and blackheads than dry or normal skin.

Sensitive skin is easily burned by the sun and irritated by chemicals found in many commercial skin products that may cause rashes or blotching.

Peachy Keen Complexion Cream

This wonderful rich combination is easily made. You'll find it helps give your complexion that fabled glow. And you can't find anything like it in the stores.

1 ripe peach
Heavy cream

1. Mash the peach by hand or puree it in a food processor.

2. Add enough cream to the pulp to give you a soft, creamy mixture. Spoon into a clean glass jar with a tight-fitting lid and store in the refrigerator.

3. Once a day, apply the mixture to your face and massage in.

Artichoke Facial

Artichoke conditions dry or damaged skin. It reduces flaking and restores suppleness. Enjoy making this recipe in your kitchen laboratory, but watch out for the "choke!"

1 fresh artichoke heart, well cooked, or canned hearts in water, not oil

2 teaspoons light oil (avocado, olive, or canola)

1 teaspoon vinegar or fresh lemon juice

1. Mash artichoke heart in a ceramic bowl. Mix in oil and vinegar or lemon juice. Stir well until a smooth paste is formed.
2. Massage on face and neck. Let sit 10 to 15 minutes. Rinse off with warm water and pat dry.

Basic Skin Toner

A gentle cleanser or first step in your daily ritual. You can custom-design this basic skin toner to suit your skin type. See the box on page 254 to choose the essential oils that are right for you.

1 teaspoon dried chamomile

1/3 cup boiling water

2 drops essential oil

1. Place the chamomile and boiling water in a cup. Cover and allow to steep for 15 minutes. Strain the liquid through a fine sieve into a sterile 4-ounce glass bottle that has a tight-fitting lid. When cool, add the essential oil and shake well to mix. Allow to stand for 48 hours, shaking periodically.
2. Pour the liquid through a paper coffee filter into a sterile glass bottle. Cap the bottle and store in a cool, dark place.
3. Apply daily with a cotton ball.

fixed oil vs. essential oil

Olive oil, almond oil, and vegetable oils are all derived primarily from seeds. They are "fixed oils" that are nonvolatile. Essential oils, distilled from leaves or flowers, are volatile and flammable. They evaporate even at low temperatures, and they are potentially toxic if they are inhaled or if they are used incorrectly.

Most essential oils must be diluted in a fixed, or "carrier," oil before they are applied to the skin. The exceptions are lavender and tea tree essential oils, but even they should be used sparingly.

Cucumber Astringent

Straight from your garden or the grocer's counter, you can make this skin bracer in a jiffy. In summer you'll find this a refreshing and light treat for your skin. But any time of year, a simple cucumber astringent will perk you up.

1 cucumber

1. Peel the cucumber and puree it in a food processor. Apply the puree to your skin using a cotton pad, gently swathing your face. Rinse off with cool water.
2. Refrigerate any leftovers in a clean, covered container. It should keep for a day or two.

Egg-White Toner
For the price of an egg, you can make this one-ingredient toner that leaves your skin feeling tight and silky smooth.

1 egg white

1. Clean your face thoroughly using any natural cleanser.
2. Whisk the egg white just before applying it to your face. Leave it on for about 15 minutes.
3. Wash off with tepid water and pat skin dry.

Lemon Skin Toner
You can toss this toner together in just a few seconds from items you have in your pantry. Total cost: just pennies. Most toners purchased at the cosmetics counter run more than $6 a bottle.

2 ounces lemon juice
4 ounces distilled water
3 ounces witch hazel

1. Combine all ingredients. Pour into a clean bottle or decorative cosmetics container. Shake well before using. Apply with a clean cotton ball.
2. Keep in the refrigerator indefinitely.

One-Minute Substitute

Instant Grape Cleanser for Your Face
Here's a sweet way to clean and refresh your skin. Split 3 or 4 large green or red grapes, remove any seeds, and rub the fleshy interior on your face and neck. The grapes condition your skin and reduce dryness, restoring suppleness. Rinse with cool water and gently pat skin dry.

Facial Cleansing Mask
This simple recipe is aimed at deep cleansing and is especially suited for young faces and the treatment of oily skin.

1 packet dry yeast
3 drops lemon juice
2 teaspoons water

1. In a small bowl, mix the yeast, lemon juice, and water vigorously until a thick paste forms. If necessary, add more water to achieve the correct consistency for applying to the face.
2. Pat the mixture on the face, avoiding the eyes. Allow to sit for 10 to 15 minutes. Rinse off with warm water. Pat skin dry.

Green Clay Purifying Face Mask

Green clay—also known as bentonite— is the most commonly used clay in face masks. It can absorb large quantities of water. In this mask, it is used to draw out excess sebum and dirt from deep down, making the mask suited to oily complexions. Green clay powder can be purchased online or in health food stores for about $5 for 8 ounces, which would be enough clay for 16 masks. Palmarosa is an essential oil available at health food or "new age" shops.

1 teaspoon apricot kernel oil
2 drops palmarosa
1 tablespoon green clay
Warm water

1. Clean your face thoroughly using any natural cleanser. In a small dish, mix the apricot oil and the palmarosa together. Put the green clay in a small bowl and stir in the apricot oil mixture. Add just enough warm water to make a spreadable paste. With your fingers, work the mixture thoroughly to incorporate all the ingredients.

2. Apply the mask immediately, avoiding the eyes. Let it sit for 10 to 15 minutes. As the moisture evaporates, you will feel the mask tighten.

3. Rinse the mask off with warm water, pat skin dry, and follow with an application of toner and then of moisturizer.

Yogurt and Oatmeal Deep-Cleansing Facial

Imagine! You can mix up this deep-cleansing face mask for less than 50 cents. Your face and your pocketbook will thank you.

1 tablespoon finely ground oatmeal
1 tablespoon yogurt (any kind)
1/2 teaspoon honey

1. Before starting, clean your face thoroughly with any natural cleanser so that you can immediately apply the deep-cleansing facial mixture when it has been stirred together.

2. In a clean bowl, combine the yogurt and oatmeal and mix to a spreadable consistency. In a small glass bowl sitting in a larger bowl of hot water, warm the honey and pour it into the yogurt and oatmeal mixture. Using a spoon, blend the ingredients thoroughly.

3. Immediately apply the mask to your face, avoiding the eyes, and let it stay on for 10 to 15 minutes. Wash it off with warm water. Pat skin dry and apply a toner and moisturizer to your face.

Almond Mayonnaise Scrub

Don't be afraid of this one, but keep in mind that it is for very dry skin. Mayonnaise, which contains eggs, oil, and lemon juice, will nourish the face. The almonds will provide a mild exfoliation/dermabrasion.

1/4 cup almonds
1/8 teaspoon mayonnaise
1 teaspoon red-wine or cider vinegar
1/2 cup water

1. Clean your face thoroughly with any natural cleanser. Grind almonds in a blender or food processor until they form a meal. Whirl in mayonnaise. Set aside.
2. In a small bowl, combine the vinegar and water. Rinse your face with this mixture.
3. Now gently and thoroughly massage your face with the almond-mayonnaise scrub. Leave it on your skin for 10 minutes. Rinse off with warm water and pat skin dry.

Honey Mask

The ingredients in this mask would make up a solid breakfast, but they're nourishing for your skin too. Costing under a dollar, it's a good deal for a meal or a mask.

1/2 cup hot water
10 tablespoons quick oats
1/2 apple, cored but with peel on
2 heaping tablespoons plain yogurt
2 tablespoons honey
1 egg white

1. Clean your face thoroughly with any natural cleanser. In a small bowl, stir the oats into the hot water until you have a smooth mixture. Let stand for about 5 minutes or until the mixture thickens to a paste.
2. Put the apple, yogurt, honey, and egg white in a blender or food processor and pulse for 45 seconds just to mix. Now add oatmeal mixture and pulse for 20 seconds more.
3. Apply this mask evenly to the face, avoiding the eyes, and let sit for 15 minutes or until skin feels tight. Rinse thoroughly with warm water and pat skin dry.

Banana, Sour Cream, and Honey Face Mask

Although this sounds like the beginning of a rich dessert, it's actually an enriching mask for your face. The banana is an astringent, the honey conditions, and the sour cream allows them to work together in a mask. You could travel to a fancy spa for a treatment like this, but making it at home will cost you just a few cents. Enjoy!

1/2 banana
1 tablespoon honey
2 tablespoons sour cream

1. Clean your face thoroughly with any natural cleanser. In a small bowl, mash the half-banana. Stir in the honey and sour cream.
2. Apply to your face, avoiding the eyes, and let set for 10 minutes. Gently wipe off with a damp washcloth. Rinse clean with warm water. Pat your skin dry.

Youthful Skin Face Mask

In this variation of the banana facial mask, banana is again the astringent. It induces a tightening or tingling sensation and thereby gives the effect of decreasing the appearance of wrinkles.

1/4 cup heavy whipping cream

1 medium banana

1 vitamin E capsule, 400 IU

1. Clean your face thoroughly with any natural cleanser. In a small bowl, mash together the cream and banana. Pierce the vitamin E capsule with a needle, squeeze out the contents, and stir in.

2. Smooth onto face and neck. Leave on for 10 to 15 minutes. Remove with damp cloth. Rinse clean with warm water. Pat your skin dry.

Helpful Hint

When Vitamin E Is Called For

Several of the recipes on in this part of the book call for using vitamin E. You can buy vitamin E oil as a liquid at most drugstores, but if you only need a small amount, it's sometimes more practical to use a 400 IU vitamin E capsule. Just pierce the capsule with a needle and squeeze out the contents.

Oatmeal Exfoliant

Here's a treat for your face that might be part of a spa regimen. You can mix this up in a jiffy to use as a cleanser anytime you're in the mood. Cost to you: less than 25 cents.

2 heaping teaspoons fine oatmeal

1 teaspoon baking soda

Lukewarm water

1. Clean your face thoroughly with any natural cleanser.

2. In a small bowl, stir together oatmeal and baking soda. (The oatmeal needs to be fine; if necessary, first pulse it in a food processor or blender.) Add enough lukewarm water to make a paste. Apply to face and rub gently. Rinse and gently pat the skin dry.

One-Minute Substitute

A Quick Banana Wrinkle Fighter

Peel away the years with this easy facial treatment. Banana is an astringent that induces a tightening or tingling sensation on the skin, which decreases the appearance of wrinkles. With bananas usually selling for less than 50 cents a pound, this is a very reasonable facial treatment. Clean your face thoroughly with any natural cleanser. Mash 1/4 of a ripe banana until very creamy and spread it all over your face, avoiding the eyes. Leave on for 15 to 20 minutes. Rinse with warm water and then splash cold water on your face. Gently pat your skin dry.

Mask for Oily Skin

This combination of brewer's yeast and yogurt deep-cleanses oily skin without over-drying. The inexpensive homemade mask leaves skin feeling fresh and revitalized, just as a $30 salon mask treatment does.

1 teaspoon brewer's yeast
1/3 cup yogurt or as needed

1. Clean your face thoroughly with any natural cleanser. In a small bowl, mix the brewer's yeast with the yogurt to make a thin paste. Pat this mixture onto the oily areas of your face. Allow the mask to dry for 15 to 20 minutes.

2. Rinse with warm water. Splash with cool water. Gently pat dry.

Strawberry Yogurt Mask

If you grow strawberries in your garden, pluck a few to use in this treatment. Your face will thank you for this gentle, delicious treat that leaves the skin smooth and refreshed.

1 handful ripe strawberries
1 tablespoon ground almonds
2 tablespoons yogurt

1. Clean your face thoroughly with any natural cleanser. In a small bowl, mash the strawberries and almonds until completely blended together. Stir in the yogurt to make a spreadable paste.

2. Apply immediately or refrigerate and use within 1 day on a clean face.

how to apply a face mask

Women have used face masks for centuries to clean and tone the skin and give it a glowing vitality. Face masks give their best results if used regularly—once a week is not too often.

1. To make the process easier, sit or stand in front of a mirror. Cover your shoulders with a clean towel and have a damp washrag or hand towel ready for wiping up any drips.

2. Apply the mask with a clean cotton ball or with your fingers. The mask should cover your face from the hairline to the chin, missing only the area around the eyes.

3. Leave the mask on for 15 minutes the first few times you use it. Later, if your skin is not irritated and you like the mask's effects, you can slowly increase the time to 30 minutes. To best enjoy the facial mask, lie down, shut your eyes, and relax while the mask is working.

4. When the time is up, remove the mask with your fingers over a basin. If the mask has dried, splash warm water on your face and try again to remove the mask with your fingers. Then use a wet washcloth to remove the last residue of the mask. Finally, splash your face with cool water, pat the skin dry, and apply a toner.

Galen's Cold Cream

1 ounce beeswax, grated or shaved

1/3 cup light olive oil

2 tablespoons distilled water or rose water

3 drops geranium essential oil

As old as the hills, this recipe for cold cream is believed to have been devised by the Greek philosopher and doctor Galen in the 2nd century C.E. It is still every bit as effective today and will cost you pennies compared to the name brands at cosmetics counters. A 1-ounce bar of beeswax can be bought online for as little as 85 cents.

1. In the top of a double boiler, over simmering water, melt the beeswax.

2. In a small saucepan over low heat, heat the oil slightly and then pour it into the melted wax. Using a fork, beat this mixture until combined.

3. Now heat the water or rose water in the saucepan and then stir it into the oil and wax mixture, one drop at a time. Remove from heat and stir until the mixture is cooled and thick. Stir in the essential oil.

4. Using a wooden spoon, put the mixture into a clean 5-ounce widemouthed jar with a tight-fitting lid. Store in a cool, dark place for several months.

care for lips and mouth

Honey Lip Balm

4 ounces extra-virgin olive oil

3 ounces grated or shaved beeswax

1 ounce honey

1/2 capsule vitamin E, 400 IU

You'll get a kick out of making lip balm at home. You'll feel a little bit like a mad scientist, and a little bit like a truly creative cook. The following three formulations will cost about a dollar or so each, and provide a lot of lip gloss or balm for the buck. Consider dividing the lip balm mixture into several small containers, so that you can carry some with you.

1. In a microwave or the top of a double boiler, melt the beeswax and oil together. *Do not boil.* If the mixture starts to boil, remove from heat and allow it to cool. Once the beeswax and oil are blended, stir in the honey. Then pierce the vitamin E capsule with a needle, squeeze out half the contents, and stir in. Pour the resulting mixture into clean containers with tops.

2. Let the lip balm sit at room temperature for 48 hours until it arrives at the proper consistency for spreading. You can carry a small container of lip balm around with you during the day, but you may find it keeps better in the refrigerator overnight.

Cocoa Lip Balm
Remember, although this concoction smells sweet, it is not a food product. If you plan to give it to a child, label it accordingly and explain how to use it.

4 ounces extra-virgin
  olive oil

3 ounces beeswax,
  grated or shaved

1/2 teaspoon cocoa powder

1/2 capsule vitamin E, 400 IU

1. In a microwave or the top of a double boiler, melt the beeswax and oil together. *Do not boil.* If the mixture starts to boil, remove from the heat and allow it to cool. Once the beeswax and oil are blended, stir in the cocoa powder. Pierce the vitamin E capsule with a needle, squeeze out half the contents, and stir it in. Pour the resulting mixture into clean containers with tops.

2. Let the lip balm sit for 48 hours at room temperature until it arrives at the proper consistency for spreading. You can carry a small container of lip balm around with you during the day, but you may find it keeps better in the refrigerator overnight.

Chocolate Chip Lip Balm for Kids
When you cook up this little treat in your kitchen, you may be tempted to eat it, but this yummy-smelling lip balm is not edible. Be sure to label it as lip balm and explain to young children what it is.

4 ounces extra-virgin
  olive oil

3 ounces beeswax, grated or
  shaved

1/2 capsule vitamin E,
  400 IU

3-6 chocolate chips

1. In a microwave or the top of a double boiler, melt the beeswax and oil together. *Do not boil.* If the mixture starts to boil, remove from the heat and allow it to cool. Once the beeswax and oil are blended, pierce the vitamin E capsule with a needle, squeeze out half the contents, and stir in. Stir in the chocolate chips and pour the resulting mixture into clean containers with tops.

2. Let the lip balm sit for 48 hours at room temperature until it arrives at the proper consistency for spreading. You can carry a small container of lip balm around with you during the day, but you may find it keeps better in the refrigerator overnight.

One-Minute
Substitute

A Fast, Hard-Working Mouthwash
For fighting bacteria and removing food particles caught in your teeth, this inexpensive recipe is about as effective a mouthwash as you can get. It uses the standard 3% hydrogen peroxide sold in drugstores. Hydrogen peroxide, however, may irritate sensitive teeth or delicate tissue in the mouth, so this rinse should not be used more than three times a week. In a cup, mix 2 tablespoons of hydrogen peroxide solution with 2 tablespoons of water. Swish the mixture in your mouth for 30 seconds, then spit it out—don't swallow it.

Refreshing Mouthwash

For just a few cents you can cook up a potful of this rinse that tastes good and can be safely used as often as you like. Unlike more expensive commercial mouthwashes, it has no alcohol.

1 cup water

2 tablespoons angelica seeds

Dash of peppermint oil or lemon verbena

1. In a small saucepan over medium heat, bring the water to a boil. Remove from the heat. Stir in the angelica seeds and peppermint oil or lemon verbena. Let the mixture sit for 10 minutes. Strain off and discard the solids.

2. Store the liquid in a clean, covered container in the refrigerator and use every day. It should keep indefinitely.

Spicy, Minty Mouthwash

This simple recipe offers a kick that will make your mouth feel wonderful for hours. Use it as often as you like—it's very inexpensive and doesn't burn like commercial mouthwashes with alcohol in them.

1 cup water

1 teaspoon whole cloves

1 teaspoon ground cinnamon

1 teaspoon peppermint extract

2 teaspoons parsley

1. In a small saucepan, bring the water to a boil over medium heat. Remove the pan from the stove and stir in the cloves, cinnamon, peppermint extract, and parsley. Let mixture sit for 10 minutes. Strain off the solids.

2. Pour the liquid into a clean, tightly covered container and store in the refrigerator, where it will keep indefinitely. Use as a gargle and mouthwash.

Bacteria-Fighting Citrus Mouthwash

Fight the damaging bacteria that dwell in your mouth with this lemon-tasting mouthwash with an alcohol base that acts as a disinfectant. It is as effective as any mouthwash you can buy and much less expensive. Rinse and swish or gargle, but don't swallow the liquid.

3/4 cup vodka

30 drops lemon essential oil

25 drops bergamot essential oil

1 1/4 cups distilled water

1. Place the vodka and the lemon and bergamot essential oils in a sterilized 16-ounce glass bottle with a tight-fitting lid. Shake the mixture vigorously to combine.

2. Add the distilled water and shake until well blended. Leave in the refrigerator for 1 week to mature, shaking from time to time.

3. To use, shake the bottle and mix 1 part of the mixture with 3 parts lukewarm distilled water in a small drinking glass. Rinse, but do not swallow the mouthwash.

Toothpaste

We've grown accustomed to some highly sweetened commercial toothpastes. And at $3 or $4 a tube, that acquired taste can add up to a nice chunk of change over the course of a year. Once you perfect your own homemade toothpaste recipe by adjusting the ingredients to your liking, you should be able to keep a family of four in toothpaste for less than $2 a year.

1/2 cup baking soda

2 teaspoons salt

3 teaspoons glycerin

10 or more drops pepper-mint or wintergreen flavoring

1 drop food coloring *(optional)*

Warm water

1. In a small bowl, mix the baking soda and salt. Add the glycerin, flavoring, and if desired, 1 drop blue or green food coloring. Add warm water, a drop at a time, until the texture and consistency seem right. Spoon the mixture into a clean squeeze bottle or any convenient, clean container with a tight lid.

2. You may have to adjust the amount of glycerin to arrive at a consistency that suits you. This toothpaste will keep indefinitely in a covered container.

shampoos, conditioners, and rinses

Beer Shampoo

This concoction will leave your hair with wonderful body. The proteins from the malt and hops in the beer coat the hair and build it up, helping to repair damage.

3/4 cup beer

1 cup shampoo (any kind)

1. In a nonreactive pan, boil the beer until it reduces to 1/4 cup. Cool the beer and add it to the 1 cup of shampoo in a clean bottle with a tight cap.

2. Wash your hair as usual.

One-Minute Substitute

A Quick, Sweet-Smelling Vinegar Hair Rinse

Pick up a bottle of raspberry or plum vinegar the next time you go shopping. Expect to pay about $2.50 for an 8-ounce bottle. It can do double duty in the kitchen. Use a few tablespoons for this recipe and the rest for salad dressings.

Rather than prepare ahead of time, simply bring a clean 1- or 2-cup measuring cup with 2 to 3 tablespoons of scented vinegar into the shower. After shampooing, add water, and rinse your hair with the solution. You can use this every time you shampoo, if you like.

Vinegar restores the proper acidic pH balance to hair. This rinse will remove remnants of shampoo and give your hair more shine.

Your Own Beauty Products   **663**

Dandruff Treatment

Over-the-counter dandruff treatments can be very costly, starting at about $6 for a 10-ounce bottle. You can create this herbal remedy for less than a dollar.

2 teaspoons dried rosemary
2 teaspoons dried thyme
2/3 cup boiling water
2/3 cup cider vinegar

1. Place the herbs in a heatproof ceramic bowl. Pour in the boiling water. Cover and allow to steep for 15 to 20 minutes.

2. Strain the liquid into a clean, 10-ounce bottle that has a tight-fitting lid. Add the vinegar and shake. Store in a cool, dark place.

3. After shampooing, rinse hair thoroughly and then massage a small amount of the herbal treatment into the scalp. Between shampoos, massage a small amount into the scalp before going to bed.

Sun-Streaking Rinse

This is a rich hair dressing that provides sheen and elegance to tired hair. People with light-colored hair will find it helps them get clean, honest-looking highlights that they might otherwise pay $30 to $40 for at a salon. It can also be used as a pressing oil for hair straightening.

Juice of 1 lemon
2 teaspoons chamomile tea

1. In a small bowl, mix the lemon juice and tea. To achieve blond highlights, use an inexpensive straw hat with lots of holes in it. Pull strands of hair you would like to lighten through the holes with a crochet hook or pencil.

2. Douse the strands with the rinse. Sit in the sun for 1 1/2 hours.

what herbs in hair rinses do		
	Catnip	Believed to promote hair growth
	Chamomile	Keeps scalp and hair follicles healthy
	Comfrey	Soothes and heals scalp irritations
	Elder berries	Traditionally used to add color to gray hair
	Lemongrass	Tones the scalp
	Nettle	An astringent that helps relieve skin irritations and itching
	Parsley	Helps relieve skin irritations
	Rosemary	Believed to enhance color of dark hair and help control dandruff
	Sage	An astringent for oily hair and a benefit for damaged or fragile hair
	Thyme	Has antiseptic, tonic, and astringent properties
	Yarrow	Acts as a tonic for the hair

Chamomile Shampoo

This mild shampoo leaves your hair clean and healthy. The recipe gives you a chance to use those leftover slivers of soap you wonder why you save. Forget the well-advertised shampoos that cost $4 or $5 a bottle. You need only one tablespoon of this inexpensive shampoo per washing.

1 handful fresh or dried chamomile flowers
1 1/4 cups boiling water
3 tablespoons pure soap flakes or leftover slivers of soap
1 tablespoon glycerin
5 drops yellow food coloring

1. Place the flowers in a heatproof bowl and add the boiling water. Let stand for 15 minutes, then strain into another heatproof bowl.
2. Clean out the first bowl. Combine in it the soap flakes and the chamomile mixture and let them stand until the soap softens—a few minutes. Beat in the glycerin and food coloring until well blended.
3. Pour the mixture into a clean 14-ounce bottle with a tight-fitting lid. Keep in a cool, dark place.

Thick Hair Conditioner for Everyone

This two-ingredient conditioner offers a protein boost for your hair that in turn will make it feel thicker and more luxuriant. You don't need to go to an expensive hair salon to revitalize your hair.

1/2 ripe avocado
1/4 cup coconut milk, or as needed

1. In a small bowl, mash the avocado with a spoon. Mix in the coconut milk to form a thick gel-like substance.
2. Apply the entire recipe to clean hair and comb through. Leave the conditioner on the hair for 10 to 15 minutes. Rinse thoroughly.

Salad Dressing Conditioner

This treatment will leave your hair feeling cleansed and enriched. The conditioner will perform as well as drugstore conditioners that cost many times more.

2 tablespoons olive oil
1 tablespoon lemon juice
1/2 teaspoon apple cider vinegar
1 egg

1. In the container of a blender, combine the oil, lemon juice, vinegar, and egg and whirl until blended. Alternatively, whisk vigorously until combined.
2. Use the entire batch to condition hair after a regular shampoo. Leave the conditioner on the hair for 10 to 15 minutes. Rinse clean.

Shampoo Residue Remover for Blond Hair

Mix up this cleansing rinse that will leave your blond hair shining for just pennies.

1 part lemon juice
4 parts water

1. Combine lemon juice and water in a clean container. Shake to mix.

2. Use as a final rinse after a regular shampoo. Don't rinse it out.

Instant Dry Shampoo

This homey, penny-pinching recipe is tailor-made for that moment when you need a quick pick-me-up or you haven't got time to wash your hair.

1 tablespoon cornstarch or finely ground oatmeal

1. Sprinkle small amounts of cornstarch or oatmeal onto the hair, lifting it up in sections to let the powder get to the scalp. Rub the shampoo through the hair to absorb excess oil.

2. Comb the hair to remove tangles, then spend 5 to 10 minutes brushing (depending on the length and thickness of the hair) to remove all traces of the powder and prevent the suggestion of dandruff. Shake and blow on your hairbrush to clean it while you brush your hair.

body care treatments

Warm Herbal Body Treatment

This warm, scented spa-style treatment will relax and rejuvenate you—for the cost of a few tea bags!

8 cups water
4 chamomile tea bags or other gentle herbal tea
3 peppermint tea bags
Sprigs of fresh rosemary or sage *(optional)*

1. In a large saucepan, bring the water to a boil. Remove it from the heat and add the tea bags and herbs. Cover the pan and steep the tea for 10 to 15 minutes. Once the tea has cooled to a comfortably warm temperature, remove the tea bags and herbs.

2. Drop several clean but dispensable hand towels into the tea (the towels will be stained). Let them soak up the mixture, and then wring them out. Wrap your upper arms and legs with the tea-soaked towels. You may also place a soaked towel on your torso, but don't put one on your face.

3. Lie down on a protected bed, couch, or pad and rest for 10 to 15 minutes. Remove the towels and relax while cooling off for another 10 to 15 minutes. Shower off the residue.

Caution: Heat treatments such as this are not recommended for people with high blood pressure or heart problems.

Creamy Citrus Moisturizer

This creamy moisturizer will leave your skin soft and silky for less than a dollar. You can't buy a commercial moisturizer for anywhere near that.

1 egg yolk
2 tablespoons lemon juice
1 cup olive oil

1. In a medium bowl, whisk the egg yolk, lemon juice, and olive oil together until the mixture reaches a creamy consistency. Thin with more lemon juice as desired.

2. Massage into your skin as an intense moisturizing treatment before a shower or bath. Apply a light coating on your hands, arms, legs, and face. Gently massage into nails and cuticles. Apply about a tablespoon to each foot. Gently massage your toes, one by one, and then the arch of your foot, moving to the heel. Relax and allow the moisturizer to soak in for 10 to 15 minutes. Wipe away the excess and then step into the shower or tub to complete the treatment.

3. Store any leftovers in the refrigerator for a day or two.

Glorious Green Aloe Moisturizing Lotion

For about $1.50 you can cook up this delightful body lotion that has aloe vera, an antioxidant, as its primary ingredient. You scoop the gel out of aloe vera leaves or you can buy it at a health food store.

1 cup aloe vera gel
1 teaspoon vitamin E oil (if necessary, break several capsules)
5-10 drops essential oil of your choosing
3/4 ounce cosmetic-grade beeswax, grated or shaved
1/2 cup vegetable oil

1. In a medium bowl, stir together the aloe vera gel, vitamin E, and essential oil. Set aside.

2. In the top of a double boiler over simmering water, melt together the beeswax and vegetable oil. Stir until smooth and well blended. Remove from heat.

3. Slowly and continuously pour the melted mixture into the bowl with the aloe vera mixture, using a handheld electric mixer at slow speed to combine. Run a clean rubber spatula around the rim of the bowl to incorporate all the ingredients. Continue mixing until all the ingredients are blended.

4. Pour the final mixture into one sterilized 13-ounce jar or two sterilized 6-ounce jars with tight-fitting lids. You can use sterilized canning jars, if you have them. Keep the lotion in the refrigerator for up to 6 weeks.

the best body
oil for your
skin type

To make body oil, put 4 teaspoons almond oil in a sterile glass jar with a tight-fitting top. Add the appropriate drops of essential oils listed below for your skin type, shake, and pour a little into your palm, so that you can apply it to the rest of your body. Each blend will give you four body rubs.

Normal skin: 8 drops lavender

6 drops geranium

2 drops chamomile

Dry skin: 8 drops patchouli

4 drops geranium

2 drops carrot

Oily skin: 10 drops lemon

6 drops geranium

4 drops sandalwood

Sensitive skin: 3 drops geranium

2 drops patchouli

Shaving Gel for Women

Using just four ingredients you probably already have at home in ample supply, you can make your very own shaving gel that is just right for shaving legs and underarms. It's a good recipe to make in a pinch, but it will also help you cut one more expense from your weekly shopping bill.

2 tablespoons conditioner (preferably the same brand as the shampoo used)

2 tablespoons shampoo

1/2-1 teaspoon baby oil

1 teaspoon hand cream

1. Start with a clean bottle with a secure cap. Pour 2 tablespoons conditioner into the bottle, then add 2 tablespoons shampoo. Mix together. Add the baby oil and then the hand cream. Secure top and shake until all the ingredients are well blended. Let mixture sit for about an hour before using.

2. Lather legs or underarms with the gel, shave, and rinse skin thoroughly. The shaving gel should keep for about a month in the bathroom. If the mixture separates, just shake it up before you use it.

Summer Body Splash

Refresh yourself with a splash of this delicate mixture of fruit and flower scents just perfect for hot summer days and nights.

1/3 cup vodka

10 drops lavender essential oil

5 drops lime essential oil

5 drops lemon essential oil

5 drops lemongrass essential oil

2 cups distilled or boiled water

1. Pour the vodka and essential oils into a sterilized 20-ounce bottle with a tight-fitting stopper. Stopper the bottle and shake for several minutes. Add the distilled or boiled water and shake for several minutes more. Set aside for at least 48 hours or up to 3 weeks.

2. Place a paper coffee filter in a sieve and drip the liquid through the filter into a ceramic or glass bowl. Now pour the liquid back into the large bottle or into a few smaller sterilized bottles. Keep one bottle in the refrigerator and store the others in a cool, dark place until needed.

Helpful Hint

What Is a Cool, Dark Place?

When you make home remedies and beauty products, you are usually told to store them in a cool, dark, dry place. Where is that? If you seal things in amber or opaque containers, that takes care of dark (most homemade potions are weakened by exposure to sunlight). A cool, dry place could be the linen closet or a shelf in a clothes closet that is not near any heat pipes, or a basement cupboard if the basement is dry. A safe last resort is the refrigerator.

Simple Fragrant Body Splash

If you have a favorite perfume oil that you'd like to wear in a lighter concentration, you'll love this easy recipe. Keep this spritzer in your purse for a pick-me-up on a warm day.

1 cup water

5-7 drops perfume oil

1. Have on hand a clean 8-ounce spray bottle. Pour the water into the bottle and drip the perfume oil drops into the water. Cover the top with your thumb and shake well.

2. Screw the top on and your body splash is ready.

Citrus Cologne Splash

Make this cooling scent at home for a few cents.

1 lime

1/2 cup rubbing alcohol

3 teaspoons lemon extract or orange extract

1. Juice the lime. Strain out the pulp. Combine the alcohol, lime juice, and lemon or orange extract in a clean bottle with a tight-fitting lid. Shake well.

2. Dab on pulse points. You may transfer the splash to a spray bottle. Store the splash in the refrigerator.

Cellulite Massage Oil

Include this massage oil—along with regular exercise and a healthy diet—in your tool kit to help lessen cellulite. A regular massage with this oil may help increase circulation and break down fatty deposits.

2 tablespoons almond oil

1/2 teaspoon jojoba oil

1/2 teaspoon carrot oil, available through mail order

14 drops geranium essential oil

6 drops lemongrass essential oil

4 drops cypress essential oil (available through mail order)

1. Combine all ingredients in a 1 1/2- to 2-ounce sterilized glass jar with a tight-fitting lid. Shake vigorously.
2. After a bath or shower, pat your skin dry and massage a small amount of the oil on cellulite-affected areas, using circular movements. Use 1/4 to 1/2 teaspoon, depending on the size of the area you are treating. Apply only once a day.

Almond Exfoliating Body Scrub

Scented, gritty body scrubs are all the rage. Here's a recipe you can make at home for about 50 cents.

1/4 cup coarse sea salt

1/4 cup baby oil

1/2 teaspoon almond extract, vanilla extract, or lightly scented perfume oil

1. In a small bowl, stir the salt and baby oil together until the oil is thoroughly incorporated into the salt. Add the extract and stir until it, too, is incorporated.
2. Use in the shower, after you are thoroughly wet. Apply with your hands, a washcloth, or a body puff scrubber. Massage in and rinse off.

Simple Sugar Scrub for Dry Skin

Here's another yummy body scrub that costs less than a dollar for three to four uses. For dry skin, this cannot be duplicated without spending at least 10 times as much.

1 cup brown sugar, white sugar, or a mix

1/2 cup olive, grapeseed, or other oil

2 drops vanilla or almond extract *(optional)*

1. In a medium bowl, combine the sugar and oil. Mix with a wooden spoon until you achieve a pastelike blend. Add extract if desired and stir until incorporated.
2. Transfer to a clean, airtight glass container to slow breakdown of the oil.
3. In the shower, massage this mixture gently over damp skin. It will exfoliate and moisturize at the same time. Do not use on broken, irritated, or scarred skin. Avoid the eyes. This is an especially oily mixture, so it is really best for dry skin.
4. Store mixture in the refrigerator for 6 months to a year.

Cranberry Sugar Scrub

The beauty of sugar scrub recipes is the way they offer up scent while managing to exfoliate, nourish, and polish the skin. Here is another spa-quality product you can make in your own kitchen.

1/2 cup frozen cranberries

1 teaspoon vegetable glycerin

1/4 cup sweet almond oil

1/4 cup sugar

2 drops orange essential oil

2 tablespoons oat powder (whirl oatmeal in blender if needed)

1. In the container of a food processor, combine cranberries, glycerin, and almond oil and whirl for 30 seconds—just enough to blend the ingredients without turning the berries to pulp. You want to keep the mixture thick.

2. Transfer mixture to a bowl and stir in the sugar. Stir in the essential oil. Add just enough of the oat powder to create a cohesive mixture that you can apply to your skin.

3. In the shower, rub the mixture on your skin. Massage in and remove with warm water.

Body Powder

This is a fresh-smelling and silky after-shower powder that you can use every day for a pittance. For a more feminine product, use just lavender and rose essential oils.

1/2 cup arrowroot

2 tablespoons white cosmetic clay

7 drops lavender essential oil

5 drops clary sage essential oil

2 drops patchouli essential oil

1. In a medium bowl, mix the arrowroot with the white cosmetic clay. Add the essential oils and mix well with your fingers.

2. Store in a tightly covered container for a couple of days to allow the powder to absorb the oils, then use all over your body as desired.

Body Spray

You can't buy a more refreshing body spray than this citrusy mixture that smells good, tones the skin, and feels delightfully cool.

1 tablespoon finely chopped orange peel

1 tablespoon finely chopped lemon peel

3 tablespoons plain vodka

1 tablespoon witch hazel

1 cup water

5 drops lemon verbena essential oil

10 drops bergamot essential oil

10 drops orange essential oil

1. In a small jar with a tight top, add orange and lemon peels to the vodka. Cover and leave for a week in a cool, dark place.

2. Strain the liquid into a clean spray bottle. Add the witch hazel, water, and the essential oils. Shake well and use as needed. Store in the refrigerator for up to two weeks.

Deodorant

Here's a serious homemade underarm deodorant that won't stain your clothes or strain your pocketbook.

2 ounces distilled witch hazel

1 ounce sage alcohol-based herbal extract

10 drops grapefruit-seed extract

10 drops clary sage essential oil

5 drops patchouli essential oil

1. In a small spray bottle, combine all the ingredients.

2. Shake well and spray under arms as needed.

bath products

Bubble Bath for Kids

This simple recipe provides a scented, bubbly bathful of suds you know are safe for your child and, as a bonus, helps you recycle extra shampoo. As always, parents should supervise children's use of such products. Beware of slippery tubs. Bubble baths are fun, but children shouldn't use them daily. Too much of a good thing could irritate sensitive skin.

1/2 cup shampoo

3/4 cup water

1/4 teaspoon table salt

1. In a medium bowl, mix shampoo and water. Gently stir until blended. Add salt. Stir until mixture thickens.

2. Pour through a funnel into a clean bottle with a tight cap. This bubble bath will keep safely for months in the bathroom.

Bubble Bath or Conditioning Bath

For an inexpensive, fun, and squeaky-clean bubble bath, this recipe gives you lots of bubbles and cleans up the tub as well. To be extra safe, test the solution on your child's inner arm to make sure he or she is not allergic to the solution. As always, parents should handle bubble bath products. Keep out of children's reach.

2 ounces gentle dishwashing solution

5-6 cups water

1 ounce glycerin

1. In a small bucket, swish all the ingredients together, altering the balance as you see fit. Pour into a bathtub of warm water for long-lasting bubbles. You may want to bring a bubble wand to the tub.

2. Keep an eye on children in the tub, which may be extra slippery with the bubble bath. Infants and very young children should not take bubble baths.

Bath Gel

This recipe is especially suited for children or adults with sensitive skin. It's easy to make and costs only about 50 cents for an 8-ounce jar. Wrap a grosgrain ribbon around the jar and you've got a delightful homemade gift.

- 1/2 cup distilled or bottled water, not tap water
- 1 packet unflavored gelatin
- 1/2 cup baby shampoo

1. In a small saucepan, bring the water to a boil. Add gelatin and stir until it is dissolved. Remove from heat. Slowly stir in the baby shampoo. Let this mixture cool until it's tepid enough to put in a clean, decorative widemouthed jar with a tight-fitting top.
2. Place jar in the refrigerator to set the gel.
3. Use a few teaspoons of gel per bath. Bath gel should keep up to a month in the refrigerator.

Liquid or Gel Soap

This bath or hand soap is easy to cook up and is a good way to use up old slivers of bar soap. Transfer the liquid soap to an empty pump container and you can supply your bathroom for just a portion of the price you'd pay at the store.

- 2 cups soap flakes or grated bar soap
- 1/2 gallon water
- 2 tablespoons glycerin

1. In a large pot or Dutch oven, combine all the ingredients. Cook over low heat, stirring occasionally, until the soap flakes have dissolved.
2. Transfer the mixture to a clean 1/2-gallon container and cover tightly. For a thinner gel soap, increase the water to 1 gallon.

Almond Rose Soap

Here's a simple method of soap-making using just a few basic tools. You'll create a fragrant soap that gently cleans.

- 2 tablespoons dried red rose petals
- 8 ounces pure soap flakes
- 2/3 cup boiling water
- 1/2 cup rose water
- 2 tablespoons ground almonds
- 9 drops geranium essential oil

1. Pound the rose petals with a mortar and pestle. In a large bowl, combine the ground petals, soap, and water and stir until smooth. If the soap starts to solidify, place the bowl over near-boiling water.
2. Stir in the rose water and ground almonds. Allow to cool. Stir in the essential oil.
3. Shape mixture into six balls and flatten them slightly. Allow the soap to harden between sheets of wax paper. Keep unused soap in a cool, dark place until needed.

Cinnamon Soap
You'll enjoy making this rich, spicy soap, which gives you another opportunity to use up leftover soap scraps.

2 pounds leftover soap

1 tablespoon spring water

1 teaspoon glycerin

1/2 teaspoon cinnamon essential oil

1 tablespoon sweet orange essential oil

10 drops clove bud essential oil *(optional)*

1. Coarsely grate the scraps of soap into a large mixing bowl. Add the spring water, glycerin, and essential oils. Mix well.

2. Cover the bowl with a clean cloth and allow it to stand for about 15 minutes, until the soap is slightly soft and pliable. (If your soap scraps are fairly new, they may be soft and not need much softening time.)

3. Scoop the mixture up by the handful and press or roll it into small balls. Compress it tightly. Place on wax paper. Allow the soap balls to dry and harden for a day or two.

Strawberries and Cream Bath Bags
Here's a charming idea you can make for about a dollar that provides a relaxing and soothing bath. The oatmeal mixture may help relieve dry or itching skin. For extra-sensitive skin, reduce or eliminate the essential oil. Dress up this bath product by scooping it into attractive cloth bags bought at a crafts store to create your own inexpensive version of high-end bath goodies.

1/2 cup oatmeal (regular or quick)

1/2 cup powdered milk

4 tablespoons almond meal (if necessary, whirl almonds in blender, coffee grinder, or food processor)

16 drops strawberry essential oil

1. In a small bowl, combine oatmeal, powdered milk, and almond meal, stirring to mix well. Stir in essential oil until blended. Divide mixture among three pretty cloth bags, and tie them at the top. Tie a generous loop of string or ribbon to the top of each bag.

2. When ready to use, hang the bag from the tub faucet by its loop. When you fill the tub, the water will run over the mixture inside the bag, dispersing it into the tub.

3. Keep bags in a cool, dark place until ready to use.

Bath Bag
This is a most inexpensive luxury for your bath. It makes you smell good afterward, but it is also delightful while you soak.

1 large handful mixed herbs (rosemary, lovage, lavender, lemongrass, sage, parsley, or peppermint)

Cheesecloth

1. Place the herbs of your choice in a doubled square of cheesecloth. Gather up the corners of the cheesecloth and tie securely.

2. Toss herb bag into a hot bath to soften and scent the water. Once you're in the bath, rub it all over your skin, paying particular attention to areas where odor is a problem.

Cinnamon Oatmeal Milk Bath

Mixing up this pleasantly scented bath will give you a double benefit. You'll gain as much pleasure making the concoction as you will from soaking in it. The combination of powdered milk, oatmeal, and cornstarch will leave you feeling silky and soft. The cinnamon will gently warm you and offer up a soothing aroma.

1 cup powdered milk
1/2 cup baking soda
1/2 cup finely ground oatmeal
2 teaspoon cornstarch
1 teaspoon cream of tartar
1 teaspoon cinnamon

1. Place all ingredients in a food processor and whirl to combine. Transfer into a clean, tightly covered, moisture-proof container, where it will keep indefinitely.
2. Add about 1/2 cup of the Cinnamon Oatmeal Milk Bath to a full tub of warm water and enjoy the soak.

Make It a Gift

Women's Bath Basket

Buy four brightly colored washcloths. Use each to wrap a home-made bath product: Almond Rose Soap, Delicately Scented Bath Powder, Bath Cookies, and Eucalyptus Foot Lotion, for example. Be sure each is labeled with ingredients and storage instructions. Nestle the bath treats in a nice basket that could hold extraneous bath supplies and attach a card with a large bow.

Gentle Milk Bath

You can shake up a soothing milk bath anytime you want to escape into a warm tub. Milk will leave your skin smooth and silky.

1/3 cup powdered milk
3 tablespoons cornstarch
1-2 drops essential oil of your choice

1. Pour the powdered milk and cornstarch into a clean jar with a tight top. Shake well. Add the essential oil and shake to thoroughly incorporate. If the mixture clumps, use your fingers to dissolve the lumps.
2. For a bath, put the mixture under the running water. Splash around with your hand to disperse it in the tub.

Note: You may double or triple this recipe and store it indefinitely by omitting the oil. Store the combined powdered milk and cornstarch in an airtight container; use 1/2 cup for each bath. Add the essential oil to the tub separately after swishing in the combined powders.

Magic Fruity Bath Salts

For about $1.35 you can mix up a quart of colorful, soothing bath salts. They're every bit as good as any you'd find in boutiques or on pharmacy shelves selling for anywhere from $3 to $12.

4 cups Epsom salts

1 envelope unsweetened Kool-Aid or equivalent, any flavor

1. Pour half the Epsom salts into a clean one-quart container. Empty the pouch of soft drink into the salts. Cover and shake until combined.

2. Add the rest of the salts and continue shaking. Your mixture will be subtly colored, but the "magic" colors will appear as you toss the salts into the warm tub.

3. Use up to a half-cup of bath salts per bath. Water will be scented and colorful. For a more dramatic appearing display, double or triple the recipe, but use several different-colored (flavored) packets of drink mix and layer the crystals and salt in a clear glass jar. Don't shake to mix. (Be sure to purchase the unsweetened drink mix.)

Store in a covered container. Keeps indefinitely.

Bath Cookies

If you like experimenting with recipes in the kitchen, you'll get a real kick out of making these "cookies" for the tub. Bakers will recognize the steps in dough-making, rolling, and baking, but there's a twist! Make one batch for yourself and another for friends.

2 cups fine sea salt

1/2 cup cornstarch, plus more for rolling dough

1/2 cup baking soda

1 tablespoon dried, chopped lavender or sage *(optional)*

2 eggs

2 tablespoons vegetable oil

1 teaspoon vitamin E oil (if necessary, break open several capsules)

8 drops essential oil or perfume oil of your choosing

1. Preheat oven to 350°F. In a large bowl, combine salt, cornstarch, and baking soda. Stir in chopped herbs, if using. Stir in eggs, vegetable oil, vitamin E oil, and essential oil and keep stirring until you form a dough.

2. Rub cornstarch on a rolling pin and spread some on a work surface. Roll the dough out to about 3/4 inch. Cut into shapes with cookie cutters or a biscuit cutter. Place your "cookies" on an ungreased cookie sheet about 1 inch apart. Bake for 10 to 12 minutes. Cool and store in a tight-topped cookie tin in a cool, dry place.

3. When ready to use, place one or two of your bath cookies into the tub as the water runs.

Easy Bath Powder

This simple combination creates a refreshing finish to the shower or bath and costs just pennies to make.

1 cup powdered arrowroot

1 cup cornstarch

1/4 cup baking soda

In a medium bowl, stir together all the ingredients. Store in an airtight container. Should keep indefinitely.

Basic Bath Powder

For an after-bath or after-shower touch, this fragrance-free home-made powder is so natural, it's a safe bet your great-grandmother used it. Keep a container of this mixture in your bathroom. Apply with a powder puff or sprinkle it on from a shaker-top jar.

1/2 cup baking soda
1/2 cup cornstarch

In a small bowl, stir both ingredients to combine. Store in a wide-mouthed glass jar or plastic container or keep in a shaker-top jar. Should keep indefinitely.

Delicately Scented Bath Powder

This variation provides a lightly scented powder suitable for adults. While alum is used as an antiperspirant and deodorant for adults, it is best to use a simple sprinkle of cornstarch on baby's skin.

2 tablespoons crumbled dried chamomile flowers
1/4 cup cornstarch
1 tablespoon orrisroot
1/2 teaspoon alum

1. Combine ingredients in a bowl and mix well. Let stand a few days.
2. Sift mixture through a flour sifter. Pour into a powder shaker or other container. Should keep indefinitely.

nail, hand, and foot care

Gardener's Hand Cream

This hand cream is especially good for those hard-working hands. You will spend just a dollar or so to make the entire recipe, but because you are using unpreserved vegetable oils, if you don't have a cool, dark place to store the hand cream or a friend to share with, consider making only half this recipe at a time. To make calendula tea, pour a cup of boiling water over half a teaspoon of dried calendula flower petals and let it steep until cool.

3 tablespoons beeswax, grated or shaved
1/2 cup sesame oil
1 tablespoon coconut oil
1 teaspoon honey
2 tablespoons calendula tea
3 drops lavender essential oil
1/2 teaspoon baking soda

1. In a small microwave-safe bowl, mix all the ingredients. Set the microwave to a medium heat and cook 30 seconds or until beeswax is melted. Remove from oven with hot pads and allow to cool.
2. Pour mixture into a widemouthed, sterilized jar with a tight top. Store in cool, dark place until ready to use.

Cuticle Cream *Here's a spa treatment you can make in the comfort of your own kitchen.*

3 tablespoons paraffin

1/2 cup mineral oil

1 tablespoon coconut oil

1 tablespoon glycerin

1. In the top of a double boiler over simmering water, combine the paraffin with the oils. Stir until paraffin is melted and the mixture is blended. Stir in the glycerin and remove the pan from the heat. Let mixture cool.

2. Apply cooled cream to cuticle area. Rub in and allow to rest for ten minutes or so.

3. Trim cuticles with a cuticle tool. Massage away cream by applying a gentle body or hand lotion and rubbing lightly, then rinsing with warm water.

Warm Oil Hand Treatment *Manicurists charge $15 to $35 for hot oil hand treatments. Here is a delightfully simple recipe you can create for about 50 cents or less.*

1 tablespoon olive or other cooking oil

1 teaspoon almond extract *or* 1 drop lavender essential oil *(optional)*

2 small plastic bags that will fit over your hands

1. Place the oil in a microwave-safe dish and heat it on medium-high for a few seconds until it is warmed, not hot. Add almond extract or lavender, if desired. Stir.

2. Rub the oil on your hands, massaging your fingers and palms. Cover your hands with the plastic bags and wrap a clean hand towel over the bags. Sit comfortably for about 5 minutes.

3. Remove the bags and rinse your hands with warm water, massaging away the oil. Gently pat dry with the towel and apply a light hand lotion.

Cornmeal Hand Scrub *This gentle massage scrub costs about a nickel to make and leaves your hands smooth and soft.*

1/4 cup cornmeal

3 tablespoons milk

1 drop almond oil (or almond extract)

1. In a small saucepan, mix the cornmeal with the milk. Heat the mixture over a low flame on the stovetop until it forms a paste. Remove from heat and stir in the almond oil. Allow to cool.

2. Spread mixture on hands and allow to sit for 10 minutes. Gently scrub your hands with the mixture and then rinse off with warm water.

Love Your Feet Cream

Our feet take a lot of abuse. Here's a special treatment to apply to dry, cracked feet that will leave them soft and pretty and costs about one-tenth the price of a visit to the salon for a pedicure.

1 ounce grated or shaved beeswax

3/4 cup almond oil

1. Place the beeswax and almond oil in the top of a double boiler over simmering water. Stir together until they are blended and the wax has melted. Remove from heat and pour into two 4-ounce sterilized containers with tight tops.

2. Allow mixture to cool before applying to feet. Spread on feet at night before bedtime. Wear a pair of clean cotton socks over the cream. In the morning, your feet will be much softer.

Soothing Footbath

This relaxing foot soak will work wonders on your entire body. Use a large dishpan or kiddie tub if you don't have a special foot tub.

1 tablespoon sea salt

2 drops lavender essential oil

1 drop rosemary essential oil

1 drop bay essential oil

1 drop geranium essential oil

Rose petals *(optional)*

1. Fill the soaking pan or tub with enough warm water to cover the feet.

2. Stir in the sea salt until it dissolves. Use your toes to stir, if you wish. Add the essential oils, mixing them well. Float rose petals on the surface.

3. Soak your feet in the basin for 10 minutes, or until the water has cooled off. Pat your feet dry with a towel.

Eucalyptus Foot Lotion

Use this rich and refreshing foot lotion to follow the Soothing Footbath (above) or simply to salve sore feet.

1 tablespoon almond oil

1 teaspoon avocado oil

1 teaspoon wheat germ oil

10 drops eucalyptus essential oil

1. Put all the ingredients in a small, sterilized glass bottle with a tight-fitting stopper. Shake the liquid vigorously until it is completely combined.

2. Store the bottle in a cool, dark place. Shake well before using.

Refreshing Foot Spray

This clean, fresh blend is great for hot summer days. Carry a little spray bottle with you and spritz it on tired feet.

3 tablespoons witch hazel

1 tablespoon rose flower water, orange blossom water, or distilled water

1/8 teaspoon glycerin

10-15 drops of essential oil of your choice

Pour all ingredients into a clean spray bottle and shake. Will keep for two months in plastic container.

Strawberry Foot Scrub

Can't get to the spa for a luxury treatment for those tired feet? Work this simple and sweetly scented natural scrub into your feet and feel like a queen.

2 teaspoons coarse salt

2 tablespoons olive oil

8 fresh strawberries

1. Pour salt into a mixing bowl. Add the oil and stir to combine. Remove caps from strawberries and slice or chop them. Add strawberries to the salt and oil mixture and mash with a potato masher or fork. The resulting mixture should be chunky but well blended.

2. Rub this mixture onto your feet, massaging the balls of the feet and the heels. If desired, use a body puff or foot brush. Rinse off and coat feet with a gentle lotion.

Makes enough for one treatment.

Leg Massage Cream

Treat yourself to a massage from your knees to your toes with this easy-to-make cream especially for the legs.

3 tablespoons anhydrous (water-free) lanolin

3 tablespoons olive oil

2 tablespoons apricot oil

1. Put all the ingredients together in the nonreactive top of a double boiler over simmering water. Heat and stir with a wooden spoon until the lanolin has liquefied.

2. Pour the mixture into a sterilized 4-ounce jar with a tight-fitting lid and allow to cool. Keep in a cool, dark place.

just for men

Rosemary Shaving Soap for Men

Rinse your face with fresh water, then lather up your beard with this fragrant soap before shaving. Be sure to thoroughly rinse off the lather.

2/3 cup rose water

4 ounces pure soap flakes

4 drops rosemary essential oil

3 drops lemon essential oil

2 drops bay essential oil

1 drop sage essential oil

1. Warm the rose water in a nonreactive saucepan over low heat. Place the soap flakes in the top of a double boiler over simmering water. Stir the warmed rose water into the flakes to moisten. Keep stirring the mixture until the soap has melted to a smooth gel (if necessary use a potato masher to dissolve the soap). Remove from the heat and cool to lukewarm.

2. Stir in the essential oils and spoon the soap into a sterilized shallow 7-ounce glass jar with a tight-fitting lid. Set aside to harden for 3 to 5 days. Keep handy in a cool, dark place.

Lightly Scented Aftershave

Aftershave splashes serve two purposes: to soothe the just-shaved beard area and to offer a pleasant scent. Instead of purchasing costly scented aftershaves, make this at home for less than $2 per cup.

1/2 cup witch hazel

1/2 cup rose water

Combine the two liquids in a sterilized jar. Splash on face directly after shaving. Keep tightly covered. Should keep indefinitely on bathroom shelf.

Shaving-Cut Lotion

Apply a drop of this simple, inexpensive, and effective lotion to stop bleeding and prevent infection in the event of a razor nick.

4 teaspoons witch hazel lotion

13 drops lavender essential oil

7 drops geranium essential oil

Put all ingredients in a sterilized 1-ounce glass bottle with a tight-fitting lid. Shake well to combine. Keep in a cool, dark place. Shake before using.

Aloe Aftershave Gel

This alcohol-free gel is suitable for men or women because it refreshes and is safe for sensitive skin. See if you don't love it as much as anything you can buy. Aloe vera gel is available in health food stores—or you can scoop it out of the leaves of a plant.

1/2 cup aloe vera gel

1 1/2 tablespoons distilled water

1 tablespoon witch hazel

10 drops essential or fragrance oils of your choice

1. Combine all the ingredients in the container you'll store the gel in. Stir until well mixed. Cover container with a tight-fitting lid.
2. Keep in a cool, dark location. Should keep indefinitely.

Muscle Rub

This salve really does wonders for hard-working muscles. Massage into stressed, stiff, and aching shoulders, neck, back, or feet. (This is not recommended for pregnant women.)

1 teaspoon lanolin

1 1/2 ounces extra-virgin olive oil

1/4 ounce beeswax, shaved or grated

2-3 drops arnica essential oil

6 drops ginger essential oil

3-4 drops lemon essential oil

1. In an ovenproof glass measuring cup with a pour spout, combine the lanolin, olive oil, and beeswax. Place the cup in a hot-water bath until the wax is nearly melted. At this point, remove the cup from the water bath and stir the mixture with a clean utensil to evenly mix the ingredients.
2. Let the mixture cool. When the mixture begins to harden around the edges of the cup, add the essential oils and stir to incorporate them.
3. Pour into a sterile widemouthed jar and allow to cool before capping. Store in a cool, dark place for several months.

Your Own Beauty Products **681**

for digestive distress
Soothing Tea for Heartburn
Stomach-Calming Tea
Lemon Settler for Motion Sickness
Hiccup Reliever
Anti-Diarrhea Tea
Electrolyte Drink for Diarrhea
Laxative
Herbal Tea for Flatulence
Hemorrhoid Pads

for colds, congestion, and fever
Chest Rub for Bronchitis
Another Chest Rub
Chest Compress
Mustard Seed Plaster
Mustard Powder Plaster
Cough Suppressant Tea
Cough Suppressant Medicine
Steam Cough Relief
Cough Drops
Gargle Solution
Slippery Elm and Marshmallow Tea
Steam Treatment for Congestion
Herbal Inhalant
Sore-Throat Lozenges
Decongestant Salve
Humidifier Booster
Saline Spray for Clogged Sinuses
Drops for Earache
Fever Tea
Spray for Fever

for bug bites, hives, and itching
Insect Repellent
Soothing Gel for Insect Bites
Essential Oil Itch Soother
Poison Ivy Lotion
Poison Ivy Drying Paste
Healing Oil Bath
Healing Calendula Lotion
Skin Salve for Eczema or Dermatitis
Honey Ointment

Anti-Itching Solution for Hives
Oatmeal Bath for Hives
Anti-Itch Wrap

treatments for skin outbreaks
Acne Facial Scrub
Cleansing Liquid for Acne
Acne Cleansing Pads
Overnight Acne Cream
Hot Compress for Boils
Antibacterial Drawing Paste
Antibacterial Oil
Ringworm Paste
Dandelion/Fig Wart Remover
Herbal Wart Remover

for cuts, bruises, and burns
First-Aid Antiseptic
Calendula Ointment
Healing Ointment
Cleansing Soap
Compress for Bruises
Anti-Bruising Oil
Oil Rub for Burned Skin
Soothing Oil for Burns
Burn Spray
Antiseptic Lotion for Burns
Sunburn Cooler

foot care products
Athlete's Foot Powder
Antifungal Foot Ointment
Antifungal Solution
Corn Plaster
Essential Oil Corn Remover
Salicylic Acid Corn Remover

for mouth and lip irritations
Healing Balm for Chapped Lips
Cold Sore Ointment
Mouthwash for Cold Sores
Cold Sore Paste

dental care products
Mouthwash
Mints
Toothpaste
Antibacterial Mouthwash
Gum Tonic
Super Dental Floss
Toothache-Relieving Rinse
Toothache-Relieving Dental Paste

for joint and muscle aches
Hot Pepper Rub
Massage Cream
Quick-and-Dirty Muscle Rub
Muscle Soak
Liniment
Cold Pack for Strains and Sprains
Castor Oil Rub for Back Pain

for women's problems
Muscle Relaxant for Cramps
Hot Compress for Cramps
Anti-Cramp Tea
Ginger Tea for Morning Sickness
PMS Tea
Yeast Infection Cream

headache treatments
Headache Compresses
Chamomile Tea
Lemon Balm Tea
Migraine Tea
Headache Massage
Headache Oil with Vitamin E

for anxiety and fatigue
Catnip Anti-Anxiety Tea
Hops Anti-Anxiety Tea
Calming Tea for Insomnia
Sleep Pillow
Herbal Milk Bath for Sleeplessness
Relaxing Aromatic Bath
Invigorating Oil for Fatigue
Energy Tea for Fatigue

Healthy Home Remedies

In a time of soaring health care costs—when a single trip to the doctor's office can cost hundreds of dollars and a visit to the hospital emergency room can balloon into the thousands—it is comforting to know that there are many everyday health problems that you can safely and successfully treat with homemade remedies. As you use the recipes on the following pages, you will be happy to discover that they can make a real difference in how you or a family member feels and in when you start to mend without a budget-busting consultation at a medical facility—or spending a small fortune at the drugstore.

From heartburn and motion sickness to constipation, colds and sore throats to earaches and fever, hives and rashes to acne and warts, cuts and bruises to minor burns, cold sores to gum disease and toothaches, sprains to muscle aches, yeast infections and PMS to headaches, insomnia, fatigue, and many, many more conditions, there are effective home remedies in this chapter that you can make and apply yourself. And all have been checked and approved by an experienced professional.

Many of these homemade recipes use herbs and other natural ingredients that were known to our ancestors and have an honorable place in the history of healing. Many modern medicines were discovered, after all, when scientists took plants that were recognized by herbalists as having special healing properties to the lab for testing. The healing ingredients were then extracted and tested and later manufactured. And with many of these recipes, you are simply going back to the original natural source.

for digestive distress

Soothing Tea for Heartburn
Licorice, ginger, and chamomile are traditional, easy-to-make, and inexpensive digestive tract soothers that still work wonders for occasional flare-ups of heartburn.

1 cup water

1 teaspoon grated licorice root

1 teaspoon chopped fresh ginger

1 teaspoon dried chamomile flowers

1. In a small pan, bring the water to a boil. Add the licorice and ginger. Simmer for 15 minutes. Remove from heat and add chamomile. Cover and steep for 10 minutes.

2. Strain into a teacup and drink.

Stomach-Calming Tea
If you have indigestion, this therapeutic infusion will likely tame your outraged stomach as well as any patent medicine you can buy.

1 cup boiling water

1 teaspoon dried peppermint

1 teaspoon dried chamomile

1. In a small pot, pour boiling water over the dried peppermint and chamomile. Cover and steep for 10 minutes, then strain into a teacup.

2. Drink up to three cups a day to help ease intestinal cramps.

One-Minute Substitute

Quick Antacid from Your Spice Shelf

Some common kitchen spice seeds contain oils that soothe spasms in your stomach and relieve nausea—without costing too pretty a penny. Just chew 1 teaspoon of aniseed, dill, or caraway seeds for a minute, then spit them out without swallowing any. Repeat three times a day.

Lemon Settler for Motion Sickness
While over-the-counter motion-sickness remedies can make you sleepy, ours just take away the sick feeling. This is a tummy-soothing drink.

Juice of 1 lemon

1 cup boiling water

1 teaspoon honey

1 crushed sprig spearmint or peppermint

1. In a large cup, combine lemon juice, boiling water, and honey. Stir to mix and add spearmint or peppermint.

2. Sip as needed. Keep warm in a thermos when traveling.

One-Minute Substitute | **Chew Ginger to Settle Your Stomach**
Ginger is a traditional tummy settler for nausea and motion sickness, and crystallized ginger—the candy version of it—may save a trip. Just chew on a lump of crystallized ginger as needed. Keep a packet in the car or your purse so you always have it handy.

Hiccup Reliever

You can't even find a remedy for hiccups in the drugstore, but you can make one yourself.

2 teaspoons to 1 tablespoon sugar or dry drink mix (cocoa or Ovaltine)

Swallow the dry sugar or drink mix, which isn't easy. Trying to get it down will short-circuit the hiccups.

Anti-Diarrhea Tea

This tea will settle an irate digestive system and help you back to health. It costs nothing if you have raspberries or blackberries in your garden. If your diarrhea persists for more than 24 hours, however, see a doctor.

2 teaspoons dried raspberry and/or blackberry leaves
Boiling water

1. In a teacup, steep the berry leaves in freshly boiled water for at least 10 minutes. Strain.
2. Drink a small cup 3 times a day along with other fluids to prevent dehydration.

making an infusion

Making an herbal infusion is similar to making a cup of tea. Place 3 rounded teaspoons (1/2 ounce) fresh herb leaves or 1 rounded teaspoon dried herb leaves in a teacup. Pour 1/2 cup boiling water over the leaves, cover with a saucer, and let steep for 5 or 10 minutes. Strain the drink while hot—or let it cool if you're going to use it as part of a lotion or gargle with it. Infusions may be stored in the refrigerator for up to 24 hours.

Electrolyte Drink for Diarrhea

Diarrhea can drain your body of liquids and electrolytes quite quickly and quite dangerously. This easily made, inexpensive juice drink helps maintain your body's equilibrium. If your diarrhea persists for more than 24 hours, however, see a doctor.

1 cup apple juice
2 cups water
1/2-1 teaspoon salt
Juice from a lemon or a lime

1. In a pitcher, combine apple juice, water, salt, and the lemon or lime juice. Store in the refrigerator.
2. Drink throughout the day to maintain hydration and proper balance of electrolytes.

Laxative
You don't have to buy expensive psyllium fiber supplements to treat temporary constipation.

1-3 teaspoons psyllium husks

Warm water

1. Stir psyllium husks into an 8-ounce glass of warm water and drink once a day. Follow with a glass of plain water.
2. Drink 6 to 8 additional glasses of water throughout the day.

One-Minute Substitute

Grandma's Always Ready Laxative
This old-fashioned penny-pincher's remedy for constipation sounds simple because it is. Just take 1 to 2 teaspoons castor oil on an empty stomach. It should get things moving within 8 to 10 hours.

Herbal Tea for Flatulence
It's embarrassing to have flatulence and embarrassing to have to buy something to treat it. Instead, make the following tea in the privacy of your home.

1 teaspoon dried chamomile

1/2 teaspoon dried peppermint

1 teaspoon dried catnip

1 teaspoon dried basil

2 crushed fennel seeds

1/2 teaspoon dried marjoram

1. In a large cup, mix the herbs. Pour in 6 to 8 ounces of boiling water and steep, covered, for 10 minutes. Strain and drink tea.
2. Drink 3 or more cups a day.

Hemorrhoid Pads
These work just as well as the commercial brands.

1 ounce witch hazel

5 drops cypress essential oil

3 drops geranium essential oil

5 drops lavender essential oil

2 tablespoons aloe vera gel

Cotton cosmetic pads

1. In an open-mouthed jar with a tight-fitting lid, combine the witch hazel, essential oils, and aloe vera gel. Saturate several cotton cosmetic pads in the liquid and refrigerate for at least an hour.
2. Use a pad on the affected area when it burns and after each bowel movement. Store in the refrigerator for several days.

for colds, congestion, and fever

Chest Rub for Bronchitis
The essential oils in this easy-to-make and easy-to-pay-for rub are therapeutic. You cover them with flannel and a hot pad to warm your chest and help you absorb the essential oil.

- 30 drops massage or carrier oil such as almond, jojoba, or avocado oil
- 5-10 drops eucalyptus or wintergreen essential oil

1. In a small bowl mix the carrier oil with the essential oil. Rub the mixture onto your chest.

2. Cover your chest with a cotton towel or piece of flannel, then put a heating pad or hot-water bottle on top of the flannel and snuggle under the blankets.

Another Chest Rub
A warm, homemade chest rub can relax you and calm your cough without bothering your pocketbook.

- 12 drops eucalyptus essential oil
- 8 drops hyssop essential oil
- 4 drops peppermint essential oil
- 2 tablespoons almond or olive oil

1. In a small dish, mix essential oils with the almond or olive oil.

2. Rub the mixture onto your chest and cover with a damp, warm flannel (try warming the damp flannel in the microwave). Leave on until the warmth fades.

Chest Compress
This warm, soothing compress will make you relax while it helps you to breathe.

- A handful of dried, chopped mullein or dried, chopped lobelia
- 1-2 cups boiling water

1. In a bowl, steep the mullein or lobelia in boiling water for 10 minutes.

2. Saturate a hand towel in the warm liquid, wring it out, and place on your chest. Cover with a warm towel and place a heating pad on top of that.

Mustard Seed Plaster

It's old-fashioned, but sometimes it's these kinds of remedies that are the best. And you are not risking the family fortune to try it.

2 or more tablespoons olive oil

1/3 cup mustard seed

2 tablespoons grated beeswax

Cloth to cover chest

1. Put 2 tablespoons olive oil and the mustard seed into a blender and blend. Continue adding olive oil until you have a nice, thick liquid.

2. Pour the mixture into the top of a double boiler over low heat; add the beeswax and heat, stirring, until the wax melts. Spread the cloth on a flat surface. Once the mustard-wax mixture is warm and can be spread, apply it to the cloth and let it cool to room temperature.

3. Place the cloth salve-side-down on your chest and cover with a T-shirt or old flannel, then apply external heat on top with a heating pad or hot-water bottle. You should start to feel warmth seeping into your chest in about 10 to 15 minutes. Leave on another 15 minutes. You can store the plaster in the fridge for several days; when needed, remove and let warm to room temperature before using.

Mustard Powder Plaster

You can also make an inexpensive, effective mustard plaster using a strong mustard powder such as Coleman's.

1 tablespoon mustard powder

2 tablespoons flour

1. In a small bowl, mix the mustard powder with the flour. Add enough water to make a paste.

2. Spread the paste over half of a dishtowel. Then fold the towel in half, covering the paste, and apply to chest. Don't apply the mustard paste directly onto the skin. Check chest skin often and remove the mustard plaster if there are signs of irritation.

Cough Suppressant Tea

Now that we know that those commercial cough syrups are pretty useless when it comes to most coughs, why waste your money? Here's a nicer, cheaper alternative.

4 fresh sage leaves or 1 teaspoon dried

Boiling water

In a standard teacup, steep the sage leaves in freshly boiled water for at least 20 minutes. Strain and drink hot or cold.

Cough Suppressant Medicine

You will appreciate onions, garlic, ginger, and honey all the more after they conspire to stop your coughing. And you don't have to worry about ingredients that your body doesn't need or that counteract the suppressing effect as you do with many commercial cough medicines.

1 large onion, finely diced

2 cloves garlic, finely diced

2 tablespoons finely diced fresh ginger

Honey

1. In a small saucepan, combine onion, garlic, and ginger. Add honey to cover and cook over very low heat for 30 minutes. Then mash together and let cool. Strain and store in a clean jar with a tight-fitting lid in the refrigerator.

2. Take one teaspoon every 15 to 30 minutes.

Steam Cough Relief

Sometimes an herbal steam treatment will do more to relieve a cough than any mentholated ointment you can buy.

4 cups water

2 drops thyme essential oil

4 drops eucalyptus essential oil

2 drops hyssop essential oil

1. In a saucepan over medium heat, heat the water until nearly boiling (but don't boil). Pour into a heat-safe bowl and add the essential oils.

2. Hold your head about 8 inches above the water, drape a towel over your head and the bowl to make a tent, and breathe in deeply until the water cools. Keep your eyes closed throughout.

Cough Drops

Do a little steeping and straining, boiling and stirring, rolling and cooling. Voilà! Your very own cough drops at half the price and just as effective as commercial ones. You need a candy thermometer to make these.

2 ounces dried or 6 ounces fresh horehound leaves

3 1/2 cups dark brown sugar

20 drops eucalyptus essential oil

20 drops tea tree essential oil

1. In a saucepan, pour 3 cups boiling water over the horehound leaves and steep for 30 minutes over low heat. Strain into another saucepan and add the brown sugar; stir until the sugar dissolves.

2. Bring the mixture to a boil and boil until it reaches 295°F on a candy thermometer. Stir in the eucalyptus and tea tree oils. Let cool slightly, then, using buttered hands, roll into small balls and let the balls harden on wax paper. Wrap them individually in plastic wrap and use as needed.

One-Minute Substitute

Pepper Spray for a Raw Throat

This quick and easy spray is an antiseptic and a painkiller that costs almost nothing to make. In a clean 8-ounce spray bottle, combine 1 tablespoon of cayenne pepper with just enough water to almost fill the bottle. Shake well and use as a spray to numb the back of your throat. You can also use it for gargling. Just don't get it near your eyes.

Healthy Home Remedies   **689**

Gargle Solution
This old-fashioned gargle will make your throat feel much better, and it costs very little.

2 heaping tablespoons brown sugar

1/2 teaspoon salt

1/4 teaspoon baking soda

1 quart warm water

1. In a jar with a tight-fitting lid, combine the brown sugar, salt, baking soda, and warm water. Shake well before each use.

2. Gargle with up to 1/2 cup of this mixture as often as needed.

Slippery Elm and Marshmallow Tea
The tea is slippery and the herbs soothing, so they ease throat pain as well as any commercial products for a great deal less.

2 teaspoons powdered slippery elm bark

2 teaspoons powdered marshmallow root

6 ounces boiling water

In a cup, place the slippery elm and marshmallow root. Pour in the boiling water and steep until cool. Strain into a teacup and drink. Store in refrigerator and gently reheat as needed.

Steam Treatment for Congestion
Aromatic herbs and humidity can do wonders for a stuffed-up head. This treatment takes only minutes to put together, and the results are priceless.

3 tablespoons finely chopped fresh thyme, sage, peppermint, eucalyptus, or pine needles

Boiling water

1. Put the herbs in a medium bowl and add boiling water.

2. Lean over the bowl with a towel draped over your head and the bowl and inhale for 10 minutes. Repeat 2 or 3 times a day as needed.

Herbal Inhalant
You can make your own inhalant quickly and safely for pennies.

1/4-1/2 teaspoon rock salt

2-4 drops peppermint essential oil

2-4 drops eucalyptus essential oil

2-4 drops wintergreen essential oil

1. Put the rock salt in the bottom of a small glass bottle or jar with a tight-fitting lid. Add the oils.

2. Carry with you and sniff as needed to open clogged nasal passages.

Sore-Throat Lozenges

These lozenges are called pastilles, and are made with dried plant ingredients. They are cheap, easy to make, and very effective.

1/4 cup violet petals

1/4 cup rose petals

Honey or maple syrup

1 teaspoon dried marshmallow root

Confectioners' sugar *(optional)*

1. With a mortar and pestle, crush the violet and rose petals until you get a fine powder. Mix with just enough honey or maple syrup to form a ball and add marshmallow root. If the mixture is too liquid, add more herbs or powdered sugar until it can hold its shape.

2. Form into small balls about the size of a large pea and place on a greased cookie sheet. Leave 24 to 48 hours or until they harden, then wrap each individually in plastic wrap and store in a cool, dry place.

Decongestant Salve

This rub can give that stuff in the dark blue bottle a run for its money.

4 ounces olive oil

1/2 ounce peppermint oil

1/2 ounce eucalyptus oil

1/2 ounce wintergreen oil

1/2 ounce grated beeswax

4 drops tincture of benzoin

1. In the top of a double boiler over low heat, heat the oils. Add the beeswax and tincture of benzoin and stir until the beeswax is melted and the oils are well mixed.

2. Pour mixture into a clean, widemouthed jar with a tight top and allow to cool. Put under your nose or rub on your chest as a decongestant. You can keep this mixture in a cool, dark place for up to two weeks.

One-Minute Substitute

A Quick Decongestant to Carry with You

The good news about this decongestant is that it doesn't come with a list of warnings! Just put 1 drop of tea tree, peppermint, or rosemary essential oil on a clean handkerchief and carry the handkerchief with you. Inhale as needed.

Humidifier Booster

Getting a good night's sleep is probably the best thing you can do for a cold. This recipe allows you to breathe and sleep through the night.

2-4 drops peppermint essential oil

2-4 drops eucalyptus essential oil

2-4 drops wintergreen essential oil

Cotton ball

1. In a small bowl, mix the oils. Dip a cotton ball into the mixture and put it near the vent of a steam humidifier.

2. Place the humidifier and the cotton ball near your bed when you have a cold.

Saline Spray for Clogged Sinuses

Why pay good money for something that is essentially salt and water? Make your own saline spray.

1/4 teaspoon table salt

1 cup distilled water, warmed to a comfortable temperature

1. Add the salt to the distilled water and stir until it dissolves.

2. To get the solution into your nose, use an ear bulb syringe (like the kind used to clean out a baby's nose), a neti pot (an Indian sinus cleaning tool available in health food stores), or a waterpick on the lowest setting (you'll need a special adapter for this). Flush your nasal passages two to three times a day.

Drops for Earache

In winter weather when earaches are more prevalent, it is smart to keep these bargain ear drops on hand in the refrigerator for emergencies.

1 clove garlic, crushed

2 tablespoons fresh or dried mullein flower

1/2 cup olive or almond oil

1. In a clean jar with a tight-fitting lid, combine the garlic and mullein flower. Cover with the oil, seal the top, and shake to blend. Store in a cool, dark place and shake daily.

2. Make sure the herbs remain under the oil for two weeks, then strain and store the oil in a clean jar with a tight-fitting lid in the refrigerator.

3. To treat an earache, let the oil come to room temperature or run it under warm water. Dispense two or three drops at a time with a sterile eye dropper. Gently massage the ear to help the oil make its way through the ear canal.

Fever Tea

You can certainly take Tylenol or Motrin, but this tea will make you feel better without putting any additional strain on your liver.

Yarrow

Linden flowers

Chamomile

Spearmint

Elder flowers

1 cup boiling water

1. In a small bowl, mix equal amounts of dried, crushed yarrow, linden flowers, chamomile, spearmint, and elder flowers.

2. Combine 3 teaspoons of this mix in a large cup, and add boiling water.

3. Cover and steep for 10 to 15 minutes. Strain and drink hot. After drinking, get under the covers to induce sweating.

Spray for Fever

Spraying pulse points with a cool, soothing solution is said by many to bring down a fever quicker than any pill you can buy. Whether it does work that well or not, it feels great when you are hot and feverish. The pulse points are the places on the body where you can easily feel your heart rate when you touch them with your fingers—typically inside your wrists, just under each side of the jaw, and the back of the knees.

- 1/4 cup rubbing alcohol
- 1/4 cup witch hazel
- 3 drops peppermint essential oil
- 2 drops lavender essential oil

1. In a clean spray bottle, combine the rubbing alcohol, witch hazel, and essential oils. Shake to mix and then chill in the refrigerator.

2. Spray onto pulse points to reduce fever, avoiding eyes and mouth.

for bug bites, hives, and itching

Insect Repellent

The best way to treat bites is to avoid getting bitten in the first place. But forget spraying poisons on yourself. The essential ingredients of this homemade insect repellent have been shown in numerous studies to keep stinging insects—notably, mosquitoes—far, far away. Keep in mind, however, that if you're in an area with a high rate of mosquito-transmitted diseases, such as West Nile disease, you may need stronger protection.

- 15-20 drops eucalyptus essential oil
- 15-20 drops lemon essential oil
- 15-20 drops lemongrass essential oil
- 15-20 drops citronella essential oil
- 1 ounce carrier oil (olive oil or any massage oil)

1. In a small pitcher, mix the essential oils with the carrier oil.

2. Put into a spray bottle and use as needed. Do not use on small children or infants.

Soothing Gel for Insect Bites

Once you've been bitten, you need something to soothe the itch. This easy, inexpensive mixture will do it.

- 10-20 drops of a combination of lavender, tea tree, chamomile, cedarwood, and/or eucalyptus essential oils
- 1 ounce aloe vera gel or chamomile or calendula cream

1. In a small bowl, mix essential oils into the gel or cream.

2. Smooth over itchy/painful area. If you make more than you need, you can store the mixture in a clean jar in a cool, dark place for a week.

Baking Soda Paste for Itches
Here is an incredibly easy itch reliever that costs just pennies.
In a small bowl, mix 1/4 teaspoon baking soda (or meat
tenderizer) with a little ice water to make a paste. Then
spread the paste over the bite area. Repeat as necessary.

Essential Oil Itch Soother

Instead of messy, expensive anti-itch salves, try this homemade soother, which can be made for under $1.

1 drop lavender, rose, chamomile, or tea tree essential oil

Cold water

1. Fill a bowl with enough cold water to moisten a small washcloth or cotton pad. Swirl the essential oil through the water; then soak the cloth or pad.
2. Squeeze gently to remove any excess water and apply the cloth to the skin. Hold in place with your hand for as long as possible, or cover with plastic wrap and leave in place for about an hour.

Poison Ivy Lotion

The key to healing poison ivy is to dry it up. To make it less annoying, a coating of a heavy lotion keeps it from itching. This may be just as messy as calamine lotion, but it is a lot cheaper.

1/2 teaspoon salt

1/2 cup water

Bentonite clay

12 drops lavender essential oil

12 drops peppermint essential oil

1. In a small bowl, dissolve the salt in the water and add enough bentonite clay to make a creamy mixture. Stir in the lavender and peppermint essential oils.
2. Spread over the affected area.

Poison Ivy Drying Paste

This easily made, inexpensive paste may coat and stick to the skin better than a lotion.

1 tablespoon bentonite clay or finely ground oatmeal

10 drops lavender, chamomile, cypress, and/or geranium essential oil

Water

1. In a small bowl, put enough bentonite clay or finely ground oatmeal to cover the affected area. For each tablespoon of powder, stir in 10 drops of one or more of the essential oils. Moisten the mixture with water to allow for easy application and spread over the affected area.
2. Cover loosely and allow to dry. Rinse off and reapply as needed.

Healing Oil Bath
Dry, irritated skin is the greatest culprit with either eczema or dermatitis. Store shelves are stocked with dozens of creams and lotions, but the natural way is less expensive.

6-8 drops pine, geranium, or lavender essential oils

1. Add essential oil to a hot bath. Swirl to disperse the oil, then get in and soak for about 10 minutes.
2. Carefully get out of the bath (it will be slippery) and massage in any oil still left on the skin. Don't take this bath more than once every 24 hours.

Healing Calendula Lotion
Be sure you have Calendula officinalis flowers from your garden or a health store for this lotion for treating eczema or dermatitis; they are the ones with the therapeutic effect.

Calendula flower petals

1. Crush several calendula flower petals between your fingers (or with a mortar or pestle) until the petals are juicy.
2. Rub both petals and juice onto the skin.

Skin Salve for Eczema or Dermatitis
Here is another treatment for rough, dry, irritated skin that outperforms the store-bought versions.

1 ounce grated beeswax

1 cup untoasted sesame oil

1/2 teaspoon tincture of goldenseal

1/2 teaspoon tincture of barberry root

8 drops tea tree essential oil

8 drops chamomile essential oil

1. In the top of a double boiler over low heat, melt the beeswax, stirring occasionally. Stir in the sesame oil.
2. In a small dish, mix tincture of goldenseal and barberry root. Add the tea tree and chamomile essential oils.
3. Stir this mixture into the beeswax-oil mixture. Apply as needed.

Honey Ointment
The honey in this ointment serves as a humectant to draw in moisture, which eases the skin irritation produced by eczema and dermatitis.

1 ounce grated beeswax

1 cup untoasted sesame oil

1/3 cup honey

1 capsule vitamin E, 400 IU

60 drops rose, geranium, chamomile, lavender, or bergamot essential oils in any combination

1. In the top of a double boiler over low heat, melt the beeswax, stirring occasionally. Stir in the sesame oil. Remove from the heat and let cool slightly, then add honey. Pierce the vitamin E capsule and squeeze in the contents. Add up to 60 drops of essential oils.
2. Pour mixture into a clean jars or jars with tight-fitting lids and use as needed to keep skin smooth and hydrated.

Healthy Home Remedies

Anti-Itching Solution for Hives
You can buy pricey salves at the drugstore to tame the itching of hives, but this easy, pennies-a-pop solution is just as effective.

20-30 drops lavender
essential oil

Bowl cold water

1. Stir the lavender essential oil into the bowl of cold water.
2. Dip a cloth into the liquid and apply directly to the hives to reduce inflammation.

Oatmeal Bath for Hives
You know the brand that's famous for its oat-based products. Now you can make your own.

1 handful of rolled oats

1/2 handful dry powdered
milk

1/2 handful chamomile

1/4 handful calendula and/or
lavender

Double-ply square of
cheesecloth

1. Place the oats, milk, chamomile, and calendula or lavender on the cheesecloth square. Tie the ends together to make a bag.
2. Run a warm (not hot) bath. Put the bag under the spout while the water is running. Leave it in the bath and allow the water to cool. (If the water is too hot, it will make the hives worse.)
3. Get into the tub and soak, squeezing the bag over your skin to reduce itching.

Anti-Itch Wrap
Cheaper than cortisone salves, but quite effective, this herbal wrap solution will make life worth living again for people with irritating rashes.

1/4 cup apple cider vinegar

1/4 cup witch hazel

2 cups cold water

4 drops lavender essential oil

2 drops chamomile essential
oil

2 drops bergamot essential oil

2 teaspoons baking soda

Clean cloths

1. In a large bowl, mix the vinegar, witch hazel, and 2 cups cold water. In a separate small bowl, mix the essential oils with the baking soda. Stir the baking soda mixture into the water mixture.
2. Soak a cloth in the cool solution and wrap it over the itchy area for 20 minutes at a time or until the cloth begins to dry. Keep the solution chilled in the refrigerator for up to two weeks.
3. May be repeated three times a day.

One-Minute
Substitute

Using Essential Oil to Soothe Rashes
Lavender and tea tree essential oils have soothing properties that can alleviate as well as heal rashes. Try this simple solution before buying expensive ointments. Put 1 drop of lavender or tea tree essential oil directly on the rash, gently smoothing it over the surface. To treat a large area, apply a blend made by mixing 3 drops of either essential oil in 2 teaspoons light olive oil.

treatments for skin outbreaks

Acne Facial Scrub
For a homemade version of an acne-relieving exfoliant that won't break the bank, try this. For more information on green clay powder, see Green Clay Purifying Face Mask, page 242.

2 cups rolled oats

1/2 cup almonds

2 tablespoons dried lavender

1 tablespoon dried peppermint

1 tablespoon calendula leaf

1/2 cup green clay powder

1. In a coffee grinder or blender, grind the oats, almonds, lavender, peppermint, and calendula leaf

2. Add the clay and mix thoroughly, then put in a clean covered container and keep in a cool place. You can keep this scrub for up to three months.

3. To use, in a small open dish, make a paste by mixing a teaspoon of the mixture with water. Massage the paste onto your skin. Let dry, then rinse well.

Cleansing Liquid for Acne
Toners are primarily just water with a few other ingredients, yet they can cost more than $5 a bottle. Instead, make your own (see Making an Infusion, page 271). Dab an affected area three times a day, or use over your whole face after washing.

1 cup distilled water

1 teaspoon dried thyme

1 teaspoon dried calendula flowers

1 teaspoon dried lavender

1 teaspoon dried yarrow

1/4 cup witch hazel

5-10 drops tea tree essential oil

1. In a small pan, bring the distilled water to a boil. Add the thyme, calendula, lavender, and yarrow. Remove from heat and steep covered until cool.

2. Strain and mix strained liquid with the witch hazel. Add the tea tree essential oil, shake, and apply to affected areas with a cotton pad.

3. Store the leftover liquid in the refrigerator and use within two weeks.

Acne Cleansing Pads
Forget those high-priced acne pads that come impregnated with the medicine. Just make your own!

2 cups distilled water

1 tablespoon dried yarrow

1 tablespoon dried chamomile

15 drops tincture of benzoin

6 drops peppermint or wintergreen essential oil

Cosmetic pads

1. In a small pan, bring the distilled water to a boil. Add the yarrow and chamomile. Remove from heat after two to three minutes and steep, covered, for half an hour. Strain and add the tincture of benzoin and peppermint or wintergreen essential oil. Mix well and pour into a sterilized jar with a tight-fitting lid.

2. Put several cosmetic pads in with the liquid. Refrigerate and use as needed.

Healthy Home Remedies **697**

Overnight Acne Cream

Those little tubes of overnight acne medicine can set you back a pretty penny. Instead, try this homemade paste.

4 drops tea tree oil

1 teaspoon cosmetic clay

1. In a small dish, mix the tea tree oil and the cosmetic clay, and just enough water to make a thick paste.
2. Dab onto blemishes and leave on overnight.

Hot Compress for Boils

This gentle treatment will help relieve the boil in a lovely, aromatic way.

4 teaspoons hot water

2 drops lavender, lemon, tea tree, sage, or clove essential oil

1 cotton ball or gauze pad

1. Put the hot water in a bowl. Swirl your chosen essential oil through the water, then soak the cotton ball or gauze pad in the solution.
2. Gently squeeze out excess fluid and apply the cotton ball or pad directly to the area of the boil. Cover with plastic wrap and secure with a bandage or tape. Leave in place for at least an hour. Repeat twice a day.

Antibacterial Drawing Paste

This therapeutic paste works best if it is applied after putting a hot compress (above) on the boil for 15 minutes.

5 drops total tea tree, lavender, and/or spikenard essential oils

Slippery elm powder or green clay powder

1. Mix essential oils with enough slippery elm powder or green clay powder to generously cover the affected area.
2. Apply the moist powder to the boil and cover with a bandage for 24 hours.

Antibacterial Oil

You don't want a boil to get infected; this antibacterial oil protects you from that. You should, however, test it on a small area of normal skin first to make sure it's not irritating to your skin.

1 tablespoon carrier oil

20 drops tea tree essential oil

20 drops lavender essential oil

10 drops thyme essential oil

1. In a small bowl, combine the carrier oil with the essential oils. Mix well.
2. Hold a hot compress (above) on the boil for 10 minutes, then apply a small amount of the antibacterial oil and cover with a dressing. Repeat every few hours.

Ringworm Paste
Save yourself a trip to the doctor for a prescription with this antifungal paste. If it's not better in a week, see a doctor.

1 tablespoon mustard seeds
Water
1-2 drops sage and/or thyme essential oil

1. Crush the mustard seeds with a mortar and pestle. Stir in enough water to make a paste, then add the essential oil or oils.
2. Apply to the affected area and cover with a light bandage. Reapply once a day until the infection clears.

Dandelion/Fig Wart Remover
Here's an easy wart remover straight from the backyard that won't cost you a thing.

Freshly cut dandelion stalks or fig leaves

1. Use the milky sap that exudes from the dandelion stalks or fig leaves and apply directly to the wart once or twice a day for several days or until the wart pulls away from the skin. Keep the sap away from the skin around the wart, and from sensitive areas such as the eyes.
2. If you are using this treatment on a child, cover the wart area with a bandage to prevent spreading the sap to sensitive skin.

Herbal Wart Remover
Warts are mysterious—they come and go seemingly without reason. You usually don't need a dermatologist or an expensive patent medicine to make them disappear.

1 drop tea tree, lemon, clove, thuja, or thyme essential oil
1 drop almond or olive oil
1 strip bandage

1. Soak the wart in warm water for 15 minutes. Towel off excess water.
2. In a small dish, combine the essential oil with the almond or olive carrier oil. Test this oil mixture on a patch of skin to make sure it isn't irritating.
3. Apply the oil mixture to the wart and cover with the strip bandage. Reapply every 24 hours.

for cuts, bruises, and burns

First-Aid Antiseptic
Here is an all-natural solution with germ-killing properties that will help soothe a minor cut or abrasion. Be sure to wash the affected area well before applying it.

2 ounces Calendula Ointment (below)

40 drops lavender essential oil

20 drops tea tree essential oil

10 drops chamomile essential oil

10 drops lemon essential oil

1. In a small sterile jar with a tight-fitting lid, combine the calendula ointment with the essential oils, mixing thoroughly.

2. Apply a small amount to the cleaned injury. Keep the remainder in a cool, dark place for up to two weeks.

Calendula Ointment
Use the old-fashioned calendula flower (Calendula officinalis) for this therapeutic salve that has many uses.

3 tablespoons fresh calendula petals

1/3 cup light olive oil

2 tablespoons chopped beeswax

1 capsule vitamin E, 400 IU

1. Put the calendula petals in a double boiler and crush slightly with the back of a spoon. Add the olive oil and simmer for two hours over low heat.

2. Strain the liquid into a bowl, pressing against the strainer with the back of a spoon to extract all the oils.

3. Return the liquid to the double boiler. Over medium heat, add the chopped beeswax and stir until it melts. Remove from the double boiler and beat the mixture until it cools and becomes creamy and thick. Pierce the vitamin E capsule with a needle, squeeze in the contents, and mix.

4. Spoon into a sterilized 4 1/2-ounce jar with a tight top, seal, and keep in a cool, dark place for up to two weeks.

Healing Ointment
You can have this ointment on hand to treat everyday cuts and scrapes as they arise, just as you would a tube of pricey commercial antiseptic.

1-1 1/2 ounces grated beeswax

1 cup olive or almond oil

2 capsules vitamin E, 400 IU

30 drops tea tree essential oil

20 drops spike lavender or French lavender essential oil

10 drops chamomile essential oil

10 drops fir essential oil

1. In the top of a double boiler over low heat, melt the beeswax. Stir in the olive or almond oil. Remove from the heat. Pierce each vitamin E capsule with a needle and squeeze the contents into the mixture. Then stir in the essential oils.

2. Pour into a small sterilized jar with a tight-fitting lid and store in a cool, dark place. Use as needed on wounds. Should last a year.

Cleansing Soap
Here is an antiseptic soap you can trust to clean out wounds properly and stave off infections. It smells good and costs very little.

Liquid castile soap

Lavender essential oil

Rosemary essential oil

Tea tree essential oil

1. To the castile soap, add lavender, rosemary, and tea tree essential oils (10 drops total per 2 ounces of soap). Dilute with more soap if skin is especially sensitive to any of the essential oils.

2. Use to clean off cuts and abrasions.

Compress for Bruises
A wet compress can relieve some of the pain of a bruise and help the healing process. This simple formula will have you feeling better in no time and for very little money.

1/4 cup water

1/4 cup witch hazel or cider vinegar

2 drops lavender essential oil

2 drops rosemary essential oil

2 drops peppermint or juniper essential oil

1. In a bowl, mix the water, witch hazel or vinegar, and the essential oils. Soak a flannel cloth in the liquid, wring it out until nearly dry, and then place over injured area.

2. Cover with plastic wrap so the skin absorbs the essential oils and cover the whole thing with a towel. Apply the compress for 30 minutes up to three times daily.

Anti-Bruising Oil
Use this rub very, very gently to help in the healing process.

10 drops rosemary essential oil

10 drops peppermint essential oil

10 drops juniper essential oils

30 drops carrier oil (olive or almond).

1. In a small bowl, mix the essential oils with the carrier oil.

2. Massage the mixture gently into bruised areas every two hours.

One-Minute Substitute

Two Quick Treatments for Burns

Aloe vera gel is a traditional and effective salve for burns. And it costs you nothing if you have aloe vera as a houseplant. Pull a leaf off the plant and with a small spoon, scoop out the clear gel. Apply directly to the burn.

Lavender essential oil provides relief from minor burns, including sunburn. Just apply several drops of the oil directly to the burn.

Oil Rub for Burned Skin
This mixture gives relief. And you can safely use it several times a day.

1 drop tea tree essential oil

1/4 cup organic olive oil

1. In a small dish, dilute the essential oil with the olive oil.

2. Gently massage the mixture over the burned area.

Soothing Oil for Burns
If the burn area is large, you may need to double the ingredients for this soothing oil.

2 capsules vitamin E, 400 IU

5 drops lavender essential oil

1. Pierce each vitamin E capsule with a needle and squeeze the contents into a small dish. Stir in the lavender essential oil.

2. Gently massage into the skin.

Burn Spray
Applying a spray doesn't hurt the burn the way massaging in an oil might. This cool mixture offers relief and healing at very little cost.

1 ounce ice water

1 ounce aloe vera gel

25 drops total lavender, chamomile, spearmint, and yarrow essential oils

1 capsule vitamin E, 400 IU

1. In a small spray bottle, mix the ice water, aloe vera, and essential oils. Pierce the vitamin E capsule with a needle, squeeze its contents into the mixture, and chill.

2. Shake before use and spray over burned area. Keeps in the refrigerator for several days.

growing your own aloe vera

You can buy an aloe vera plant at any garden shop or nursery. Aloes like warmth, so in most areas, it is safer to keep the plant potted and place it near a sunny window than to plant it outdoors. (You can move the pot outdoors during the summer months.) Repot an aloe vera in a wide rather than a deep pot; it has shallow, spreading roots. Use one with a drainage hole and fill it with a good potting mix (page 377) with extra perlite. Don't overwater this succulent plant. Let its soil dry completely between soakings. Fertilize it yearly, in the spring, with a half-strength 10-40-10 fertilizer mixture. When you need some aloe vera gel, just cut a lower leaf off the plant and squeeze it.

Antiseptic Lotion for Burns
Nobody wants a burn to become infected. Here's a quick remedy that costs only pennies.

1 handful dried plantain leaves

1/2 cup hot water

10 drops tea tree essential oil

1. In a blender, add a handful of dried plantain leaves to about 1/2 cup hot water. Begin blending, slowly adding water or plantain leaves as necessary until the mixture becomes thick, like oatmeal. Mix in the tea tree oil.

2. Spread mixture over affected area. You can refrigerate the remainder for several days.

Sunburn Cooler
Brew a pot of regular tea (Lipton, Salada, or a store brand will do fine). The tannins in the tea help soothe the burning feeling.

3 tea bags or 3 tablespoons loose tea

Boiling water

1. In a teapot, place the tea. Pour in boiling water, cover, and steep 5 minutes. Cool.

2. Use a cloth or cotton ball to dab the sunburn with cooling tea.

foot care products

Athlete's Foot Powder
Dr. Scholl doesn't have a lock on the foot care market. Not when you can make your own antifungal foot powder. It can also be used for jock itch.

1/2 cup arrowroot or cornstarch

2 tablespoons white cosmetic clay

10 drops cypress essential oil

10 drops lavender essential oil

3 drops clove essential oil

5 drops tea tree essential oil

5 drops thyme essential oil

1. In a small container with a tight-fitting cover, mix the arrowroot or cornstarch with 2 tablespoons cosmetic clay. Add the cypress, lavender, and clove essential oils and mix. To make the powder antiseptic, add the tea tree and thyme essential oils.

2. Let the powder sit for a couple of days to absorb the oils, then dust on your feet once or twice a day. Keeps in a dry, covered container for several weeks.

Antifungal Foot Ointment

Treating a fungus with your own aromatic home-made ointment is much pleasanter than paying big bucks for a commercial antifungal ointment. Organic light olive oil is available in health food stores and many supermarkets.

3 tablespoons organic light olive oil

1/3 ounce finely chopped beeswax

50 drops of tea tree, geranium, lavender, pine, myrrh, or peppermint essential oil (or any combination)

1. In the top of a double boiler, warm the oil over simmering water. Add the beeswax to the warmed oil and stir until it melts. Remove from the heat and stir until it cools. Then beat in essential oil.

2. Spoon the ointment into a small, sterilized, widemouthed jar with a tight-fitting lid. Keep in a cool, dark place. Massage a small amount into the affected area twice a day. The ointment should keep for several weeks.

Helpful Hint

Getting Ointment to the Right Consistency

When making ointments, if the salve is too watery, reheat and add more beeswax. If it's too thick, reheat and add more oil.

Antifungal Solution

Use this solution to wipe down areas affected with fungal outbreaks twice a day. It's effective and inexpensive. Before applying this solution, wash the affected area with tea tree soap (available in health food stores).

1-2 tablespoons dried thyme

1-2 tablespoons dried eucalyptus

1-2 tablespoons dried lavender

1. In a large cup, combine the herbs. Cover with 8 ounces of boiling water and steep, covered, for 10 to 15 minutes. Strain and cool.

2. Soak a clean cotton cloth in the solution and apply twice daily to the skin (after your shower in the morning and before bed). You can also use this solution to soak your feet.

One-Minute Substitute

A Quick and Cheap Antifungal Footbath

Here's an easy, pennies-a-pop, footbath to make up in a hurry. Fill a basin with warm water and add 2 or 3 drops of mustard oil or 1 teaspoon of powdered mustard, such as Coleman's. Soak your feet for at least half an hour. The mustard helps kill the fungus. Rinse your feet and dry thoroughly.

Corn Plaster *This homemade corn plaster is very effective and costs only pennies.*

1 banana skin or fig skin or pulp of a squeezed lemon

1 small dandelion leaf or garlic clove, crushed

1. Scrape the inside of the banana or fig skin until you have about a teaspoonful of the pulp. Alternatively, you can use the flesh of a squeezed lemon.

2. In a small dish, mix the pulp with the dandelion or garlic to make a paste. Apply paste directly to the corn, binding in place with a small adhesive bandage.

3. When the skin is soft, gently rub the top layer of the corn away with an emery board.

4. Repeat the entire process daily until the corn disappears. For several days after the corn is gone, massage the area with a small amount of Calendula Ointment (page 286).

calendula treatments for blisters

Here are two ways to make use of the healing properties of calendula when treating blisters. Which you use depends on whether the blister is open or still intact.

• For open blisters, make an infusion of dried calendula flowers (see Making an Infusion, page 271). Dab on and let dry.

• For other foot blisters, apply a small amount of Calendula Ointment (page 286) to a clean piece of gauze, and cover the blister. Remove when you're not wearing shoes.

Essential Oil Corn Remover *Here's an easy, inexpensive way to take care of a corn.*

1 drop clove or tea tree essential oil

2 drops olive oil

1. In a small dish, dilute the essential oil with the olive oil. Spread over corn.

2. Cover the corn with a sterile strip bandage. Repeat application and change bandage daily until corn disappears.

One-Minute Substitute

Treating a Blister with Essential Oil
Here's a quick fix for a blister that costs pennies. Just place 1 drop tea tree or lavender essential oil on the blister and gently massage it in. Make sure you don't break the skin and don't use tea tree oil on open blisters.

Salicylic Acid Corn Remover
Most commercial corn removers have salicylic acid as their main ingredient—the same ingredient in aspirin. Here's how you can make your own salicylic acid remover.

5 aspirin tablets, 325 mg (adult)

1/2 teaspoon lemon juice

1/2 teaspoon water

1. In a small bowl, with the back of a spoon, crush the aspirin into a powder. Add the lemon juice and water and stir until the mixture forms a paste.

2. Dab the paste onto the corn and cover with plastic wrap, then place a heated towel over the wrap to help the paste penetrate more deeply. It will take several applications over several days before the corn falls off.

for mouth and lip irritations

Healing Balm for Chapped Lips
During winter this homemade lip balm will keep your lips from cracking and peeling, if you use it faithfully. With its lovely smell, it is a true bargain.

4 tablespoons almond oil

1 tablespoon grated beeswax

1 teaspoon honey

1 capsule vitamin E, 400 IU

10 drops chamomile essential oil

10 drops orange essential oil

10 drops wintergreen essential oil

5 drops lavender essential oil

1. In the top of a double boiler, warm the oil, the beeswax, and the honey over low heat until the wax melts. Remove from heat. Pierce the vitamin E capsule with a needle and squeeze its contents into the mixture.

2. Stir in the essential oils. Store in a cool, dark place and use by dipping a finger into the balm and smoothing it on your lips.

One-Minute Substitute | **Quickly Soothe a Canker Sore with Aloe Vera**
Instead of buying balm in the drugstore to coat that painful mouth sore, make your own instantly. All you need are a cotton swab and an aloe vera leaf. Dry the sore area with a cotton swab, then squeeze a bit of gel from the aloe vera leaf over the area. Repeat as often as necessary.

Cold Sore Ointment

This is really more of a liquid than an ointment, but it works the same way. The jojoba oil serves as a carrier oil.

5 drops lemon balm essential oil

1 drop lavender essential oil

1 drop chamomile essential oil

1 drop bergamot or rose essential oil

10 drops jojoba oil

1. In a small, clean jar with a tight-fitting lid, dilute the lemon balm and the lavender, chamomile, bergamot or rose oil essential oils in the jojoba oil (which serves as a carrier oil).

2. Smooth over the affected area several times a day.

Mouthwash for Cold Sores

This is a simple, certainly inexpensive, mouthwash that helps to heal annoying cold sores as fast as possible.

6 ounces water

3-4 drops clove or tea tree essential oil

1. In a clean jar with a tight-fitting lid, mix the water with the essential oil.

2. Swish the mixture in your mouth for 30 seconds, then spit it out. Cap bottle and keep mixture on the counter. Repeat mouthwash several times a day.

One-Minute Substitute

A Fast Cold Sore Preventive

You probably can't even find a cold sore preventive at your local CVS or Walgreens. If you feel one coming on, here's what to do. Apply 1 drop of lavender or lemon balm essential oil to the area where you feel the cold sore forming. Then hold an ice cube on top of the area for 10 minutes. This should either prevent the outbreak altogether or at least reduce its severity. Repeat the whole procedure several times a day.

Cold Sore Paste

This soothing, not-so-costly paste smothers the irritation of a cold sore and helps to heal it.

1 teaspoon finely chopped licorice root or rhizome

3 ounces distilled water

Slippery elm powder, as needed

Goldenseal powder, as needed

1. In a small saucepan, combine licorice root and distilled water. Bring the water to a boil, then simmer for 10 minutes. Strain into a clean bowl. This makes a strong licorice decoction.

2. In a small, clean container with a tight-fitting lid, mix equal amounts of slippery elm and goldenseal powder and moisten with the licorice decoction.

3. Apply the paste to the sore area to control pain and increase healing. Store extra paste in the refrigerator or dilute with water and use as mouthwash.

dental care products

Mouthwash
You don't need to spend upward of $4 a bottle for artificially flavored mouthwash that is primarily alcohol.

1 teaspoon vegetable glycerin

1 teaspoon aloe vera gel

10 drops peppermint, wintergreen, or spearmint essential oil

1 1/2 cups water

1. In a clean jar with a tight-fitting cap, mix vegetable glycerin and aloe vera gel with the essential oil you have chosen. Add water and shake well. Use as a gargle.

2. Store in a covered jar and shake well before using.

Mints
Instead of sugary candy, chew on breath-freshening herbs and spices.

1-2 fresh leaves spearmint, peppermint, fennel, or parsley

1/4 teaspoon fresh or dried caraway, cardamom, or fennel seeds

Chew on the herb leaves or seeds for two or three minutes. Spit out and discard.

Toothpaste
Although we can't say 4 out of 5 dentists recommend it, we do know this home-made version will cost you far less than any of the commercial brands that fill drugstore shelves. The tea tree oil provides an additional antiseptic boost to help prevent gum disease.

3 tablespoons baking soda

Water

10 drops tea tree essential oil

10 drops peppermint essential oil

1. In a small bowl, mix the baking soda with just enough water to make a paste. Add the tea tree and peppermint essential oils.

2. Use paste to brush your teeth and tongue. Cover the remaining paste and use for the next couple of days.

One-Minute Substitute

Fast Toothache Relief with Clove Oil

Until you can get to the dentist, try this quick numbing trick. Put 1 drop of oil of cloves on a cotton swab, dip the swab in water, and then rub on the aching tooth and gum area.

Antibacterial Mouthwash
Used regularly, this mouthwash can help kill the germs that cause gum disease for a lot less than commercial mouthwashes.

2 cups distilled water

2 tablespoons green tea

2 tablespoon dried, crumbled peppermint, spearmint, or rosemary

10 drops tincture of benzoin or 1 teaspoon tincture of myrrh

1. In a saucepan, bring the water to a boil. In a pint jar with a tight-fitting lid, mix the green tea and peppermint, spearmint, or rosemary. Pour in the boiling water, let cool, cover, and steep overnight in the refrigerator.

2. Strain into a clean bottle with a tight-fitting lid. Add the tincture of benzoin or the tincture of myrrh and shake to mix.

3. Use 2 tablespoons at a time as a mouthwash for sore and/or bleeding gums. Swish and spit without swallowing.

Gum Tonic
This will treat bad gums with respect without running up your grocery bill.

1 dropperful of goldenseal tincture (about 20 drops)

2 drops myrrh essential oil

1 ounce hot water

1. In a glass, combine the goldenseal tincture and myrrh essential oil. Dilute with the hot water.

2. Swish around your mouth and spit.

Super Dental Floss
There may be antiseptic dental floss on the market, but it will cost more than this and may not even work as well.

10 drops goldenseal tincture

3 drops myrrh essential oil

2 drops tea tree essential oil

Dental floss

1. In a small container, combine the goldenseal tincture, myrrh essential oil, and tea tree essential oil. Cut off enough dental floss to clean between your teeth and dip it into the mixture.

2. Use the dipped floss to clean between your teeth. Make a fresh batch every time you want to floss your teeth.

Toothache-Relieving Rinse
To quell the pain until you can get to a dentist, try this inexpensive rinse.

1 1/2 teaspoons whole cloves

1 cup boiling water

1. In a small pot, place the cloves. Pour in boiling water and steep for 10 minutes. Strain into a glass.

2. Rinse your mouth with the warm infusion.

Toothache-Relieving Dental Paste
Some people don't like cloves and need another way to relieve dental pain without using expensive pain pills with lots of side effects. Try this.

2 tablespoons powdered ginger

2 tablespoons red cayenne pepper

Water

1. In a small dish, mix powdered ginger and red cayenne pepper with enough water to make a paste.
2. Saturate a cotton ball with the paste and put on the painful tooth. Keep the paste off your gums, because it may be irritating to gums.

for joint and muscle aches

Hot Pepper Rub
The capsaicin in hot peppers has begun to be appreciated as a pain reliever even by commercial drug companies. Make your own for lots less.

2 tablespoons ground cayenne pepper

1/2 cup Glorious Green Aloe Moisturizing Lotion (page 253) or any commercial moisturizing lotion

1. In a small bowl, combine the cayenne pepper with the moisturizing lotion.
2. Massage the mixture into the painful area, being careful to wash your hands afterward before touching your face or eyes.

Massage Cream
This soothing, painkilling massage cream will take care of sore muscles and your bank balance.

2 teaspoons grated beeswax

1 tablespoon coconut oil

4 tablespoons cayenne-infused oil

10-15 drops wintergreen essential oil

2 tablespoons ginger tincture

2 tablespoons water

2 tablespoons aloe vera gel

1/2 teaspoon borax

1/4 teaspoon powdered vitamin C (from drugstore or health food store)

1. In the top of a double boiler over low heat, mix the beeswax and coconut oil and stir until the beeswax has melted. Stir in the cayenne-infused oil and the wintergreen essential oil.
2. In a separate pan, heat the ginger tincture to evaporate as much alcohol as possible, then add the water, aloe vera gel, borax, and vitamin C and bring to 160°F to 175°F on a candy thermometer. Place the ginger tincture mixture in a blender and whirl at high speed as you add the beeswax-oil mixture. Pour the resulting cream into a clean jar with a tight-fitting lid.
3. Massage cream into sore joints as needed. Keep refrigerated for 4 to 6 weeks.

Quick-and-Dirty Muscle Rub

Again, capsaicin comes to the rescue of tense and tired muscles that need a good massage in a hurry without costing an arm and a leg.

5 drops cayenne-based hot sauce

3-5 drops peppermint essential oil

15 drops massage oil or olive oil

1. In a clean small jar, combine hot sauce, peppermint essential oil, and massage or olive oil and mix thoroughly.
2. Rub the mixture into the affected area by hand or with a cotton ball. This may initially irritate the skin, but the irritation will disappear as the painkilling becomes more effective.
3. Clean your hands with soap and water after each application and avoid touching your eyes.

Muscle Soak

A luxurious hot soak with beneficial herbs is priceless for relieving tight muscles and joints. You can make your own bag of just the right herbs.

1/2 cup baking soda

10-20 drops essential oil of eucalyptus, peppermint, juniper, or pine

1/2 cup Epsom salts

1 tablespoon juniper berries

1 tablespoon dried rosemary leaves

1 tablespoon dried chamomile flowers

1 tablespoon dried eucalyptus leaves

2 teaspoons dried lemon balm leaves

2 teaspoons dried peppermint leaves

1 two-ply square cheesecloth

1. In a small dish, place the baking soda and add the essential oils; mix until the baking soda has absorbed the oils. In a bowl, combine the Epsom salts, herbs, and baking soda mixture. Place in middle of cheesecloth and tie up the ends to make a bag.
2. Hold beneath the running water until tub fills, then massage your body with the bag and let it float in the tub. Soak until water cools.

Liniment

This is a traditional remedy for man and beast, and nothing on the market loosens tight joints and offers relief any better.

4 teaspoons castor oil

2 tablespoon glycerin

2 tablespoon aloe vera gel

2 tablespoons cayenne tincture

20 drops wintergreen essential oil

1. In a clean glass bottle with a tight-fitting stopper, combine the castor oil, glycerin, aloe vera gel, cayenne tincture, and wintergreen essential oil. Shake well.
2. Massage over sore joints as needed. Refrigerate for up to 6 weeks.

Cold Pack for Strains and Sprains

There are all kinds of clever products on the market to use as cold packs. This one is flexible, reusable, and very, very inexpensive.

3 parts water

1 part rubbing alcohol

1 plastic zip-close freezer bag

1. Combine the water and rubbing alcohol in the freezer bag and freeze.

2. Wrap the frozen pack in a towel and apply to the hurting joint. The alcohol keeps the pack flexible.

Castor Oil Rub for Back Pain

You don't have to pay for a special tube of rubbing cream for back pain. Instead, try this easily made rub.

5 drops ginger essential oil

5 drops peppermint or wintergreen essential oil

2 drops camphor essential oil

2 drops rosemary essential oil

1 ounce castor oil

1. In a small bowl, mix together the essential oils and the castor oil.

2. Rub into the painful area and cover with a piece of flannel or an old T-shirt, then put a heating pad over the cloth for 15 to 20 minutes to help the rub soak in. You can double the recipe for larger areas.

for women's problems

Muscle Relaxant for Cramps

Forget the pills marketed just for cramps. Try this less expensive, easy-to-make remedy instead. These tinctures are available in natural food stores.

1/2 teaspoon valerian tincture

1/2 teaspoon cramp bark tincture

Take a dose of valerian tincture and a dose of cramp bark tincture every one to two hours. These are both natural muscle relaxants.

Hot Compress for Cramps

You can enhance the help of a heating pad by using a touch of ginger and oil.

2 tablespoons castor oil

10 drops ginger essential oil

In a small dish, mix castor oil and ginger essential oil. Spread the oil mixture over your abdomen, cover with a cotton or wool flannel cloth, then apply a heating pad for 20 to 30 minutes.

Anti-Cramp Tea

This combination of herbs can safely relax cramps and reduce your discomfort.

1 cup boiling water

1/4 teaspoon dried raspberry leaves

1/4 teaspoon dried chamomile flowers

1/4 teaspoon crushed fennel seeds

1/4 teaspoon dried spearmint leaves

1. In a large cup, pour 1 cup of boiling water over the raspberry leaves, chamomile, crushed fennel seeds, and spearmint. Steep 10 minutes and strain into a teacup.

2. Drink for relief when the cramps hit.

Ginger Tea for Morning Sickness

Here is a simple preparation that will calm your stomach in the morning and reduce nausea without making you sleepy.

1 cup boiling water

1/2 teaspoon minced fresh ginger

1. In a large cup, pour the cup of boiling water over the ginger. Steep 10 minutes, strain into a container, and refrigerate.

2. Sip in the morning when you wake.

PMS Tea

This tea is designed to help regulate hormone levels for all types of premenstrual syndrome without harming your stomach or liver.

1 tablespoon chopped dried dandelion roots and/or leaves

1 tablespoon chopped dried burdock root

4 cups water

1 teaspoon chopped dried black cohosh rhizome or root

1 teaspoon dried cramp bark

1 teaspoon grated orange peel

1 teaspoon chopped dried licorice root

1. In a pot, combine the dandelion roots and/or leaves and burdock root with the water. Add the black cohosh, cramp bark, orange peel, and licorice root. Bring to a boil, reduce the heat, and simmer, uncovered, 40 minutes. Cover and steep for 15 minutes. Strain into a clean container with a tight-fitting lid.

2. Drink 1/2 to 1 cup hot or cold as needed throughout the day. Refrigerate remainder.

Yeast Infection Cream

1 capsule acidophilus bacteria

3 tablespoons plain organic yogurt with active cultures

You don't need those expensive over-the-counter yeast infection remedies. You can make this in no time and for very little money. You can buy capsules of acidophilus bacteria—the bacteria used to make yogurt—in health food stores.

1. In a small dish, open the capsule and mix the bacteria and the yogurt.
2. Apply inside the vagina with a medicine syringe at night and wear a pad to prevent leakage.

headache treatments

Headache Compresses

Enough chilled lavender toilet water to soak 2 washcloths

2 washcloths

There's a whole host of treatments beyond pills. But you won't find them in your local drugstore. To ease tension after a hard day, try this cool compress.

1. In a small bowl, pour in the toilet water. Soak both washcloths in the toilet water and squeeze out the excess.
2. Lie down with a towel behind your neck. Place one wet washcloth on your forehead and the other cloth at the base of your skull. Relax for at least 15 minutes, preferably in a darkened quiet room.

Chamomile Tea

3 teaspoons dried chamomile

1 cup boiling water

1 teaspoon honey *(optional)*

Taking a break in a busy schedule can relieve some of the tension that causes many headaches. Chamomile tea—inexpensive and easy to make—is particularly soothing to frazzled nerves.

1. In a small pot, place chamomile. Pour in boiling water and steep for 5 minutes. Strain into a teacup.
2. Take a few minutes to sip the hot tea slowly while sitting in a quiet spot. Sweeten with a teaspoon of honey if desired.

Lemon Balm Tea

3 teaspoons dried lemon balm

1 cup boiling water

1 teaspoon honey *(optional)*

Lemon balm is another soothing tea herb that can relax away headaches for pennies with little fuss.

1. In a small pot, place lemon balm. Pour in boiling water and steep for 5 minutes. Strain into a teacup.
2. Take a few minutes to sip the hot tea slowly while sitting in a quiet spot. Sweeten with a teaspoon of honey if desired.

Migraine Tea

These vicious headaches are difficult to treat with pills. This inexpensive tea, served in a quiet, darkened room, can be very calming.

- 2 1/2 cups water
- 9 teaspoons dried lady's mantle leaves
- 3 teaspoons dried mint leaves

1. In a saucepan, bring the water to a boil. Add the herbs and boil for 20 minutes. Remove from heat and steep for 10 minutes. Strain into a teacup.
2. Drink 1 cup slowly in a quiet, darkened room.

Headache Massage

The combination of fragrant aroma and gentle massage can bring a throbbing head back to health without jeopardizing your stomach or liver as many headache pills do.

- 10 drops massage oil
- 3 drops peppermint essential oil
- 2 drops lavender essential oil
- 1 drop lemon, orange, or lime essential oil

1. In a small bowl, mix the massage oil and the essential oils.
2. Dip your fingers into the oil and then massage the oil into the temples, along the hairline, and along the base of the skull, being careful not to get any oil in the eyes.
3. Wash your hands thoroughly after each application.

Headache Oil with Vitamin E

Here is another aromatic solution for safely massaging away a headache.

- 15 drops lavender essential oil
- 7 drops wintergreen essential oil
- 1 1/2 tablespoons almond or olive oil
- 1 capsule vitamin E, 400 IU
- Bowl hot water

1. In a small dish, combine the essential oils with the almond or olive oil. Pierce the vitamin E capsule with a needle and squeeze the contents into the dish.
2. Warm the oil mixture by putting the dish in a bowl of hot water before using. Dab your fingers into the fragrant oil and gently massage your temples and the back of your neck. Wash your hands thoroughly after each application.

for anxiety and fatigue

Catnip Anti-Anxiety Tea

You can ask your doctor for a prescription for an anti-anxiety medication, or you can make a cup of catnip tea (yes, they make it for humans too) and sip it several times a day.

- 2 teaspoons dried catnip
- 1 cup boiling water

1. In a teapot, steep catnip in boiling water for five to seven minutes. Strain and drink.
2. Serve yourself catnip tea three times a day.

Healthy Home Remedies   **715**

Hops Anti-Anxiety Tea
Your cat is casting jealous glances at your catnip tea. So try hops, the critical ingredient in beer, instead.

2 teaspoons dried hops

1 cup boiling water

1. In a teapot, steep hops in boiling water for five to seven minutes. Strain and drink.
2. Serve yourself hops tea three times a day.

Calming Tea for Insomnia
All those over-the-counter sleep aids are just repackaged antihistamines. Instead, try this natural (and less expensive) alternative.

Boiling water

3 teaspoons dried chamomile or lemon balm

1. In a small pot, pour boiling water over chamomile or lemon balm. Steep 10 minutes, strain, and drink an hour before bed.
2. Once you start falling asleep more easily, cut the amount of herb in half.

One-Minute Substitute	**Lavender Rub for Insomnia** Massage a single drop of lavender essential oil into each temple before going to bed.

Sleep Pillow
This aromatic small pillow will work its wonders—with no side effects—on your sleep habits.

4 tablespoons sweet woodruff

2 tablespoons lemon balm

2 tablespoons lavender

1 tablespoon chamomile

1 tablespoon hops

1 tablespoon rosebuds

10-15 drops chamomile essential oil

10-15 drops lavender essential oil

10-15 drops clary sage essential oil

10-15 drops marjoram essential oil

1 tablespoon powdered or freshly grated orrisroot

1 small zippered pillowcase

1. In a large bowl, mix the woodruff, lemon balm, lavender, chamomile, hops, and rosebuds. In a separate small bowl, mix the essential oils with the orrisroot. Stir this mixture into the large bowl.
2. Fill the pillowcase, zip it, and add it to your bed pillows for sweet dreams.

Herbal Milk Bath for Sleeplessness

What is more relaxing than a nice soak in a soothing herbal bath? And there are no bad aftereffects in the morning.

1/2 handful lavender

1/2 handful chamomile

1/2 handful rose petals

1/2 handful dry powdered milk

Double-ply square of cheesecloth

1. Place the lavender, chamomile, rose petals, and powdered milk on the cheesecloth and tie the ends to make a bag.
2. Place under the spigot of the tub while the water is running. Start with warm water but allow it to cool before getting in. The cool water helps lower your body temperature, important for sleep.
3. Soak for 15 minutes while listening to relaxing music or a relaxation tape.

Relaxing Aromatic Bath

Here's another way to get sleepy or anxiety-free without any pills. Keep the water relatively cool to maintain a low body temperature, important for sleep.

10 drops lavender, rose, geranium, and/or bergamot essential oil.

1. Add the essential oils to a cool bath.
2. Soak for 15 minutes while listening to relaxing music or a relaxation tape.

Invigorating Oil for Fatigue

These essential oils have fragrances that help to stimulate you and keep your mind alert.

Eucalyptus essential oil

Juniper essential oil

Grapefruit essential oil

Clary sage essential oil

Ginger or peppermint essential oil

Rosemary essential oil

1. In a clean small spray bottle, mix 2 parts eucalyptus, 2 parts juniper, 2 parts grapefruit, 1 part clary sage, 1 part ginger or peppermint, and 2 parts rosemary essential oils. Shake to mix.
2. You can use this spray in a variety of ways: Spritz an entire room when you feel tired and need to keep reading. Spray a cloth, hold it up to your nose, and breathe deeply. Rub into your hands. Use in a diffuser or humidifier.

Energy Tea for Fatigue

This tea is a real homemade pick-me-up that beats the pricey specialty teas you find at the grocery.

1 teacup boiling water

1/2 teaspoon dried rosemary leaves

1/2 teaspoon dried ginseng root

Honey *(optional)*

In a teacup, make an infusion of boiling water, dried rosemary leaves, and dried ginseng root. Sweeten with a bit of honey, if you like, and drink as often as necessary.

inside this chapter

dog food

Calcium-Rich Dog Food

Low-Fat Chicken and
Rice Dog Dinner

Delectable Dog Biscuits

Dog Slaw

Lucky Liver Snaps

Sweet Breath Dog Treats

Doggie Birthday Cake

canine care products

Brush-and-Go Dry Dog Shampoo

Minty Skunk Cure

Cocktail Flea Dip

Flea-Begone Bandanna

Flea Powder

Ear Mite Oil

Firm Stool Fix

cat food

Wholesome Kitty Dinner

Tuna Treats

Catnip Crackers

Quick Fish Stick Treats

Sardine Balls

Melon Squares

Cat Grass Buffet

feline care products

Baby-Fresh Litter

Dry Cat Shampoo

Fragrant Flea Treatment

Tick Removal from Cats

treats for birds

Pet Bird Honey Treats

Pet Bird Snacking Salad

Sweet and Crunchy Bird Muffins

Finch and Canary Treat

Parrot Pops

Wild Bird Food

Premium Wild Bird Mix

Healthy Hummingbird Nectar

food for exotic pets

Guinea Pig Salad

Hamster Fruit Cup

Gerbil and Rabbit Salad

Pet Rodent Tabbouleh

Turtle and Reptile Treat

Aquarium Fish Treats

Wholesome Natural Pet Care Products

Our animal companions provide us not only with comfort and amusement but also with an uncritical devotion and loyalty that is difficult to obtain

elsewhere. And a loving pet provides therapy that instantly lifts its caretaker's spirits. So all of us who love pets tend to be suckers for buying them expensive treats and toys. As this chapter will show you, however, you don't have to spend a fortune to keep your pet—dog, cat, bird, hamster, guinea pig, gerbil, rat, turtle, or fish—well fed, healthily groomed, and happily occupied.

You can indulge your pets with nutritious meals that they will gobble up eagerly and healthy treats that they can enjoy without jeopardizing their health and well-being. None of these foods will strain your budget and most are actually fun to make. And it is always reassuring to know exactly what goes into your pet's food. In the recipes that follow, you will find not only healthy everyday foods and treats but also special-occasion treats such as a dog's birthday cake, feline catnip crackers, and parrot pops.

You will also find great recipes for natural wet and dry shampoos, flea dips, breath-saving dog biscuits, even a formula for dealing with skunk spray. For backyard bird lovers, there are recipes for inexpensive seed combinations you can mix to feed wild birds outside your window. And for young families, there are salads and treats for gerbils, hamsters, turtles, and other childhood favorites.

dog food

Calcium-Rich Dog Food

This easy-to-make recipe appeals to dogs and strengthens their bones. Although it is not inexpensive, it costs less than canned dog foods and you can vouch for the quality of its ingredients.

1 pound ground chicken or hamburger

4 cups cooked oatmeal or brown rice

1/2 cup bread crumbs

1/4 cup vegetable oil

1 tablespoon bonemeal (available at garden centers)

1 pet vitamin, crushed

1/2 cup shredded cheddar cheese

1. In a skillet over moderate heat, brown meat, stirring frequently. Remove from heat.

2. Stir in other ingredients and enough water to keep the mixture from being crumbly.

3. Cool and store in the refrigerator for one week or in the freezer for up to three months.

Feed according to weight of dog. Feed a 5-pound dog 1/2 cup daily; double the serving for every 5 pounds. Monitor your dog's weight and adjust portions to avoid obesity.

Makes 6 cups

Low-Fat Chicken and Rice Dog Dinner

If you want a nutritious beef- and-wheat-free diet for your pet, this combination will satisfy its appetite and may even keep its weight under control. This is also an economical dog food with fresh ingredients.

3 pounds chicken, with skin and bone

1 1/2 cups cooked oatmeal or brown rice

1 pint fat-free cottage cheese

1 dog vitamin

1. Poach, bake, or microwave chicken until well done. Cool and cut into 1/2-inch cubes. Drain and reserve pan juices to use as soup stock. Discard bones. Cook oatmeal or rice according to package directions and let cool.

2. In a large bowl, mix together cubed chicken and grains. Crumble vitamin and stir it in. Drain cottage cheese and fold it into the mixture.

3. Store in a covered container in the refrigerator for up to one week.

Feed according to weight of dog. Feed a 5-pound dog 1/2 cup daily; double the serving for every five pounds. Monitor your dog's weight and adjust portions to avoid obesity.

Makes 12 servings, 1/2 cup each

Delectable Dog Biscuits

The combination of dog food and oatmeal makes these biscuits a healthy and much-desired treat for your dog. You are assured of good ingredients and a better price than commercial dog biscuits. For a nutritional boost, add a crumbled dog vitamin.

2 pounds Calcium-Rich Dog Food (opposite) or canned dog food

1/4 cup whole wheat flour

3/4 cup oat bran

1 cup rolled oats

1 dog vitamin, crushed *(optional)*

1/4 cup Parmesan or cheddar cheese, shredded *(optional)*

1/2 cup vegetable oil

1. Preheat oven to 250°F.
2. Mix dog food, flour, bran, rolled oats, vitamin (if desired), and cheese (if desired for a flavor boost).
3. Add oil slowly, mixing dough to a consistency that can be rolled and cut with a cookie cutter.
4. Roll and cut or mold biscuits; place on an ungreased baking sheet. Bake for 3 1/2 hours, or until hard.
5. Cool and store in a covered canister in refrigerator for one week, or in a freezer for up to one month.

Makes 16 medium biscuits

homemade comforts for a new puppy

Puppies suffer from separation anxiety when they first leave their mother.

• To ease the transition, ask the breeder to put an old T-shirt or other piece of clothing into the puppy's box for a few days. When you bring the puppy home, bring along the clothing with the smells it recognizes and put it into the puppy's new bed.

• Along with this security blanket, add something that smells of you, so that the pup will soon get used to its new home.

• Another helpful transition aid is an old-fashioned ticking alarm clock, which emulates the mother's heartbeat.

• Also try filling an old sock with dried beans and microwaving it for a few seconds to create a soft, warm "body" for the puppy to snuggle up to.

Dog Slaw

Here's a dietary supplement for your dog, such as you will only find at very expensive pet emporiums. Making your own costs less than a dollar per serving. Dogs like carrots, which aid in digestion, freshen breath, and provide vitamins. The yogurt is digestion-friendly.

1 cup shredded carrots, raw

1/3 cup brown raisins

1/2 cup fat-free plain, live-culture yogurt

1/4 cup salad oil

1. Mix carrots and raisins in a bowl and set aside. In a second bowl, stir together the yogurt and salad oil. Pour this mixture over the slaw and toss.
2. Store in a covered container in the refrigerator for up to three days. Serve 1/4 cup every day along with meals or as a treat.

Makes 4 servings

Wholesome Natural Pet Care Products

Lucky Liver Snaps

The secret of many successful show and obedience trainers is nothing more than a little chewy liver nibble that dogs can't resist. Try it—your pet will jump through hoops for this homemade treat that has much more liver flavor than the store-bought kind.

1 pound beef or chicken livers
1 egg
1 cup flour
1/4 cup bran meal
3/4 cup cornmeal
1 tablespoon garlic powder

1. Preheat oven to 400°F. Chop raw livers, and then liquefy them in a blender. Add egg, pulse to blend, and then pour mixture into a mixing bowl. Stir in flour, bran, cornmeal, and garlic powder.

2. Spread mixture evenly into 9 x 13-inch greased sheet-cake pan and bake for 15 minutes.

3. While still warm, cut sheet into 1-inch squares. Turn squares out onto baking rack to cool and harden.

4. Store cooled treats in a plastic zip bag in the freezer to preserve freshness for up to three months. Serve either frozen or at room temperature.

Makes 117 liver snaps

Sweet Breath Dog Treats

Puppies often have "puppy breath" that they naturally outgrow by the age of 6 months. If an adult dog has occasional bad breath, this tasty recipe will combat the problem. If bad breath persists, however, it may be a sign of dental or digestive problems that a vet should treat. Here is a specialty dog biscuit that you don't have to shell out a fortune for at a pet store.

1 tablespoon activated charcoal (available in fish section of pet shops)
1/2 cup whole wheat flour
1 cup white flour
1/4 cup bran cereal
1/2 cup cornmeal
4 tablespoons vegetable oil
1 egg
1/2 cup chopped fresh basil, wintergreen, or mint
1/2 cup chopped fresh rosemary or thyme
1 cup of acidophilus milk

1. Preheat oven to 400°F. Process charcoal in coffee grinder until finely ground. Mix flour, bran, cornmeal, and charcoal together in a bowl. Stir in other ingredients.

2. Form into bite-size patties and place on a greased cookie sheet. Bake 20 minutes, or until dry and hard.

3. Store in a covered container in the refrigerator for one week, or in the freezer for up to three months.

Makes 24 medium biscuits

One-Minute Substitute

A Quick Water Bowl for Dog Walkers

Pick up an inexpensive plastic shower cap (or save a free one from a hotel) to use as a portable pet water dish. Stick it in your pocket when walking your dog, and when needed, pull it out and fill it from a water bottle or the nearest faucet or water fountain.

Doggie Birthday Cake

People do like to make a fuss over their dogs. For a birthday or adoption anniversary, you can go to a very fancy pet store and spend a lot of money or you can make up this nutritious treat (to be meted out during the week) for a few dollars. Here's a cake that you can feel good about offering him.

1 small package cornbread mix or 1/3 cup flour

1/3 cup cornmeal, bran, or rolled oats

1 1/2 teaspoons baking powder

1/2 teaspoon garlic powder

1 pound ground chicken

2 tablespoons honey

1 large egg

1/4 cup live-culture plain yogurt

4 teaspoons vegetable oil

1 container (4 ounces) whipped cream cheese

Delectable Dog Biscuits, as needed to decorate cake (page 307)

1. Preheat oven to 350°F. In a medium bowl, stir together dry ingredients. Make a well in the center and add chicken and wet ingredients. Stir just until mixed (or substitute cornbread mix made according to directions and combined with chicken).

2. Pour into greased cake pan and bake for 25 minutes or until chicken is done and a toothpick inserted in the center of cake comes out clean.

3. Turn out onto a cake rack to cool.

4. Frost with cream cheese (thin, if needed, with a little milk) and decorate with dog biscuits. Refrigerate in a covered container for up to one week.

Makes one cake with 4 to 6 servings

canine care products

Brush-and-Go Dry Dog Shampoo

You can save $5 a pop by substituting this single ingredient for a commercial dry pet shampoo. Although your pet will still need the occasional soap-and-water shampoo to remove ground-in dirt, dry shampoo will keep your dog clean and fresh smelling during cold weather or when you're traveling.

1 box (1 pound) baking soda

1. Test for sensitivity by rubbing a little baking soda into your dog's coat between the ears (where it can't be licked off). Wait 5 minutes and check for reddening or other signs of irritation. If there are none, proceed.

2. Rub baking soda into the dog's coat, working it in all the way to the skin. Be careful to avoid eyes, nose, mouth, and ears. Allow soda to remain in coat for a full minute to absorb oil and odor.

3. Brush fur with a pet brush until all the baking soda and debris are removed.

Makes one or more shampoos, depending on the size of dog

Minty Skunk Cure

When a skunk sprays your dog, confine it outdoors and run to the bathroom supply cabinet for help. Speed is important: Dried skunk essence is harder to remove and lingers longer.

1 or more large tubes traditional-formula white toothpaste (colored or gel pastes can discolor fur)

1 bottle dog shampoo

1/4 cup cider vinegar

1. Work toothpaste into the dog's fur from head to tail, nose to toe. Allow toothpaste to air-dry for 20 minutes.

2. Wet the dog and apply dog shampoo, working up a full lather.

3. In a large bucket, combine vinegar with 1 gallon of warm water. Rinse the dog with this solution (double it for a big dog) and dry as usual.

4. Repeat treatment as needed.

Makes one treatment

Cocktail Flea Dip

To check for fleas, comb your pet over a sheet of white paper: If black specks (flea frass) drop onto the paper, treat the animal at once with this dip (double it for large pets). There are many expensive flea dips on the market but this one—pennies a pop—works without harsh chemicals. To get rid of flea eggs—and future infestations—wash the animal's bedding and vacuum your house thoroughly.

2 tablespoons vodka or dry vermouth

1 3/4 pints water

1. In a 2-quart saucepan, stir alcohol into water and bring to a boil.

2. Remove from heat, cover pan, and allow solution to steep for two hours.

3. Rub cooled solution into pet's fur, rinse, and comb out.

Makes one treatment

Flea-Begone Bandanna

Here's a safe, renewable, flea-repelling bandanna to make for your dog that is much healthier for the dog and anyone who plays with it than expensive toxic flea collars. It's prettier too. The active ingredients are essential herb oils, which smell good to us, but fleas and mosquitoes can't stand them. Herbal oils are readily available at health food stores.

1 cotton bandanna (color and pattern of your choice)

1 small vial rose geranium essential oil

1 small vial lavender essential oil

1. Sprinkle several drops of each oil on the bandanna.

2. Roll the bandanna and tie it loosely around your dog's neck.

3. Launder the bandanna; retreat with oil when the scent fades.

Note: If your dog won't wear a bandanna, dab oil between its shoulder blades where it can't be licked off. Don't get oil near a dog's eyes, nose, or mouth.

natural ways to make fleas flee

Consider aromatic leaves, wood shavings, and soap the first defense in your arsenal of flea repellents.

• Fill small drawstring bags (available at cooking supply and natural foods stores) with fresh or dried chamomile leaves, walnut leaves, or cedar shavings, and tuck them into your dog's bedding (where they can't be chewed) to repel fleas.

• Sprinkle garlic powder or mix a crushed garlic clove into your dog's food to ward off fleabites. Both garlic and chamomile are attractive flowering perennials, so for a free supply, try growing these herbs in your flower or vegetable beds.

• Sprinkling brewer's yeast on your pets' food daily is also generally thought to help them repel fleas.

Brewer's yeast is available at health food stores.

• Soap kills fleas on contact. When bathing your dog, begin by lathering the neck area first and then work your way toward the tail, because fleas tend to congregate around the neck.

• After rinsing, rub apple cider vinegar through the fur to repel fleas, and add a teaspoonful of cider vinegar to the dog's drinking water.

Flea Powder

This inexpensive powder will leave your dog fresh smelling and free of pesky fleas. It is safe to apply as often as needed. Mix and match the oils according to your own scent preference. Commercial flea powders cost much more and contain toxic chemicals.

1 box (1 pound) baking soda

10 drops peppermint, lavender, rosemary, cedar, eucalyptus, or rose geranium essential oil

1. Empty baking soda into a mixing bowl, sprinkle with your personal blend of oils, and stir to blend.

2. Work treated baking soda into your pet's fur, beginning at the neck (where fleas congregate) and working toward the tail. Keep the powder away from nose, mouth, eyes, and ears.

3. Allow the powder to remain on the dog for 10 minutes, then comb or brush it out, along with dirt and fleas.

Makes one treatment

Note: If you have a large dog, you may need to make two or more recipes.

Helpful Hint

Easy Way to Remove Burrs and Gum from Fur

Burrs and chewing gum can be nearly impossible to comb or shampoo out of a pet's tangled fur. To make burrs easier to comb out, coat them with vegetable or mineral oil. Allow the oil to soften the burr for a few minutes, and then comb it out. To remove chewing gum, work creamy-style peanut butter into the gum until it dissolves, then comb out.

Ear Mite Oil

Ear mites can lead to serious infections and problems, including hearing loss in dogs. You can head off problems—and expensive vet bills—with this simple treatment. If you are too late and the problem persists, consult a veterinarian. It could be a yeast infection and not mites at all.

1 vitamin E capsule, 400 IU
1/4 cup mineral oil

1. Pierce a vitamin E capsule with a needle and squeeze the contents into a small dropper bottle. Add oil and shake. Store at room temperature.
2. To apply, hold the bottle in your hand for a few minutes to warm the oil. Put two or three drops of warm oil into the dog's ear canal and massage gently for a count of ten. Allow the dog to shake its head, then carefully swab oil and dirt from the ear. Repeat in the other ear.
3. Apply every other day for a full week.

Makes 1/4 cup

---

free pooper scoopers

• Save used zip-shut plastic sandwich and food storage bags to recycle as puppy poop bags. To use a bag, turn it inside out and reach inside the clean side of the bag to grab the poop. Then pull it right-side-out, zip it closed, and toss it.
• If you don't like the hands-on approach, relegate a cheap or decommissioned pair of scissors-style salad tongs to the status of pooper scooper—they work better than the real thing, and you can still make deposits into used zipper bags.

Firm Stool Fix

If your pup or dog suffers occasionally from loose or runny stools, try this cheap and easy high-fiber remedy. If the problem persists, it could indicate internal parasites and you should consult a vet.

2 teaspoons canned pumpkin
1 tablespoon cream cheese
1/4 cup corn flakes

1. In a bowl, mix pumpkin and cheese; roll into a ball and coat with corn flakes.
2. Serve as a treat.

Makes 1 treatment

cat food

Wholesome Kitty Dinner
This nutritious meat and vegetable meal will be a welcome change of pace for your cat. You know exactly what is in it, and it's budget-friendly too.

2/3 cup ground chicken or hamburger

1 jar mixed vegetable baby food

1 cat vitamin, crumbled (*optional*)

1/3 cup plain dry bread crumbs

1. In a small saucepan over medium heat, poach the ground meat in a small amount of water until medium rare. Remove from heat and allow to cool.

2. Stir together the meat, meat juices, vegetables, and vitamin, if desired. Form into bite-size balls and roll in bread crumbs.

3. Serve as much as your cat will eat in one sitting. Store the rest in a covered container in the refrigerator for up to three days.

Makes 2 or 3 servings

Helpful Hint | **Trick Your Cat into Taking Medicine**
Cats are choosy about what they eat, and often turn their noses up at the taste of medicine. If you have trouble getting yours to take its medicine, try smearing the medication on the back of a front paw—the cat will lick it off. If it is in pill form, crush the pill and mix it with a little cream cheese to make it adhere to the paw.

Tuna Treats
Cats are famous for loving tuna, and yours will jump for joy when you whip up these healthful treats that use a can of "people" tuna and a few pantry staples. As a bonus, the oil-packed tuna will help prevent hairballs. You won't find fresh treats like this at any pet store.

1 can oil-packed tuna

1/4 cup cornmeal

1/4 cup bran cereal

1 1/2 cups whole wheat flour

1. Preheat oven to 350°F. In a large bowl, mix all the ingredients together.

2. Press dough out on a floured board and cut into small cookies with a cookie cutter or pizza roller.

3. Place cookies on a greased cookie sheet and bake for 20 minutes or until light brown. Turn out onto a cake rack to cool. Store in a covered container in the refrigerator for up to a week or in the freezer for up to a month.

Makes 24 or more depending on size of cookie

Catnip Crackers

Cats will go bonkers for these catnip crackers, so save them for rainy-day treats and special occasions. You can pay a lot more for commercial cat treats, but they won't measure up to these fresh, homemade ones.

3/4 cup flour

1/2 cup whole wheat flour

2 tablespoons dried catnip (available at pet shops and in pet aisle at most supermarkets)

1/2 cup yogurt

1 egg

1 tablespoon honey

3 tablespoons vegetable oil

1. Preheat oven to 350°F. In a medium bowl, mix flours and catnip together. Stir in yogurt, egg, honey, and vegetable oil.

2. Press out dough on a floured surface and cut into tiny treats using a cookie cutter or pizza wheel. Place on greased cookie sheet and bake for 15 minutes or until golden brown.

3. Store in a covered container in the refrigerator for a week or in the freezer for up to three months.

Makes 24 or more depending on the size of crackers

Quick Fish Stick Treats

Cats and their human companions alike will love these instant treats made from inexpensive frozen fish sticks. Adding a sprinkle of garlic powder will help your cat to repel fleas, and you won't find any treats as fresh or wholesome as these in a pet store.

1 package frozen, breaded fish sticks

1/2 teaspoon garlic powder

1. Empty a box of frozen fish sticks onto a cutting board. Sprinkle with garlic powder and cut the frozen sticks into 1-inch squares.

2. Store the squares in a zipper plastic bag (along with cooking instructions from the package) in the freezer for up to three months.

3. To serve, remove a square and microwave according to package directions, cool, and serve at room temperature.

Makes approximately 36 treats

Sardine Balls

Cats will meow for the fishy flavor of these wholesome little fish balls. They're easy to make, easy on the budget, and the oily fish will help keep hairballs from forming. You won't find the likes of these in any store.

1 can (6 1/2 ounces) sardines, packed in oil

3/4 cup plain bread crumbs

1. Empty the can of sardines into a mixing bowl. Mix in 1/2 cup bread crumbs. Roll the mixture into bite-size balls. When all balls are made, roll them in the remaining bread crumbs to coat.

2. Store in a sealed container or zipper plastic bag in the freezer.

3. To serve, thaw a ball to room temperature and place in your cat's bowl.

Makes 6 or 8 treats

make your own cat toys

Cats love a variety of toys, and are especially fond of small, lightweight, flexible, and sparkly toys. Avoid a costly trip to the pet store by offering these found toys to your pet.

• Save foil wrappers from chewing gum and other snacks, and roll them into little balls for your cat to bat around.

• Twist a foil wrapper into a little "bow tie" and fasten it on the end of a piece of string, then dangle it for your cat to play with. You can even tie these string toys to doorknobs throughout the house. Your cat will love hiding behind the door and reaching around to bat at them.

• Create little rolling noisemakers by filling film canisters with nontoxic items such as pieces of breakfast cereal and chopped nuts. Your cat will spend many happy hours rolling and chasing these toys.

Melon Squares
Some cats love the flavor of melon. If yours is among them, keep some of these mixed melon treats on hand.

1/2 orange-fleshed melon
1/2 green-fleshed melon

1. Peel and cube the melon flesh as you would for a salad.
2. Store in a sealed container in the refrigerator for up to one week.
3. Serve one or two cubes as a treat daily.

Makes 1 cup

Cat Grass Buffet
House cats like green "grass" to nibble on, and this recipe offers your cat long-lasting variety for pennies. You can buy untreated sprouting grains inexpensively at health food stores or even cheaper at feed mills. Keep grains in sealed plastic containers in the refrigerator. Save an empty Parmesan cheese shaker to fill with seed mix: It makes sowing easier.

1 cup whole oat berries
1/2 cup wheat berries
1/2 cup barley seeds
1/4 cup alfalfa seeds
1/4 cup rye grass

1. Put grains into a sealed plastic container and shake to mix. Fill shallow, tip-resistant pots with potting soil and moisten with tepid water.
2. Sprinkle the grains thickly over the top of the soil and cover grains with a sprinkling of soil. Set the pots in a sunny window and water as needed to keep the soil as moist as a wrung-out sponge. When the grass is an inch tall, set a pot beside your cat's dinner dish and watch the fun.
3. For an ongoing supply, start a fresh pot of cat grass every other week.

Makes four 4-inch flowerpots of grass

Wholesome Natural Pet Care Products   **729**

feline care products

Baby-Fresh Litter

Cat litter to cover bottom of
  litter box
1/3 cup baby powder

The most effective way to prevent cat litter odor is also a money saver: Instead of throwing money away by filling the litter box to the top, pour in a shallow layer. Use only 2 or 3 inches so that the litter can air-dry rapidly. Between litter changes, you can keep even the cheapest brand of litter smelling fresh with this simple, baby-safe recipe.

1. Pour litter into cat pan to a depth of 3 inches.
2. Sprinkle baby powder over the top of litter and stir to blend. For best results, change litter at least once a week.

Makes filler for one litter box

Helpful Hint | **Clever Cat Litter Storage**

If you keep your litter box in the laundry room, bathroom, or a closet, try storing new kitty litter in an open bag at the bottom of your clothes hamper, corner of a closet, or near the washer. Not only will the litter absorb odors and help keep these rooms smelling fresh, but you'll also be reminded to change the litter every time you change clothes.

Dry Cat Shampoo

1/3 cup bran
1/3 cup cornmeal
1/3 cup rolled oats

Take the stress out of bath time for your cat by bathing it with this soothing, dry shampoo. As an added bonus, you'll save some pocket change because it's made from common pantry staples.

1. Pour grains into a microwave-safe plastic container, seal, and shake to combine. Warm in microwave set on low for 10 seconds.
2. Rub warm grains into fur. When finished, brush the meal out along with oil, dirt, and dander.

Makes 1 shampoo

Fragrant Flea Treatment

Cats can be sensitive to any flea treatment, particularly toxic commercial flea powders. So try this mixture on a small patch of skin on the cat's stomach and wait for a day to see if there is a reaction. You must also wash the cat's bedding and vacuum the house thoroughly to get rid of flea eggs.

6 drops lavender essential oil
1 tablespoon mineral oil

1. Drop the lavender essential oil and the mineral oil into a small bottle and shake to combine.
2. Warm the oil by holding the bottle in your hands for a few minutes.
3. Massage the warm oil into the neck area and the base of the tail where fleas congregate, then all parts of the cat, being careful to avoid contact with the cat's ears, eyes, nose, and mouth. Repeat treatment when the scent is no longer detectable.

Makes 1 treatment

Help Hint | **Free Disposable Cat Litter Boxes**
Why clean a smelly plastic litter box when you can get bio-friendly ones for free and toss them, dirty litter and all? Make a habit of stopping by your local convenience or beverage store and asking for empty plastic-wrapped, shallow soda boxes—the kind that hold a dozen cans of soda pop. Keep the plastic on the box while in use, pull it off and toss in the recycle bin before dumping the litter-filled box into the trash. They also make convenient toss-and-go litter boxes for traveling with your cat.

Tick Removal from Cats

Cats are sensitive to many kinds of medications and herbal treatments, including tick repellents that are safe to use on dogs. Your best bet is to watch for ticks, especially around the face, ears, and neck, and remove them according to the following recipe. It will save you a trip to the vet.

Petroleum jelly
Hydrogen peroxide

1. Coat the tick and surrounding skin with petroleum jelly applied with a cotton swab.
2. After the tick smothers, gently pull it, with the head intact, from the cat's skin.
3. Swab the area with hydrogen peroxide to disinfect it.
4. If you remove a tiny deer tick (a potential transmitter of Lyme disease), seal it in a plastic container, such as a film canister, and take it and the cat to a veterinarian for testing.

Makes one treatment

Wholesome Natural Pet Care Products   **731**

treats for birds

Pet Bird Honey Treats

Parakeets and songbirds like sweets. This calcium-rich sweet treat is an inexpensive, wholesome snack. Most of the ingredients are already in your kitchen. You can find cuttlebone and bird grit at any pet supply store or in the pet aisle of your grocery.

1/3 cup cornmeal

1/2 cuttlebone, finely ground (in coffee grinder or mortar and pestle)

1/4 teaspoon fine bird grit

1/4 cup mixed parakeet, finch, or canary seeds

1 piece spray millet, crumbled

2 tablespoons honey

1/4 cup wheat germ

1 egg

1. Preheat oven to 350°F. Place all ingredients into a bowl and mix well. If mixture is too thick to mold, add a little water. Press with hands into small logs onto a greased and floured cookie sheet.

2. Bake for 30 minutes or until lightly browned.

3. Remove from oven, and turn logs out onto a cake rack to cool. Store in covered container in the freezer for up to three months.

4. To serve, thaw a log and fasten to cage bars with a treat clip. Renew when well nibbled.

Makes approximately 12 treats

making your home safe for birds

Birds are very sensitive to environmental pollutants and poor air quality. In the 1800s canaries were routinely carried into coal mines—if a canary died, the miners knew they, too, were in danger and should evacuate.

• **Beware of household fumes.** The kitchen may seem like a friendly place for a bird, but it is actually filled with potential poisons. Nonstick pans placed over high heat can give off fumes that are toxic to birds, and it's best not to expose birds to aerosol cleaner and detergent fumes.

• **Watch the temperature.** Study references for the care needed by the type of bird you have. Most thrive in a very specific and narrow range of temperatures. Put your bird in a room where you can regulate the temperature year-round, and where there are no drafts. Place the cage well away from windows, and if possible, cover it at night with a breathable cloth cover.

• **Use a safe, secure cage.** Antique and decorative cages are often beautiful, but may have sharp edges, bars far enough apart to either trap or let birds escape, or wood bars that birds can chew through. Even worse, they may have been painted with lead-based paint. Use such cages as decorative objects, and house your birds in cages with stainless steel or nontoxic enameled bars.

• **Avoid dangerous treats.** Chocolate can be lethal to birds. Wash vegetable and fruit skins to remove pesticide residue. While it's safe to offer apples, cherries, peaches, and pears to birds, the seeds are toxic, as are all parts of avocado, onions, mushrooms, tomatoes, salt, dried beans, and rice.

Pet Bird Snacking Salad

For optimum health, offer your bird fresh or thawed frozen fruits and vegetables daily. Forget expensive dried treats from a pet shop—they can't compare in freshness, flavor, or vitamins. This salad appeals to all bird species, and is easy to put together by saving a little here and there from your meal preparations. Modify it as needed: You will learn quickly which ingredients your bird devours and which ingredients it leaves uneaten.

- 3 leaves leaf lettuce or 1/2 cup fresh spinach, chopped
- 1/2 cup fresh or frozen, thawed, broccoli florets
- 1/2 cup frozen and thawed whole kernel corn
- 1/2 apple, diced
- 1/2 segmented orange, diced
- 1/4 cup dried currants
- 1/2 cup unsalted peanuts (for large birds only)

1. Toss all ingredients in a covered bowl and store in the refrigerator for up to 5 days.
2. To serve, put 1/3 cup salad in a shallow bowl or clay flowerpot saucer in the cage. Offer daily and make new salad as needed.

Makes 6 servings

Helpful Hint | **The Easy Way to Trap Bird Ticks**

If your bird has ticks, hang a disposable white cloth (or a paper towel) on one side of its cage. The ticks are attracted to the bright object. After the ticks congregate on the cloth, remove and dispose of it in a sealed plastic bag.

Sweet and Crunchy Bird Muffins

Small-quantity corn, bran, and oatmeal muffin mixes are sold in envelopes for less than 50 cents apiece—using them as a basis for these yummy bird treats lets you whip up treats faster than you could make them from scratch—but you can substitute your favorite muffin recipe (omit salt, which can harm birds). Plus, this all-in-one treat takes the place of several pricey commercial single-ingredient treats. For variety's sake, make all three flavors at the same time and alternate the flavors you offer your bird each day.

- 1 small package of commercial corn, bran, or oatmeal muffin mix
- 1/3 cup milk
- 1 egg
- 1/4 cup applesauce
- 1/2 cup mixed dried fruits (not sugared)
- 1/2 cup birdseed mix (appropriate to the species of bird)
- 1 bird vitamin (crumbled)

1. Preheat oven to 375°F. Prepare muffin mix according to directions, substituting applesauce for oil. Stir in the dried fruit and seed.
2. Pour batter into greased muffin tins and bake according to package directions, baking for 20 minutes or until golden brown.
3. Store muffins in sealed container in the freezer for up to three months.
4. To serve, thaw a muffin and place part or all of it in the bird's cage. You can refrigerate unused portions for up to a week.

Makes 6 muffins

Wholesome Natural Pet Care Products   **733**

Finch and Canary Treat

Here's a bite-size nutritious treat that's easy to make for small songbirds like finches and canaries. It is fresher and far less expensive than store-bought treats.

1/4 cup crunchy homemade Peanut Butter (page 33) or crunchy, unsweetened, low-salt commercial peanut butter

1/2 cup high-quality finch seed mix

1/4 cup wheat germ

1. In a medium bowl, mix peanut butter and seeds together, adding more seeds if needed to make a stiff batter.

2. Pour wheat germ into a shallow saucer. Form the peanut butter mix into small balls and roll the balls in wheat germ to coat.

3. Serve one ball as a treat, in a bird-proof bowl. Store leftovers in a covered container in the refrigerator for up to one month or freeze for up to three months.

Makes 8 treats

homemade toys for parakeets and parrots

Birds in the parrot family, including parakeets, love toys, but they can be pricey, and the bigger birds can destroy them quickly. Try these time-tested, and inexpensive, homemade toys.

• Parakeets love to preen in a mirror. So, instead of paying for a fancy and often fragile bird mirror, just remove the hinge from a sturdy old compact and fasten the mirror securely to the cage bars near a perch.

• Parrots love to climb. Satisfy this urge by tying knots along a sturdy cotton rope and hanging it from the top of the cage.

• Parrots also love to bite and chew, and a dog-chew toy is often less expensive and just as long lasting as a parrot chew toy. Try a rawhide "bone," or one made from nylon.

• Both parakeets and parrots like colorful toys, so string big wooden beads onto cotton rope and hang it for them to bat around and chew.

Parrot Pops

These chewy sweet treats will keep your parrot happily occupied for hours. Whip them up inexpensively, then sit back and watch the fun.

1 cup high-quality mixed commercial parrot treats

1/2 cup round oat cereal pieces

1 cup dried mixed fruit, unsweetened

1 cup unsalted peanuts

1/2 banana, mashed

1 egg white

6 craft sticks or sucker handles (available at craft or kitchen supply stores)

1/2 cup honey

1. Preheat oven to 100°F. In a medium bowl, mix together parrot treats, oat cereal, dried fruit, and peanuts. Add banana and egg white and stir to coat.

2. Spray muffin or corn-stick tin with nonstick spray, fill compartments with mixture, insert a stick or handle in each and press to compress. Bake for two hours, or until very hard. Remove pops from pan, coat each pop with honey, place on a greased cookie sheet, return to oven and bake for another 10 minutes or until honey is dry.

3. Serve one treat at a time. Remove and discard uneaten parts after 4 hours. Store pops in a sealed container in the refrigerator for up to one month or in the freezer for up to three months.

Makes 6 treats

Wild Bird Food

Watching backyard birds brings hours of enjoyment to adults and teaches children valuable nature lessons. This easy and inexpensive recipe—better than a store-bought packet of birdseed—will attract a wide variety of colorful and interesting birds, including doves, woodpeckers, blue jays, nuthatches, chickadees, tufted titmice, cardinals, goldfinches, and many others, depending on where you live.

1/2 cup sunflower seeds
1/2 cup cracked corn
1/2 cup raisins
1/2 cup crunchy homemade Peanut Butter (page 33)

1. Mix all ingredients together in a bowl. Press the mixture into an empty suet feeder or small string bag.
2. Hang the feeder in a tree.

Makes 2 cups

One-Minute Substitute

Quick Treat for Wild Birds

Don't discard day-old doughnuts. They are great for feathered visitors to your backyard! These oily, carb-rich treats make a high-energy food that will help keep wild birds warm in winter. Just drive one or more nails into a fence post or tree trunk at eye level. Then hang a glazed cake or yeast doughnut on each nail. After you mount them, sit back and enjoy watching a congregation of hungry birds devour them.

Premium Wild Bird Mix

Avoid high-priced, and often inferior, wild birdseed blends. Buy premium individual types of seeds in bulk and mix your own feeder food for less money and greater quality. These individual seeds are available at feed, hardware, and wild-bird stores. The addition of live mealworms may entice elusive bluebirds to your feeders in the northeastern and western areas of the United States. Mealworms can be purchased at pet shops and through the Internet.

1 pound striped sunflower seeds, hulls on
1 pound black-oil sunflower seeds, hulls on
1 pound raw peanuts
1 pound dark raisins, dried blueberries, apples, or other dried fruits, chopped
1 pound cracked corn
1 small carton live mealworms

1. In a rodent-proof metal container with a tight lid, mix together the striped sunflower seeds, black-oil sunflower seeds, peanuts, fruit, and cracked corn and store in a cool area, such as the basement or garage. Store mealworms in the refrigerator according to package directions.
2. Spread one or two scoops of the seed mixture onto a tray-type feeder and sprinkle with mealworms.

Makes 5 pounds

Healthy Hummingbird Nectar

Why buy expensive hummingbird nectar when you can make your own for pennies? This nectar will attract both hummingbirds and orioles. Choose a feeder with a red base to attract the birds, so there's no need to use potentially harmful red food coloring. To prevent fermentation in hot weather, empty your feeder every three days and sterilize it by rinsing it out with boiling water.

2 cups water
1/2 cup granulated sugar

1. In a small saucepan over medium heat, bring water to a boil and then stir in sugar until it dissolves. Return solution to a boil. Remove from heat and cool, uncovered.
2. Store the nectar in a clean tightly capped jar in the refrigerator for up to one month.
3. Sterilize feeder by rinsing it with boiling water. Fill with fresh nectar and hang in the shade, at eye level.

Makes 2 1/2 cups

food for exotic pets

Guinea Pig Salad

Fresh vegetables and fruits should be essential parts of a guinea pig's diet. The dried treats sold in pet shops are good in a pinch, but they're expensive and a poor substitute for fresh treats. This is a vitamin-rich fresh salad that's easy to make and good enough to share with your guinea pig.

1/2 cup fresh spinach
1/4 cup shredded carrot
1/2 cup chopped strawberries
1/4 cup orange juice

1. Toss spinach, carrots, and strawberries in a bowl with juice.
2. Serve in a feeding bowl. Remove and discard uneaten salad after 4 hours. Store leftovers in a sealed container in the refrigerator for one day.

Makes 2 servings

One-Minute Substitute

Quick Free Playthings for Pet Rodents
Rodents have a never-ending need to chew, and they can rapidly demolish expensive store-bought toys. Save your pocketbook by collecting household "chew toys" for mice, rats, guinea pigs, and bunnies, such as empty cardboard egg cartons, rolls from paper towels, food wrap, and toilet paper, as well as small blocks of wood left from woodworking projects.

Hamster Fruit Cup

1/2 banana
1/4 cup carrot, grated
Lemon juice
1 tablespoon dark raisins
1 teaspoon honey

Experts agree that dried hamster pellets and treats do not provide a complete diet, and pet shops don't include a salad bar, but your hamster can scurry to its bowl for this budget-friendly sweet treat that you can whip up in no time, using fresh fruits and vegetables.

1. Slice banana and toss with grated carrot in a bowl, adding a sprinkling of lemon juice to keep them from discoloring. Drain juice from bowl; add raisins and honey and mash with a fork.
2. Serve half in a treat bowl, and store the remainder in a covered container in the refrigerator for one day. Remove and discard uneaten treats after 4 hours.

Makes 2 servings

Gerbil and Rabbit Salad

1/4 cup spinach or leaf lettuce, chopped fine
1/4 cup carrot, grated
1 teaspoon sunflower or pumpkin seeds, unsalted

It's important to offer pet rodents vitamin-rich fresh fruits and vegetables, and your gerbils and bunnies will welcome this healthy salad. For budget-boosting ingredients, ask for discarded outer leaves (which are more vitamin rich than inner leaves) at your produce counter, farmers' market, or a restaurant salad bar. For variety, alternate seed and nut toppings.

1. Toss vegetables together in a bowl, top with seeds or nuts, and serve in a small treat bowl. Store leftovers in a sealed container in the refrigerator for one day.
2. Remove and dispose of uneaten fresh foods after four hours.

Makes 1/2 cup

Pet Rodent Tabbouleh

1 cup bulgur wheat, uncooked
1 ounce boiling water (1 jiggerful)
1/4 cup brown rice, cooked
1/4 cup rolled oats, cooked
1/4 cup parrot seed mix
1/4 cup dark molasses
1 rodent vitamin, crushed *(optional)*
1/4 cup wheat germ

You just can't substitute dried pellets or grains from the pet store for fresh foods when it comes to feeding a balanced diet to rodents. This is a nutritious treat recipe for pet mice and rats. You can make it easy by saving plain, leftover grains from the family table.

1. Put bulgur in a bowl, add boiling water, and allow to stand five minutes. Stir in remaining ingredients to make a thick, crumbly mixture.
2. Form into small balls and roll in a saucer of wheat germ to coat.
3. Serve 1 ball daily as a treat. Discard uneaten treats after four hours. Store extra treats in a sealed container in the refrigerator for up to one week, or in the freezer for up to one month.

Makes 1 3/4 cups

Turtle and Reptile Treat

To give your pet turtle a calcium boost, try this fortified daily vegetable medley. With a few additions, this treat will also benefit iguanas and other cold-blooded vegetarian pets. Reptiles have very specific dietary needs and must be housed at the proper temperature to induce an appetite.

1/2 cup carrot, shredded

1/2 cup lettuce or spinach, chopped

1 stalk celery, chopped

1 calcium tablet, crushed

1 teaspoon alfalfa sprouts (available at pet or health food stores)

1/4 cup melon or strawberries, chopped

1. Place vegetables into a bowl, sprinkle with calcium, and toss for turtle snack. For iguanas and other reptiles, add alfalfa and fruit.

2. Serve half in a chew-proof bowl. Store the remainder in a covered container in the refrigerator for one day.

Makes 1 1/2 cups

pet emergency kit

Set a pet carrier—or a cage for birds or reptiles—where it's easy to find. Place a lightweight nylon backpack inside the carrier and fill it with the following items:

• Photocopies of your pet's license and shot records

• Address and telephone number of your veterinarian, kennel, and breeder

• Your cell phone number and another emergency contact phone number

• Identifying photos of your pet

• Food and water bowls

• Packaged food (for dog or cat), seed mixes and supplements (for birds and cold-blooded pets), and instructions for feeding

• Bottled water

• Leash (for dog or cat)

• A couple of old toys

• Pet sweater (for dog or cat)

• Litter bags (for a dog), a small bag of litter and disposable litter box (for a cat)

• Newspapers to use as carrier or cage liners

Aquarium Fish Treats

The best food for your aquarium fish is a high-quality commercial fish food formulated for the species of fish, but, for variety, they especially enjoy fresh or fresh-frozen live food and fresh vegetables. Experiment with treats listed here. Crickets, mealworms, and bloodworms are sold at pet shops.

1/4 cup spinach, pureed

1 earthworm, finely chopped

6 crickets

6 mealworms

6 bloodworms

1/4 cup raw beef liver (blended)

1 raw shrimp (blended)

1. Mix spinach plus any two other ingredients. Store a week's worth of the mix in a sealed container in the refrigerator. Freeze the rest for up to one month.

2. To serve, drop a piece of the mix the size of a pencil eraser into the aquarium. Continue until fish stop feeding. After five minutes, remove uneaten food from the bottom of the aquarium, using a siphon or cooking bulb baster.

Makes 2/3 cup

Part 3

*around the
house*

*

Spit-and-Polish
Cleaning Products

Advertisements for "new and better" cleaning supplies fill home-oriented magazines, and they virtually subsidize daytime broadcasting (that's why they are called soap operas). Many of these highly touted products do have seemingly miraculous ingredients that can make dirt vanish, but you should think twice before using these chemicals in your home, and they are often no better than traditional cleaning compounds that you can made yourself. As the recipes here show, there are many safer ways to clean everything in your house, using simple mixtures of inexpensive, everyday staples that you probably already have in your pantry.

Homemade cleaning solutions not only get the job done easily and inexpensively, but more important, they do it without harming you or your possessions. Most of these cleaning solutions have a long and honorable history—your grandmother probably used many of them. As you might expect, you'll see recipes that use many time-tested ingredients such as baking soda, vinegar, and lemon juice. But you might be surprised to know that you can still buy borax and washing soda among the laundry detergents in your local supermarket. And you might be even more surprised to find that tomato ketchup is a fine copper polish.

These homemade cleaning products are all very economical. White vinegar and baking soda, for example, are much cheaper than commercial fabric softener for keeping lint off your clothes and stopping static electricity. Old newspapers are cheaper than paper towels for cleaning windows. And dried herbs refresh your house far more inexpensively than any commercial room deodorizer.

general housecleaning

Basic Window and Glass Cleaner

Forget about all of those store-bought window cleaners. Your windows can get a professional shine for just pennies. This recipe will clean a houseful of windows. You can make a smaller batch in a quart spray bottle by mixing 1/4 cup vinegar with enough water to fill the container.

1/2 cup white vinegar

2/3 gallon water

1 clean gallon container

1 clean 32-ounce spray bottle

1. Mix the ingredients in the gallon container.
2. Fill the spray bottle and spray on windows and glass items as needed. (Save the remaining cleaner for another day.)
3. Dry glass with crumpled newspaper for added brightness—and savings!

Super Window and Glass Cleaner

The alcohol in this formula helps prevent streaking.

1/3 cup white vinegar

1/4 cup rubbing alcohol

3 1/2 cups water

1 clean 32-ounce spray bottle

1. Mix all the ingredients in the spray bottle. Shake well before using.
2. Spray on dirty windowpane or other glass surface.
3. Dry with crumpled newspaper.

Citrus Disinfectant

If you like pricey commercial orange cleaners, you'll love this fresh citrus-scented vinegar spray that is easy to make and costs less than a dollar. You can also deodorize a room by setting out a small bowl of citrus vinegar.

Peel from 1 orange, grapefruit, lemon, or lime

3 cups white vinegar

1 clean quart jar with lid

1 clean 32-ounce spray bottle

1. Combine the citrus peel and vinegar in the quart jar. Fasten the lid on the jar and store the mixture in a cupboard for two weeks, giving it an occasional shake.
2. Remove the peel from the jar, strain the vinegar, and return it to the jar.
3. To use as a spray cleaner, pour 1 cup of citrus vinegar in the spray bottle and fill with water.
4. To clean linoleum floors, add 1 cup citrus vinegar to 2 gallons water.

Tough Multipurpose Cleaner

When it comes to cleaning non-wood surfaces around your home, this cleaner is tough to beat—you might even say it's "fantastic." And it costs only pennies.

1 1/2 pints water
1/3 cup rubbing alcohol
1 teaspoon clear household ammonia
1 teaspoon mild dishwashing liquid
1/2 teaspoon lemon juice
1 clean 32-ounce spray bottle

1. Combine the ingredients in the spray bottle and shake well before each use.
2. Spray on countertops, kitchen appliances and fixtures, and tile or painted surfaces.
3. Wipe down with a clean cloth or damp sponge.

Fresh-Smelling Multipurpose Cleaner

This formula has a clean smell and works hard, despite its inexpensive ingredients. You can buy liquid castile soap at health food stores.

3 1/2 cups hot water
1/2 cup white or apple cider vinegar
1 teaspoon borax
1 teaspoon washing soda
1 teaspoon liquid castile soap
1 clean 32-ounce spray bottle

1. Fill spray bottle first with hot water; then add vinegar, borax, washing soda, and liquid castile soap. Shake well before using.
2. Spray on countertops, kitchen appliances and fixtures, and tile or painted surfaces.
3. Wipe down with a clean cloth or damp sponge.

Wall and Cabinet Cleaner

If you have dingy cupboards, this cleaning solution will deodorize them as well as wiping up the dust and dirt.

1 cup clear household ammonia
1 cup white vinegar
1/4 cup baking soda
1 gallon warm water

1. Combine the ammonia, vinegar, and baking soda in a large bucket, add water, and give it a few stirs.
2. Use a sponge or cloth rag to wash walls, ceilings, floors, or cabinets.
3. Wipe up the excess liquid with a clean cloth and allow to dry thoroughly before replacing contents.

One-Minute Substitute

Use Bread to Spot-Clean Wallpaper
Cut the crusts off a slice of white bread and roll it up into a ball. Once the bread starts to feel slightly doughy, roll it over the bad spots on the wallpaper to lift off the dirt or fingerprints. Test the bread ball first on an inconspicuous corner.

Interior Wall Cleaner

Those scuff marks and stains on your painted walls seem to appear out of nowhere. This potent cleaner will remove them without harming your paint job.

1/2 cup borax
1 tablespoon clear household ammonia
1/4 cup vinegar
1 gallon warm water

1. In a large bucket, mix all the ingredients.
2. Apply the solution to the wall with a clean sponge. Use a second clean sponge to rinse the wall with plain water.
3. To minimize streaking, start at the bottom of the wall and work up.

Herbal Carpet Freshener

Many commercial air and carpet deodorizers work to mask odors by deadening the nerves associated with your sense of smell. To truly freshen carpets around your home, try this inexpensive natural formula instead. (If you don't like the smell of lavender, you can also freshen up carpets with plain baking soda.)

1/2 cup lavender flowers
1 cup baking soda

1. In a large bowl, crush the lavender flowers to release their scent.
2. Add the baking soda and mix well. Pour the mixture into a cheese shaker or a can with holes punched in the lid.
3. Sprinkle liberally on the carpet. Wait 30 minutes; then vacuum.

Pine Floor Cleaner

You shouldn't have to spend a small fortune to give your no-wax floors a pine-fresh smell. This excellent cleaner will do the job for only a few cents a floor. Since soap flakes are not widely available, as they once were, it's usually necessary to make your own by grating a soap bar; it takes only a minute or so.

1/2 cup soap flakes
1/4 cup washing soda
1 cup salt
2 cups water
2 teaspoons pine oil
1 clean 16-ounce plastic bottle with a tight-fitting lid
1 cup white vinegar

1. To make the soap flakes, lightly grate a bar of pure soap, such as Ivory, on a coarse kitchen grater.
2. In a saucepan over low heat, combine the soap, washing soda, salt, and water and stir until the soap, soda, and salt have dissolved.
3. Remove from the heat and allow the mixture to cool until it is lukewarm. Add the pine oil. Stir well, pour into the plastic bottle, and secure the top.
4. To use, pour 2 or 3 tablespoons of the cleaner into a half-bucket of hot water, stirring well. For large areas, you may need to double the amount.
5. After cleaning, add the vinegar to a half-bucket of clean water and rinse the floor.

Spicy Carpet Freshener

Add a nice smell to your rooms while you freshen the carpets with this simple mixture.

1 cup baking soda or cornstarch

7-10 drops essential oil in your favorite scent (eucalyptus or rosewood, for example)

1. In a large bowl, combine the baking soda or cornstarch with the essential oil. Break up any clumps with a fork and stir well. Pour the mixture into a cheese shaker or a can with holes punched in the lid.

2. Sprinkle liberally on the carpet. Wait 30 minutes, then vacuum.

air fresheners

Spicy Room Freshener Spray

Why waste your money on commercial air fresheners when it's so easy to make your own favorite scents? Use this spray judiciously, however. A room should have a hint of the spicy scent, not an overpowering perfume. You can combine up to three different essential oils to create a fragrance that suits you. Other popular choices include eucalyptus, lavender, geranium, grapefruit, orange, peppermint, pine, juniper, rose, and spearmint.

1 clean 12-ounce spray bottle

1/4 cup rubbing alcohol

25 drops bergamot essential oil

8 drops clove essential oil

5 drops lemon essential oil

1 cup distilled water

1. In the spray bottle, combine the alcohol and the essential oils and shake well to disperse the oil. Add the water and shake for a minute or two more to thoroughly blend all the ingredients.

2. Let the mixture sit for a few days before using to allow the fragrance to blend and mature. A quick spritz is all that's needed to freshen a room.

Pie Spice Room Freshener

This homey and aromatic mixture can be made for pennies and makes you think an apple pie is in the oven; real estate agents sometimes suggest that homeowners put this mixture on the stove before prospective buyers come to see the house. No commercial room freshener at any price smells as good.

3 cups water

6 cloves

1 cinnamon stick

6 pieces dried orange peel

In a small saucepan, combine all the ingredients and bring to a boil over medium heat. Reduce the heat and simmer, uncovered, until your home is filled with a fresh, spicy scent. (Don't let the water boil away.)

furniture polishes

Lemon Oil Furniture Polish

Shine up your wood furniture, paneling, and knickknacks with this all-natural polish that will take you only a minute to prepare, and costs less than a bagel. Discard any leftovers and make up a fresh batch each time you want to polish your wood treasures.

1 cup olive oil
1/3 cup lemon juice
1 clean 16-ounce spray bottle

1. Combine the oil and lemon juice in the spray bottle. Shake well before using
2. Apply a small amount to a soft flannel cloth or chamois, and apply it evenly over the wood surface.
3. Use a clean, dry flannel cloth to buff and polish.

No-Fuss Furniture Polish

How would you like a furniture polish that you can just wipe on and forget? Well, your prayers have been answered—and for a lot less money than you might expect!

1/4 cup boiled linseed oil
1/8 cup vinegar
1/8 cup whisky
1 clean 16-ounce spray bottle

1. Combine all the ingredients in the bottle. Shake well.
2. Apply a small amount of polish to a clean, soft cloth and wipe on. No need to buff; the dullness evaporates along with the alcohol.

Cabinet Polish

Why burn through your household budget on furniture polish for those large wood kitchen cabinets, bookshelves, or wardrobes around your home? Here's the perfect polish to use on big jobs—and it costs a couple of pennies to make. Be sure to mix up a fresh batch for each use.

1 teaspoon lemon juice
1 teaspoon olive oil
2 cups warm water

1. Combine the ingredients in a bowl or container.
2. Dip a soft flannel cloth into the solution and wring it out. Wipe over the wood.
3. Buff and polish with a soft, dry cloth.

mold and mildew removers

Spot Mold and Mildew Remover
Mix up a batch of this powerful but benign-smelling disinfectant to get rid of small patches of mold and mildew that breed in bathroom medicine cabinets, windowsills, and other surfaces around your home.

1 cup white vinegar
2 tablespoons borax
4 cups hot water
1 clean 32-ounce spray bottle

1. Combine the ingredients in the spray bottle. Shake well.
2. Spray on surfaces where mold or mildew is forming. Wipe off mildew, but leave cleaning solution residue to keep mildew from returning.

Paint and Tile Mold and Mildew Remover
This formula will take mold and mildew off painted and tile surfaces for only pennies a pop. Be sure the room is well ventilated as you work.

1/4 cup chlorine bleach
1 tablespoon borax
1 1/2 cups water
1 clean 16-ounce spray bottle

1. Combine all the ingredients in the spray bottle and shake to mix.
2. Spray painted or tile surface and wipe off mildew and mold with a clean cloth. Rinse with clean water and dry with clean cloths.

Mold Remover for Leather and Luggage
If you discover mold on your expensive luggage or leather jacket, don't race to the dry cleaners. Instead, remove the offending growth with this simple, inexpensive mold-removal recipe.

1/2 cup rubbing alcohol
1/4 cup water
1 clean 8-ounce spray bottle

1. Combine the ingredients in the spray bottle and shake well to mix.
2. Spray affected area. Let solution set 10 to 20 minutes, then wipe off mold with a clean rag and allow the item to thoroughly air-dry.

metal polishes

Brass and Copper Paste Polish
Use this simple, nontoxic—and very inexpensive—polish to brighten up all your tarnished unlacquered brass and copperware. (Lacquered items only need dusting.)

1/4 cup flour
1/4 cup salt
1/4 cup vinegar
1/4 cup hot water
1 teaspoon lemon juice

1. In a small bowl, combine all the ingredients to form a paste.
2. Using a soft cloth, rub the mixture onto the metal surfaces to remove tarnish.
3. Rinse the object thoroughly in warm water (remember, salt is corrosive).
4. Dry with soft, clean cloths and then buff to a shine with a soft flannel cloth or chamois.

Cut-Lemon Brass and Copper Polish
Here's an even easier way to shine up unlacquered brass or copper objects—and a useful way to use up leftover half lemons.

1/2 cup white vinegar
2 tablespoons salt
1/2 lemon

1. In a saucepan over medium heat, heat the vinegar 5 minutes, then pour it into a small bowl and stir in the salt.
2. Dip the lemon into the mixture and rub it over the object, concentrating on the most heavily tarnished areas.
3. Thoroughly rinse the object in warm water and dry with soft, clean cloths. Buff to a shine with a soft cloth.

Ketchup Copper Polish
This simple polish can be a bit messy, but it works like a charm on unlacquered copper—and it's completely nontoxic. Can your old copper polish say that?

1/2-1 cup tomato ketchup
1/4-1 lemon, juiced

1. In a small bowl, combine the ketchup and lemon juice and stir to mix. How much you need of each ingredient depends on the size of the object you want to polish, but keep the ratio of ketchup to lemon juice about 8:1.
2. Spread out some old newspapers on your work surface. Rub the mixture over the copper piece's surface. Let it sit 5 to 10 minutes.
3. Thoroughly rinse the copper piece in warm water and dry with soft, clean cloths. Buff to a shine with a soft cloth.

One-Minute Substitute | **Potato Rust Remover for Tin Pans**
Tin pie plates and other kitchen utensils are subject to rust if they are not dried carefully after each washing. Here, for little more than the price of a potato, is a way to restore your tinware without harsh chemicals. Peel a potato and cut it into easy-to-handle pieces. Put some baking soda or salt in a saucer. Then dip a cut piece of potato in the soda or salt, and rub it over the rust spots. Rinse the tin utensil and dry thoroughly.

Chrome and Stainless Steel Polish

Baby the chrome and stainless steel finishes around your home with this simple one-two set of cleaners. They remove stains as well as dirt and fingerprints in no time for less than a quarter.

1/4 teaspoon baby oil
1/2 cup club soda

1. Apply a few drops of baby oil to a soft cloth or piece of flannel and wipe down the chrome or stainless steel surface. Use a second soft cloth, moistened with club soda, to rinse off the oil.
2. Dry and buff with a soft, dry cloth.

Quick and Easy Silver Shine

Want a really easy, inexpensive, and amazingly effective way to polish your silver without any smelly chemicals or commercial products? This is easier than using a silver dipping cleaner.

1 quart hot water
1 tablespoon baking soda or washing soda
1 tablespoon salt
1 sheet aluminum foil

1. Fill the kitchen sink with about 1 quart hot water.
2. Dissolve the baking (or washing) soda and salt in the water, then place the sheet of aluminum foil at the bottom of the sink.
3. Rest the tarnished silver on the foil for 10 seconds. Remove and dry with a soft flannel cloth.

Spit-and-Polish Cleaning Products   **749**

in the kitchen

Automatic Dishwasher Detergent
Even if you live in a hard-water area, this simple, inexpensive detergent recipe will give you shiny, spotless dishes.

2 cups borax

2 cups washing soda

1 clean 32-ounce plastic container with cover

1. Combine the borax and washing soda in the container and seal it tightly for storage.

2. For each load of dishes, put 2 tablespoons of the mixture in the dishwasher soap dispenser.

One-Minute Substitute

Fast, Cheap Rinsing Agent for Your Dishwasher

Here's an easy way to get those dishes sparkling in your automatic dishwasher without using any chemical rinsing agents. Just stop the dishwasher during its rinse cycle and add 1 to 1 1/2 cups of white vinegar. Or pour the vinegar into the rinse compartment beforehand (being careful not to overfill). Wash dishes as usual.

Dishwashing Liquid
This dishwashing soap for washing dishes by hand costs less than a dollar for a 16-ounce bottle and really gets your dishes clean. And unlike some of its commercial counterparts, it's mild on your hands too.

1/4 cup soap flakes

1 1/2 cups hot water

1/4 cup glycerin

1/2 teaspoon lemon oil

1 clean 16-ounce squirt bottle

1. To make the soap flakes, lightly grate a bar of pure soap, such as Ivory, on a coarse kitchen grater.

2. In a medium pitcher, pour the soap flakes into the hot water and stir with a fork until most of the soap has dissolved. Let the solution cool for 5 minutes.

3. Stir in the glycerin and lemon oil. A loose gel will form as it cools. Use the fork to break up any congealed parts and pour the liquid into the squirt bottle. Use 2 to 3 teaspoons per sink or dishpan of hot water to clean dishes.

Microwave Oven Cleaner

You don't need harsh cleansers and lots of elbow grease to clean your microwave. For the price of a lemon, some baking soda, or some white vinegar, you can just wipe away the splatters and stains inside the oven.

1 1/2 cups water

3 tablespoons lemon juice or 1 cup water

3 tablespoons baking soda or 2 cups white vinegar

1. In a microwave-safe bowl, combine the water and lemon juice, water and baking soda, or just the vinegar. Place the uncovered bowl inside the oven, and run the oven on high for 3 to 5 minutes, allowing the liquid to condense on its inside walls and ceiling.

2. Carefully remove the bowl with a towel or pot holder (it will be very hot!), and wipe the interior with a dishrag or paper towel.

Basic Oven Cleaner

Use this odorless recipe the next time you need to clean your oven, and leave those caustic chemical-based oven cleaners where they belong—on the store shelf.

2 tablespoons liquid soap

2 teaspoons borax

2 cups warm water

1 clean 16-ounce spray bottle

1/2 cup baking soda in an open bowl

1. Pour the soap and borax into the spray bottle, and add the warm water. Shake well to dissolve the borax.

2. Spray the solution on the oven's surfaces, giving special attention to dried, cooked-on spills.

3. Let the mixture set for 30 minutes to an hour, then scrub the oven surfaces with a damp scrub pad dipped in the baking soda. Rinse with clean water.

Lazy Person's Oven Cleaner

Here is the recipe for a cheap, almost effortless oven cleaner that rivals any commercial counterparts.

3/4 cup clear household ammonia

1 cup baking soda in a widemouthed dish

1. Pour the ammonia into a small bowl and leave it overnight in a closed, cool oven.

2. The next day, remove and discard the ammonia and wipe down the oven's interior surfaces with moistened paper towels or damp sponges dipped in baking soda.

Oven Floor Cleaner

This recipe is for cleaning up the oven floor after a sticky sweet pie or a too-full casserole has spilled over and caused a real mess. You don't need expensive, caustic commercial oven cleaners to deal with it. You probably already have everything you need on hand.

1/2 cup water
1-2 cups baking soda
1 teaspoon liquid detergent

1. Sprinkle water along the bottom of the oven.
2. Spread enough baking soda over the surface to coat it entirely, and sprinkle more water on top of it.
3. Let the paste set overnight. The next morning, the grease and grime will be loosened enough for you to wipe it up with damp paper towels or dishrags.
4. Once you've wiped up the core of the mess, use the liquid detergent on a damp sponge to remove any remaining residue. Rinse with water and let dry.
5. Repeat if necessary.

Garbage Disposer Cleaner

Those in-the-sink garbage disposer units are great for cutting down on bagged waste, but they can produce some unpleasant odors from time to time. Here is an easy and efficient way to get rid of any unwanted smells.

1 quart white vinegar
Ice-cube tray

1. Fill an ice-cube tray with white vinegar and freeze it. Remove cubes, place in a sealed plastic bag, and return to the freezer.
2. Once a week run 2 to 3 vinegar ice cubes through your garbage disposer.

One-Minute Substitute

Quick Garbage Disposer Sweetener
Instead of buying a commercial product to keep your garbage disposer smelling good, try this easy solution. Save leftover orange, lemon, and grapefruit peels in a sealed plastic bag in your refrigerator. Then, once or twice a week, run a few peels through the disposer.

Scouring Powder

You don't need chlorine bleach to clean stains off the nonporous surfaces in your kitchen and bathroom. This scouring powder is just as effective, a lot safer to use, and far more economical.

1 cup baking soda
1 cup borax
1 cup salt
1 clean 32-ounce plastic container with cover

1. Combine the ingredients in the container and mix well. Close the container tightly to store.
2. To clean a stained surface, sprinkle some of the powder onto a damp sponge or directly on to the surface to be cleaned. Scour, rinse, and dry.

Homemade Scrub Powder

Use this mixture to scrub off grease and grime from your stainless steel and enameled cookware. (If you use baking soda on aluminum cookware, it may cause darkening.) You don't need pricey commercial products.

2 1/2 cups baking soda
1 1/2 cups salt
2 tablespoons cream of tartar
1 clean 32-ounce plastic container with lid

1. Mix the ingredients well, and store in a tightly sealed plastic container.
2. To use, pour 2 to 3 tablespoons of powder onto cookware and scrub with a brush or nylon scrubber that's been slightly moistened with water. Rinse well and dry with a soft cloth.

Steel Wool Soap Pads

Those popular prepackaged steel wool soap pads are great for getting tough stains and cooked-on foods off your pots and pans, but they can be rough on your hands. These homemade steel wool pads work just as well, and are easier on both your wallet and your skin.

1 bag steel wool pads (available at hardware stores)
3 tablespoons Homemade Scrub Powder (above)

1. If you've purchased large pads, use a sharp scissors or shears and carefully cut them into rectangles approximately 3 inches long by 2 inches high.
2. Spread a layer of scouring powder over the cooking surface, moisten the steel wool pad with warm water, and scrub away stains. Rinse well with water. Dry with a soft, absorbent towel.
3. To make your pads last longer, squeeze out remaining water and keep them in a bowl lined with aluminum foil.

in the laundry

Fabric Softener

Here's a simple recipe for keeping your fabrics soft and fluffy. It's a lot gentler on your clothes than commercial fabric softeners, and much easier on your wallet as well.

1/4 cup baking soda
1/2 cup white vinegar

1. Fill the washing machine with water.
2. Add the baking soda and then the clothing.
3. During the final rinse cycle, add the vinegar (pour it into the softener dispenser if your washing machine has one).

Laundry Soap

This basic laundry soap gets clothes as clean as those fancy single-name commercial cleaners; it just costs a lot less.

1/2 cup soap flakes
1/2 cup baking soda
1/4 cup washing soda
1/4 cup borax.
1 clean 16-ounce plastic container with lid

1. To make the soap flakes, lightly grate a bar of pure soap, such as Ivory, on a coarse kitchen grater.
2. In a large bowl mix all the ingredients together. Store in a tightly sealed plastic container.
3. Use about 1/2 cup of the mixture instead of detergent in each load of laundry.

Stain Remover

Stains are always easier to get out if you treat them before they set (club soda is effective for lifting many types of stains before they dry). You can also use other ingredients found around your home to remove many common types of stains (see Removing Common Stains, below).

1/3 cup clear household ammonia
1/2 cup white vinegar
1/4 cup baking soda
2 tablespoons liquid castile soap
1 1/2 quarts water
1 clean half-gallon (64-ounce) recycled plastic container
1 clean 16-ounce spray bottle

1. Mix all the ingredients in a 1/2-gallon container. Pour some of the solution into the spray bottle. Shake well before each use.
2. Spray liquid onto the stain and let set 3 to 5 minutes. Launder as usual.

removing common stains

Automotive Oil and Grease Stain Remover

1 liter cola

For severe stains, soak the garment in cola overnight. Rinse and launder the next morning.

Grass and Bloodstain Remover

1 teaspoon 3% hydrogen peroxide
1/4 teaspoon clear household ammonia

Mix the ingredients in a small bowl. Rub the mixture on the stain. As soon as the stain fades, rinse and launder.

Perspiration Stain Remover

1 cup white vinegar
1/4 cup salt
2 quarts warm water

Mix the ingredients in a bucket and soak garment for one hour before washing.

Red Wine Remover

1 tablespoon borax
2 cups warm water

Dip garment in solution, let it soak for one minute, then launder.

Tomato Sauce Remover

1/2 cup 3% hydrogen peroxide
3 cups water

Mix ingredients in a dishpan or bucket. Soak garment in the solution for 30 minutes before laundering.

Whitening Yellowed Whites

1/2 cup white vinegar
6 cups warm water

Mix ingredients in a dishpan or bucket. Soak clothes overnight and launder the next morning.

One-Minute
Substitute

Vinegar: Fabric Softener Plus

Who would have guessed that a single cup of an everyday staple—white vinegar—which costs about a quarter, could do everything that many people use a fabric softener, a color setter, a disinfectant, and a bleach to do? Just add 1 cup distilled white vinegar to your washer's rinse cycle, and it will kill any bacteria in the wash, set the color of newly dyed fabrics, keep clothes lint- and static-free, brighten small loads of white clothes, and eliminate the need for fabric softeners.

Washer Disinfectant

Just because your washer sees a lot of soap and water doesn't mean it doesn't get dirty. Use this simple recipe to disinfect it twice a year. This rinse also removes some of the built-up soap scum from your washer's hoses, so it may even spare you a visit from your local repairman.

2 cups white vinegar
2 cups bleach

1. Let the tub fill with water, then add the vinegar. Let it soak for 1 hour, then restart and let it run through a complete cycle.

2. Repeat process using the bleach.

in the bathroom

Multipurpose Disinfectant Cleaner

Here's a good all-purpose disinfectant that is as easy to use and effective as any commercial bathroom cleaner but much less expensive.

2 teaspoons borax
1/2 teaspoon washing soda
2 tablespoons lemon juice
4 tablespoons white vinegar
3 cups very hot water
1 clean 24-ounce spray bottle

1. Combine the borax, washing soda, lemon juice, and vinegar in the spray bottle.

2. Slowly add the hot water, then vigorously shake the bottle until the powdered ingredients have dissolved. Shake the bottle before each use.

3. Spray on tile and ceramic surfaces and wipe with a damp, clean cloth.

Soft Scrub

You don't need to buy special cleaners for your vulnerable kitchen and bathroom surfaces. This homemade soft scrub gets out tough stains on surfaces that are easily scratched, including ceramic sinks and countertops, and costs just pennies per cleaning job.

1/4 cup borax

1/2 teaspoon vegetable-oil-based liquid soap (such as Murphy's Oil Soap)

1/2 teaspoon lemon juice

1. In a small bowl, combine the borax and liquid soap to make a smooth paste.

2. Stir in the lemon juice and mix well.

3. Place a small amount of the paste onto a clean, damp sponge, apply to the surface, then rinse off and dry surface with a clean rag.

Eucalyptus Tile Cleaner

This fresh, tangy powder will leave your kitchen and bathroom tiles as shiny and clean as any commercial cleaner and for less than half the price.

1/2 cup soap flakes

1 cup chalk or diatomaceous earth

1 cup baking soda

1 teaspoon essential oil of eucalyptus

1 clean recycled 16-ounce jar with metal top

1. To make the soap flakes, lightly grate a bar of pure soap, such as Ivory, on a coarse kitchen grater. Then, in a small bowl, crush the soap flakes with the back of a spoon until powdered (or whirl them in a blender).

2. Mix in the chalk or diatomaceous earth and the baking soda, breaking up any lumps.

3. Sprinkle the essential oil over the surface of the powdered mixture and stir it with the spoon. Continue stirring for several minutes to disperse the oil throughout the mixture, then spoon the mixture into a screw-top jar or can with several holes punched in the lid.

4. Cover the holes with masking tape to keep the powder dry between uses. Let the mixture sit a week before using to be sure the essential oil has been thoroughly absorbed. Sprinkle surface with powder, scrub with a damp sponge, and rinse with clear water. Dry with soft towel.

Nontoxic Bathroom Cleaner

This is a terrific deep-cleaning cleanser for any bathroom surface. It cuts through soap scum and mildew as well as any commercial bathroom product and costs just pennies.

1 2/3 cups baking soda

1/2 cup liquid soap

1/2 cup water

2 tablespoons white vinegar

1 clean 16-ounce squirt bottle with closing cap

1. Mix baking soda and liquid soap in a bowl. Dilute with water and add the vinegar. Stir the mixture with a fork until any lumps have been dissolved. Pour the liquid into the bottle. Shake well before using.

2. Squirt on area to be cleaned. Scrub with a nylon-backed sponge. Rinse off with water. Keep cap on between uses.

Showerhead Cleaner

Use this "explosive" mix to blast away mineral deposits blocking up your showerhead. You don't need the plumber at $75 an hour to clean out your showerhead. Use this recipe to do it yourself.

1/4 cup baking soda

1 cup vinegar

1 plastic sandwich bag

Adhesive tape or a large bag tie

1. Pour the baking soda and vinegar into the bag over a sink. Wait a minute or two for the foaming to stop and then place the opened end of the bag over the showerhead, which should be submerged in the solution.

2. Secure the bag to the showerhead stem with the tape or bag tie. Let the showerhead soak in the solution 1 to 1 1/2 hours. Wipe off showerhead with a soft cloth.

Nontoxic Rust Remover

Commercial rust removers are among the most toxic compounds found around the home. But here's a completely safe and surprisingly effective way to give rust stains on bathtubs and sinks the brush-off.

1 lime (a second one may be needed for some jobs)

1/4 cup salt

1. Squeeze the lime over the rust spots, then cover the moistened area with salt.

2. Let the mixture set 3 to 4 hours.

3. Use a nylon scrubber to scrub the mixture off. The rust will be gone.

Nontoxic Toilet Bowl Cleaner

Clean and sanitize your toilet bowl without harmful chlorine! For no-scrub convenience, simply pour in this mixture and leave overnight. No commercial product at any price matches that.

1 cup borax

1/2 cup white vinegar

1. Flush the toilet to wet the sides of the bowl.

2. Sprinkle the borax around the toilet bowl; then liberally drizzle some vinegar on top. Let the toilet sit undisturbed for 3 to 4 hours before scrubbing with a toilet brush.

Tougher Toilet Bowl Cleaner

For tougher jobs, try this potent paste that still has no chlorine and costs much less than commercial toilet bowl cleaners.

2/3 cup borax

1/3 cup lemon juice

1. In a small bowl, combine the ingredients to form a paste.

2. Apply the paste to the toilet bowl using a sponge or rag. Let the paste set for 2 hours, then scrub off. Flush the toilet.

Spit-and-Polish Cleaning Products   **757**

Drain Opener

Commercial drain cleaners are not only extremely toxic; they can actually harm the pipes in your home with repeated use. Don't bother with those caustic cleaners; use this simple, inexpensive, and safe way to unclog drains instead.

1/2 cup baking soda
1 cup vinegar
1 teapot boiling water

1. Pack the drain with the baking soda, then pour in the vinegar.
2. Keep the drain covered for 10 minutes, then flush it out with boiling water.

One-Minute Substitute

Fast and Easy Drain Freshener
Here's an easy way to eliminate drain odors while maintaining the proper pH and health of your septic system. Run warm tap water for several seconds, then pour 1 cup baking soda into the drain. Wait an hour and flush with a teapot of boiling water. For best results, repeat once every two weeks.

Septic Tank Activator

If you detect a persistent unpleasant odor from your septic tank, it's probably due to a "die-off" of sewage-digesting bacteria. Before you call in your local septic tank specialist, try using this simple recipe to give the little beasties a boost.

2 cups sugar
1 quart simmering water
2 cups cornmeal
2 packages dry yeast powder

1. Dissolve the sugar in a saucepan of simmering water and cool to lukewarm. Mix in the cornmeal and the yeast.
2. Once the solution has been mixed, flush it down the toilet (flush twice, if necessary). For best results, do this before turning in for the night, or when there will be no activity in the bathroom for several hours.

cleaning the car

Basic Car Wash

Taking your car to a commercial car wash can be a costly habit to maintain—and the results are never as satisfying as when you do it yourself. This soap is tough on grime but gentle on your car's finish and your wallet.

1/2 cup mild liquid dish soap
1/2 cup baking soda
1 gallon warm water

1. Mix ingredients in a clean gallon container. Shake until all the baking soda is dissolved.
2. To use, mix 1 cup solution in a pail of warm water.

Upholstery Shampoo

Use this shampoo on a regular basis to freshen up fabric interiors that get a lot of use. It's much cheaper than commercial upholstery cleaners, and does the job just as well.

6 tablespoons soap flakes
2 tablespoons borax
1 pint boiling water

1. To make the soap flakes, lightly grate a bar of pure soap, such as Ivory, on a coarse kitchen grater.
2. In a large bowl, mix the soap flakes and borax together. Slowly add the boiling water, stirring well to thoroughly dissolve the dry ingredients.
3. Let cool, then whip into a foamy consistency with an eggbeater.
4. Brush dry suds onto the furniture, concentrating on soiled areas. Quickly wipe off with a damp sponge.

Vinyl and Leather Interior Cleaner

Put the life back into your car's vinyl or leather interior with this fresh-scented polish without paying auto-parts-store prices.

2 tablespoons vegetable-oil-based soap (such as Murphy's Oil Soap)
1/4 cup olive oil
1 teaspoon lemon essential oil (available at aroma-therapy or health food stores)

1. Mix the ingredients well in a small bowl, and apply with a sponge.
2. Wipe off with a soft cloth.

Windshield Cleaner

You shouldn't drive with a dirty windshield, and you shouldn't have to buy a commercial windshield cleaner either. Fill up a spray bottle with this solution and keep it in your trunk (along with some old newspaper to wipe off the grime). It will also keep steam and frost from forming on your car's windshield. Be sure to wipe off any solution that gets on rubber or plastic gaskets or wipers with a damp cloth, because prolonged contact with alcohol may damage them.

3 cups glycerin
1 cup rubbing alcohol
2 cups water
1 clean 32-ounce spray bottle

Combine the liquid ingredients in the spray bottle and shake well before using.

Spit-and-Polish Cleaning Products   **759**

Useful House and Garden Products

Running a household is a challenge. These days, just keeping a house operating smoothly takes a fat billfold and ingenuity. But you can lessen the drain and

strain with some of the easy-to-make products in this chapter. Here you will find time-honored recipes for wallpaper pastes and strippers, furniture stains, and other useful household compounds. You will also find safe natural ways to keep your home pest-free, along with ideas and recipes for providing fun for children—and adults—with busy hands. And you can make them all with a minimum of money and a maximum of good results.

Keeping your yard and garden beautiful and productive without spending a fortune or using a lot of questionable chemical compounds is also a major concern of most householders. There are recipes and formulas here for keeping your garden weed-free without using expensive manufactured herbicides and for making your own organic compost and natural soil conditioners and fertilizers. The many recipes for homemade garden pest controls will provide you with a choice of effective solutions to classic garden problems that neither cost very much nor taint the atmosphere. Just using ingredients that you already have in your kitchen, you can foil everything from black spot on your roses to slugs in the marigolds—and keep rabbits and deer out of your vegetable patch or shrubs. You will also discover some useful seed and potting mixes and other natural products that you can make to give your indoor plants a boost.

household compounds

Fabric Paste

Covering a less than perfect wall with an attractive fabric is an old decorating trick that you probably already know. Using liquid starch as your glue may surprise you. It's now cheap and easy to add some color to a wall, under the wainscoting, or inside an alcove.

Fabric to cover the area
Bottled liquid starch

1. Select a fabric that is medium to light weight. Cut the fabric to the lengths needed and soak the cut pieces, one at a time, in a tub filled with liquid fabric starch.

2. Press the fabric to the wall as you would if wallpapering, smoothing out wrinkles, and allow it to dry.

3. When you want to remove the fabric, simply pull it away from the wall and rinse away any starch that remains on the wall with a sponge or wet towel.

Wallpaper Stripper

Removing old wallpaper is never fun, but you can make it easier by heating up your own homemade stripper. For a large room, make up batches of the stripper so that it always goes on hot.

Wallpaper scoring wheel or wire-bristle brush
1 1/3 cups very hot water
2/3 cup liquid fabric softener
Sponge
Paint roller
Wallpaper scraper or putty knife

1. Score wallpaper lightly with scoring tool or wire-bristle brush so that stripper solution will be absorbed beneath the paper's water-resistant surface.

2. In a bucket, mix hot water and fabric softener. Apply this stripper to small areas with a sponge. You can cover larger areas with a paint roller soaked in the hot solution.

3. Allow stripper to soak into wallpaper for 20 minutes, then scrape paper off the wall with a wallpaper scraper or putty knife, being careful not to gouge the wallboard or plaster underneath.

4. Reapply stripper solution to stubborn spots, or if stripping multiple layers of paper. When paper is removed, rinse the wall with a sponge and clean water, and allow it to dry before priming to paint, or applying new paper.

Oil-Paint Stain

This stain is perfect for coloring wooden picture frames because you can use the exact colors of a painting to make the artwork coordinate with the frame, thinning the pigment to allow the natural wood grain to show. If you want traditional wood colors, choose raw umber (equivalent to walnut), burnt umber (mahogany), and yellow ocher (golden oak).

Artist's oil paints in tubes
   (one or more colors, as
   needed)
Turpentine

1. Mix equal parts oil paint and turpentine in a clean, wide-mouthed jar. Test the hue and opacity of the stain on a scrap of wood. This flexible stain can be easily modified. If it is too opaque, add turpentine; if it is too transparent, add more oil paint. If you want a unique shade, mix paints as needed. Be sure to mix enough stain for the entire project, as it is hard to duplicate a custom stain if you run short.

2. Brush the stain on the wood and allow it to dry to the touch before varnishing. If you want more grain to show, wipe the freshly stained wood with a clean, lint-free cotton cloth (such as an old T-shirt) moistened with turpentine.

One-Minute Substitute

Fast Fix for Furniture Scratches

You don't have to refinish a piece of wooden furniture, trim, or floor just because it has a few scratches. (In the case of an antique, refinishing can actually reduce its value.) Here is an easy, inexpensive way to disguise a scratch. Get a children's crayon in a color that closely matches the wood's finish. Burnt sienna, sienna, and yellow ocher are among the most useful colors. Then just rub the sharpened crayon over the scratch and buff to blend it in. If you want permanent coverage, and the piece is less valuable, use a felt-tip marker instead; then apply paste wax as directed to add sheen.

Varnish-Based Stain

Some wood species, such as maple, are so hard that they don't absorb stain satisfactorily. If you find that this is the case, you can still "stain" a piece of furniture by tinting the sealer and varnish with the wood stain of your choice. This custom-tinted varnish recipe solves the problem as no commercial product can, and is a little less expensive to boot.

Varnish

Paint thinner

Stain

1 varnish-quality natural- or nylon-bristle brush

Extra-fine sandpaper

Tack cloth

1. Stir together 1 part varnish, 1 part paint thinner, and 1/2 part stain in a widemouthed jar to create a tinted sealer coat. Stir slowly to avoid bubbling. Brush onto a smoothly sanded piece of wood and allow to dry overnight before varnishing.

2. Sand the sealed piece of furniture lightly and wipe down with a tack cloth. To deepen the stain color, add stain, as desired, to tint the varnish in the can. When mixing the color, remember that the color will deepen with each coat of varnish. Test the color on a scrap of wood or inconspicuous part of the project before proceeding. When the color is right (it should be transparent enough to allow wood grain to show through), brush varnish onto the entire piece, taking care to avoid drips or streaks. Allow varnish to dry overnight.

3. If a second coat of varnish is needed, repeat Step 2. Allow the varnished piece to dry for 2 days before using.

four unexpected uses for vinegar

Shock Cure

If you struggle with static electricity around the house in winter, try this simple, cheap vinegar cure.

1. Mix 1 cup white vinegar with 1 cup water in a 16-ounce or larger spray bottle.

2. Spritz a dust cloth with the solution and wipe plastic tabletops, venetian blinds, and upholstery to remove dust and discourage it from coming back on static currents.

Glue Begone

You don't need to buy small bottles of expensive glue removers—you can wipe stubborn adhesive tags from store-bought products with a little household staple.

1. Dip a clean cloth into white vinegar and rub it over glue spot until it loosens. Remove the glue with a dry corner of the cloth. Use a plastic spatula to lift any stubborn spots.

2. Rinse spot with a clean, damp cloth, and polish with a dry cloth.

Hand Deodorizer

There is nothing more irritating than a strong fish, onion, or garlic smell that sticks to your hands. Here's the cheap and easy answer.

1. Wash your hands with soap and water as usual, pour vinegar over your clean hands, and rub it in for a few seconds.

2. Rinse and dry hands as usual.

Mineral Deposit Remover

If you live in an area with hard water, sooner or later you'll notice that your coffee maker takes longer to brew and the coffee doesn't taste as good, your rug steamer doesn't work as well as it did, and your steam iron may stop steaming. Here's how to make them all like new again.

1. To clean coffee makers, steam-cleaning machines, and steam irons, pour 1/2 cup (or more as needed to fill reservoir) white vinegar into the water reservoir, turn the machine on, and allow it to run until all of the vinegar passes through.

2. Follow up by filling the reservoir with clean water and running the entire reservoir of clean water through the machine to rinse out the vinegar residue. Repeat with a coffee maker, if needed.

Nontoxic Stain for Children's Wood Projects

If you have a child who is old enough for simple woodworking projects, or for painting precut blocks and plaques, you'll want to try this recipe. It gives you brightly colored, safe stains that cost pennies compared to a few dollars for a name-brand counterpart.

1/3 cup powdered tempera paint

1 cup water

Widemouthed quart jar

Paintbrush

Nontoxic spray or brush-on, water-based varnish

1. Pour powdered paint into jar. Add water, screw on cap, and shake to mix.

2. Apply to wood with a paintbrush and allow the project to dry overnight.

3. Paint details and allow to dry overnight. Varnish with a water-based, nontoxic varnish, according to package directions, to preserve the color and add an attractive glossy surface. Dry as directed before using.

Test for Finish Remover

With this simple process, you'll be able to determine the kind of finish used on a piece of furniture, and the type of stripper you'll need to buy, saving both time and money. When working with chemical finish removers, use eye protection, rubber gloves that are designed for this use, and work in a well-ventilated place, such as a garage with opened doors.

Nail-polish remover
Cotton balls

1. Saturate a cotton ball in nail-polish remover and hold it briefly against an inconspicuous part of the furniture, such as the bottom of a chair runner, side of a drawer, or back of a table leg.

2. If the furniture finish becomes sticky or begins to dissolve, it is a lacquer-based finish like shellac or oil-based varnish, and you should buy a liquid furniture refinisher or denatured alcohol to remove the finish.

3. If the covering is unaffected by nail-polish remover, it is a plastic-based varnish, such as polyurethane, and you should strip it with paint remover.

Leaking Toilet Test

Toilets can leak undetected, leading to an expensive waste of water, and sometimes ruined floors. You don't need a plumber to find out. Here's how to test a toilet for leaks yourself.

10 drops food coloring

1. Add food coloring to the tank on the back of the toilet and leave it for 1 hour.

2. When the hour is up, examine the water in the toilet bowl. If colored water has leaked into it, you need to replace the toilet-tank ball. Buy a replacement at a hardware store and, following directions on the package, put in the new ball.

3. If colored water has leaked onto the floor, you likely need a new wax ring under the toilet. Replacing this takes some strength—a porcelain toilet bowl is heavy to lift—so you may want a plumber to do this job. It's not hard to do: Shut off the water supply to the toilet (the shutoff valve is usually on the wall at the base of the toilet). Flush the toilet, and when it is empty, unscrew and lift the toilet from the floor. Buy a replacement wax ring to match the worn one under the toilet. Install the new wax ring and set the toilet back in place, screw it down, and turn the water back on. Repeat the food coloring test to make sure the leak is stopped.

craft-making supplies

Craft Paste
Flour paste is a time-honored favorite for paper crafts like decoration making and papier-mâché. It is easy and cheap to make at home.

> 1 quart water
> 1/4 cup salt
> 1 1/2 cups white flour (more or less as needed)

1. In a saucepan, bring the water to a boil, and then remove from heat.

2. Stir in salt and add flour a little at a time, stirring constantly to prevent lumping, until the mixture reaches the consistency of very thick gravy. Cool and use.

3. Store leftover paste in a sealed container in the refrigerator for up to 5 days. Discard paste if mold forms or it smells spoiled.

Pottery Glue
Use this traditional homemade recipe to make durable glue for repairing broken pieces of crockery or china.

> 1 1/2 teaspoons glycerin
> 4 1/2 teaspoons gum arabic
> 1/4 teaspoon water
> Rubber bands *(optional)*
> Duct tape *(optional)*

1. In a small bowl, mix glycerin, gum arabic, and water thoroughly and store in a small, sealed bottle.

2. Coat both sides of the surfaces to be glued with the mixture and clamp them together with strong rubber bands or duct tape until glue dries (about 1 hour).

3. Wash mended objects carefully by hand; do not place mended pieces in a dishwasher or stove.

Paper Glue
This inexpensive homemade glue is more transparent than flour paste and is good for gluing pieces of paper together where looks count, such as scrapbooking or making greeting cards.

> 1 cup cornstarch
> 3 cups water
> 4 tablespoons light corn syrup
> 2 teaspoons white vinegar

1. Mix and cook 1/2 cup cornstarch, 1 1/2 cups water, and other ingredients over medium heat until thickened. Remove from heat.

2. In a separate bowl, stir together the remaining 1/2 cup cornstarch and 1/2 cup water. Blend into heated mixture. Store in a sealed container in the refrigerator for up to 2 months.

Homemade Art Chalk

Whether you need an ongoing supply of chalk for the family note board or simply want to supply budding artists with an endless supply of sidewalk chalk, here is an easy and inexpensive way to make your own chalk.

Cardboard toilet-tissue tubes or plastic taper candle molds (available at craft stores)

Masking tape

Wax paper

1 1/2 cups plaster of paris

3/4 cup water

Disposable milk or ice-cream carton

Paint stir stick

3 tablespoons powdered tempera paint color (or mix 4 teaspoons colored paint and 4 teaspoons white paint for pastel colors)

1. Cover one end of each mold (toilet-tissue tubes for fat sidewalk chalk and taper candle molds for chalkboard-size chalk) with masking tape to prevent leaks. Line the molds with wax paper so that the finished chalk will release easily.

2. In a disposable container, stir the plaster of paris and water together slowly with a paint stirring stick. Divide the solution into two or three containers if you are making more than one color of chalk. Add paint powder to each container and stir to color evenly.

3. Set wax-paper-lined molds upright on a flat surface, fill with chalk mix, and tap the sides of the mold to release air bubbles. Allow chalk to air-dry for 3 days before unmolding. The chalk should slide out of the cardboard tubes and candle mold.

4. Make up a new batch as needed until all desired colors are made.

Homemade Play Clay

This simple, money-saving recipe is great for making children happy on a rainy afternoon, but it is also the basis of Christmas tree ornaments, beads, and other sophisticated crafts. The recipe makes doughlike "clay" that bakes hard in the oven, and can be painted and coated with a craft varnish for a permanent and professional finish.

4 cups flour

1 cup salt

1 1/2 cups water

1. Preheat oven to 350°F. Mix ingredients together and knead for 5 minutes. You can divide the dough into portions and add drops of food coloring at this point, or model the white "clay" and paint the finished piece. Put unused clay into sealed plastic bags and use within 4 hours of mixing.

2. Place finished pieces on a cookie sheet and bake for 1 hour (until hard).

Finger Paints

You can feel good about giving little artists finger paints that you make yourself from kitchen pantry staples that you know are safe—and washable.

1/2 cup cornstarch

2 cups cold water

6 small plastic containers with snap-on lids

Food coloring kit

1. In a small saucepan, combine the cornstarch and water. Bring to a boil over high heat, stirring constantly until thickened. Remove from heat and let cool to room temperature.

2. Divide cornstarch mixture evenly among the containers. Put several drops of food coloring into each container and stir to distribute colors evenly.

Play Bubbles

Bubbles are a great party starter for kids of all ages, and this easy recipe makes lots of bubbles. Use your imagination—you can create bubble blowers out of open-ended cookie cutters and empty juice cans with both ends cut out. Instead of blowing bubbles, hold these blowers and whisk them through the air to release streams of bubbles.

1/2 cup dishwashing detergent

1 1/2 cups water

2 teaspoons sugar

1 teaspoon glycerin

1. In a medium bowl, slowly mix the ingredients, using a spoon or whisk to avoid foaming.

2. Pour the mixture into shallow bowls, dip blowers into the bowls, and wave them through the air to make big bubbles.

Vegetable Easter Egg Dyes

You can make your own colorful Easter egg dyes from vegetable juices for pennies. To make patterns on the already hard-cooked eggs, draw the design with a nontoxic wax pencil or crayon and then dip the eggs into hot dye long enough to color the egg without melting the wax. For a lacy pattern, soak a piece of fabric lace in melted paraffin and wrap around an egg while the wax is still soft. Put the wrapped egg in a spoon and dip into hot dye just long enough to color it. Remove the egg, and peel the fabric off to reveal a lacy colored pattern.

Peels of two or more onions

1/2 cup frozen spinach, thawed

1 fresh beet

1. For yellow eggshells: In a saucepan of water, boil onion peels for 20 minutes or until the water turns yellow. Remove peels, add eggs, and boil for 5 minutes. Remove eggs and set aside to cool.

2. For green eggshells: In a saucepan of water, boil spinach for 20 minutes, or until the water turns green. Strain out spinach and return green water to saucepan, add eggs, and boil for 5 minutes. Remove eggs and set aside to cool.

3. For red eggshells: Cut the beet into small pieces and put in a saucepan of water, boil for 20 minutes, or until the water turns red. Remove beet pieces, add eggs, and boil for 5 minutes. Remove eggs and set aside to cool.

basic flower drying

Dried flowers can make a very natural-looking floral arrangement that will last you a long time. And if you do the drying yourself, the cost is minimal. Some candidates can come from your own garden and others you can find elsewhere. If you like roses, for example, you can often get wilted ones from a florist at no cost. (They won't look wilted when they are dried.) Try to get a dozen or more flowers with stems. Besides roses, other flowers that can be successfully dried this easy way are hydrangeas, strawflowers, Queen Anne's lace, and baby's breath. Here's how to proceed:

1. Remove the leaves from the stems. Then bundle the stems together in groups of six with a rubber band. Hang the bundle upside down by string from a rod or a clothesline in a dry, warm place, such as a closet or the attic. The stems are hung upside down so that the flowers don't flop over during drying.

2. Leave bundles for a week or two or until the flowers are dry to the touch.

Drying Medium for Preserving Flowers

Many flowers dry better in a drying medium, which you can make yourself much more economically than if you buy it. Most flowers dry best and last longest when they are picked fresh and are just beginning to open. This drying medium will dry many kinds and colors of flowers and buds, although you must re-create their stems with floral wire and floral tape. To preserve their color, display dried flowers out of direct sunlight.

1 pound borax
1 pound cornmeal
1 1/2 teaspoons salt
Flowers and flower buds
Artist's brush with
  pointed tip

1. Preheat oven to 200°F. In an open casserole, mix borax, cornmeal, and salt. Bake uncovered for 30 minutes, stirring occasionally, to completely dry the contents.

2. Pour half of the drying mixture into a shoebox or plastic storage container. Set aside the remainder of the drying mixture.

3. Make a shallow well in the center of the mix. Trim the stem of a bud or flower to 1 inch long. Hold the flower and trickle cornmeal mix between its petals to fill the blossom. Place the flower into the well in the container of mix, stem-end-down. Repeat with as many flowers as will fit in the container.

4. Pour the remainder of the mix over all flowers until they are buried. Set the container in a warm, dry, dark place, such as a closet, for two weeks.

5. After drying, remove flowers carefully from the mix and brush cornmeal mix from petals with an artist's brush. Fasten flowers and buds for arrangements onto floral wire stems with floral tape. You can hot-glue short stems to wreaths and gift packages.

Potpourri Mixes

A bowl of fragrant, flowery potpourri can fill a room with the essence of summer—even in the dead of winter. Make potpourri to perfume your own home—or as homemade gifts. If you don't have a garden, ask your florist for past-their-peak flowers, such as lavender, statice, and roses, and lemon leaves that you can dry (see Drying Medium for Freezing Flowers, page 357).

3 cups dried flower petals, herb leaves, and small pine cones *(optional)*

3 tablespoons dried orrisroot (available at craft or herb stores)

10 drops essential oil (one type or a blend of your choosing)

1. In a large bowl, mix flower petals, herb leaves, small pine cones, if using, and orrisroot together.
2. Sprinkle essential oils over the dry ingredients and stir to distribute the fragrance.
3. Display in an open bowl out of direct sunlight, and add a couple drops of oil, as needed, to refresh the fragrance.
4. Store, or give as a gift, in a sealed glass or plastic container.

Bayberry Wax for Candles and Soap

For many, the spicy fragrance of bayberry candles brings warm holiday memories. It is easy to make traditional bayberry wax for candle or soap making if you have access to a bayberry, or wax myrtle, shrub (Myrica cerifera).

Bayberries
Water
Strainer

1. Pick bayberries in November. Put berries into a pan of water large enough to accommodate the quantity you've picked. Bring water to a boil, reduce heat, and simmer until the solution is thick and syrupy.
2. Strain the berries and seeds from the solution. Allow the solution to cool in a heatproof bowl. When the bayberry wax floats to the top of the liquid and solidifies, lift it off and store it in a sealed container in the refrigerator until you have collected enough to dip or mold candles.

Molded Candles

If you love making candles, you may want to invest in metal molds for tapered candles. You can, however, make many molded candles in containers that you already have around the house. A soup can, for example, will mold a fine pillar candle. Look around and see what other shapes you have. Buy wicking, paraffin, and mold seal at a craft shop or on the Internet.

1 packet wicking

1 10-pound block paraffin

Crayons (colors of your choice)

Scented oil (scent of your choice)

Molds

Nonstick cooking spray

1 packet mold seal

1. Cut wicking 4 inches longer than the height of the mold. Melt some of the wax in a double boiler over very low heat and soak the wicks in melted wax until saturated. Lay the wicks out straight on a piece of wax paper to cool and dry.

2. Lightly spray the inside of each mold with nonstick cooking spray, and if it doesn't have its own seal, use a mold seal product.

3. Stick the wick to the bottom of the mold with a bit of mold seal. Tie the other end to a small stick or skewer, pull the wick taut and lay the stick across the mouth of the mold.

4. Melt the rest of the wax in a double boiler. Never let the wax exceed 200°F (use a candy thermometer to check the temperature). Use pot holders or mitts to handle hot wax to prevent burns. Lower the heat, add crayon bits and a few drops of scented oils, and stir to distribute evenly.

5. Pour wax into molds, stopping 1/2 inch from the top. Place the molds in a pan of cold water (use pot holders), taking care not to splash water into the mold. Let cool 1 hour.

6. When the mold is cool, remove the candle. Trim the wick and smooth the bottom of the candle by standing it in a pot of warm water. If you used a 2-part mold, trim any ragged seams with a paring knife.

Rolled Beeswax Candles
Candles rolled from sheets of beeswax are simple to make and long-burning. They make elegant gifts.

Sheets of beeswax (as many as the number of candles desired)

Wicking

1. Cut wicking 3 inches longer than the sheets of beeswax.
2. Melt a small amount of beeswax in a double boiler over low heat. Soak wicks to saturate in wax, remove, and stretch out straight on a sheet of wax paper to cool.
3. Warm beeswax sheets until malleable with an electric hair dryer set to its lowest setting. Lay a prepared wick on the edge of a sheet of beeswax, placed on a flat surface. Roll the beeswax sheet tightly and evenly around the wick until it is as thick as desired.
4. Trim excess beeswax off with a utility knife, and seal the candle seam with a heated butter knife. Repeat steps for remaining candles.

household pest repellents

Cockroach Repellent
Cockroaches are attracted to damp areas, but they'll stay away if you use this inexpensive solution. Remember to store pest treatments, such as this, in capped and labeled bottles in a childproof cabinet.

1 metal coffee can with plastic lid

1 old-style beer-can opener (that cuts a V notch)

2 tablespoons borax

1 tablespoon flour

1 tablespoon sugar

1. Punch holes around the base of an empty coffee can, using a beer-can opener. Label the can with a sign that reads "Cockroach Killer."
2. In a small bowl, mix the ingredients together. Put in the coffee can, snap on the lid, and place it under the sink or wherever you've seen roaches. Lock the undersink cabinet if you have children or pets.
3. Refill the can, or create additional cans as necessary.

Moth Repellent Cedar Sachets
You can have the benefits of a moth-repellent cedar closet or cedar-lined drawers at a fraction of the cost of the real thing with these fragrant cedar sachets.

2 pairs colorful adult or baby socks

1 bag cedar shavings (sold at pet shops as hamster bedding)

Satin or grosgrain ribbon

Clothes hanger

1. Fill socks with cedar shavings—adult-size for closets and baby-size for drawers.
2. Tie the tops of the socks closed with coordinating ribbon.
3. Tie large sachets to clothes hangers and hang in closets to freshen air and repel moths. Tuck the little ones into lingerie and sweater drawers.

Homemade Flypaper

Why buy flypaper when you can make your own? All you need is a brown paper bag, a little sugar, and some corn syrup.

3 1/2 ounces corn syrup
1 tablespoon brown sugar
1 tablespoon white sugar
6 strips brown paper
  (cut from a paper bag)

1. Combine the syrup and sugars in a shallow bowl.
2. Poke a hole at the top of each strip of brown paper. Soak paper in the syrup mixture overnight.
3. Scrape paper strips across the edge of the saucer to remove excess syrup and hang the finished flypaper strips near windows and doors.
4. Replace when strips are covered with insects.

Pungent Moth-Repelling Bundles

Moths dislike the strong fragrance of certain herbs. They also avoid cupboards that are regularly aired out, so every once in a while leave your closet or dresser drawers cracked open for a day, and make an herbal repellent.

1 small bundle southern-
  wood, camphor, tansy, or
  sweet woodruff
1 rubber band
String
1 coat hanger

1. Bind together a small bundle of fresh herbs (one kind or a blend) by fastening a rubber band around the stems.
2. Tie a bundle to an empty coat hanger and hang it in the closet among woolen clothes, or tuck it under drawer-liner paper in a drawer containing woolens.

Aromatic Moth-Repelling Sachets

This sachet containing lavender and elder flowers makes a nice gift, and will also keep your drawers fragrant and moth-free.

10 inches fine material, such
  as silk or nylon netting
Dried lavender flowers
Dried elder flowers

1. Fold the fabric with right sides together and cut to create an 8 x 8-inch square plus a 1/2-inch seam allowance on all four sides. Sew three seams.
2. Turn the pouch right side out, and fill with flowers. Tuck the remaining seams inside and stitch the bag closed by hand.
3. Place in drawers or chests with woolens to repel moths

Ant Traps
Here's an easy, inexpensive way to round up the ants that begin to invade your house each summer.

3 cups water

1 cup sugar

4 teaspoons boric acid

Cotton balls

3 clean 8-ounce screw-top jars

Old-style beer-can opener (that cuts V notches)

1. In a pitcher, mix the water, sugar, and boric acid together. Loosely pack the jars half-full of cotton balls, and saturate with the solution.

2. Pierce jar lids with the can opener, making two or three holes just large enough to admit ants.

3. Place the baited jars where ants are active, but make sure jars are out of the reach of pets and children. Attracted by the lethal sugar and boric acid mixture, ants will crawl into the traps.

Helpful Hint | **How to Keep Pet Food Ant-Free**
Placed on the floor, pet food bowls are like a natural magnet for ants. Here's a simple, totally nontoxic way to keep ants away. Set an empty pie pan where you usually feed your pet. Fill the pet's dish with food and set it into the pie pan. Pour water into the pie pan, filling it to the rim. Ants and other crawling insects cannot cross this "moat" to reach the pet food.

Carpet Flea Remover
If fleas hitchhiked indoors on your pet, try this simple, effective, and cheap fix for freshening and debugging your carpets, using your vacuum.

3 mothballs

Duct tape

1. Cut a small slit into the disposable vacuum bag liner and drop in mothballs. Seal the slit with a piece of duct tape. If you have a bagless vacuum, simply drop the balls on the floor and vacuum them up, or open the canister and drop them in.

2. Vacuum as usual. Fleas that are vacuumed up will be killed by the mothballs in the bag or canister. Drop in new mothballs when you change the disposable bag or empty the canister.

garden helpers

Spot Weed Killer

Weeds that pop up between flagstones and in cracks of the sidewalk are hard to dig out of the small crevices. Kill weeds in your terrace or walkway by dousing them with this simple laundry-room solution.

Household bleach
Boiling water

1. Prepare a solution of 5 percent bleach and 95 percent boiling water.

2. Douse weeds with the solution, wait a day and check for withering. If the weeds resist, increase the percentage of bleach and repeat.

Helpful Hint | **How to Protect Plants When Spot-Treating Weeds**
It's difficult to spot-treat weeds that sidle up to your favorite garden plants without killing the good plants. Here's how to keep the weed killer on the weed and off your prized peonies: Cut the bottom out of a large, 2-liter clear plastic soda bottle or 1-gallon milk jug and remove the cap. To isolate a weed for treatment, set the bottomless jug over it, stick the weed-killer spray applicator into the cap opening and spray. Be sure to label the bottomless bottle with the pesticide being used and to store it in a locked cabinet with other pesticide equipment.

Red Clay Stain Remover

If you garden in an area with clay soil, you know all too well how its red color stains your clothes. Set aside an old pair of jeans just to garden in. When they're caked with mud, use this simple recipe to keep stains off the clothes you wash them with.

1 part table salt
Vinegar

1. Drape muddy jeans over the back of a lawn chair or lay them out on a picnic table and rinse vigorously with a garden hose.

2. In a small jar, add vinegar to the salt, a little at a time, to make a paste. Rub the paste into the mud stains, allow to sit for 20 minutes, then launder as usual.

Useful House and Garden Products   **777**

Rust Remover

Vinegar makes an inexpensive rust remover for old hinges, screws, and metal lawn furniture that have started to rust from outdoor exposure.

White vinegar
Steel wool
Paper towels

1. Fill a widemouthed jar half-full of vinegar, drop in small rusty parts, screw the lid on, and soak for a few days until rust loosens. Remove the objects, rinse, and carefully dry.

2. Soak a paper towel in vinegar and lay it over furniture surfaces to loosen rust. If the rust is stubborn, cover the saturated towel with plastic wrap to keep the towel damp. Set the piece out of direct sunlight for a few days. Remove the wrapping, steel-wool the spot smooth, rinse, dry, and paint if desired.

Fire Starters

If you use this simple recipe to make your own fire starters, you'll never have to dash to the hardware store at the last minute when you'd rather be enjoying your patio fire pit or charcoal grill.

Scraps of particleboard or kindling
1 pound paraffin wax
Cake cooling rack

1. Melt paraffin in the top of a double boiler over low heat or in a slow cooker set on low heat.

2. Dip wood scraps into the melted wax to cover completely, remove, and set on the cooling rack to harden.

3. When the wax cools, store the waxed scraps in an old coffee can in a cool place. To use, place one or two scraps at the bottom of your fire pit or charcoal grill and stack logs or charcoal over them. Use a long-handled match to light the waxed starters, which will act as long-burning igniters for your fire.

Whitewash

Whitewash is a wood coating that has been used for hundreds of years. In the days when paint was an expensive luxury, whitewash was popular for painting farm buildings and fences. Whitewash has no binders and will slowly wear away in rain, which is why it was routinely painted on greenhouse roofs to shade plants in summer. To finish a traditional project, or to shade your greenhouse, try this simple recipe. While whitewash must still be mixed by hand, the ingredients, including color tints, are sold at concrete supply stores.

1 cup table salt
2 cups hydrated lime
1 gallon water or milk

1. Stir ingredients together slowly in a metal bucket, taking care not to splash. Add more lime or water as needed to achieve the color and consistency of milk. For a more permanent paint, substitute fresh milk for water.

2. Allow mixture to cool before painting on wood and allow it to air-dry.

Caution: Mix whitewash outdoors; wear protective eye goggles and old clothes. Be careful not to splash the mixture on your skin when mixing, and rinse it off right away if it does get on your skin. Mix whitewash in a metal bucket, because it heats up as the ingredients combine and may affect a plastic container.

Water Repellent for Exposed Wood

Try this recipe for a long-lasting, waterproof coating for decks, shutters, and other wooden items that are exposed to the elements. If you plan to stain the wood, do so before applying the water repellent. If you want to paint or varnish, apply the water repellent first and allow it to dry before painting or varnishing.

1 quart exterior varnish (spar or polyurethane)
1 clean 1-gallon paint can
1 cup grated paraffin wax
1 stirring stick
Mineral spirits
Paintbrush or roller

1. Pour varnish into can. Add wax and stir slowly until wax dissolves.

2. Add mineral spirits until the can is full, and stir slowly to mix all ingredients, without creating air bubbles.

3. Brush or roll the treatment onto raw or stained wood and allow to dry for 4 hours before using, painting, or varnishing.

4. If you want to paint the wood, prime with oil primer after the water repellent dries, allow primer to dry as directed on package label, then paint.

garden soil care

Compost

Compost is the best all-natural soil amendment you can use. It contains valuable plant nutrients and plant disease-fighting organisms, and it also makes soil moisture-retentive and easier to till. Best of all, compost is free when you make your own. You can make compost in a bin (3 feet square is ideal) or simply pile the ingredients on the ground. If you turn the pile periodically, it will break down faster, but even if you pile it and leave it for a year, it will break down.

6 parts dried (brown) plant material (dry leaves, straw, sawdust, paper)

1 part fresh (green) plant material (grass clippings, vegetable scraps, coffee grounds, horse, cow, or chicken manure)

1. Put a layer of brown material directly on the ground, then add a layer of green material. Continue to layer brown and green material to a height of 3 feet. Water with a hose as needed to keep the pile as moist as a wrung-out sponge.

2. To speed up decomposition, use a hay fork to puncture and turn the pile to allow air into its center. In rainy weather cover the pile with a tarp to prevent saturating it.

3. If the pile becomes smelly, it is too wet—mix in more brown ingredients. When the pile looks like rich, crumbly black soil and has a sweet, earthy fragrance, it is ready to use in the garden or as mulch.

Helpful Hint

An Inexpensive, Very Helpful Soil Test

A complete soil test—available from your local Cooperative Extension office or your state agricultural university—costs less than $20 and is the best investment you can make in your garden. The results will provide an exact prescription for fertilization, liming, and adding trace elements. Knowing what your soil needs allows you to furnish your plants with ideal conditions with no wasted effort. For testing locations and to order a kit by mail, check the government pages of your phone book or do an Internet search.

Green Manure Soil Conditioner
Often called green manures, these annual crops thrive in cool weather, protecting garden soil from erosion and weeds.

> Hairy vetch or
> winter rye seeds

1. After clearing vegetables or annual flowers from a bed in fall, sow hairy vetch or winter rye seeds in cleared beds according to package directions.

2. In early spring, three to four weeks before planting time, dig the green manure right into the soil. As it decomposes, it adds humus to the soil and acts as fertilizer for the coming season's crop.

Seaweed Soil Conditioner
Seaweed is actually higher in nitrogen and potassium than most animal manures, and is also a rich source of trace elements. Many municipalities with beaches are glad to have you haul it away.

> Seaweed

1. To cleanse seaweed of salt, pile it where runoff will be directed to a storm drain, such as on your driveway. Allow several rains to rinse away the sea salt, then add the seaweed to your compost pile or dig it into garden beds in the fall.

2. To make seaweed tea, steep an old pillowcase filled with seaweed in a bucket of water for a week. Remove and discard the bag, dilute the liquid to the color of weak tea, and water plants with it.

water-wise gardening techniques

You can save water and still have a beautiful garden. All it takes is noting moist and dry areas of your property and choosing the right plant for the right place.

Think of your yard as radiating outward from your house like a bull's-eye target. The wettest areas are closest to the house—particularly around outdoor faucets where water drips, and the next wettest area is within reach of a 50- or 100-foot garden hose. Beyond the reach of your hose are the driest areas.

For efficient water use and healthy plants, grow water lovers like ferns and woodland perennials near the house, and select drought-tolerant perennials with deep roots that can reach groundwater, such as coneflower, rudbeckia, and ornamental grasses, outside the reach of your garden hose.

If you live in a mild-winter climate, consider water-conserving garden plants that are native to South Africa, Australia, and the Mediterranean. Or select plants that are native to your region, which are naturally adapted to your local soil and rainfall.

Wood-Ash Potassium Boost

Wood ashes from a fireplace or woodstove (not coal or charcoal ashes) are a free source of the plant nutrients potassium, calcium, and phosphorus. They can also be used, like lime, to decrease soil acidity. Benefits of treating soil with ashes include improved hardiness and flavor of fruits. Be sure to apply in small amounts or compost well before applying to keep the caustic ashes from burning plants. Water-soluble nutrients can leach from ashes, so be sure to use fresh ones that have not been exposed to rain.

1. Apply 5 to 10 pounds of ashes per 100 square feet of garden in the fall.
2. To reduce soil acidity, use as a substitute for ground limestone: Apply up to twice as much wood ashes as limestone package recommends, and allow ashes to weather over the winter before planting.

Helpful Hint | **Fertilizer, Free for the Asking**

Healthy plants are naturally resistant to insects and diseases, and natural fertilizers are the best way to ensure healthy plants and a balanced garden ecosystem. No matter where you live, good sources of fertilizer, free for the hauling, are available at farms and from neighbors who have pet rabbits or chickens. All you have to do is ask for animal manure to enrich your compost.

Coffee Grounds Fertilizer

Acidic coffee grounds make an excellent soil conditioner or mulch for acid-loving plants like conifers, azaleas, and rhododendrons. You can often have as much of the used grounds as you need, free for the taking, from chain coffeehouses.

1. Apply a 3-inch-thick mulch of coffee grounds around the base of acid-loving plants, leaving a 6-inch ring of bare soil around the trunk of the plant to discourage trunk-eating insects and voles that like to nest in mulch.
2. For a complete fertilizer, 2-4-2 analysis, mix 4 parts coffee grounds with 1 part composted wood ashes, and work into soil in autumn.

garden pest fighters

Blood Meal Rabbit Repellent

They may be cute, but when bunnies munch on your prized garden produce or gnaw the bark of young trees, they wear out their welcome. Blood meal is an organic fertilizer that is high in nitrogen, the nutrient most needed by green plants. But more important, rabbits associate the smell of blood meal with predators, and will avoid gardens treated with it.

Blood meal

1. Sprinkle over the soil around garden perimeters and in garden beds according to package directions.
2. Reapply after heavy rains.

Helpful Hint | **Use Fencing to Keep Rabbits Out**
Use fence wire or hardware cloth with holes small enough to discourage chewing and exclude the tiniest rabbit. Wrap young tree trunks with hardware cloth to keep rabbits from gnawing the bark. To protect a vegetable garden, staple chicken wire that has small holes along the inside of your garden fence. For most effective control, bury the fencing a foot deep to keep rabbits from digging under it.

White Flag Deer Repellent

Deer flash the white undersides of their tails as a warning signal when predators or other dangers are near. Frighten deer away from your garden by duplicating this reaction with flags you can make from recycled materials.

Stakes (2 or 3 feet tall)

Several white plastic grocery bags or rags (such as strips torn from old white T-shirts)

1. Hammer stakes that are nose-high to a deer into the ground around your garden at 6-foot intervals.
2. Tie grocery bags to the stakes so that wind will billow them out, or tie strips of white fabric long enough to flutter in the wind.

Soap Deer Repellent

Deer dislike the smell of deodorant soap. Scraps collected and tied into an old sock make a long-lasting, environmentally safe protection for prized shrubs, flowers, and vegetables. Fresh bars of soap make an even stronger deterrent. One bar can protect a 9-square-foot area, so space bars as needed to protect vulnerable plants.

Several bars or scraps of deodorant bath soap (not floral scented)

Long nail (12 penny), or drill with 1/8-inch bit, or old socks

String

1. Remove soap from wrapper, make a hole in one end of a bar with the nail or the drill, and run a piece of string through the hole. If using soap scraps, drop them into the toe of an old sock and tie the open end shut with string.

2. Tie soap (or soap-filled sock) to the branch of a shrub or tree with string or attach to a stake in the garden bed. Replace when soap is diminished by rain.

Stink 'Um Deer Spray

Deer have sensitive noses, and are repelled by animal odors, especially that of spoiled eggs. Whip up this stinky brew and deer will soon be feeding elsewhere.

1 egg

1 cup water

1/4 cup garlic juice

1 tablespoon liquid dish detergent

Scrap of panty hose

Rubber band

1. In a blender, mix egg, water, and garlic juice. Stir in detergent to avoid foaming. Pour solution into an open container and set in an out-of-nose-range spot outdoors to age for 3 days.

2. Cover the siphon of a spray bottle with a scrap of panty hose held on with a rubber band to prevent clogging. Fill spray bottle with Stink 'Um and spray vulnerable plants. Repeat applications after rains.

Repellent for Four-Footed Pests

Whether it's raccoons treating your trash like an all-you-can-eat buffet or mice looking for a barbecue-grill condo, you can get four-footed pests to scram with a couple of inexpensive household products.

Ammonia

Water

Mothballs

1. In a spray bottle, mix a solution of half water and half ammonia. Liberally spray trash cans or other areas visited by animal pests. If trash cans sit outside, swab them out with full-strength ammonia after every emptying.

2. Place a handful of mothballs in a shallow dish or pan and set into an unused barbecue grill to repel mice, opossums, and raccoons. Remove the mothballs when the grill is in use. Tuck a few mothballs into patio furniture cushions before storing them over the winter to repel nesting mice. Be sure to keep mothballs, which are toxic, out of the reach of children and pets.

A Quick Slug and Snail Barrier

When you don't have time to set elaborate traps for these garden pests, make an unbroken ring of wood ashes around your favorite flowers. Snails and slugs will turn away from caustic ashes. Make sure to reapply the ashes after a rain.

Slug and Snail Trap

Slugs and snails devastate prized garden plants by chewing round holes in the leaves, leaving telltale shiny slime trails. They climb up into plants like hostas and marigolds to feed after sundown, and in the morning, crawl down to hide in mulch or garden debris. Here's a nontoxic recipe for catching them.

1 or more clear plastic
  drinking-water bottles and
  caps
1 teaspoon dry yeast
1 teaspoon sugar
1 cup tepid water
Stale beer *(optional)*

1. Mix yeast, sugar, and water together and allow it to rest for 5 minutes. Pour just enough yeast solution (or stale beer) into an empty drinking-water bottle, so that when you lay it on its side the liquid does not run out.

2. Lay the bottle on its side under a plant that shows slug damage or place under a vulnerable plant as a preventive measure. Slugs and snails will be attracted by the yeasty odor, crawl in, and drown.

3. Check the bottle daily, and when full, replace the cap, throw it away, and make a new trap. Make as many as you need—these traps may not be beautiful, but they look better than the skeletal remains of a slug-eaten plant in the garden.

Easy Earwig Trap

These fearsome-looking insects can be identified by the pincers at the ends of their tails. Although they don't hurt people, these nocturnal feeders can nibble plants overnight. Try this nontoxic control made with recycled newspaper.

Several sheets of used
  newspaper
String

1. Roll several thicknesses of newspaper into a tight cylinder and secure with string. Dampen the rolled paper and place on the soil near eaten plants.

2. Check the roll each morning to see if earwigs are hiding inside. If so, dispose of them in a securely tied trash bag and set out a new roll. Continue this routine until earwigs are under control.

Homemade Insecticide

When aphids, whiteflies, and other insect pests become a problem in the garden or on your houseplants, don't rush to the market for an expensive spray. Make your own from these kitchen-tested ingredients. Store all garden treatments, such as this, in a capped and labeled bottle in a childproof cabinet.

10 garlic cloves

1 tablespoon vegetable or mineral oil

3 cups hot water

1 teaspoon dishwashing soap (not laundry or dishwasher detergent)

1. In a blender, puree the garlic, skin and all, and oil.
2. Strain mixture through a sieve into a quart jar. Add water and dishwashing soap. Cap the jar and shake gently to mix.
3. Decant the mixture into a spray bottle (you can clean and reuse a cleaning product spray bottle). Spray infested plants, making sure to cover both sides of the leaves. Apply every 3 days for a week to control hatching insect eggs. Repeat as needed after rains or when problems arise.

Alcohol Insect Treatment

Rubbing alcohol is a time-tested treatment for soft-bodied garden pest insects like aphids and mealybugs. Traditionally, it was advised that you dab it onto individual insects with a cotton swab, but this is a time-consuming task. Try this speedy spritz instead.

1 cup rubbing alcohol

1 cup water

1. Combine the alcohol and water in a spray bottle and shake to combine.
2. Before treating, spray one leaf of the infested plant as a test to make sure there are no reactions, such as browning. If not, spray the entire plant, including undersides of leaves and flower buds. Avoid spraying open flowers, which may turn brown if treated with alcohol.
3. Repeat every other day for 3 days to kill hatchlings. Monitor plants and spray again as needed. Label the bottle and store it out of the reach of children and pets.

outsmarting stinging insects

You can avoid attracting stinging insects, such as bees, yellow jackets, and mosquitoes, by being careful about what you wear or how you smell while gardening or sitting on the patio. Here are some suggestions.

- Stinging insects that strike during daylight hours are attracted to flower colors—red, pink, yellow, orange, and purple—so wear clothes in cool shades of blue, green, black, gray, or white for yard and garden work.
- Many stinging insects are also attracted to floral and fruity scents, so forgo perfume, scented shampoo, scented hair conditioners, and scented lotions.
- These insects are often repelled by herbal scents. Wear a broad-brimmed hat and tuck sprigs of rosemary or chrysanthemum or marigold flowers into the brim to repel insects. Or, if you don't want to wear a hat, put the sprigs into the pocket of a T-shirt.

Aspirin Systemic Insecticide

Plant experts have experimented successfully with watering plants with aspirin-water as a systemic insecticide and promoter of plant growth. Plants naturally produce some salicylic acid, which aspirin contains, as a natural protection. When watered with the aspirin solution, treated plants absorb extra salicylic acid, which helps them repel sucking insects, and they produce strong, healthy growth.

3 regular-strength aspirin (325 mg)
5 gallons water

1. In a large watering can, stir aspirin into water until dissolved. Water plants as usual with treated water or put it in a spray bottle and use as a foliar spray.
2. Treat plants twice monthly with aspirin water.

Antifungal Compost Tea

Compost is not just a great soil conditioner and fertilizer. It also contains beneficial organisms that resist soil-borne fungal diseases. To discourage formation of fungus on plants, such as brown patch, sooty mildew, and powdery mildew, make a "tea" treatment using common garden compost.

1 gallon container compost
1 burlap bag or old pillowcase
String
3 gallons water

1. Place compost in the bag, tie the bag shut with string, and drop it into a bucket of water.
2. Set the bucket in a sunny spot, and steep the bag in the water for 2 or 3 days—until the water turns dark brown.
3. Remove the bag of compost (use the contents as mulch). Dilute the remaining solution with water to the color of weak tea. Spray it on roses, rudbeckia, phlox, and other plants that are susceptible to fungal infections. Repeat twice monthly during the growing season to prevent outbreaks.

Baking Soda Fungal Fix

When a baking soda solution is applied to fungus-prone plants, such as roses and bee balm, before signs of mildew appear, it can prevent diseases including powdery and sooty mildew and black spot. And because this spray is cheap and easy to make, you can keep it on hand and apply as needed. To further discourage fungal diseases, keep plant leaves as dry as possible by watering the soil without splashing the leaves, and mulch plants with disease-fighting compost.

1 teaspoon baking soda

1 teaspoon liquid dish-washing soap (do not use laundry or dishwasher detergent)

1 quart warm water

Pour ingredients into a large spray bottle and shake to mix. Spray both sides of leaves and stems.

Bug Blaster Soap Spray

Dishwashing soap is harmless to the environment and is safe to use in the house. Outdoors it also makes an effective control for soft-bodied insects, such as caterpillars, thrips, aphids, and mealybugs, because soap breaks down their protective coverings, causing the pests to dehydrate.

1 tablespoon liquid dish-washing soap (do not use laundry or dishwasher detergent)

1 gallon water

1. Pour soap into water and stir to dissolve. Fill a spray bottle and test-spray one or two leaves of an infested plant. Wait a day, and if the leaves are not damaged, spray the entire plant. Be sure to coat the stems as well as both sides of the leaves.

2. Repeat the treatment twice a week until the pests are no longer visible. Then repeat as often as needed.

Catnip Bird Repellent

There are times when you may want to attract birds to your garden. In the spring, when they are feeding nestlings, birds can rid your garden of harmful insects. But later on, if they decide to eat your freshly planted corn and vegetable seeds, you will want to discourage them. Here's how.

Catnip plants or seeds

1. Plant catnip plants or seeds near, but not right next to, vulnerable garden seeds and seedlings.

2. The catnip will draw neighborhood cats, which in turn will scare the birds from your garden.

Rhubarb Insect Solution

3 stalks rhubarb with leaves
1 gallon water

Rhubarb is an attractive perennial plant that not only makes good pies but also makes an insecticide that is toxic to sucking insects. This recipe is for ornamental plants only. Do not spray on herbs, fruits, or vegetables, because rhubarb leaves are toxic to humans.

1. Chop rhubarb leaves and stems. In a stockpot, combine rhubarb and the water. Bring to a boil, reduce the heat, and simmer, uncovered, for 1 hour.
2. Cool to room temperature, and strain liquid into a spray bottle through a funnel. Spray on infested plants at 3-day intervals for 10 days. Repeat as necessary.

Ammonia Plant Conditioning Spray

1 part household clear ammonia
1 part liquid dishwashing soap (do not use laundry or dishwasher detergent)
7 parts water

Ammonia is a concentrated form of nitrogen, which is the nutrient most needed by green plants. You can make an inexpensive all-purpose fertilizer and insecticidal spray using ammonia and soap. The soap helps the ammonia stick to the leaves and also kills soft-bodied insects. Mix as much as you need for garden plants and lawns. Store all garden treatments, such as this, in a capped and labeled bottle in a childproof cabinet.

1. In a large container combine the ingredients.
2. Fill a spray bottle and apply mixture to stems and both sides of leaves for garden plants. Use a hose-end applicator to spray the lawn.

Helpful Hint | **Use Scented Mulch to Keep Insects Away**
Trimming herbs frequently, especially removing flower stalks, helps them maintain lots of tender, flavorful new growth. Sprinkle the sprigs and flowers that you don't use in the kitchen along garden paths as aromatic and insect-repelling mulch.

Oil Spray Insecticide Concentrate

Some plant pests and fungal infections are hard to eradicate because they have shells or waxy coatings that protect them from traditional treatments. You can, however, smother tough-shelled scale, the eggs of many insects, and even mildew infections by coating them with oil. Store all garden treatments, such as this, in a capped and labeled bottle in a childproof cabinet.

1 tablespoon liquid dishwashing soap (do not use laundry or dishwasher detergent)

1 cup vegetable oil

1. In a pint container, combine soap and oil to form a concentrate. Store it in a sealed, labeled container.

2. To apply, mix 1 or 2 teaspoons concentrate with 1 cup water in a spray bottle and apply to stems and both sides of plant leaves. Reapply after it rains.

Insect Repellent

Insects won't bug your next patio cookout if you try this fragrant, non-toxic herbal fix.

Sprigs fresh rosemary

Sprigs fresh basil

Sprigs fresh thyme

1. When you remove food from the grill, spread out a handful of pungent culinary herbs on the top rack of the grill where they will smoke, but not burn.

2. Allow the herbs to cook and release their insect-repelling fragrances.

houseplants

Sterile Seed-Starting Mix

Mature plants develop defenses against many kinds of insects and diseases, but fragile seedlings can be wiped out by soil-borne diseases or insects. Use this money-saving recipe to make a sterile potting medium for sprouting garden seeds, and also for making potting soil to protect valued houseplants.

1 part sifted garden soil

2 parts sphagnum peat moss

2 parts coarse sand

1. In a large container, mix all ingredients together.

2. To sterilize, moisten and place ingredients in a shallow baking pan with a baking potato and bake at 200°F until the potato is done. This is a smelly process, ideal for doing on an outdoor grill.

Helpful Hint | **How to Overwinter Herbs Indoors**

To preserve culinary herbs for use in winter, dig the plants from the garden in August and transfer them to pots. Place the pots on a sunny windowsill indoors. For best results, select vigorous but compact plants and use 6-inch clay pots.

Lightweight Seed Mix
This mix is made of sterile materials bought at a garden center and does not need to be baked.

1 part vermiculite
1 part milled sphagnum
  moss
1 part perlite

1. In a large container, mix all the ingredients together.
2. Moisten with warm water before using

Flowerpot Sterilizer
Just because a flowerpot is used and dirty, you don't need to toss it. Whether clay, plastic, or ceramic, the pot can be superficially cleaned with a strong blast from a garden hose. If the pot has white, crusty mineral deposits, scrape them off with an old knife (scraping clay pots will sharpen the knife). When the pot is free of dirt and minerals, sterilize it to kill insect eggs and plant diseases.

1 part household bleach
10 parts water

1. Mix the bleach and water, making enough to fill a tub that is deeper than the largest pot you want to sterilize.
2. Place the cleaned pots in the tub and allow them to soak for 20 minutes.
3. Remove sterilized pots, rinse again with clear water, and set them in the sun to dry. They are now ready for new plants.

General Purpose Potting Mix
The compost in this mix contributes disease-fighting microorganisms and nutrients to help mature indoor and patio potted plants thrive.

1 part perlite
1 part finished compost
1 part topsoil

1. Mix all ingredients together and store in a waterproof, sealed container.
2. To modify this mix to suit succulents, cacti, and other plants that need sharply drained soil, increase the perlite to 2 parts, or add 1 part builder's sand to the original recipe.
3. Before filling a large pot, invert several small plastic pots on the bottom of the larger pot, then fill with soil. The air space beneath the small pots will aid drainage and lighten the overall weight of the pot.

reblooming holiday houseplants

When you receive a special flowering plant as a gift, it can be heartbreaking to have to toss it after the holidays, but it doesn't have to end this way. With a little effort, you can keep these plants from year to year, and get them to rebloom.

Amaryllis. After blooming, set the plant in a sunny spot and water as usual, letting it die back naturally, as you would for any bulb. This will occur sometime between late spring and early summer. Remove the withered foliage. Put the plant in a cool (about 55°F), dark place (such as a closet or garage), and do not water it. In August, bring the plant out into the light and warmth. Water and fertilize it, and flowers should appear in time for the holidays.

Poinsettia. As the length of the day increases in spring, poinsettias will stop blooming, but their foliage will remain fairly attractive. They can be placed outside in the warm months, but be sure to do a hard pruning in midsummer (cut stems back to 2 inches above the soil). During September and October, put the plants on a strict light schedule: 14 hours of total darkness at night, 10 hours of bright light during the day. Any light at all during the dark period can disturb the cycle, which is why some people place the plants under garbage cans or in a closet at night. Once the flower heads have formed, you can bring the plants back into normal conditions.

Booster for Early Spring Flowers
Get a jump on spring by forcing branches of flowering shrubs and trees to bloom early indoors. In late winter, watch for flower buds to swell on forsythia and on quince, ornamental cherry, and dogwood trees. Prune enough branches to fill a tall vase.

1 1/2 gallons warm water (110°F–115°F)

1 three-gallon bucket

1 cotton ball

Sudsy ammonia

1 plastic garbage bag

1. Cut stems, crush the cut ends with a hammer, and place them in the bucket of warm water.

2. Saturate a cotton ball in sudsy ammonia and drop it into the bucket.

3. Set the bucket of stems in a clean garbage bag, tie it closed, and set it in a warm place indoors until the buds begin to open. Then arrange the stems in a vase of clean water and set out in a room for a long-lasting bouquet.

Helpful Hint

How to Create a Lush Indoor Garden

If you display your houseplants all in one area, you will get a lush effect, and the plants will benefit from the heightened humidity gained by grouping the pots of moist soil.

In a sunny corner of a room, place a large trash bag on the floor and cover it with attractive, weatherproof decking, tiles, or an outdoor rug that coordinates with the room's décor. Arrange the potted plants on the covering, with the shorter ones at the front and rows of successively taller ones behind. For extra protection, set water-collecting saucers under each pot. To increase humidity, include a few vases or decorative bowls filled with pebbles and water. To add to the garden effect, you can include a small figure, such as a bird, child, or frog statue, if you want.

Repellent for Houseplant Pests
If you have a houseplant that is bothered by aphids, mealybugs, or other insect pests, you can banish them with this simple, no-mess recipe.

6 mothballs

1 large clear plastic dry-
cleaning bag

1 twist tie

1. Set the infested plant, pot, saucer and all, into the dry-cleaning bag. Moisten the soil, drop mothballs into the bag, and tie the bag closed with a twist tie.
2. Set the bagged plant in a bright place that is out of direct sunlight for a week. At the end of the week, remove the plant and put it in its usual home, and dispose of the bag and mothballs. Repeat the treatment as needed until pests are gone.

Houseplant Food
For an easy organic food for houseplants, try this recipe for "manure tea."

2 bucketfuls fresh horse or
cow manure or 1 bucketful
poultry manure

1 burlap bag

Rope

1 barrel or garbage can

Water

1. Dump manure into the burlap bag. Tie the bag shut with one end of a long rope and place it in an empty barrel or garbage can.
2. Fill the barrel or garbage can with water and leave the bag to steep for a week, using the rope occasionally to jerk it up and down and mix the liquid.
3. Thin the "tea" to the color of weak tea and apply monthly to the soil around houseplant roots. Keep reserved tea in labeled jars with tight lids out of the way of children and pets.

index

A

Acid, for jam, 490

Acidophilus, *Yeast Infection Cream*, 714

Acne remedies, 697–698

Activated charcoal, *Sweet Breath Dog Treats*, 722

Air fresheners, 745

Alcohol. *See* Rubbing alcohol; Wine and spirits

Almond extract, *Almond Exfoliating Body Scrub*, 670

Almond oil
Anti-Wrinkle Eye Cream, 652
body oil, 668
versus essential oil, 654
Eucalyptus Foot Lotion, 679
Healing Balm for Chapped Lips, 706
Love Your Feet Cream, 679
Orange and Almond OilDressing, 450
Rich Neck Moisturizer, 653

Almonds
Acne Facial Scrub, 697
Almond Mayonnaise Scrub, 657
Almond Rose Soap, 673

Aloe vera
Aloe Aftershave Gel, 681
for burns, 701
Burn Spray, 702
for canker sores, 706
Glorious Green Aloe Moisturizing Lotion, 667
growing, 702
Hemorrhoid Pads, 686
Soothing Gel for Insect Bites, 693

Aluminum foil
as cat toys, 729
Quick and Easy Silver Shine, 749

Amaryllis care, 792

Ammonia
Ammonia Plant Conditioning Spray, 789
Booster for Early Spring Flower, 792
buying, 435
Interior Wall Cleaner, 744
Lazy Person's Oven Cleaner, 751
precautions for, 436
Repellent for Four-Footed Pests, 784
Stain Remover, 754
Tough Multipurpose Cleaner, 743
Wall and Cabinet Cleaner, 743

Angelica, *Refreshing Mouthwash*, 662

Aniseed, as antacid, 684

Antacids, spices as, 684

Ant control, 776

Antifungal remedies
for garden, 787–789
medicinal, 699, 703–704

Anxiety remedies, 715–716

Appetizers and snacks. *See also* Dips
Antipasto Platter, 557
Chicken Liver Paté, 558
Chicken Nuggets, 553
Country Pork Sausages, 559
Deviled Eggs, 560
French Fries, 551
Globe Artichokes in Olive Oil, 561
Ham, Pork, and Veal Terrine, 558
Marinated Goat Cheese, 561
Oven-Baked French Fries, 551

Pizza, 552
Potato Chips, 550
Pretzels, 550
Quesadillas, 563
Spinach-Feta Phyllo Triangles, 562
Zucchini Strips, 563

Apples
Apple and Raisin Muffins, 522
Apple Butter, 447
Apple Ginger Jelly, 494
Electrolyte Drink for Diarrhea, 685
freezing, 502
Holiday Wassail, 577
Hot Mulled Cider, 577
Perfect Apple Pie, 539
Pet Bird Snacking Salad, 733

Appliances, 429

Apricots
Dried-Apricot Jam, 490
freezing, 502

Arnica, *Muscle Rub*, 681

Arrowroot
Athlete's Foot Powder, 703
Body Powder, 671
Easy Bath Powder, 676

Artichokes
Artichoke Facial, 654
Globe Artichokes in Olive Oil, 561

Asparagus, freezing, 499

Aspirin, *Aspirin Systemic Insecticide*, 787

Athlete's foot remedies, 703–704

Avocado oil
Anti-Wrinkle Eye Cream, 652
Eucalyptus Foot Lotion, 679
Rich Neck Moisturizer, 653